Outcome After Head, Neck and Spinal Trauma

Outcome After Head, Neck and Spinal Trauma

A Medicolegal Guide

Edited by

Robert Macfarlane MD, FRCS
Department of Neurological Surgery,
Addenbrooke's Hospital,
Cambridge, UK

David G. Hardy, FRCS
Department of Neurological Surgery,
Addenbrooke's Hospital,
Cambridge, UK

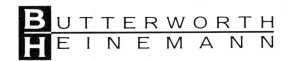

Butterworth-Heinemann
Linacre House, Jordan Hill, Oxford OX2 8DP
A division of Reed Educational and Professional Publishing Ltd

Ɒ A member of the Reed Elsevier plc group

OXFORD   BOSTON   JOHANNESBURG
MELBOURNE   NEW DELHI   SINGAPORE

First published 1997

British Library Cataloguing in Publication Data
Outcome after head, neck and spinal trauma: a medicolegal guide
  1 Head – Wounds and injuries   2 Neck – Wounds and injuries
  3 Spine – Wounds and injuries   4 Traumatology
  I Macfarlane, Robert   II Hardy, David G.
  617.1

ISBN 0 7506 2178 8

Library of Congress Cataloging in Publication Data
Outcome after head, neck and spinal trauma: a medicolegal guide/
  edited by Robert Macfarlane, David G. Hardy.
  p.   cm.
  Includes bibliographical references and index.
  ISBN 0 7506 2178 8
  1 Head – Wounds and injuries – Prognosis.   2 Neck – Wounds and
  injuries – Prognosis.   3 Spinal cord – Wounds and injuries –
  Prognosis.   4 Personal injuries – Trial practice.   5 Forensic
  neurology.   I Macfarlane, Robert, M. D.   II Hardy, David G.
  [DNLM: 1 Head Injuries – diagnosis   2 Prognosis.   3 Neck –
  injuries.   4. Spinal Cord Injuries – diagnosis.   5 Spinal Injuries –
  diagnosis.   WE 706 094]
  RD521.094   96–9270
  617.5′ 1044–dc20   CIP

Composition by Genesis Typesetting, Rochester, Kent
Printed and bound in Great Britain by The Bath Press

Contents

Section II: Ophthalmology

Section III: Ear, nose and throat

Section IV: Maxillofacial trauma

Section V: Spinal trauma

Section VI: Peripheral nerve injury

Contributors

Marcus D Atlas MBBS FRCAS
Consultant Otologist
St Vincent's Clinic
Sydney, NSW
Australia

R H Ballagh MD FRCS(C)
Consultant Otolaryngologist
Royal Victoria Hospital
Ontario
Canada

J C Benjamin FRCS FRCS(Ed)
Consultant Neurosurgeon
Regional Centre for Neurosurgery and Neurology
Oldchurch Hospital
Romford
UK

G E Berrios MA (Oxon) MD FRCPsych FBPsS
Consultant and University Lecturer in
Neuropsychiatry
Department of Psychiatry
University of Cambridge
Cambridge
UK

Paul F Bradley MD BDS FRCS FDS
Professor
Royal London Hospital Medical College Dental
School
London
UK

Hugh Cannell OStJ RD and bar MD(Lond)
MSc(Wales) FDSRCS(Engl) LRCP(Lond)
MRCS(Engl) DPMSA(Lond)
Reader, University of London and Honorary
Consultant in Oral and Maxillofacial Surgery,
London Hospital Medical College
Department of Oral and Maxillofacial Surgery
Royal London Hospital Medical College Dental
School
London
UK

John L B Carter FRCS FDS RCS
Consultant in Oral and Maxillofacial Surgery
Royal London Hospital Medical College Dental
School
London
UK

Bhupal P Chitnavis BSc MBBS FRCS
Specialist Neurological Registrar
King's College Hospital
London
UK

J D A Clark MD FRCP
Consultant Physician
West Suffolk Hospital
Suffolk
UK

G Rees Cosgrove MD FRCS(C)
Assistant Professor of Surgery, Harvard Medical
School
Department of Neurosurgery
Massachusetts General Hospital
Boston MA
USA

Brian H Cummins ChM FRCS
Consultant Neurosurgeon
Department of Neurosurgery
Frenchay Hospital
Bristol
UK

M J Davies MB BS FRACS
Senior Registrar
Department of Neurosurgery
The Royal London Hospital
London
UK

Richard F Edlich MD PhD
Distinguished Professor of Plastic Surgery and
Biomedical Engineering
Department of Plastic Surgery
University of Virginia School of Medicine
Charlottesville VA
USA

O M Edwards MD FRCP
Consultant Physician
Department of Medicine
Addenbrooke's Hospital
Cambridge
UK

Randolph W Evans MD
Chief of Neurology Section, Park Plaza Hospital;
Clinical Associate Professor, University of Texas
at Houston Medical School
Houston TX
USA

John E Fenton Bsc FRCSI
Fellow in Otology
St Vincent's Clinic
Sydney NSW
Australia

Gregg A Ferrero MD
Assistant in Orthopedics
Department of Orthopedic Surgery
Georgetown University Medical Center
Washington DC
USA

Stewart Flemming FRCS
Consultant Plastic and Hand Surgeon
St Andrew's Hospital
Billericay
UK

David M Frim MD PhD
Chief, Pediatric Neurosurgery
University of Chicago
Chicago, IL
USA

B P Gardner MA BM BCh(Oxon) MRCP(UK)
FRCS
Consultant in Spinal Injuries
National Spinal Injuries Centre
Stoke Mandeville Hospital
Aylesbury
UK

J R W Gleave MA BMBCh(Oxon)
MA(Cantab) FRCS
Emeritus Consultant in Neurosurgery,
Addenbrooke's Hospital
Cambridge
UK

Peter J Hamlyn BSc MD FRCS
Consultant Neurosurgeon
Department of Neurosurgery
St Bartholomew's Hospital
London
UK

David G Hardy FRCS
Consultant Neurosurgeon
Department of Neurosurgery
Addenbrooke's Hospital
Cambridge
UK

Robin J Hennessy MD
Attending Plastic Surgeon
Presbyterian Hospital
Charlotte NC
USA

Argye E Hillis MA
Associate Research Scientist
Department of Cognitive Science
Johns Hopkins University
Baltimore MD
USA

Peter J A Hutchinson BSc FRCS
Registrar
Department of Neurological Surgery
Addenbrooke's Hospital
Cambridge
UK

Bryan Jennett CBE MD FRCS
Emeritus Professor of Neurosurgery, University
of Glasgow
Glasgow
UK

B E Kendall FRCP FFR
Consultant Neuroradiologist
Lysholm Radiology Department
The National Hospital for Neurology and
Neurosurgery
London
UK

T T King FRCS
Consultant Neurosurgeon
Department of Neurosurgery
The Royal London Hospital
London
UK

Graham R Kirkby MBBS FRCS FRCOphth
DO
Consultant and Ophthalmic Surgeon to
Birmingham and Midland Eye Hospital;
Birmingham General Hospital and the Queen
Elizabeth Hospital
Birmingham
UK

Richard J Kryscio PhD
Professor and Chair
Department of Statistics
University of Kentucky Medical Center
Kentucky KY
USA

John P Lee FRCS FRCOphth FRCP
Consultant Ophthalmic Surgeon
Moorfields Eye Hospital
London
UK

F A Lenz MD PhD FRCS(C)
Associate Professor of Neurosurgery Johns
Hopkins University School of Medicine
Department of Neurosurgery
Baltimore MD
USA

Robert Macfarlane MD FRCS
Consultant Neurosurgeon
Department of Neurosurgery
Addenbrooke's Hospital
Cambridge
UK

Ian S Mackay MBBS FRCS
Consultant ENT Surgeon, Royal Brompton
Hospital and Charing Cross Hospital
London
UK

Hanno Millesi MD
Medical Director, Vienna Private Hospital;
Chairman, Ludwig Boltzman Institute for
Experimental Plastic Surgery
Vienna
Austria

Scott R Millis PhD ABPP AB MA Dip Clin
Neuropsychol
Chief, Rehabilitation Psychology and
Neuropsychology
Rehabilitation Institute of Michigan
Detroit MI
USA

D A Moffat BSc FRCS
Consultant Otoneurosurgeon
Department of Otolaryngology
Addenbrooke's Hospital
Cambridge
UK

Raymond F Morgan MD FACS
Distinguished Professor and Chair
Department of Plastic Surgery
University of Virginia School of Medicine
Charlottesville VA
USA

Nguyen D Nguyen MD
Resident in General Surgery
University of Virginia School of Medicine
Charlottesville VA
USA

Nandagudi S Niranjan MS FRCS FRCS(Plast)
Consultant Plastic and Reconstructive Surgeon
St. Andrews Centre for Plastic Surgery
Essex
UK

John S Norris FRCS
Senior Neurosurgical Registrar
Regional Centre for Neurosurgery and Neurology
Oldchurch Hospital
Romford
UK

John A Persing MD FACS
Professor and Chief
Section of Plastic Surgery
Department of Surgery
Yale University School of Medicine
New Haven CT
USA

J D Pickard MA MChir FRCS FRCS(Ed)
Bayer Professor of Neurosurgery
Department of Neurosurgery
Addenbrooke's Hospital
Cambridge
UK

Robert P Rapp Pharm D
Professor and Director of Pharmacy Practice and
Science
University of Kentucky Medical Center
Kentucky KY
USA

Geoffrey E Rose MS MRCP FRCS FRCOphth
Consultant Ophthalmic Surgeon
Moorfields Eye Hospital
London
UK

Mitchell Rosenthal PhD
Professor and Associate Chairman of Physical
Medicine and Rehabilitation, Adjunct Professor
of Psychology, Wayne State University;
Vice-President, Research and Education,
Rehabilitation Institute of Michigan
Detroit MI
USA

R M Rudd MD MRCP
Consultant Physician
Department of Respiratory Medicine
London Chest Hospital
London
UK

N J C Sarkies MA MRCP FRCS FRCOphth
Consultant Ophthalmic Surgeon, Addenbrooke's
Hospital, Cambridge and Hinchingbrooke
Hospital, Huntingdon
UK

P M J Scott FRCS
Senior Registrar ENT
Southampton General Hospital
Southampton
UK

Spiros Sgouros FRCS
Birmingham Neuroscience Centre
Queen Elizabeth Hospital
Birmingham
UK

O C E Sparrow MMed FRCS FRCS(SA)
Consultant Neurosurgeon
Wessex Neurological Centre
Southampton General Hospital
Southampton
UK

Nicholas Stafford MBChB FRCS
Professor
Department of ENT and
Head and Neck Surgery
Hull Royal Infirmary
Hull
UK

P Teddy MA DPhil BM BCh(Oxon) FRCS
Consultant Neurosurgeon
National Spinal Injuries Centre
Stoke Mandeville Hospital
Aylesbury
UK

Sam W Wiesel MD
Professor and Chairman, Department of
Orthopedic Surgery
Department of Orthopedic Surgery
Georgetown University Medical Center
Washington DC
USA

The late Bernard Williams ChM MD FRCS
Consultant Neurosurgeon
Syringomyelia Clinic
Midland Centre for Neurosurgery and Neurology
West Midlands
UK

Harold A Wilkinson MD PhD
Professor
Division of Neurosurgery
University of Massachusetts Medical Center
Worcester MA
USA

Byron Young MD
Johnston-Wright Chair of Surgery
Department of Surgery
University of Kentucky Medical Center
Kentucky KY
USA

Mark A Young MD
Assistant Professor
Instructor in Rehabilitation Medicine
The Johns Hopkins Hospital
Baltimore MD
USA

Preface

The burden on physicians to provide medical reports for accident victims becomes ever greater in our increasingly litigious society. In some cases, reports will require no more than a factual statement of the injuries sustained, the extent of any residual disability, and the presence or absence of any cosmetic deformity. Others will require an opinion about the likely mechanism of injury, the significance of any pre-existing medical conditions, and some measure of the severity of subjective complaints. Even greater difficulty may be encountered when, in order that an interim financial settlement can be agreed, the clinician is required to predict the likely long-term prognosis at a time when the patient has yet to achieve ultimate recovery.

Information on prognosis after various forms of cranial and spinal trauma is to be found scattered in countless journals and textbooks. The primary aim of this volume is to bring together this knowledge, and to provide a comprehensive reference source for further reading. Surprisingly perhaps, there are little or no hard data available on outcome for a wide range of conditions, particularly in the fields of plastic and maxillofacial surgery. We have encouraged authors wherever possible to state when this is the case. As a consequence, some chapters are devoted more to the classification and treatment of injury than they are to prognosis.

We hope that this book will be of interest to doctors and personal injury lawyers involved in assessment following medical injuries, and help to promote an understanding of the difficulties that clinicians may encounter when attempting to provide dogmatic statements on outcome. Because of differences in the legal systems throughout the world, details of case law are not included. For the same reasons, we have not attempted to provide advice on how a medical report should be presented, or how physicians should conduct themselves in a court of law. The issue of nonaccidental injury in children is not addressed separately. It is a clinical and legal minefield, requiring extensive experience, and cannot be addressed adequately in a single chapter. Readers are advised to consult a specialized text on the subject.

We are grateful to the many contributors who have devoted their time and energy to distil years of experience into what we hope will become a useful publication for those involved in assessing and compensating the victims of cranial or spinal trauma. We are indebted to Sheila Sellars, Catherine Zank-McKelvey and Anne Davies at Butterworth-Heinemann for their advice and encouragement during the preparation of this book.

Robert Macfarlane
David G Hardy

To Claudia, Rebecca, and Rosemary.

Section I

Head injury

1

Assessment and prediction of outcome after head injury

Bryan Jennett

Unlike injury elsewhere in the body, when damage is usually maximal immediately after impact, injuries to the head that are initially mild may rapidly develop serious complications that can lead to death or lasting disability due to secondary brain damage. Conversely, some patients who are initially in coma regain consciousness and proceed to make a complete recovery. It can therefore be important for legal purposes clearly to define the relationship between the initial severity of injury and the outcome. It is for example misleading to maintain that a patient has sustained a severe injury when in fact the severity of brain damage is wholly due to complications. From a liability viewpoint, however, there may be no argument that the complications and their effect on outcome were all consequences of the injury, however mild it was. Sometimes an attempt is made to ascribe contributory liability for the consequences of an accident or assault to inadequate medical care, on the grounds that complications were not recognized or treated sufficiently expeditiously. This argument is seldom accepted, as the chain of causation has not been broken. On the other hand, when medical negligence is alleged, the likely outcome if management had been better becomes the crux of the case, and it is this on which the lawyer wants the doctor to report.

Early complications

In order to understand the implications of these relationships it is necessary to outline the nature of early complications and their consequences. Those that can lead to secondary brain damage may be intracranial or extracranial. The former include acute intracranial haematoma, brain swelling, intracranial infection and early traumatic epilepsy.

By far the commonest is an acute intracranial haematoma, which is found in over 75% of patients who deteriorate into coma after having been talking at some stage after injury (Jennett, 1991). Although such haematomas are more common in patients who are in coma from the outset, about 50% of those operated on for removal of a blood clot have talked, and about one in six are recorded as being fully conscious and orientated when presenting at the hospital after injury (Jennett, 1991). It is such apparently mildly injured patients who are at most risk of being sent home from accident departments. This can result in delayed recognition of the signs of an intracranial haematoma developing and so of expeditious surgical evacuation. It is therefore important to recognize which of the many mildly injured patients who attend accident departments are at risk of developing an intracranial haematoma, in order to keep them under observation or to refer them for further investigation. This is because, once a haematoma develops, a patient may deteriorate rapidly due to brain compression, and, unless there is prompt surgical evacuation, death or disability results. In a large series of patients who had been fully conscious before developing an intracranial haematoma that needed surgical evacuation, almost 25% had a poor outcome: death or severe disability (Miller et al., 1990).

Table 1.1. Risk of acute haematoma for different presenting patient types after head injury (in accident department) (expressed as a ratio)

	Adults (1:–)	Children (1:–)
All cases regardless of fracture or conscious state	348	2 100
No skull fracture		
Fully conscious	7 900	13 000
Impaired consciousness	180	580
Coma	27	65
Skull fracture		
Fully conscious	45	157
Impaired consciousness	5	25
Coma	4	12

Based on data from Teasdale et al. 1990.

Statistical analysis of large numbers of head-injured patients in accident and emergency departments and of patients operated on for an acute haematoma indicates two important risk factors: state of consciousness and the presence of a skull fracture (Table 1.1). While children have a lower risk of haematoma than adults, the same risk factors apply. It is clear from this analysis that the presence of a skull fracture in patients who are fully conscious greatly increases the risk that a haematoma will develop; such patients should be kept under observation for 24 hours. If there is any impairment of consciousness and also a fracture, then a CT scan of the head is always indicated. Acute intracranial haematomas may be extradural or intradural; the latter may be either subdural or intracerebral, or a combination of both. Although extradural haematomas more commonly occur after initially mild injuries, and intradural after more severe trauma, there is considerable overlap. Moreover, the resulting cerebral compression is equally dangerous, and both need urgent surgery. Clinical suspicion that a haematoma is developing depends mainly on detecting a deteriorating consciousness level; this is best done by repeated assessment using the Glasgow Coma Scale, which is now widely used by all those who care for head-injured patients.

Brain swelling without a discrete haematoma is a complication of cerebral contusion and can lead to steady and rapid deterioration for which no surgical treatment is useful. Medical management aimed at reducing raised intracranial pressure may save the situation but is not always effective.

Intracranial infection is a risk of open injury, either a compound depressed fracture of the vault or a fracture of the skull base associated with a dural laceration. A compound depressed fracture of the vault underlying a scalp laceration may be overlooked as many of these patients have not suffered loss of consciousness, and are regarded as having only a scalp laceration. Dural penetration is even more easily overlooked if there has been a puncture wound from a sharp object such as a knitting needle or the axle of a toy vehicle in a child. The consequence of failing to recognize such an injury is that formal debridement of the wound is not undertaken and there is a risk of intracranial infection (meningitis or brain abscess). The risk of meningitis after basal skull fracture may persist for years. When meningitis then occurs, its connection with a previous head injury may not be recognized, although suspicion may be aroused if there are recurrent attacks. Clinical evidence of a skull base fracture in the acute stage includes periorbital or retro-auricular haematoma, and CSF leakage from the nose or ears. If a CSF leak persists for more than a week surgical repair of the dural tear is usually recommended.

Early epilepsy (defined as a seizure in the first week after injury) occasionally takes the form of status epilepticus and, especially in children, this can result in secondary hypoxic brain damage even after an injury that was initially only mild.

Extracranial complications that may cause secondary brain damage by reducing oxygen supply to the brain include respiratory insufficiency due to airway obstruction or chest injury, and low blood pressure due to shock. The effect of each of these may be aggravated by low haemoglobin due to blood loss. Whilst airway obstruction and failing respiration may occur as a direct consequence of the head injury alone, shock and blood loss are almost always associated with other, extracranial, injuries. Early treatment of these complications by endotracheal intubation, mechanical ventilation and replacement of blood loss are essential if secondary hypoxic brain damage is to be prevented.

Significance of skull fractures

There has been considerable controversy in recent years about the relevance of discovering a skull fracture to the management of head injuries. Thousands of mildly injured patients attend accident and emergency departments every year, many with scalp lacerations, but with no evidence of brain damage. Only 1–2% of these patients will have a fracture, but, when this has occurred, there is an increased risk of an acute intracranial haematoma or intracranial infection. If a fracture can be excluded, most of these mildly injured patients can safely be sent home. Radiologists have been critical of routine use of skull radiographs in accident and emergency departments, as most of these prove to be normal. Moreover, they point out that most patients with a fracture recover without incident, whilst some severely injured patients may have no fracture. Accordingly, they have devised criteria that identify those patients most likely to have a fracture: the so-called 'high-yield' criteria. However, many of these patients are the more seriously injured who would need to be admitted to hospital in any event. Indeed, in these patients it may be more appropriate to defer radiological investigation. In many of these a CT scan of the head may be a more useful investigation.

The discovery of a skull fracture is of most significance in the patient who is walking and talking on arrival and for whom admission (or keeping in a short stay observation ward) would not be required unless a fracture had occurred. In practice, in the UK only about half the patients attending accident and emergency departments after recent head injury have skull radiographs. Guidelines have been produced recently to set out the indications for this investigation (Group of Neurosurgeons, 1984; Bullock and Teasdale, 1990). In practice the junior staff, who make most decisions in accident and emergency departments, may not be skilled in the interpretation of skull radiographs, and a number of false positive and false diagnoses may occur, as subsequent review of films by trained radiologists has revealed. However, even in the USA where there are many more neurosurgeons and many more CT scanners, some of which are available to accident and emergency departments, only a small proportion of attenders have a scan. In the UK plain radiographs are an important triage tool in selecting which patients should have a CT scan. However, as more CT scanners become available in general hospitals that are without neurosurgeons or neuroradiologists, similar problems may arise with the interpretation of CT scans of the head. To overcome this, a number of neurosurgical units have installed telephone link lines that enable images to be transmitted from general hospitals for interpretation by experts. Another problem arising from the increased availability of CT scanners in local hospitals is that their use may delay the transfer of a deteriorating patient whose greatest need is to reach a neurosurgeon as quickly as possible.

Classification of outcome

The most widely used scale for measuring outcome after severe head injury is the Glasgow Outcome Scale (Jennett and Bond, 1975), which recognizes four grades of survivors (Table 1.2). This scale assesses the overall social functioning of the patient rather than defining specific disabilities. The disabilities that may occur after head injury

Table 1.2. PTA and outcome in 243 severe head injuries

Duration of PTA (weeks)	% of patients for each PTA category	% outcomes for each PTA category		
		SD	MD	GR
<1	9	0	9	91
1–2	17	0	18	82
2–4	22	2	40	58
>4	52	28	46	26

SD, severe disability; MD, moderate disability; GR, good recovery.

may be both mental and physical, and it is the combination of the two that makes the sequelae of severe head injury so disabling. All studies of such patients show that the mental disabilities are more of a handicap than the physical, yet these disorders of memory, cognition and behaviour are easily overlooked. This is because patients themselves often lack insight into their problems. Assessment should always include a careful questioning of the patient's relatives or other carers. Even patients who have no persisting neurological deficits (of cranial nerves, language function or the limbs) often have personality and behavioural disorders that make for social difficulties and an inability to return to work. When both mental and physical sequelae occur the mental disorders often limit the value of physical rehabilitation because lack of motivation and impaired memory impair the patient's co-operation.

Categories on the Glasgow Outcome Scale

Good recovery indicates either resumption of normal activities or the capability of doing so. These patients may however have minor abnormalities such as anosmia, mild personality changes, or cognitive deficits.

Moderate disability indicates clear-cut sequelae, which do not, however, prevent a patient from being independent (capable of living alone and using public transport unaided). Such sequelae include limb weakness, mild dysphasia, hemianopia, weakness in one or more limbs and various cranial nerve palsies.

Severe disability is an important category to recognize. It is defined as occurring when a patient is dependent on someone else for at least some activities in each 24 hours. Clearly this covers a wide range of dependency, from requiring someone for help with toileting, feeding and dressing, to needing help only in organizing daily activities when impaired by memory, cognitive and behavioural problems. These may make it impractical for such a patient to live alone. 'Independence' therefore indicates a greater degree of recovery than 'independence for self-care' or 'activities of daily living', criteria frequently used by geriatricians and rehabilitationists for those patients who are able to cope with various activities, but only within a sheltered environment such as institutional care, or living with caring family members continually at home.

Vegetative survival indicates a patient who is awake and demonstrates periods of eye opening but who is not aware and shows no psychologically meaningful responses to external stimuli and no speech. Such patients may have a wide range of reflex responses (withdrawal of limbs, grimacing to painful stimuli, or startle reactions to sudden sound). These are sometimes optimistically interpreted as conscious meaningful behaviours by family members or inexperienced nursing staff. Such patients are dependent for adequate nutrition on a gastrostomy or nasogastric tube.

Time scale of recovery

Most of the recovery occurs within the first 6–12 months after severe injury. In a series of patients whose outcome was eventually good recovery or moderate disability after one year, two-thirds had reached this category within three months and 90% by six months (Jennett *et al.*, 1981). This is not to deny that improvement within the grades of moderate or severe disability may not occur after one year, but there is little chance of a patient changing to a different category on the Glasgow Outcome Scale. It is therefore unfair to hold out false hopes of substantial late recovery, or to postpone legal settlement for years in the hope of further improvement that is likely to affect the degree of disability.

The prognosis of those patients categorized as being in the vegetative state is of particular concern. Although recovery is possible in the first few months, often this is only to a state of severe disability. Although traumatic cases more often recover than non-traumatic, it is considered even in these cases that after a year there is no realistic possibility of even limited recovery (Multi-Society Task Force on PVS, 1994). It is now widely accepted that it may be appropriate to withdraw life-sustaining treatment from such patients, as they gain no benefit from prolonged survival, and have no possibility of suffering during the withdrawal of treatment (Jennett, 1992). However, most such patients remain for years in long-term institutions or at home with live-in carers. This latter arrangement is usually possible only as a consequence of large financial awards for personal damages. As vegetative patients are unaware of their surroundings it is doubtful if awards to make this possible are justified, although patients' families may claim that they are. In view of the uncertainty of the duration of survival (see below) such awards are now commonly made as structured settlements.

Expectation of life

Most severely disabled survivors are young and their expectation of life appears to be reduced only by about five years (Roberts, 1979). However, those who are very dependent may be at increased risk of respiratory complications, when 10 years reduced life expectancy is perhaps more realistic. For vegetative patients, mean survival periods of 3–4 years have been calculated (Multi-Society Task Force on PVS, 1994), but these studies usually include not only traumatic cases but those with anoxic brain damage or other progressive pathologies. For traumatic cases who have already survived a year, many survive for 5 years or more and there are reports of these patients living for 10, 20 or even 40 years. However, the probability of these patients surviving more than 15 years has been calculated as being between 1 in 15 000 and 1 in 75 000 (Multi-Society Task Force on PVS, 1994).

Prognostic factors

Although the severity of brain damage, either primary or secondary, is the most important predictor of outcome, age is also a major factor. With the same degree of brain damage, children more often recover better than adults, and younger adults recover better than those who are older. This relationship between outcome and age is continuous, and without any obvious step changes with any particular age. Thus, the older the patient, the lower the probability of good recovery.

The severity of brain damage at initial presentation is commonly judged by the Glasgow Coma Score. This score is from 15 for fully alert to 3 for the deepest coma. Patients scoring 8 or less are considered to be severely injured, 9–12 as moderately injured, and 13 or more as mildly injured. Only 5% of injuries are judged as severe on presentation at hospital by this classification and 85% are mild. However, as already explained, a number of those who are less severely injured may suffer complications that lead to secondary brain damage that will leave them disabled. Of survivors of severe brain injury almost two-thirds become independent. Of these, about half make a good

recovery when assessed six months after injury, whilst almost a third are severely disabled and only 3% are vegetative.

The other common measure of severity of brain damage is the duration of post-traumatic amnesia (PTA). The advantage of this measure is that it can be assessed months after injury when the patient is seen for a legal report, by directly questioning the patient. PTA is defined as the interval between injury and when the patient regains continuous ongoing memory. It is ascertained by asking the patient how long it was before they realized where they were and what had happened. This is always considerably later than when the relatives report that the patient has 'woken up' and begun to speak, because there is always then a period of confusion for which the patient is subsequently amnesic. With this measure, it is not necessary to make an accurate assessment in order to define broad categories of severity of brain damage. A PTA of less than an hour indicates mild injury, of 1–24 hours moderate injury, of 1–28 days severe injury, and of over 28 days very severe injury. There is a good correlation among severe injuries between the length of PTA and the outcome grade at six months (Table 1.2); no one with a PTA of less than two weeks was severely disabled, whilst more than a quarter of those with a PTA of more than four weeks made a good recovery. It is therefore not possible to make an accurate prediction of ultimate disability when a patient initially emerges from PTA. If, however, at this stage there are marked physical disabilities such as severe dysphasia or hemiplegia, then some degree of permanent disability is likely. If cognitive psychological tests are performed, persisting abnormalities are almost always found if PTA exceeds three weeks, even though many of these patients may achieve good recovery.

Other factors that indicate the likelihood of permanent disability are complications such as acute intracranial haematoma requiring evacuation (especially if the patient is in coma before surgery), and the occurrence of systemic complications likely to have caused secondary ischaemic brain damage. The presence or absence of a skull fracture is of little prognostic significance for ultimate recovery. Its significance is in predicting the early complications of intracranial haematoma or infection.

An interim assessment of outcome after severe injury should be deferred until at least six months after injury and definitive opinion postponed until 12–18 months. However, after mild injuries, the sequelae can usually be assessed at six months, as by this time most patients in this category will have recovered.

References

Bullock R, Teasdale G. (1990) Head injuries I and II (ABC of Major Trauma). *Br Med J* **300**: 1515–18, 1576–79.

Group of Neurosurgeons. (1984) Guidelines for initial management after head injury in adults. *Br Med J* **288**: 983–85.

Jennett B. (1991) Epidemiology of severe head injury: socio-economic consequences of avoidable mortality and morbidity. In Scriabine A, Teasdale GM, Tetterborn D, Young W eds. Nimodipine: pharmacological and clinical results in cerebral ischaemia Berlin: Springer-Verlag 228–294.

Jennett B. (1992) Letting vegetative patients die: ethical and lawful and brings Britain into line. *Br Med J* **305**: 1305–06.

Jennett B, Bond M. (1975) Assessment of outcome after severe brain damage. *Lancet* **i**: 480–84.

Jennett B, Snoek J, Bond MR *et al.* (1981) Disability after severe head injury: observations on the use of the Glasgow Outcome Scale. *J Neurol Neurosurg Psychiatry* **44**: 285–93.

Miller JD, Murray LS, Teasdale GM. (1990) Development of a traumatic intracranial haematoma after minor head injury. *Neurosurgery* **27**: 669–73.

Multi-Society Task Force on PVS. (1994) Medical aspects of the persistent vegetative state (Part 2). *N Engl J Med* **330**: 1572–79.

Roberts AH. (1979) Severe accidental head injury: an assessment of longterm prognosis. London: MacMillan.

Teasdale GM, Murray G, Anderson E *et al.* (1990) Risks of acute traumatic intracranial haematoma in children and adults: implications for managing head injuries. *Br Med J* **300**: 363–67.

2

Scalp injury

Robin J Hennessy, John A Persing, Raymond F Morgan

Introduction

The skin is the largest organ of the body. Its structure varies according to its function and location. The scalp is specialized for the important function of providing a protective cover for the calvarium and brain. In addition, the scalp and hair serve a secondary role in defining the aesthetic characteristics of an individual's facial image.

Neurosurgeons, plastic surgeons, and, to some extent, general surgeons, are confronted with scalp defects that pose difficult reconstructive problems. The goal of this effort and good outcome is when restoration of the functional cover occurs, while at the same time an aesthetically pleasing result is achieved. The scalp is in a vulnerable, exposed position and therefore is especially prone to injury. Scalp laceration is the most common head injury requiring operative care. In the usual situation, primary healing results and complications are infrequent. The most difficult therapeutic challenges for scalp coverage are caused by avulsion injuries with loss of major segments of the scalp, thermal or electrical burns, postradiation injuries, congenital deficiency, and defects secondary to neoplastic processes.

History of scalp loss and soft tissue cover

As early as 3000 BC, Egyptians recognized that the uncovered and unprotected skull threatened life. Throughout recorded medical history, including Biblical medical references, scalp losses have been mentioned as a form of social punishment, displayed as trophies of the vanquished, or used as a means of marking slaves. Death often occurred secondary to generalized sepsis due to osteomyelitis or virulent intracranial infections, or both.

Although there are earlier references to similar treatment by Celsus and Ambroise Pare, the medical treatment of the denuded calvarium was first recorded by Augustin Belloste in Paris in 1654 (Celsus, 1493; Koss *et al.*, 1975; McGrath, 1983; Pare, 1634). Belloste perforated bone down to the diploe to develop 'external' granulation tissue that was subsequently covered by epithelium. This technique was passed on and used by many.

Harvey Cushing studied scalp injuries during World War I and established principles regarding the management of combined cranial and scalp injuries (Cushing, 1918). His principles emphasized early cleansing, debridement and primary closure of scalp wounds. He also introduced the principle of early wound closure by the use of tripod incisions and outlined scalp flaps to achieve wound closure.

Anatomy

Scalp layers

A thorough knowledge of scalp anatomy is important in order to understand the operative management and repair of scalp deformities. The scalp functions as a protective and nutritive layer for the cranium. It is rich in skin adnexae and is the thickest integument in the body. The scalp consists of five layers: the skin, subcutaneous layer, epicranium, subepicranium and pericranium (Figure 2.1).

The skin, which is the superficial layer of the scalp, is composed of thick epidermis and dermis. Scalp thickness varies from 3 to 8 mm. The upper neck and occipital areas are the thickest, with thinning over frontal, mastoid and temporal areas. The average thickness of skin elsewhere on the body is 1–2 mm but ranges from 0.5 mm in the eyelid to 3–6 mm in the infrascapular region.

The subcutaneous layer is made up of dense connective tissue and fat. The septa of the superficial fascia lie in this layer, which binds the skin tightly to the underlying galea aponeurotica and the occipitalis and frontalis muscles. Also, coursing through this level are numerous main and anastomotic blood vessels and nerves, as well as epithelial and adnexal structures.

The epicranium is composed of paired occipitalis and frontalis muscles, joined by the galea aponeurotica. The galea is made up of a flat central tendon attached anteriorly to the belly of the frontalis muscle and posteriorly to the occipitalis muscle. The anterior insertions of the galea are into the upper eyelids and into the subcutaneous tissue over the eyebrows and nose. Posterior insertions are into the lambdoid ridge of the occiput and the external occipital protuberance. Laterally, the definitions of the galea are indistinct, but it courses into the temporal area to the upper attachments of the helix of the ear and is continuous with the superficial musculoaponeurotic system layer of the face (Horowitz *et al.*, 1984). The galea is the layer

of tensile strength of the scalp. If it is not repaired, contracture of its attached muscles may develop and result in a depressed appearance of the scalp wound (Dingman and Johnson, 1977).

The subepicranium, also known as the cavum subgalea, is the fourth layer of the scalp and consists of loose areolar connective tissue as well as small vessels and emissary veins. This layer provides scalp mobility and allows the superficial veins of the scalp to communicate with the intracranial venous sinuses. This is also the usual plane of scalp avulsion or the site of haematomas and purulent infections (Mathes *et al.*, 1981).

The pericranium is the deepest layer of the scalp and is adherent to the skull. The pericranium of the cranial vault is thought to be different from periosteum elsewhere in the body, as much of the skull is formed by membranous bone. The pericranium contains many small capillaries that pass through the underlying bone, and it is intimately attached to the outer table of the skull, especially at the suture lines. It is this layer that is able to support split thickness skin grafts in the absence of more suitable scalp tissue (Converse, 1955; Dingman and Johnson, 1977; Edlich *et al.*, 1984). Histologically, the pericranium consists of two adjacent layers: an outer layer of fibrous connective tissue that is well vascularized and innervated and an inner layer of dense elastic fibres. When the latter is stripped from the surface of bone, a layer of osteoblasts adheres to the fibres. As humans age, the pericranium thins and becomes less vascularized and the osteoblasts attenuate to a thin epithelial layer.

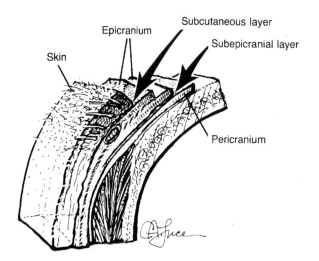

Figure 2.1. Scalp layers: skin, subcutaneous layer, epicranium (paired occipitalis and frontalis muscle with galea aponeurotica), subepicranium and pericranium.

Blood supply

The scalp is extremely vascular and is supplied by five paired arteries of the external and internal carotid systems passing into the subcutaneous tissue (second layer) from the periphery to the vertex (Figure 2.2). The arteries richly anastomose with each other so that collateral sources of vascular supply are abundant. This feature of scalp anatomy allows for significant variability in flap design to cover scalp defects. These anastomoses, however, vary in degree with increasing age. Corso (1961) demonstrated a paucity of midline vascular anastomoses after the sixth decade. Therefore, flaps designed to cross the midline should be planned with great care in the older patient.

Scalp vessels are supported by multiple fibrous tissue connections that impede retraction following severing; thus, there is a tendency toward profuse bleeding when cut. The occipital artery, the superficial temporal artery, and the posterior auricular artery run superficial to the galea high in the neck. The supraorbital artery is a terminal branch of the internal carotid artery and may anastomose with the external carotid through the angular artery. The supraorbital artery perforates the galea at the supraorbital ridge. As most head injuries are frontal, this vessel is usually not available for reconstructive procedures in patients with acute trauma. It may be useful, however, for later reconstructive options.

The veins of the scalp parallel the arterial supply. Unlike the arterial tree, they communicate intracranially via the diploic and emissary veins to the cavernous, superior sagittal, sigmoid and transverse sinuses. Haemorrhage can be profuse from these channels. Consistent extracranial to intracranial venous connections occur in the parietal region adjacent to the sagittal sinus and in the retromastoid area. Extracranial infection may lead to intracranial infection via these veins, causing sinus thrombophlebitis and meningitis.

Lymphatics

The scalp contains abundant lymphatic channels but no lymph nodes. Posterior scalp drainage is to the occipital nodes through the postauricular and superior cervical nodes. Anterior scalp drainage is to the preauricular and parotid nodes. In the temporal and parietal regions, drainage is into

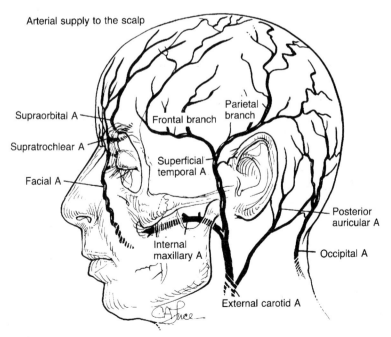

Figure 2.2. Arterial supply to the scalp is supplied by five paired arteries of the external and internal carotid systems.

the superficial parotid, superficial cervical, retro-auricular or deep cervical nodes.

Nerves

The occipitofrontalis muscle and the auricular muscles are innervated by the seventh cranial nerve. Sensation is primarily from the fifth cranial nerve and partially from the cervical plexus (C2–C3). The anterior two-thirds of the scalp is supplied by the fifth cranial nerve and the posterior one-third by the cervical plexus. Anteriorly, the supratrochlear, supraorbital and frontal branches arise from the first division of the fifth cranial nerve, the zygomaticotemporal nerve from the second division, and the auriculotemporal nerve from the third division. Posteriorly, the greater occipital nerves arise from the posterior branch of C2 and C3, and the lesser occipital nerve arises from C3.

General management

Treatment considerations

The initial assessment of the scalp defect must take into consideration a number of factors, including: size, depth and condition of the wound; location of the scalp defect; mechanisms of injury; age and general condition of the patient; and possibilities for camouflage.

Estimation of the size of the wound

An accurate measurement of the dimensions of the wound is essential. Small wounds (2–4 cm wide) may be closed by undermining skin edges and releasing skin tension by scoring the galea. Moderate-size wounds may require local flaps, such as those described by Orticochea, to close defects in the scalp measuring up to 10 × 14 cm, or tissue expansion techniques may be used (Manders *et al.*, 1982; Orticochea, 1967, 1971). Larger defects or total loss of the scalp often require the use of microvascular free flap transfers.

Depth of the wound

One of the most important determinations to be made regarding reconstruction of scalp defects is the level (or depth) of the scalp loss. Optimally, one would like to replace 'like tissue with like'. Therefore, the level of injury would dictate the thickness of the material to be used for reconstruction. More important, however, is the concept that certain reconstructive options are negated by a scalp defect associated with a nonvascular base. For example, a scalp defect that leaves the galea or periosteum, or both, intact may be treated immediately as well as over the long term by free grafts of skin (split or full thickness). If the pericranium is absent, however, the underlying denuded bone rarely supplies enough nutrient vessels to support a skin graft. Therefore, another preparatory procedure that fenestrates or removes the outer table of the calvarial bone in order to generate a granulation tissue bed is required prior to the application of a skin graft. Likewise, if a bony defect of the calvarium is present in addition to the scalp defect, the graft is more liable to break down (although a skin graft will survive on the dura), and the consequent lack of protection for the underlying brain requires that flap tissue with or without bone should be provided.

Condition of the wound

The time elapsed from the development of the scalp defect and the degree of bacterial contamination in the wound guide the surgeon's reconstructive options. With heavy bacterial contaminations ($>10^5$ bacteria per gram of tissue) in the wound bed, neither skin grafts nor flaps would be successful (Magee *et al.*, 1977). Increased numbers of bacteria may be reduced by antibiotic therapy or debridement, or both, prior to wound closure. A scalp laceration seen later than 24 hours after injury may be optimally treated by secondary wound contracture to avoid the possibility of wound infection due to bacterial contamination. If the number of local bacteria is low and the wound bed is sufficiently vascular, delayed primary closure may be performed (usually 4 days or more after injury) (Edlich *et al.*, 1984). In the glabrous forehead region, however, closure by secondary wound contracture may be inadvisable because of the significant emotional stress to the patient with an open wound in a highly visible area. Therefore, immediate closure after obtaining a quantitative smear of the wound bed or delayed primary closure is usually a better reconstructive option (Magee *et al.*, 1977).

Location of the scalp defect

Scalp defects are closed according to their location. Glabrous defects should be reconstructed employing nonhair-bearing skin. Nonglabrous defects optimally should be reconstructed using hair-bearing local scalp flaps. This procedure may also be limited in the anterior scalp, compared with the posterior scalp, because of the possibility of distortions of the forehead hairline.

Mechanisms of injury

Knowledge of whether the scalp defect was caused by crush injury, avulsion, scald or electrical burn, radiation injury, or other mechanisms, will influence reconstructive decisions. If a scalp defect occurred as a result of a crush injury with significant bruising to the surrounding skin, local scalp flaps would not be an immediate treatment option. Similarly, if irradiation resulted in a scalp defect, the vascularity of the local skin and pericranial tissue would be insufficient to maintain viability if the structures were to be elevated or transposed.

Age and general condition of the patient

An elderly or debilitated patient may be unsuitable for reconstructive options that require a prolonged operative or perioperative course. If the patient will not be able to withstand a lengthy operative procedure or recovery, a compromise in aesthetic outcome and durability may have to be made.

Camouflage

Sometimes, scalp defects may be managed by using adjacent tissue (often hair) to cover the defects. These defects are usually relatively minor and located more posteriorly in the scalp.

Therapeutic options

The primary goal of the reconstructive surgeon dealing with a scalp defect is to close the defect rapidly and safely and to have the end result look as normal as possible. Therapeutic options include primary or delayed closure, skin grafts, or various types of flaps.

Primary closure

The least involved and most expedient means of closure of a scalp defect is by primary coaptation of the wound edges. This may be accomplished in the majority of scalp wounds by sufficient undermining of the galea. When the need arises, scoring the undersurface of the scalp and severing the binding galea perpendicular to the direction of pull at the wound edge allows for further advancement of the wound edges and closure of the wound (see Figure 2.3). A new device used for intra-operative scalp expansion made by Life Medical Sciences

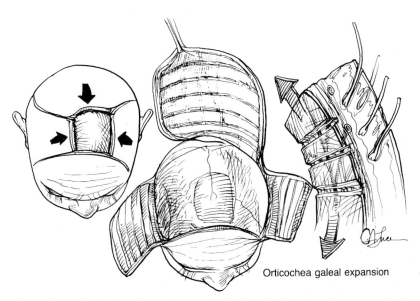

Orticochea galeal expansion

Figure 2.3. Orticochea three-flap technique and principle of incising the galea transversely in the direction of pull of the wound edge.

called Sure-Closure has shown ease in closing primary scalp defects of between 10 and 15 centimeters. The device works by a spring tension method with pins directed parallel to the wound throughout its entire length. Over a period of 5 to 15 minutes the scalp is stretched and the device is tightened up again maximally. This slow expansion is repeated 3 to 5 times over a period of 20 to 45 minutes. Reports of complications are few when only a defect of clean healthy scalp is closed by this method. This may be a worthwhile option when only a single defect is present in lieu of moving large flaps.

Results of repair are usually quite favourable and are also hidden by hair. For that reason, any type of scar revision is rarely required.

Delayed closure

If the wound cannot be closed immediately, or at least within a few hours, healing by secondary intention may be allowed to occur. If the wound bed is kept moist, epithelialization will occur readily. The disadvantages, however, are that it is lengthy, may require large amounts of dressing materials and extensive supportive care, and frequently results in a more significant aesthetic defect and an area of alopecia and a less stable scarred wound. An alternative to secondary wound closure is delayed primary closure, which, when possible, expedites the healing process. This also results in less visible scar and a higher likelihood of achieving hair growth able to camouflage the site of injury.

Skin grafts

Skin grafts may be classified according to the percentage of dermis and epidermis contained in the graft material. A graft containing partial thickness of the dermis and all of the epidermis is referred to as a split thickness graft, and one containing 100% of the thickness of both the dermis and the epidermis is called a full thickness graft. Both types have advantages and disadvantages. Both provide simple wound coverage but with visible deformity.

Split thickness skin grafts have large areas of donor sites available (e.g. buttocks, thighs, abdomen). They are the graft of choice for marginally vascularized wound beds. However, split thickness grafts contract and change pigment more often than full thickness grafts. In addition, because they contain no sweat glands, split thickness grafts may desiccate and fissure if not kept moist with lotions or creams. Most importantly, they provide a less stable coverage directly over bone than do thicker full thickness grafts or flaps.

Full thickness grafts have more limited donor sites and available skin (e.g. cervical region, groin, retroauricular areas). They tend to contract less than split thickness skin grafts but more than flap tissue. Finally, full thickness skin grafts are often a better colour match with facial skin, especially if taken in the supraclavicular region, and may retain better sensibility at the recipient site.

Both split and full thickness grafts have the same drawbacks (i.e. they are neither the same thickness as nor the exact colour of the surrounding scalp tissue). Therefore, they both provide less protection for the calvarium. Moreover, substitution of nonhair-bearing skin for areas of scalp originally covered by hair usually results in a significant highly visible and scarred aesthetic defect.

Skin grafts, however, are very useful in the treatment of the patient who is severely injured and unstable and in whom scalp loss is accompanied by retention of the periosteum. A split thickness skin graft may provide a temporary stable coverage of the cranium to prevent desiccation and subsequent loss of both the periosteum and calvarial bone. When the scalp injury includes loss of the periosteum, immediate skin grafting is usually not successful. It is first necessary to decorticate the outer table of the calvarium and allow granulation tissue to develop. Ordinarily, 2–3 weeks are required before the granulating bed can support a skin graft. This option is used less often today because of local flap and microvascular operative procedures. In such patients, wound closure takes priority over functional cover. Revisions would be staged at a later time once the patient has recovered from serious injuries.

Local flaps

Whenever possible, scalp defects should be repaired by means of local scalp flaps. No other method provides as close a colour or hair density match. Local flaps are the method of choice for coverage of small moderate-sized defects. The rich vascular network located in the subdermal plexus allows for significant variation in design of the scalp flaps (Figure 2.4).

Two major types of flaps – random pattern and axial pattern – are used on the scalp. The random flap is based solely on the vascular supply from the

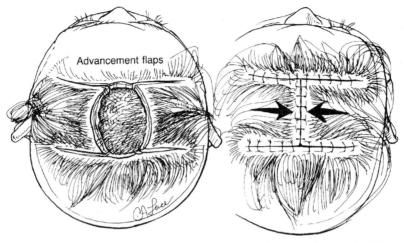

Figure 2.4. Advancement flaps. Bilateral advancement of scalp tissue adjacent to the defect may be performed with one advancement if the defect is small or in stages with progressive advancement if a larger defect exists.

subdermal plexus of vessels. There are many different types or designs, which may be broadly classified as advancement, transposition and rotation flaps. The axial pattern flap receives significant vascular input from large vessels (such as the superficial temporal artery) located adjacent to the galeal plane (Figure 2.5). Because of the vascular input directed to the flap, very long length to width ratios in flap design may be obtained (greater than 15:1). Ultimately, the axial pattern flap, like the random flap, nourishes the skin via the subdermal plexus. Where possible, incisions orientated in the direction of hair follicle growth

facilitate hair growth, the end result being far superior with less visible scarring and alopecia.

Random Pattern Flaps

Advancement flaps

Advancement flaps are the simplest in design and execution (see Figure 2.4). They are useful for relatively small defects in which the edges of the defect may be mobilized sufficiently to coapt the wound margins. The flaps are mobilized in the cleavage plane of the loose areolar connective

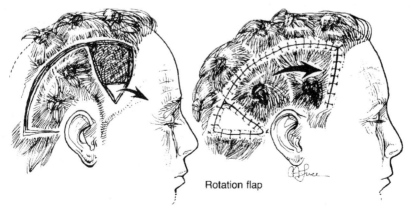

Rotation flap

Figure 2.5. The rotation flap is usually semicircular in shape. It is designed adjacent to the defect and rotated about a fixed pivot. Here the superficial temporal artery provides an axial blood supply as well.

tissue between the galea and periosteum. Scoring of the galea may be helpful in reducing skin tension, but care should be taken to avoid cutting major vessels located just superficial to the galea that supply the subdermal plexus.

Transposition flaps

The usefulness of a transposition flap is in the redirection of skin tension and coverage of un-stable wounds (Figure 2.6). A scalp defect may be large and orientated in a direction in which skin tension is too great to allow for direct wound closure. In another direction, however, skin laxity may be present. Ordinarily, the transposition flap transfers skin from a region of relative excess to an area of skin deficiency. If the excess laxity of skin is great enough, the donor defect may be closed primarily. If, however, the wound edges at the donor site are unable to be closed primarily, skin graft coverage of the donor site may be performed. The need for skin grafts at the donor site is relatively high in scalp wounds, but the transposi-tion flap is still quite useful in situations in which the surgeon is trying to re-establish the anterior hairline and the donor site can be hidden by more posteriorly located hair (see Figure 2.5).

Rotation flaps

Rotation flaps are usually used to close triangular defects in the scalp (see Figure 2.5). A curvilinear incision is extended from the base of the defect outward. The scalp is mobilized in the subgaleal plane and is rotated into the defect. These flaps should be broad based and, if possible, should include major supplying vessels of the superficial temporal or postauricular arteries. The flaps should fill the defect with very little tension. Often, a 'back-cut' into the flap is needed to close the donor defect. At other times, if skin laxity is sufficient, the donor defect may be closed by a V-Y advancement of the surrounding scalp. There are myriad variations in the design of these general categories of flaps, but the general principles are basically the same.

Axial pattern flaps

The axial pattern flap offers perhaps the greatest variation in design, as the aforementioned random pattern flaps may also include axial pattern vessels. This provides greater ability to 'tailor-design' flaps to the defect site because the vascular input is more abundant. One of the interesting and useful variations in the design of the axial pattern flap is

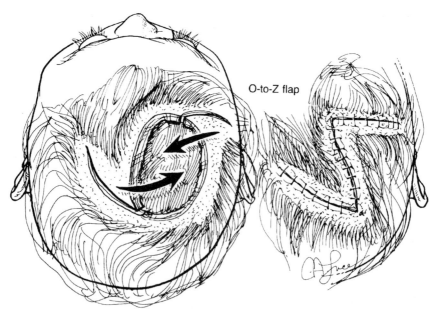

O-to-Z flap

Figure 2.6. Bilateral transposition flaps demonstrate the redirecting skin tension to allow wound closure. This also demonstrates an 'O' shaped defect being converted to a 'Z' shaped flap closure.

the island pedicle flap. This flap is based on a vascular (artery and vein) pedicle without overlying dermis or epidermis. Extremely long length to width ratios may be obtained because, regardless of how long the flap is relative to its width, sufficient blood supply will be present as long as the vascular pedicle is in line with the donor skin. The advantage of this type of flap is that tissue may be transferred to other locations on the scalp without the excess bulk or 'dog ear' deformity caused by nonisland flaps. Therefore, only the tissue needed to fill the defect is transferred. The selection of the flap design is dependent on a number of variables, as described previously, but additional variability is offered by the choice of which individual scalp tissue layers are used. The scalp may thus be transferred as a subunit such as the galea alone, the periosteum alone, or the galea plus subcutaneous tissue; the temporalis fascia may also be transferred, with subsequent skin grafts placed on top of the transferred flap tissue to cover problem wounds (Argenta *et al.*, 1985; Fonseca, 1983; Mathes *et al.*, 1981). Relatively large defects of the scalp may be covered by local scalp flaps, as evidenced by the Orticochea's 'banana peel' flaps (Figure 2.3). Using a three- or four-flap technique, defects of up to 10×14 cm at the vertex of the scalp have been closed primarily by this technique (Orticochea, 1967).

More recently, however, even larger defects in the scalp have been covered by the use of soft tissue expanders, which stretch the adjacent scalp to provide almost limitless amounts of scalp tissue (Figure 2.7). The major advantage that this technique has compared with distant flap coverage is that it replaces 'like tissue with like'. The disadvantages are that scalp stretching is occasionally painful and requires time. When immediate coverage of the brain or denuded bone is needed, this technique is not useful.

To provide immediate tissue coverage for large defects of the scalp, distant tissue is used, requiring microvascular transfer.

The most frequently employed flaps for whole scalp coverage are the latissimus dorsi and omental flaps. They provide a broad, relatively flat surface on to which skin grafts may be placed. These flaps have readily identifiable vascular pedicles that may be anastomosed to a number of external carotid artery branches in the scalp. Unfortunately, there is no good substitute for the hair-bearing scalp elsewhere in the body; however, for the forehead region, both radial forearm and scapular flaps have provided excellent aesthetic substitutes (Alpert *et al.*, 1982; Chicarilli *et al.*, 1986; McGrath, 1983). The disadvantages of microvascular free flap transfers are that they are often lengthy procedures and frequently do not replace 'like tissue with like'.

Scalp defects

Laceration

Scalp lacerations may be linear, sharp, irregular or stellate, trapdoor or multiple. If they extend across

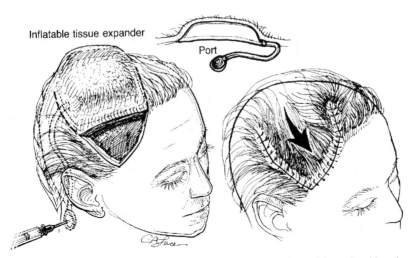

Figure 2.7. Soft tissue expansion allows for coverage of larger defects of the scalp with scalp tissue, therefore optimally replacing 'like tissue with like'.

the galea, muscle pull may result in gaping of the wound. Bruising, abrasions or contusions can occur in association with an underlying haematoma. A small haematoma may resorb in several weeks; a large haematoma may require needle aspiration or incision with its extraction if symptomatic. The principal complications of scalp lacerations are haemorrhage and infection. The majority of scalp lacerations heal without incident. Keloids are an unusual problem, which occur more commonly in dark skinned individuals and are more of a problem in the posterior neck. Treatment by injection of Kenalog and/or excision and compression or silastic sheeting are most effectively employed.

Contusion

Scalp contusions usually involve a crush injury to a localized area with abrasion. As for skin contusions elsewhere on the body, treatment involves cleansing and removal of any particulate matter. Acute debridement is performed only if extreme crushing and avulsion of tissue has occurred. Daily cleansing and application of topical antibacterial agents are usually sufficient to promote rapid re-epithelialization and healing. Scarring may be more prominent, especially if the degree of contusion is significant. This would most commonly result in hair follicle attrition and alopecia. Treatment requires either a zig-zag excision and/or flap advancement to camouflage if it is severe.

Avulsion

Scalp avulsion is a major injury with a high associated morbidity rate secondary to cranial exposure with desiccation and eventual necrosis and osteomyelitis. The development of microvascular procedures has allowed successful initial replantation or subsequent one-stage reconstruction of the scalp using free flap techniques (Alpert *et al.*, 1982; Mathes *et al.*, 1981). The scalp will avulse if a strong shearing or tearing force is applied to lift the scalp at the loose areolar tissue plane layer between the galea and periosteum. If the force is transmitted so that the shear is progressive, it may extend until the points of facial attachments are reached at the supraorbital ridge, zygoma and occipital mastoid region (Alpert *et al.*, 1982).

There are many reports of successful scalp replantation. The first milestone was established in 1976 by Miller and co-workers, who successfully replanted a totally avulsed scalp and documented subsequent normal hair growth and function of the frontalis muscle (Miller *et al.*, 1976). Reinnervation of the scalp is a common outcome and painful neuroma is unusual, the exception being the occipital nerve, which is quite large and has more of a tendency to be painful posteriorly, as significant motion occurs around this area. Immediately after a scalp avulsion injury, haemorrhage may be profuse and must be controlled and the patient's blood volume restored. Preoperative skull and cervical spine radiograph films are required, and the exposed calvarium must be kept moistened. The avulsed scalp is kept moist in a container with iced saline for transport to a centre where a microsurgical team is available for replantation. Extended periods of ischaemia have been tolerated with ultimate success, particularly if the part has been cooled, but no author has yet established the maximal ischaemia for survival. If replantation is not available or not possible, immediate coverage must be undertaken and eventual reconstruction planned to minimize morbidity. After the avulsion, coverage may be provided by skin grafts or harvesting skin from the avulsed scalp fragments or using defatted scalp or other biological dressings (Koss *et al.*, 1975; Osborne, 1950).

Once the acute problem has been managed, the next goal is to provide full thickness, well vascularized coverage to prevent repetitive ulcerations, which may potentially lead to osteomyelitis. If a large portion of scalp remains with normal vascular supply, a variety of local flaps have been used to establish a hairline. For large midscalp defects, Orticochea designed a three- or four-flap 'banana peel' method to divide and share the remaining scalp, and skin graft the newly created defects (Orticochea, 1967, 1971).

Radiation induced injuries

Scalp injuries induced by ionizing radiation may produce a chronic radiodermatitis or radionecrotic ulcer. The lesions are often the secondary sequelae of tumour therapy but may be the result of past treatment for conditions such as ringworm, when overlapping fields and poorly controlled doses were used (Dingman and Johnson, 1977). Robinson (1975), Malbec and co-workers, and many others, have reported late sequelae of radiation injury in which chronic ulceration may be complicated by subsequent malignant degeneration (Malbec *et al.*, 1963; van Swieten, 1754).

Of primary concern in the operative management of these scalp defects is the underlying pathology of scalp tissue induced by radiation. Injury is extensive. Fibrinoid necrosis of vessel walls occurs in both superficial and deep tissues of the scalp. This usually precludes using primary closure skin grafting or using local flaps to cover the defect. These methods may fail because of the poorly vascularized bed and surrounding tissue; they are fraught with complications (DiMeo and Jones, 1984; Dingman and Johnson, 1977; Mathes *et al.*, 1981; Robinson, 1975).

Serafin and co-workers (1982) emphasized the use of a well vascularized pedicle or distal free flaps, employing pattern cutaneous and myocutaneous flaps after irradiation (Serafin *et al.*, 1982). However, patient selection is critical and should be considered in deciding on the treatment modality. If symptoms are minor and the patient is extremely frail and debilitated, symptomatic management with regular dressing changes may be the best plan of treatment. However, when selecting a free flap for coverage, it should be remembered that overall time in the operating room and subsequent hospitalization may be less for a single extensive procedure than for several less than satisfactory 'minor' operations.

Burns

Burns of the scalp are still another challenge in patient care that may face the surgeon. There are essentially four main types of burn injury to the scalp: scald injury from hot liquids; thermal burns from fire; electrical burns; and chemical burns. Additionally, burns are classified as superficial and possibly healing with only local care, or deep to bone or meninges and requiring operative excision and grafting or a major reconstructive procedure.

Electrical or thermal burns involving only the scalp may be managed by the same technique as soft tissue burns of other areas of the body. Operative or spontaneous debridement followed by coverage with a split thickness graft will provide good restoration of function. An eventual good cosmetic result may require subsequent advancement and rotation of scalp flaps.

If the burn extends to include the pericranium, the arterial supply to the outer cortex of the skull is also destroyed, with resultant devitalization. These patients were formerly treated by removing the outer table of the skull with a drill to allow granulation tissue to form. Eventual split thickness skin grafting was then possible. This solution is temporary, however, as the skull contour predisposes to ulceration of the epithelium after even minimal trauma. Eventual replacement of the skin graft with a well padded, full thickness flap has now become a functional requirement.

Summary

The scalp is a well vascularized, highly specialized tissue that is very tolerant of injury. When scalp defects do occur, multiple local and distant treatment methods are available to provide satisfactory coverage of the open wound and protection of the skull and brain. Co-operation among surgical specialists dealing with these patients allows for their optimal care.

References

Alpert BS, Buncke HJ, Mathes SJ. (1982) Surgical treatment of the totally avulsed scalp. *Clin Plast Surg* **9**: 145–59.

Argenta LC, Friedman RJ, Dingman RO, *et al.*, (1985) The versatility of pericranial flaps. *Plast Reconstr Surg* **76**: 695–702.

Celsus AC. (1493): *De medicina*, vol. 3. Spencer WG (1938), translator. Cambridge, MA: Harvard University Press, 501–503.

Chicarilli ZN, Ariyan S, Cuono CB. (1986) Single state repair of complex scalp and cranial defects with the free radial forearm flap. *Plast Reconstr Surg* **77**: 577–85.

Converse JM. (1955) Surgical closure of scalp defects. In: Kahn E, Bassett RC, Scheider RC, Crosby ED, editor. *Correlative neurosurgery.* Springfield, IL: Charles C. Thomas, 262–74.

Corso PS. (1961) Variations of the arterial, venous and capillary circulation of the soft tissues of the head by decades, as demonstrated by the methyl methacrylate injection technique, and their application to the construction of flaps and pedicles. *Plast Reconstr Surg* **27**: 160–84.

Cushing HA. (1918) A study of a series of wounds involving the brain and its enveloping structures. *Br J Surg* **5**: 555–684.

DiMeo L, Jones BM. (1984) Surgical treatment of radiation-induced scalp lesions. *Br J Plast Surg* **37**: 373–78.

Dingman RO, Johnson HA. (1977) Surgery of the scalp. *Surg Clin North Am* **57**: 1011–22.

Edlich RF, Friedman HI, Haines PC, Rodeheaver GT. (1984) Biology of wound repair: its influence on surgical decision. *Facial Plast Surg* **1**: 169–80.

Fonseca JL. (1983) Use of pericranial flap in scalp wounds with exposed bone. *Plast Reconstr Surg* **72**: 786–90.

Horowitz JH, Persing JA, Nichter LS, Morgan RF, Edgerton MT. (1984) Galeal-pericranial flaps in head and neck reconstruction: anatomy and application. *Am J Surg* **148**: 489–97.

Koss N, Robson MC, Krizek TJ. (1975) Scalping injury. *Plast Reconstr Surg* **55**: 439–44.

McGrath MH. (1983) Scalping: the savage and the surgeon. *Clin Plast Surg* **10**: 679–88.

Magee C, Haury B, Rodeheaver GT, Fox J, Edgerton MT, Edlich RF. (1977) A reported technique for quantitating wound bacteria count. *Am J Surg* **133**: 760–62.

Malbec EF, Quaife JV, Vieyra-Urquiza HA. (1963) Carcinoma complications in radiodermatitis. *Plast Reconstr Surg* **32**: 447.

Manders EK, Graham WD, Schenden MJ, Davis TS. (1982) Skin expansion to eliminate large scalp defects. *Ann Plast Surg* **9**: 131–44.

Mathes SJ, Vasconez LO, Rosenblum ML. (1981) Management of the difficult scalp and intracranial wound. *Clin Plast Surg* **8**: 327–32.

Miller GDH, Anstee EJ, Snell JA. (1976) A successful replantation of an avulsed scalp by microvascular anastomoses. *Plast Reconstr Surg* **58**: 133.

Orticochea M. (1967) Four-flap scalp reconstruction technique. *Br J Plast Surg* **20**: 159–71.

Orticochea M. (1971) New three-flap scalp reconstruction technique. *Br J Plast Surg* **24**: 184–88.

Osborne MP. (1950) Complete scalp avulsion: report of cases. Experimental basis for production of free hair-bearing grafts from avulsed scalp itself. *Ann Surg* **132**: 198.

Pare A. (1634) *The collected works of Ambroise Pare*, 1st English edition Johnson T, translator. (1968) London: Milford House, 371.

Robinson DW. (1975) Surgical problems in the excision and repair of radiated tissue. *Plast Reconstr Surg* **55**: 41–49.

Serafin D, Deland M, Lesesne CB, Smith PJ, Noell KT, Georgiade N. (1982) Reconstruction with vascularized composite tissue in patients with extensive injury following surgery and irradiation. *Ann Plast Surg* **8**: 35–54.

Van Swieten GF (1754) *The commentaries upon the aphorisms of Dr Herman Boerhaave, concerning the knowledge and cure of the several diseases incident to human bodies*. London: John and Paul Knapton.

3

Skull fracture and cranial defects

Brian H Cummins

The importance of a skull fracture

Like beauty, the importance of a fractured skull is in the eye of the beholder. The victim may be blissfully unaware of it, until clear fluid drips from his nose. The neurosurgeon may simply note a linear crack on his way to the brain. The lawyer may regard 'a hairline fracture' as a major event in itself, particularly if, by mismanagement, it was not identified earlier.

The doctor preparing a report for the legal profession, whether concerning the trauma itself, or in cases of alleged negligence, should be aware of this wide variety of perceptions. He must also be aware of the frequently difficult circumstances that accompany radiological confirmation of a fracture, as well as the evolving pattern of head injury management that now dictates a scan in preference to a simple radiograph. This opinion, like that of a judge, must weigh these factors in the balance, since it will be on the authority of the doctor that legal events may proceed.

Be that as it may, a skull fracture is without doubt evidence that the head has been hit fairly hard and its proven presence is an indication for admission to hospital for observation in case of the development of an intracranial haematoma. Before ubiquitous CT scanning, a skull radiograph was the sieve through which the admissible sheep were separated from the dischargeable goats; this is still valid practice.

The work of the Glasgow group, led by Bryan Jennett (1980), gave great weight to this argument. They stressed that a radiologically proven fracture is an indicator that raises the chance of an intracranial haematoma 20 times in the comatose. This led to a proliferation of skull radiographs for trivial injuries for 'medicolegal' reasons and to the consequent reaction from the radiologists who were anxious to curtail waste. A series of options were presented ranging from 'radiograph none' to 'radiograph all' head injuries, however slight (Royal College of Radiologists, 1983). Mindful of the importance of balancing the clinical value of the examination against limited resources, and casting aside fear of legal repercussion as not germane to the issue, a group of neurosurgeons published, after lengthy debate, guidelines for skull radiography and consequent admission, which have served well despite the dawn of the CT scanning era (Group of Neurosurgeons, 1984). Contrary to expectations, adherence to these guidelines, particularly if reduced to an algorithm for the guidance of junior staff, cut in half not only the number of skull radiographs performed but also admissions of patients to hospital, resulting in major cost savings (Table 3.1).

Thus, clinical judgement backed by sound guidelines takes precedence. A skull fracture whether clinically perceived (boggy haematoma, cerebrospinal fluid leak, bleeding from nose or ear, subconjunctival haematoma or black eye without

Table 3.1. Changes in clinical management due to guidelines established half way through 1984

	1975–6	*1982–3*	*1983–4*	*1984–5*
All cases to A/E	50 628	46 864	48 539	49 966
Head injury to A/E	4 250	3 824	3 734	3 625
Head injury admitted	996	983	729	414
Head injury to ITU, NSU	32	41	36	27
Skull radiograph	2 549	2 402	1 566	1 259

In this series, no acute intracranial haematoma was missed. (ITU = intensive therapy unit; NSU = neurosurgical unit.)

local trauma) or identified on radiography, should require admission for observation, regardless of the neurological state.

Various difficulties in identification of skull fracture

Since a fracture of the skull gives such weight to clinical management, it is evident to any lawyer that its identification by radiography is equally important and should be easily revealed by routine examination. Doctors know to their cost that full many a crack is borne to blush unseen and that even to the most experienced eyes a simple radiograph of the skull may bristle with uncertainty; interpretation can be difficult in trauma for the following reasons.

1. In 1976, a research team from the National Institutes of Health USA (Webber and Folio, 1976) radiographed nine cadaver skulls with lateral and Towne's views, then fractured each in the occipital or temporoparietal area with a lead hammer, producing both linear and depressed fractures of varying sizes, before taking the same radiograph films again. The films were presented as two pairs from each cadaver to six radiologists, three of whom had more than 10 years' experience. Of the 216 decisions concerning the presence or absence of a fracture, 41 were attributed to the wrong radiograph film. The more experienced radiologists fared no better than their juniors. Large depressed fractures were missed. (These radiographs were taken in ideal conditions with very still patients.)
2. Over half of all skull radiographs on the acutely injured will be performed in the evening or at the weekend, when most such injuries occur. The majority of these will first be interpreted by a junior accident service doctor, not expert in

radiological analysis. It can be assumed that the error rate will be high. In my experience, a skull radiograph is difficult to be certain about, while a CT scan is relatively easy. A CT scan may not reveal a fracture, but it does establish what is more important, and what the skull radiograph can give only a clue to: the presence or absence of freshly spilt blood within the cranial cavity. If it is clinically important to establish a basal fracture of the skull, then bone setting windows of the CT scan should be performed. In a restless patient, a CT scan may require an anaesthetic, as there is no justification for a poor quality scan, and the airway must be protected.

For this reason alone, clinical judgement is paramount, the skull radiograph becoming less important as the availability of CT scans in district general hospitals increases. At present, acute MRI scanning is rare, because of the slowness of the machines and the lack of availability of nonmagnetic anaesthetic apparatus, but things will probably change as the machines improve and hospitals have to decide whether they want an MR or a CT scanner to do the routine work. Curiously, because MRI is poor at delineating bone, if it becomes an alternative to CT scanning, then accident departments may be thrown back upon the straight skull radiograph for their head injury triage.

3. Emergency radiograph examinations of the skull are often carried out in less than ideal circumstances. The patient may be confused or drunk. A blurred image from patient movement is worse than useless. Bitter experience in Bosnia taught me that straight radiographs of the skull (the only available diagnostic tool) were of little use in the pursuit of indriven metal and bone, unless there were true AP and true lateral views so that some co-ordinates were possible. A lateral view must not be taken with

the head twisted sideways on a possibly fractured neck. The development of powerful portable radiograph machines and well trained radiographers now ensures excellent quality films in most British accident and emergency departments. Other countries are not so fortunate and radiographs from abroad may therefore give little useful information.

Clinical expertise therefore remains at the core of skull fracture identification. It must be remembered that, apart from a fractured base of skull with cerebrospinal leak or cranial nerve disruption, a fracture of the skull is only of importance as testimony to the violence of the injury to the brain beneath it and the possibility that it confers on the development of intracranial haematoma. The brain injury and indeed the intracranial haematoma is best demonstrated by clinical observation and CT or MRI scanning.

Types of skull fracture and their legal significance

Patients who have sustained a skull fracture will have almost certainly been concussed and, even if conscious, may still be in the post-traumatic amnesic phase when first examined. If the fracture is at the site of a single blow to the head, the overlying scalp may be lacerated as its indicator. Where there is no laceration there is usually a bruise, although the skin may not discolour for some hours after injury. It does not take an extradural haematoma to produce a boggy swelling of the scalp; a simple linear fracture will produce a definite soft indentible swelling, which is more easily felt than seen, particularly in patients with a good head of hair and of the black races. Such a swelling demands an radiograph examination of the skull unless the depth of coma requires a CT scan instead.

Despite the violence required to fracture the skull, it is not common for a simple linear fracture to cause severe headache. If the patient complains of a bad headache, a scan must be done. Severe headache, particularly if accompanied by persistent vomiting, frequently means blood spilt inside the skull.

Most linear fractures seen on skull radiographs seem to be produced by torsion of the thinnest parts of the cranium on its thicker base, so that there is usually an oblique temporal fracture heading down to the sphenoidal ridge across the main middle meningeal artery branches. In many post-mortems, an apparently small temporal linear fracture will go right across the sphenoid bone in the midline in front of the anterior clinoid processes.

More posteriorly, a temporal fracture may extend into the petrosal bone. This may be evident clinically by a bleeding ear, a facial weakness, or the late development of a bruise behind the ear over the mastoid process (Battle's sign).

Occipital linear fracture

An occipital linear fracture should be viewed with suspicion. It is rarely seen in high speed vehicle accidents (unless the victim has been carrying a loose cargo of hard objects), but is commonly present in the elderly or the bibulous who fall, hitting the backs of their heads against the unyielding pavement. Such violent deceleration not only fractures the back of the skull by direct blow (coup) but more importantly, by rebound, bruises the anterior parts of the brain, particularly the frontal and temporal poles (contrecoup) (Figure 3.1).

A 5-feet-tall granny will hit the back of her head against the floor at about 12 miles an hour, her wrists in such a fall being unlikely to save her. A linear fracture to the occiput may be evidence of troubles to come. Even if not confused on first examination, the patient may become so, with the delayed development of a frontal intracerebral haematomata, particularly when the clotting mechanisms of the blood have been disordered. Alcoholics fall down often. There is an increasing population of predominantly elderly people who also fall frequently, who are on an anticoagulant therapy. Aspirin is so commonly used as to be disregarded by the public as a drug, but may produce long-lasting problems of bleeding after both operation and trauma. Such patients' relatives should be warned of the possibility of a slow decline in conscious level, even after discharge, although the majority will show symptoms within the first day after injury. It is not all that common for chronic subdural haematomas to have a recognizable generation by head injury, but it is probable that an unrecorded minor blow to the head is the genesis of most. The antique pachymeningitis haemorrhagica interna of alcoholics was almost certainly the chronic subdural haematoma induced by a tipsy stumble.

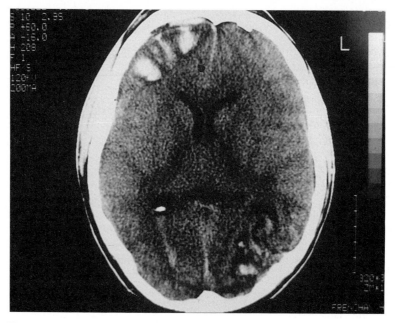

Figure 3.1. Occipital and frontal contusions following a heavy blow to the occiput. A coup–contrecoup injury.

Contrecoup

Contrecoup usually causes more cerebral damage than a direct blow. It is capable of producing dysphasia from right sided temporal fractures and epilepsy from frontal contusion in occipital fractures.

Most occipital fractures will cross the transverse sinus, but this seems rarely damaged or subject to thrombosis in simple linear cracks. In young people, an extradural haematoma may compress the posterior fossa when the dura and the transverse sinus have been wrenched off the undersurface of the fractured skull. In these rare cases, the rapidity of the depression of consciousness and cessation of respiration may be precipitous.

Transverse fractures

Transverse fractures from parietal to frontal bones seem to be produced by the peculiarity of the object hitting the skull (a pavement or edge of a wall) and are commonly accompanied by a similarly shaped scalp bruise or laceration. Such long fractures crossing the motor strip are often atten-ded by considerable local cerebral cortical contusion, producing contralateral upper limb weakness of such severity that it can mimic a brachial plexus lesion, distinguishable only later as the reflexes become brisk while the paresis remains severe. Fortunately, such pareses usually recover, although many months may pass before supple strength returns.

Bilateral coronal fractures

Bilateral coronal fractures cross the sagittal sinus and are usually produced by high speed crashes or falls from high places. The victim is unconscious from the time of the injury. Here, extradural haematoma is less common than acute subdural haematoma caused by avulsion of the cerebral veins off the sagittal sinus. Such rapidly developing haematomas may be difficult to detect clinically if the patient is deeply unconscious from the beginning. Here, the clue of the fracture should require frequent CT scanning or intracranial pressure monitoring. Frequently in intensive care situations a combination of both is performed and this is probably the optimal, but not the required, management.

Frontral linear fractures

Frontral linear fractures are less common than they were in countries where the seat belt laws are respected. The 'stove-in' forehead and rearranged orbits are now rarely seen in a society that has learned to protect itself from traumas of its own manufacture. Helmets for the riders of motor-cycles, horses or pedal cycles reduce the risk of fracture of the skull. However, it is most important to stress to lawyers that the absence of a fracture of the skull means little if the artificial cranium of the helmet itself is smashed. The same degree of violence will have been applied to the head, although vitiated. The absence of a fracture, like the dog who did not bark, may conceal the familiar diffuse axonal injury with long-term brain dis-organization. When a linear frontal fracture does occur, its relationship to the frontal and ethmoidal air sinuses is of importance. It is useful to look for fluid levels on the lateral radiograph films, although the sinuses are usually plugged with haematoma at first. Cerebrospinal fluid rhinor-rhoea may come later.

With frontal and indeed occipital fractures, it is important to test for the sense of smell as soon as the patient has come out of the amnesic state and the nose is clear from blood clot. In these sophisticated days, the inability to smell and taste is a considerable disadvantage. In certain occupa-tions, anosmia is a distinct health hazard. An absent sense of smell, a poor memory and a gas cooker can, at home, be a lethal combination.

Compound fractures of the skull

These can range from the gaping hole left by an axe and holes drilled by missiles to penetration of infant skulls by household objects such as pencils and toys. While a high velocity bullet has only to touch the skull tangentially to explode it and the brain beneath, the majority of martial and civilian open fractures are of relatively low velocity, even if of savage intent. Consciousness may not be lost.

I have seen a rapier thrust through the orbit transfix the brain and the patient puzzled at the fuss. A 16-year-old boy shot himself with an airgun and cycled 10 miles to the nearest hospital to have a radiograph examination, which showed the bullet on the opposite side of the head; this was disbelieved and RIGHT substituted for LEFT in crayon on the film. A suicidal man solemnly drilled holes through his head with a do-it-yourself drill before reporting, quite intact, to his local accident department. Radiography did not disclose the holes and he was admitted to the psychiatric unit as depressed. Two weeks later he was hemiplegic with a cerebral abscess. He made a full recovery after surgery and lost his depression.

Always treat seriously a history of possible penetration of the skull. A straight radiograph may not show the minute fracture, but a CT scan will reveal the track of the penetration.

Axe injuries of the skull can be surprisingly benign unless they cross a major sinus. The danger is of past, present and future bleeding, and resuscitation should be prompt and adequate with only emergency clamping of major bleeding ves-sels before definitive surgery is undertaken with adequate blood available for transfusion. Even a major venous sinus tear is capable either of being sutured or plugged, provided that: the anaesthetic conditions are good; the position of the head is neutral and does not twist the veins of the neck, allowing the head to be elevated or depressed at will; blood is available; bone is sacrificed liberally around the damaged dura; and the operating table is tilted to allow a gentle lapping of blood out of the hole rather than a heart-sinking gush. The head should not be raised too high or air embolism may ensue. The dura should always be closed or patched.

In cases like this, a good operation note is of inestimable value if only for the coroner. Appar-ently trivial scalp lacerations in children may produce a fleck of pinkish grey cerebral cortex at the surface of the wound, even in an alert child. The child's skull and dura mater are very fragile and can be lacerated by minor trauma. This evidence of cerebral disruption demands neuro-surgical attention.

Nonaccidental injuries to infants

Subdural haematomas from child abuse are now less common than they were 20 years ago. Skull fractures are frequent, but not usually accompanied by subdural haematomas, although cerebral con-tusion can often be demonstrated on CT scan. A history of trivial causation ('fell off settee on to carpeted floor') combined with skull fracture, multiple bruises (frequently of different ages) and occasionally limb fracture, lead to the sad con-clusion of nonaccidental violence. All of the convoluted, but necessary, social service and police investigations should then be initiated if the child and its siblings are to be protected.

Basal fractures of the skull

The history of the mechanism of trauma should be sought in all cases of head injury, since it is, if not clouded by amnesia, a very good indicator of the vectors of violence applied to the head. This is particularly true in fractures of the base of the skull, whose long-term problems are of cerebrospinal fluid leakage and cranial nerve damage. There is an uncommon but interesting variety of injury, in which the distortion of the skull has been relatively slow, usually by a ponderous mass squashing the head, as when a car settles on top of the patient on hard ground.

Many fractures of the base of skull are undetectable, except by clinical supposition, yet their consequences are important. A medical report must seek and detail these.

The most common basal fracture of the skull is probably an extension of a linear fracture of the calvarium which itself may be identified by radiography. The clinical features of the case will give the clue to its basal extension.

Cerebrospinal fluid rhinorrhoea may come from the frontal ethmoidal or sphenoidal sinuses. It may be detected early with fluid levels in the affected sinus on radiograph examination. It may, on the other hand, be very difficult to pin down and require sophisticated scanning with radio-opaque dye. Occasionally, a fractured petrous temporal bone, with lacerated dura over it, will leak cerebrospinal fluid via the middle ear to the eustachian tube and out through the nostril. Persistent leakage should be stopped surgically. The sense of smell should be tested before operation and if it still exists, warning should be given that the sense of smell is unlikely to remain after frontal operation. Anosmia is a considerable disability.

Cerebrospinal fluid otorrhoea usually stops spontaneously, but is evidence of a petrous temporal bone fracture. A Battle's sign of delayed spreading haematoma over the mastoid process is usually present the following day. Unilateral deafness and facial weakness are common, the latter often delayed by up to a week after injury. This must be anticipated. There is usually recovery of facial, if not full auditory, function. Operative decompression is not often practised in Britain, there being no observable difference from a conservative non-operative therapy. The role of steroids is debatable.

Tinnitus, deafness and troublesome vertigo are often the long-standing sequelae of a skull base fracture. It is common for the first few months to be the worst, but in a few patients symptoms may persist for years. In this situation an opinion from an otolaryngologist with access to sophisticated electrophysiological testing should be recommended, both as a base line and as a follow-up report. The tell-tale sign of corneal opacity attests to an undiscovered facial weakness early in the course of the illness.

The optic nerve may be seriously disordered by basal and orbital fractures. This is difficult to be certain about when the patient is unconscious, since, in this sort of injury, the oculomotor nerve is often also injured, with a pupillary paresis. If the patient is not totally blind, the outcome is often a nondescript lack of visual perception with a very pale optic disc. Careful fundoscopy should be made in any examination for a medical report. It is surprising how pale optic discs are in patients who simply complain 'my eyesight is not what it was'.

Orbital fractures are often complex and may be the result of localized trauma such as from a boot or a clenched fist. Traumatic mydriasis should not be the excuse for failing to diagnose an extradural haematoma. The horrors of seriously disrupted orbits and frontal bones have largely been dispelled by good helmets and seat belts.

When it is possible to be sure about the co-operation of the patient, the visual fields should be tested, since optic chiasm injuries are not uncommon in anterior basal skull fractures. The provider of a medical report may be the first to determine partial visual loss and indeed, retrospectively, an accompanying diabetes insipidus, which may trouble patients for some months after injury. Here sexual dysfunction is often an undisclosed concomitant, there being little cause to enquire about it in hospital. The victim is usually patient enough to wait for many months for return of normal sexual function and thereafter may become too inhibited to talk about it.

If a basal fracture around the clinoid process is suspected, an adequate coronal CT scan should be performed in the early days after injury. It is uncommon to have to remove bone chips from the optic foramen and dubious whether any good comes of it. Most optic nerve disorders, unless complete, will improve with time, but the victim may be left with inadequate vision. This should be documented at various stages. An expert ophthalmological report should be requested, particularly when visual fields need to be plotted accurately.

The causes of diplopia, which can accompany orbital fracturing, may be hard to elucidate clinically particularly if there is an accompanying brain stem injury. In these circumstances, there is often a mixture of oculomotor, trochlear and abducens disorder. Simple failure to elevate a single eye may indicate the possibility of a 'blow-out' fracture of the floor of the orbit, with entrapment of the inferior rectus muscle. This may be seen on skull radiography as a 'tear drop' into the antrum.

The trigeminal nerve is occasionally involved in a large basal fracture, usually of the crush variety. In this situation it often accompanies a facial nerve paresis and may not be detected until serious corneal damage has occurred. Intensive care units are usually skilled at protection of the cornea in unconscious patients, but the return to a ward with unskilled nurses and doctors who are unaware of the potential damage to the eye, is frequently the beginning of the little grey band across the clear cornea, if not overt conjunctivitis, which is easier to spot. Disorders of the lowest cranial nerves are very rare and are usually accompanied by brain stem disorder, which makes their elucidation difficult.

Where fracture of the base of skull is suspected, the provider of a medical report should look carefully for the cranial nerve disorders that may persist. It is important to liaise with the patient's general practitioner if such defects are newly discovered. It is wise to include other experts in one's opinion, particularly from the ophthalmological and otolaryngological field.

Depressed fractures

Although they may be associated with the extreme violence of a motor vehicle crash, when there is usually cerebral disruption, the majority of depressed fractures are caused by local low velocity blows of a foot, a hammer or, in these affluent days and usually amongst children, a golf club. There may be no clear recollection of the blow, no amnesia and no evidence of brain disorder. If the dura is penetrated, there is a long-term risk of epilepsy, which is much greater than if it is not (Jennett, 1975), but there is no proof that surgery will decrease this risk. Indeed, there is recent evidence that operation increases the risk of complications of infection, epilepsy and cerebral disorder, so that it is at least arguable that a clean compound depressed fracture should simply have the scalp sutured and be left alone. Probably this is the fate of many such fractures treated in accident and emergency departments and, to my knowledge, the neurosurgical units are not overloaded by the consequences of apparent neglect. If recognized, a CT scan should be performed to identify any underlying brain damage and indicate the extent of bone injury. Infants with simple 'pond' fractures can almost certainly be left for nature to remould the calvarium.

Nevertheless, a careful history should be taken of the genesis of the fracture. I would still be very uneasy about leaving bits of indriven skull in the brain. When there is the slightest chance of contaminated soft material unidentifiable by radiograph examination, which is lodged within the brain, the fracture should be expeditiously explored.

The Vietnam war confirmed what every military surgeon has discovered, that indriven bone and soft material produces an abscess unless removed, and that the risk of infection is less the more expeditiously and rigorously they are extirpated. Personal recent experience in Bosnia has shown the fatal effect of cerebral fungation from infected wounds. Following Hammon's advice: do a good biplanar radiograph examination and CT scan, get in early, suck out the whole track with the bone fragments until the brain does not fall in to block the track, and then close the dura. As long as the bone and bits of material, including hair, have been removed, the metal, which may have gone very deep or indeed right across the brain, can be left alone. It is not a good idea to recommend MRI scanning in such cases, although the metal of most missiles is not magnetic.

Skull defects

Holes in the head are more unsightly than dangerous and the majority will soon develop a thin calcification over the dura, which is protective. Indeed, the concavity produced by a long-standing cranial defect may have a calcified saucer adherent to the dura or underlying brain if the dura was left open at the initial operation. Removal of this is hazardous and conducive to compressive haematoma. Such an operation should not be undertaken lightly and the complications should be discussed fully with the patient and the relatives.

Like much of surgery, 'if twere done then twere best done quickly', and unsightly cranial defects should not be left to calcify as a saucer unless the condition of the patient forbids operation, or if it has been decided by the patient that the cosmetic defects are discountable. From time to time, a patient will have a change of mind and opt for the cosmetic closure of the defect, particularly if it is associated with tenderness and discomfort around the perimeter. In such a case, the simplest procedure, leaving the adventitious covering of the brain intact, has always seemed to me the best option. The bone effect can be filled in with tantalum mesh and acrylic, titanium plate or partial thickness of bone taken from the skull. Bone from the skull is less stable immediately and risks being reabsorbed. Mooring wires should avoid the frontal sinus. It is rarely a good idea to put a lot of plating into a freshly contaminated wound, however clean it seems to have been made. I have seen on many occasions one or all of the tiny plates form a septic focus.

On balance, it is best to operate on obtrusive cranial defects as soon as the patient's clinical state and the condition of the wound permit, and to avoid unnecessary operation on long-standing cosmetic calcified defects.

Growing skull fractures

Otherwise known as a leptomeningeal cyst, the 'growing' fracture is a very uncommon complication of paediatric head injury. Matson (1969) recorded only 17 cases, all in patients under the age of six years. The pathology is of a diastatic fracture producing an underlying dural laceration, which is combined with some distending force, such as a growing brain or hydrocephalus. Rarely does it occur beyond the age of three years, and around 75% of patients are less than one year of age (Luerssen *et al.*, 1994). The mean age in Matson's series was 10.5 months, although one patient was 12 years of age at the time of injury. An enlarging mass and palpable cranial defect develops some weeks or months after the initial injury, and may be associated with seizures or the development of neurological deficit. Rarely does the condition regress spontaneously, and progressive herniation of brain tissue is usually accompanied by resorption of the bony margins. However, a few patients have been reported in whom there was no progression of the defect, or any neurological deficit (Vas and Winn, 1966; Addy, 1973). Treatment is by dural repair with an autograft, combined with cranioplasty in all except very young children.

References

Addy DP. (1973) Expanding skull fractures of childhood. *Br Med J* **iv**: 338–39.

Group of Neurosurgeons. (1984) Guidelines for initial management after head injury in adults. *Br Med J* **288**: 983–85.

Jennett B. (1975) *Epilepsy after non-missile head injuries*, 2nd edition. London: William Heinemann.

Jennett B. (1980) Skull X-rays after recent head injury. *Clin Radiol* **31**: 463–69.

Luerssen T, Eisenberg HM, Levin HS. (1994) Late complications of head injury. In: Cheek WR, editor. *Pediatric Neurosurgery: Surgery of the developing nervous system*, 3rd edition. Philadelphia, PA: Saunders, 297–306.

Matson DD. (1969) Neurosurgery of infancy and childhood, 2nd edition. Springfield IL: Charles C. Thomas, 304–11.

Royal College of Radiologists. (1983) Patient selection for skull radiography in uncomplicated head injury. *Lancet* **i**: 115–18.

Vas CJ, Winn JM. (1966) Growing skull fractures. *Dev Med Child Neurol* **8**: 735–40.

Webber RJ, Folio J. (1976) Radiographic detectability of occipital and temporo-parietal fractures induced in cadaver heads. *J Trauma* **16**: 115–23.

4

Penetrating and perforating cranial trauma

Robert Macfarlane

Introduction and definitions

Missile wounds to the head are often termed 'penetrating', whilst puncture or stab wounds may be referred to as 'perforating'. As well as the risks of infection and haemorrhage, the possibility of retained foreign bodies and deep-seated parenchymal injury set these apart from other compound fractures of the skull. Penetration is particularly common when objects striking the cranium are less than two square inches in cross-section (Gennarelli, 1990).

A wound is described as compound if there is a scalp laceration in the vicinity of the fracture, or if the scalp is intact but the fracture involves the paranasal air sinuses. A skull fracture is defined as depressed if the outer table of one or more of the fractured segments lies below the level of the inner table of the intact surrounding skull. An underlying dural laceration is unlikely in such cases if the bone has been depressed by less than 3 mm (McLaurin and Towbin, 1990).

Pathophysiology

Missile injuries

A detailed account of the pathophysiology of missile wounds to the brain can be found in Hopkinson and Marshall (1967), and Cooper (1982). In brief, a number of factors govern the extent of injury. Because the kinetic energy of a projectile is related to the square of its velocity, the speed at the moment of impact is of critical importance (DeMuth, 1963). However its mass, its type of movement ('yaw': deviation about the horizontal axis of the projectile, and 'tumble': deviation about the vertical axis), the angle at which it strikes the head (angle of incidence), the degree of fragmentation, the nature of the structures that it encounters, and the tendency for the projectile to deform and thereby increase its presenting area (mushrooming) are other important variables. The bullets from military weapons are usually jacketed with steel and retain their shape on entering the skull, whilst civilian bullets are often soft and are therefore more prone to deform or shatter. The pattern of injury produced by a shotgun varies with the distance between the muzzle and the victim. When the distance is greater than 10 metres the wound is composed of multiple holes whilst, at less than five metres, the impact site is solitary and large, containing not only the pellets, but wadding from the shell (Bakay and Glasauer, 1980).

Penetration of the head by a bullet from a military rifle with a high muzzle velocity (>2400 ft s^{-1}) is generally incompatible with survival (Cooper, 1982). An instantaneous rise in intracranial pressure accompanies the shock wave, and is transmitted down the neuroaxis to the brain stem, resulting in herniation (Freytag, 1963). As a consequence, the majority of reports detailing the management and outcome of combat wounds relate to shrapnel injury. Many civilian wounds are produced by handguns with low muzzle velocities (<1000 ft s^{-1}). The presence of smoke on the skin is evidence that the victim was shot at very close range, whilst fragments of burnt powder may be evident if the muzzle is close but somewhat further from the scalp. The projectile may be spent and lodge within the brain, it may ricochet off the contralateral side of the skull creating a second track (Figure 4.1), or it may exit the cranium. In a series of 254 civilian firearm injuries, 82% left a single track within the brain, whilst 18% created two or more tracks from ricochets (Freytag, 1963).

Impact with the skull comminutes the bone and forces fragments inwards (spallation). Substantial injury to the cortex and white matter may occur even in the absence of bone penetration, such as when a missile strikes the skull tangentially (Gade *et al.*, 1990). The scalp injury in this instance is frequently a 'gutter' laceration (Adeloye and Odeku, 1971). This may be associated with a linear skull fracture, or fragments of the inner table of the skull may penetrate deep into the brain in the absence of a fracture of the outer table (Matson, 1958). An important consequence of this is that there may be substantial brain injury in the presence of seemingly trivial scalp trauma, and with no skull fracture apparent at the time of wound exploration (Adeloye and Odeku, 1971).

There are three velocity-dependent mechanisms by which brain parenchyma is damaged by a missile (Hopkinson and Marshall, 1967). Direct tissue disruption occurs below a velocity of 320 m s^{-1}. The size of this permanent cavity is determined by the diameter of the deformed missile, its muzzle energy, and its flight characteristics (Kirkpatrick and Di Maio, 1978). Above this, shock waves are generated in front of the missile, creating pressure gradients, which disrupt tissue some distance from the track itself. Thirdly, the missile imparts radial velocity to the tissue as it forces it apart (temporary cavitation), at times creating a cavity 30 times larger than the diameter of the projectile (Butler *et al.*, 1945; DeMuth, 1969). The negative pressure within the cavity sucks debris deep within it. The cavity then collapses after 10–20 ms. However, there then follow 5–6 cycles of gradually diminishing collapse and re-expansion (pulsation) due to tissue elasticity. Under experimental conditions, intracranial pressure may rise transiently to 100 mmHg at this time (Kirkpatrick and Di Maio, 1978). High velocity missiles may cause bursting of the skull at the point of exit as a result of the associated pressure wave (Crockard *et al.*, 1974). Butler *et al.* (1945) demonstrated a massive increase in skull damage when an intact cranium was shot, when compared with the exit damage inflicted by a projectile of the same size and velocity striking an empty skull. Large calibre civilian missiles of lower velocity are more likely to possess sufficient energy to exit the skull than are small ones. Linear skull fractures radiating from the site of the entry wound are seen in 71% of cases, particularly in victims shot at close range (Freytag, 1963). Left unattended, the combination

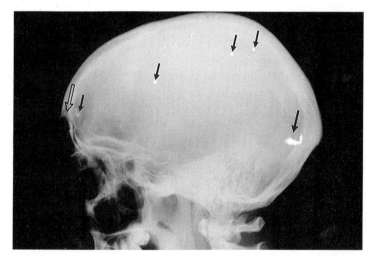

Figure 4.1. Lateral skull radiograph following a suicide attempt with a .22 calibre rifle. The entry point is via the frontal air sinus (open arrow). The bullet has fragmented, leaving metal debris along the primary missile track (small arrows), before ricocheting off the inner table of the skull vault. The large fragment has come to rest on the tentorium cerebelli (large arrow).

of devitalized tissue, haemorrhage and foreign material leads to suppuration, whilst extensive areas of gliosis may become a nidus for seizures.

Traumatic aneurysms were at one time thought to be extremely rare after missile injury. Hammon (1971a) recorded only two symptomatic cases in his series of 2187 patients. However, Haddad (1978) performed routine angiography prior to hospital discharge in 219 patients, detecting seven aneurysms and four carotico-cavernous fistulae. Histologically, all the aneurysms were false (Haddad *et al.*, 1991), and many were on a secondary branch of the middle cerebral artery. Jinkins *et al.* (1992) detected vascular injuries in 50% of the victims of civilian gunshot wounds subjected to angiography within 48 hours of the insult.

Rubber or plastic bullets ('baton rounds'), used in riot control, may caused depressed or linear skull fractures if fired from close range. Occasional reports of cerebral contusions, extensive oedema and death have appeared in the literature (Metress and Metress, 1987; Millar *et al.*, 1975).

Perforating injuries

Because of the localized nature of the injury, perforating trauma may not be associated with loss of consciousness. The apparent well-being of the patient may mislead the physician about the severity of the insult (de Villiers, 1975). This is true particularly in children, who have thin skulls and may not be able to give a good account of their injury (Figure 4.2). Sharp objects entering the orbit or nasal cavity may penetrate the cranium (Guthkelch, 1960). An intracranial foreign body was not suspected at the time of first examination in 60% of patients in one series, including a knife blade extending from the orbit to the parieto-occipital region in one, and a nail traversing the cerebellum, tentorium and occipital lobe in another (Bakay *et al.*, 1977). In a series of 22 pencil injuries to the brain, 33% of patients presented with neurological symptoms more than one year after the original insult (Bursick and Selker, 1981).

Vascular lesions are particularly common after perforating wounds. When vessel pathology was sought in a series of 109 such patients, 11 aneurysms, five carotico-cavernous fistulae, three arteriovenous fistulae, three arterial occlusions, two transections, and two cases of severe spasm were identified (Kieck and de Villiers, 1984). The total incidence of vascular pathology in patients undergoing angiography was 30%. All of the carotico-cavernous fistulae were evident within 72 hours of injury, but some aneurysms did not develop until months later. Some of these patients had negative arteriograms soon after the trauma.

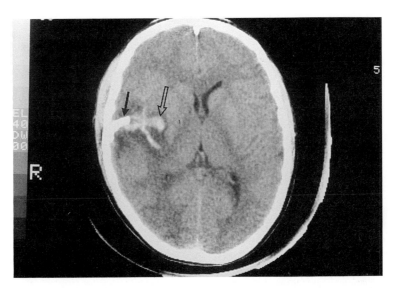

Figure 4.2. CT scan of a 17-year-old male who was assaulted with a screwdriver by his brother. The patient was sent home from the emergency department after the casualty officer failed to detect bony injury, only to present 72 hours later with a grand mal seizure. The indriven bone (closed arrow) and haematoma track from the screwdriver (open arrow) are clearly evident.

Three of the aneurysm patients died subsequently from delayed rupture. Vascular trauma is considered further in Chapter 16.

Depressed fractures

More than half the patients with depressed skull fractures are under 16 years of age (Miller and Jennett, 1968). Only 25% of patients lose consciousness at the time of their injury, and a further 25% have post-traumatic amnesia (PTA) of less than one hour (Jennett, 1975). Approximately 50–90% of depressed fractures are compound (Becker *et al.*, 1990), but the site of the laceration may be remote from the underlying calvarial fracture, due to the mobility of the scalp. Furthermore, there is a tendency for the inner table of the skull to separate from the outer table, and to be involved to a greater degree. Inspection of the outer table at the time of wound suture may therefore underestimate the degree of depression. The combination of brief or no loss of consciousness, and a lack of apparent bony injury at the time of scalp suture, is the reason why some of these injuries remain undetected initially. Significant intracranial haematomas, usually intracerebral, develop in about 7% of cases, and the major dural venous sinuses are involved in 11% (Miller and Jennett, 1968).

Investigation

Imaging should include plain skull radiographs and a CT scan. Angiography may be appropriate if the injury is close to a major vessel, and if time permits. Wooden objects in particular may be difficult to detect as retained foreign bodies. Wood is not seen well on plain radiographs. It appears as low attenuation on CT and, as such, may be mistaken for intracranial air (Jooma *et al.*, 1984; Miller *et al.*, 1977). However, assessment at high window settings may reveal a striated internal architecture, which is thought to be specific for wood (Ginsberg *et al.*, 1993). Other patients who can be difficult to assess are those who sustain perforating wounds from a thin implement that has been removed prior to hospital admission (Figure 4.2), or who suffer occult perforations that follow trauma to the orbits, nose or pharynx (Bursick and Selker, 1981; Guthkelch, 1960). Even experienced radiologists may miss large depressed fractures on plain skull radiographs (Webber and Folio, 1976).

The presence of a slot-shaped fracture is diagnostic of a stab wound (Kieck and de Villiers, 1984). Gas may be evident within the cavernous sinus on a CT scan following penetrating head injury (Rubinstein and Symonds, 1994).

Management and outcome

Depressed skull fracture

The fracture of the inner table of the skull is often larger than that of the outer table, producing injury to the brain over an area wider than might be imagined from the extent of the surface damage. Miller and Jennett (1968) reported 104 complications in a series of 400 civilian depressed skull fractures: an incidence of 26%. The results are shown in Table 4.1. The development of these complications significantly worsens outcome. When comparing those who did or did not develop complications of infection, haemorrhage or sinus involvement in association with the depressed fracture, the incidence of death was 7.7% versus 1.3%, the likelihood of persistent neurological deficit at six months was 23.1% versus 10.8%, and the incidence of late post-traumatic epilepsy was 15.4% versus 7.4% respectively in the two groups (Miller and Jennett, 1968). All of these differences were statistically significant. Occasional case reports of traumatic arteriovenous fistulae resulting from depressed fractures have been recorded (Feldman *et al.*, 1980; Nakamura *et al.*, 1966). The

Table 4.1. Complications in 104 of 400 civilians with depressed skull fracture

Complication	No. patients	% of series
Infections	38	9.5
Brain abscess	15	3.8
Meningitis	9	2.2
Wound infection	17	4.2
Fungal infection	3	0.8
Intracranial haematoma	28	7.0
Intracerebral	17	4.3
Extradural	8	2.0
Subdural	3	0.8
Venous sinus involvement	46	11.5
Sagittal sinus torn	16	4.0
Transverse sinus torn	6	1.5
Major tributary of sinus torn	6	1.5
Fracture not elevated	18	4.5

Adapted from Miller and Jennett (1968).

incidence of extradural abscess is approximately 0.25–0.4% (Meirowsky, 1965; Miller and Jennett, 1968). Haematoma evacuation and wound debridement reduce both the risk of permanent neurological deficit and the incidence of late epilepsy (Jennett and Miller 1972; Jennett *et al.*, 1974; Miller and Jennett, 1968). There is no increase in the risk of postoperative infection if bone fragments are replaced at operation, even when surgery has been delayed beyond 24 hours from the time of injury (Jennett and Miller, 1972). The risk of postoperative infection is less than 5% (Miller and Jennett, 1968). However, early cranioplasty with synthetic materials is associated with a high incidence of infective complications (Jennett and Miller, 1972).

Perforating wounds

Perforating wounds with retained intracranial wood have a particularly poor prognosis. In a review of 42 such patients, mortality was 25%, with morbidity occurring in 74% of survivors (Miller *et al.*, 1977). In a cumulative series of 22 pencil injuries to the brain in children and adolescents, 72% entered the cranium via the superior orbital plate (Bursick and Selker, 1981). The overall mortality was 36%, and permanent neurological impairment occurred in 50% of survivors, usually as a result of the initial insult. Despite antibiotic prophylaxis, 77% of patients developed septic complications.

Missile wounds

As detailed in the section on pathophysiology, missile velocity has a crucial bearing on outcome. For example, in Hammon's report on the results of 2187 penetrating brain injuries from Vietnam, the operative mortality for gunshot wounds was 22.7%, but only 7.6% for shrapnel wounds (Hammon, 1971a). Haddad (1978) recorded a mortality rate of 47.5% for high velocity injuries (muzzle velocity 700–900 m s^{-1}), and 25% for low velocity head trauma. The level of consciousness on admission is an important prognostic indicator (Rish *et al.*, 1983). Of 93 missile wounds to the head, most of which were admitted to hospital within 30 minutes of injury, 88% of patients who were conscious on admission survived, compared with 66% of those who were drowsy, and 21% of those who were unconscious (Gordon, 1975).

Decerebrate posturing carries a mortality of almost 94% (Rish *et al.*, 1983). Missile wounds involving only one lobe of the brain fare substantially better (35–45% mortality) than those that involve multiple lobes or traverse the midline (51–90% mortality) (Haddad, 1978; Hernesniemi, 1979; Raimondi and Samuelson, 1970). Early complete flaccid paralysis associated with an upper motor neurone facial weakness usually indicates extensive injury to the cortex, and has a poor prognosis compared with an early spastic paralysis, which is more likely to indicate local contusion or oedema (Matson, 1958). Delay in surgical debridement is another significant factor for a poor outcome (Raimondi and Samuelson, 1970).

The basic principles of the management of missile wounds to the brain were published by Cushing in 1918. They include debridement of the scalp, evacuation of any haematoma and devitalized brain, removal of indriven bone fragments, and watertight dural closure. The major postoperative goals are the control of intracranial hypertension, the maintenance of adequate cerebral oxygenation, and the prevention of secondary complications. Raimondi and Samuelson (1970) have reported that a delay in definitive treatment increases both morbidity and mortality. Experience from the Korean war indicated that intracerebral haematoma was present in 10% of early treatable missile wounds, but in 41% of delayed cases (Barnett and Meirowsky, 1955).

Retained fragments may have consequences other than infection. The combined effects of gravity, brain softening, and pulsation may, on occasions, cause secondary brain injury as a result of migration (Jefferson, 1917; Ott *et al.*, 1976), whilst the composition of the metal may induce a tissue reaction. Lead (e.g. gunshot), if sterile, produces only a minimal reaction, whereas copperplated missiles (e.g. most .22 calibre bullets) undergo oxidation and may create a sterile abscess or granuloma (Ott *et al.*, 1976; Sights and Bye, 1970). Copper-plated missiles are therefore more prone to migrate.

Penetrating wounds and infection

In most instances, infection is likely to manifest itself within three to five weeks of the injury (Rowe and Turner, 1945). However, infectious complications have been reported to arise several decades later (Drew and Fager, 1954; Dzenitis and Kalsbeck, 1965), particularly if there is a retained intracranial foreign body such as wood (de Villiers, 1975; Miller *et al.*, 1977). Wood is an excellent source of infection because of its soft organic nature and porosity. In combat series, the risk of late abscess formation ranges from 1.8% to 8.4% (Brandvold *et al.*, 1990; Hagan, 1971; Rish *et al.*, 1981). In general, bone fragments appear to be the most likely nidus for infection, followed by hair, skin and other foreign material (Pitlyk *et al.*, 1970). Metal fragments, however, pose less of a threat (Carey *et al.*, 1971; Hammon, 1971b). The incidence of abscess formation in one experimental model was 4% when contaminated bone was implanted into the canine cerebral cortex, but rose to 69% when scalp or fur was also included (Pitlyk *et al.*, 1970). A study of casualties from World War II indicated that the infection risk was increased tenfold by the presence of bone fragments in wounds (Martin and Campbell, 1946). Hagan obtained positive cultures from 56.4% of retained bone fragments requiring reoperation 5–54 days after injury (of which 63% cultured *Staphylococcus epidermidis*), despite patients having received antibiotics for an average of two weeks from their first surgery (Hagan, 1971). Reporting on 42 patients with retained bone fragments from combat wounds, Hammon *et al.* (1971b) noted that 16 (38%) had positive wound cultures, and a further 23 (55%) had overt infection 10–62 days after injury.

However, the risk of late infection from retained deep or inaccessible bone fragments is dependent on the timing of any primary surgery. It has been estimated that up to 75% of all indriven bone fragments are sterile initially (Carey *et al.*, 1971), and that the missile track becomes contaminated secondarily from the surface inward (Cairns, 1944). Following early surgery, but with a retained bone fragment, no complications developed within 1 year in six patients suffering a penetrating injury (Sukoff *et al.*, 1971). Isolated fragments appear to pose less risk than clusters of retained fragments, which are more likely to represent poor debridement of the missile track and, therefore, a higher risk of late sepsis (Pitlyk *et al.*, 1970). Although prophylactic antibiotics are used widely, there is no good evidence that the infection rate is lowered if the wound has been debrided adequately and a watertight dural closure obtained (Cooper, 1982). Although several series reported a reduction in the incidence of infection following the introduction of penicillin and sulphonamides, this coincided with substantial improvements in the surgical management of war wounds (Matson, 1958).

The Vietnam Head Injury Study, in a 5-year follow-up of 1221 patients (23% with retained bone fragments), found 37 abscesses, of which 11 had retained bone (a total incidence of 3–6.4% for patients with retained bone, 2.5% for those without) (Rish *et al.*, 1981). Abscesses occurred only in patients who had another major risk factor, such as a facio-orbital (i.e. air sinus) entry point, cerebrospinal fluid leakage, wound infection, prolonged coma, or multiple surgical procedures. The mortality was 54%, and significant morbidity occurred in 82% of survivors. This included seizures in 59% of patients. In an evaluation of 379 combat wounds from the Iran–Iraq war, the incidence of cerebral abscess was 1.7% in patients who did not develop a cerebrospinal fistula, and 36% in those who did develop this complication (Aarabi, 1989). The other major factor in the development of intracranial infection is the presence or absence of scalp dehiscence when retained bone fragments are present (84.6% versus 4% infection rate respectively) (Taha *et al.*, 1991).

Contrary to popular belief, the heating effect of discharging gases and the friction of the bullet against the barrel wall are insufficient to sterilize a projectile (Hopkinson and Marshall, 1967). Hagan (1971) found that all metallic fragments cultured from seven combat wounds contained bacteria. The risk of infection is related in part to the velocity of the fragment, because of the attendant damage it produces to the surrounding cerebral tissue. Hence, the risk of late sepsis in civilian practice is likely to be lower than the reports from military series. In a review of low velocity civilian wounds to the head, Raimondi and Samuelson (1970) reported no infection in 25 patients with retained metal fragments.

Brandvold *et al.* (1990) reported the results of the long-term follow-up of 46 survivors of combat wounds sustained by Israelis in Lebanon. Unlike series from Korea and Vietnam, CT scanning was used routinely, and no effort was made to locate or remove indriven bone fragments at surgery unless they were encountered readily during debridement. Although 51% of survivors had CT evidence of retained bone fragments, no relationship existed between their presence and the incidence of either infection or late epilepsy. However, cranial wounds with a craniofacial entry point pose a greater risk of infection than those that enter the vault directly (Rowe and Turner, 1945).

Of 225 consecutive patients with nonmissile depressed fractures, the risk of infection was not significantly different whether or not the bone was replaced at surgery. Infection developed in five of 109 patients in which the bone was replaced, and in five out of 56 when it was removed (Braakman, 1971). However, the study was not randomized, and it is likely that the degree of wound contamination was greater in patients in whom the bone was not replaced. Jennett and Miller (1972) reported an infection rate of 10.6% among 359 civilian compound depressed skull fractures. Replacement of the bone, even when surgery was delayed beyond 24 hours from the time of trauma, did not increase the incidence of infection (3.6% versus 4.4% when bone was removed) or epilepsy, nor did the presence of retained indriven bone fragments. Prophylactic antibiotics were thought to be of some benefit to reduce the risk of infection (1.9% versus 10% in those who did and did not receive antibiotics respectively), although the study was retrospective and nonrandomized, making firm conclusions difficult. Dural closure did not influence outcome significantly. Of compound depressed fractures treated conservatively (i.e. with wound closure alone), the incidence of septic complications was 2.8% in one series of 139 patients (van den Heever and van der Merwe, 1989).

Post-traumatic epilepsy

Missile injury

This topic is covered in detail in Chapter 8. There are few large series to document accurately the risk of late epilepsy after civilian gunshot wounds to the head, but the incidence appears to be comparable with that for military series. Reports range from 22% to 50% (Brandvold *et al.*, 1990; Crockard, 1974; Gordon, 1975). In Dodge and Meirowsky's (1952) series of patients collected from the Korean conflict who suffered tangential missile injuries to the head without penetration, 19% suffered from seizures within 14 days of injury. However, the incidence of late epilepsy in published series is dependent on the length of review. In the Vietnam Head Injury Study (421 patients) the seizure incidence was 29% at two years and 53% at 15 years (Salazar *et al.*, 1985). Prophylactic anticonvulsant medication had been administered in 95% of patients. Loss of brain volume on CT scan, early haematoma formation, and retained metal fragments were all correlated with late seizures, but tangential injury, retained bone fragments, and the development of a brain abscess did not. Approximately 70% of the patients with epilepsy experienced partial seizures. Seizure

type tended to remain relatively stable over time. Caveness *et al.* (1979) reported that one-half of patients cease to have seizures within 5–10 years of onset, and found little evidence that prophylactic anticonvulsants reduced the incidence of post-traumatic epilepsy. Raimondi and Samuelson (1970) could find no relationship between the incidence of late epilepsy and the presence or absence of retained bone fragments.

Nonmissile injury

Jennett *et al.* (1974) investigated the risk of epilepsy in 1000 nonmissile depressed fractures. The incidence of late seizures overall was 15%, but ranged from less than 4% in patients with a PTA of less than 24 hours, no early epilepsy, and no dural tear, to greater than 60% if all of these features were present. Patients below the age of 16 years with depressed fractures have a lower incidence of late seizures (6.5%) than do adults (Jennett, 1975). In nonmissile injuries with dural laceration, the incidence of late epilepsy is reported to be 21% (Jennett, 1975). After nonmissile depressed fractures, the incidence of late epilepsy in 359 patients was 20.6% in those who suffered infective complications, and 8.9% in those who did not (Jennett and Miller, 1972). Replacement of bone fragments resulted in a lower incidence of seizures (9%) than in those in whom they were removed (17%) (Jennett *et al.*, 1974). In almost half the patients in whom late epilepsy eventually develops, the first fit is delayed for a year or more (Jennett *et al.*, 1973).

Epilepsy and residual cranial defects

The effect of cranioplasty on the incidence of post-traumatic epilepsy is probably insignificant. Grant and Norcross (1939) noted an improvement of seizure control in 18 of 27 patients after the repair of cranial defects. However, Walker and Erculei (1963) followed 273 head-injured patients, of whom 68 had unrepaired defects; the remaining 205 underwent cranioplasty. There was no significant difference in the development of post-traumatic seizures between the two groups. Similar conclusions have been reached by others (Lockhart *et al.*, 1952; Mayfield and Levitch, 1945).

Repair of calvarial defects

The outer layer of the dura mater has an osteogenic capability, although much of this is lost by the age of three years. However, it is enhanced by inflammation, and older children occasionally undergo spontaneous regeneration of the calvarium after craniectomy for osteomyelitis (Delashaw and Persing, 1990). Tantalum cranioplasty at the time of debridement of nonmissile depressed fractures resulted in sepsis in two of 15 patients (Jennett and Miller, 1972). Late cranioplasty after craniectomy for wound infection also carries an increased risk of recurrent infection (17.5%).

Venous sinus injury

Reporting a series of 17 combat injuries involving the venous sinuses, Kapp and Gielchinsky (1972) ligated the anterior half of the superior sagittal sinus without mortality. Closed depressed fractures overlying the transverse sinus may result in a transient rise in intracranial pressure, which subsides usually within 10–14 days (Becker *et al.*, 1990).

References

Aarabi B. (1989) Causes of infections in penetrating head wounds in the Iran–Iraq war. *Neurosurgery* **25**: 923–26.

Adeloye A, Odeku EL. (1971) A syndrome characteristic of tangential bullet wounds of the vertex of the skull. *J Neurosurg* **34**: 155–58.

Bakay L, Glasauer FE. (1980) *Head Injury*. Boston, MA: Little, Brown, 115–28.

Bakay L, Glasauer FE, Grand W. (1977) Unusual intracranial foreign bodies. Report of five cases. *Acta Neurochir (Wien)* **39**: 219–31.

Barnett JC, Meirowsky AM. (1955) Intracranial hematomas associated with penetrating wounds of the brain. *J Neurosurg* **12**: 34–38.

Becker DP, Gade GF, Young HF, Feuerman TF. (1990) Diagnosis and treatment of head injury. In: Youmans JR, editor. *Neurological Surgery*, 3rd edition. Philadelphia, PA: Saunders, 2017–48.

Braakman R. (1971) Survey and follow-up of 225 consecutive patients with a depressed skull fracture. *J Neurol Neurosurg Psychiatry* **34**: 106.

Brandvold B, Levi L, Feinsod M, George ED. (1990) Penetrating craniocerebral injuries in the Israeli involvement in the Lebanese conflict, 1982–1985. *J Neurosurg* **72**: 15–21.

Bursick DM, Selker RG. (1981) Intracranial pencil injuries. *Surg Neurol* **16**: 427–31.

Butler EG, Puckett WO, Harvey EN, McMillen JH. (1945) Experiments on head wounding by high velocity missiles. *J Neurosurg* **2**: 358–63.

Cairns H. (1944) Penicillin in head and spinal wounds. *Br J Surg* **32**: 199–207.

Carey ME, Young H, Mathis JL, Forsythe J. (1971) A bacteriological study of craniocerebral missile wounds from Vietnam. *J Neurosurg* **34**: 145–54.

Caveness WF, Meirowsky AM, Rish BL, *et al.* (1979) The nature of posttraumatic epilepsy. *J Neurosurg* **50**: 545–53.

Cooper PR. (1982) Gunshot wounds of the brain. In: Cooper PR, editor. *Head Injury*, 2nd edition. Baltimore, MD: Williams and Wilkins, 313–26.

Crockard HA. (1974) Bullet injuries of the brain. *Ann R Coll Surg Engl* **55**: 111–23.

Cushing H. (1918) Notes on penetrating wounds of the brain. *Br Med J* **i**: 221–26.

DeMuth WE. (1969) Bullet velocity as applied to military rifle wounding capacity. *J Trauma* **9**: 27–38.

Delashaw JB, Persing JA. (1990) Cranial defects and their repair In: Youmans JR, editor. *Neurological Surgery*, 3rd edition. Philadelphia, PA: Saunders, 2290–304.

de Villiers JC. (1975) Stab wounds of the brain and skull In: Vinken PJ, Bruyn GW, editors. *Handbook of clinical neurology*, **23**. Amsterdam: Elsevier, 477–503.

Dodge PR, Meirowsky AM. (1952) Tangential wounds of scalp and skull. *J Neurosurg* **9**: 472–83.

Drew JH, Fager CA. (1954) Delayed brain abscess in relation to retained intracranial foreign bodies. *J Neurosurg* **11**: 386–93.

Dzenitis AJ, Kalsbeck JE. (1965) Chronic brain abscess discovered 31 years after intracerebral injury by missile. *J Neurosurg* **22**: 169–71.

Feldman RA, Hieshima G, Giannotta SL, Gade GF. (1980) Traumatic dural arteriovenous fistula supplied by scalp, meningeal, and cortical arteries: case report. *Neurosurgery* **6**: 670–74.

Freytag E. (1963) Autopsy findings in head injuries from firearms. Statistical evaluation of 254 cases. *Arch Pathol* **76**: 215–25.

Gade GF, Becker DP, Miller JD, Dwan PS. (1990) Pathology and pathophysiology of head injury. In: Youmans JR, editor. *Neurological Surgery*, 3rd edition. Philadelphia, PA: Saunders, 1965–2016.

Gennarelli TA. (1990) Mechanisms of cerebral concussion, contusion, and other effects of head injury. In: Youmans JR, editor. *Neurological Surgery*, 3rd edition. Philadelphia, PA: Saunders, 1953–64.

Ginsberg LE, Williams DW, Mathews VP. (1993) CT in penetrating craniocervical injury by wooden foreign bodies: reminder of a pitfall. *Am J Neuroradiol* **14**: 892–95.

Gordon DS. (1975) Missile wounds of the head and spine. *Br Med J* **1**: 614–16.

Grant FC, Norcross NC. (1939) Repair of cranial defects by cranioplasty. *Ann Surg* **110**: 488–512.

Guthkelch AN. (1960) Apparently trivial wounds of the eyelids with intracranial damage. *Br Med J* **2**: 842–44.

Haddad FS. (1978) Nature and management of penetrating head injuries during the civil war in Lebanon. *Can J Surg* **21**: 233–40.

Haddad FS, Haddad GF, Taha J. (1991) Traumatic intracranial aneurysms caused by missiles: their presentation and management. *Neurosurgery* **28**: 1–7.

Hagan RE. (1971) Early complications following penetrating wounds of the brain. *J Neurosurg* **34**: 132–41.

Hammon WM. (1971a) Analysis of 2,187 consecutive penetrating wounds of the brain from Vietnam. *J Neurosurg* **34**: 127–31.

Hammon WM. (1971b) Retained intracranial bone fragments: analysis of 42 patients. *J Neurosurg* **34**: 132–41.

Hernesniemi J. (1979) Penetrating craniocerebral gunshot wounds in civilians. *Acta Neurochir (Wien)* **49**: 199–205.

Hopkinson DAW, Marshall TK. (1967) Firearm injuries. *Br J Surg* **54**: 344–53.

Jefferson G. (1917) Removal of a rifle bullet from the right lobe of the cerebellum; illustrating the spontaneous movement of a bullet in the brain. *Br J Surg* **5**: 422–24.

Jennett WB. (1975) *Epilepsy after non-missile head injuries*, 2nd edition. London: William Heinemann.

Jennett B, Teather D, Bennie S. (1973) Epilepsy after head injury. Residual risk after varying fit-free intervals since injury. *Lancet* **ii**: 652–53.

Jennett B, Miller JD. (1972) Infection after depressed fracture of the skull. Implication for management of nonmissile injuries. *J Neurosurg* **36**: 333–39.

Jennett B, Miller JD, Braakman R. (1974) Epilepsy after nonmissile depressed skull fracture. *J Neurosurg* **41**: 208–16.

Jinkins JR, Dadsetan MR, Sener RN, Desai S, Williams RG. (1992) Value of acute-phase angiography in the detection of vascular injuries caused by gunshot wounds to the head: analysis of 12 cases. *Am J Roentgenol* **159**: 365–68.

Jooma R, Bradshaw JR, Coakham HB. (1984) Computed tomography in penetrating cranial injury by a wooden foreign body. *Surg Neurol* **21**: 236–38.

Kapp JP, Gielchinsky I. (1972) Management of combat wounds of the dural venous sinuses. *Surgery* **71**: 913–17.

Kieck CF, de Villiers JC. (1984) Vascular lesions due to transcranial stab wounds. *J Neurosurg* **60**: 42–46.

Kirkpatrick JB, Di Maio V. (1978) Civilian gunshot wounds of the brain. *J Neurosurg* **49**: 185–98.

Lockhart WS, van den Noort G, Kimsey WH, Groff RA. (1952) A comparison of polyethylene and tantalum for cranioplasty. A preliminary report. *J Neurosurg* **9**: 254–57.

Martin J, Campbell EH. (1946) Early complications following penetrating wounds of the skull. *J Neurosurg* **3**: 58–73.

Matson DD. (1958) The management of acute craniocerebral injuries due to missiles. In: Coates JB, editor in chief. *Surgery in World War II. Neurosurgery vol 1*. Washington, DC: Office of the Surgeon General, Department of the Army, 123–82.

Mayfield JF, Levitch LA. (1945) Repair of cranial defects with tantalum. *Am J Surg* **67**: 319–32.

McLaurin RL, Towbin R. (1990) Diagnosis and treatment of head injury in infants and children In: Youmans JR, editor. *Neurological Surgery*, 3rd edition. Philadelphia, PA: Saunders, 2149–93.

Metress EK, Metress SP. (1987) The anatomy of plastic bullet damage and crowd control. *Int J Health Serv* **17**: 333–42.

Meirowsky AM. (1965) Penetrating wounds of the brain. In: Coates JB, Meirowsky AM, editors. *Neurological surgery of trauma*. Washington DC: US Government Printing Office, 103–104.

Millar R, Rutherford WH, Johnston S, Malhotra VJ. (1975) Injuries caused by rubber bullets: a report of 90 patients. *Br J Surg* **62**: 480–86.

Miller CF, Brodkey JS, Colombi BJ. (1977) The danger of intracranial wood. *Surg Neurol* **7**: 95–103.

Miller JD, Jennett WB. (1968) Complications of depressed skull fracture. *Lancet* **ii**: 991–95.

Nakamura K, Tsugane R, Ito H, Obata H, Narita H. (1966) Traumatic arterio-venous fistula of the middle meningeal vessels. *J Neurosurg* **25**: 424–29.

Ott K, Tarlov E, Crowell R, Papadakis N. (1976) Retained intracranial metallic foreign bodies. *J Neurosurg* **44**: 80–83.

Pitlyk PJ, Tolchin S, Stewart W. (1970) The experimental significance of retained intracranial bone fragments. *J Neurosurg* **33**: 19–24.

Raimondi AJ, Samuelson GH. (1970) Craniocerebral gunshot wounds in civilian practice. *J Neurosurg* **32**: 647–53.

Rish BL, Caveness WF, Dillon JD, Kistler JP, Mohr JP, Weiss GH. (1981) Analysis of brain abscess after penetrating craniocerebral injuries in Vietnam. *Neurosurgery* **9**: 535–41.

Rish BL, Dillon JD, Weiss GH. (1983) Mortality following penetrating craniocerebral injuries. An analysis of the deaths in the Vietnam Head Injury Registry population. *J Neurosurg* **59**: 775–80.

Rowe SN, Turner OA. (1945) Observations on infection in penetrating wounds of the head. *J Neurosurg* **2**: 391–401.

Rubinstein D, Symonds D. (1994) Gas in the cavernous sinus. *A J Neuroradiol* **15**: 561–66.

Salazar AM, Jabbari B, Vance SC, Grafman J, Amin D, Dillon JD. (1985) Epilepsy after penetrating head injury: I. Clinical correlates: a report of the Vietnam Head Injury Study. *Neurology* **35**: 1406–14.

Sights WP, Bye RJ. (1970) The fate of retained intracerebral shotgun pellets. An experimental study. *J Neurosurg* **33**: 646–53.

Sukoff MH, Helmer FA, Plaut MR. (1971) Retained intracranial fragments following missile injuries. *Bull Los Angeles Neurol Soc* **36**: 64–71.

Taha JM, Haddad FS, Brown JA. (1991) Intracranial infection after missile injuries to the brain: report of 30 cases from the Lebanese conflict. *Neurosurgery* **29**: 864–68.

van den Heever CM, van der Merwe DJ. (1989) Management of depressed skull fractures. Selective conservative management of nonmissile injuries. *J Neurosurg* **71**: 186–90.

Walker AE, Erculei F. (1963) The late results of cranioplasty. *Arch Neurol* **9**: 105–10.

Webber RL, Folio J. (1976) Radiographic detectability of occipital and temporal-parietal fractures induced in cadaver heads. *J Trauma* **16**: 115–24.

5

Intracranial haematoma

Jonathon C Benjamin, John S Norris

Introduction

The objective of this chapter is to gauge the after-effects of traumatic intracranial haematoma. Accurate prediction enhances provision of medical care, allocates resources efficiently and provides a basis on which to rehabilitate and, if necessary, compensate the patient and counsel the family. Sir Charles Symonds, a neurologist, stated that 'it is not only the kind of head injury that matters, but the kind of head' (Symonds, 1937).

The published material on traumatic intracranial haematoma tends to discuss specific neurological deficits and mortality but not the psychological and social consequences of the condition. However, those studies that have been published do suggest that the risks of morbidity and mortality are proportional to each other.

Definitions

The intracranial compartment is the volume contained within the inner vault of the skull.

Cranial trauma may afflict all age groups, inflicting a broad spectrum of disability and, in some, mortality. In 1974 Teasdale and Jennett introduced the Glasgow Coma Score (GCS). Since the inception over 20 years ago of this simple system for correlating the level of consciousness with outcome, the GCS has stood the test of time, and studies in the mid to late 1970s (Jennett, 1975; Jennett *et al.*, 1979) have confirmed its ability to predict outcome. The Glasgow Outcome Score

(GOS) was conceived to quantify prognosis. In this scale there are five outcome categories ranging from 'good recovery' to 'dead'. A 'good recovery' is when there is resumption of pre-injury activities with no or minimal neurological deficit, and no apparent change in personality or in school performance. A moderate disability is one in which the patient is able to function independently at a reduced level because of personality, intellectual or physical differences compared with the pre-injury status. A 'severe disability' is when, as a result of physical or intellectual impairment, the patient is unable to function independently and requires substantial care at home or in an institution. The last two categories are 'vegetative' and 'dead'. Each category is given a number (5 for good and 1 for death).

Extradural haematoma

The extradural compartment is a potential space located between the vault of the skull and the dura. It is into this space that blood collects to form an extradural haematoma (EDH), typically when an injury fractures the skull vault causing bleeding from the bone, dural vessels or venous sinuses. The majority of EDHs occur beneath the squamous temporal bone when a fracture ruptures the middle meningeal artery. The ensuing haematoma, though not a 'brain injury' *per se*, has a potentially damaging effect when its mass exerts a distorting pressure on the brain and brain stem within the confines of the rigid skull. EDHs occurring at sites other than the temporal region may be due to rupture of the venous sinuses. With age, the dura becomes increasingly adherent to the skull. Consequently, EDHs are more common in younger age groups, with the exception of neonates, in whom the dura adheres to the sutures.

Subdural haematoma

The subdural space is located beneath the dura, but outside the arachnoid membrane. Following trauma, blood passes easily over the cerebral and cerebellar hemispheres, initially conforming to the surface of the brain but eventually distorting it when a sufficient volume has collected.

Subdural haematomas (SDHs) may be divided into acute, subacute and chronic. There has been much discussion over the definition of an acute SDH. They are frequently associated with parenchymal lacerations, contusions and severe primary brain injury, and therefore with neurological deficits and death. Occasionally, an acute SDH may be caused by the rupture of a single cortical vessel in the absence of significant underlying brain injury. Most authors regard acute SDHs to be those that present with clinical symptoms and signs within 72 hours of injury (Hernesniemi, 1979; McKissock *et al.*, 1960; McLaurin and Tutor, 1961). Others define 'acute' as those operated on within 24 hours (Stone *et al.*, 1983). The only factor similar in all types of SDHs (acute, subacute or chronic) are blood or blood products in the subdural space. For each type, the time course, pathogenesis, treatment and prognosis differ.

Chronic haematomas present at greater than 20 days from injury and have an incidence of 1–2/100 000/year. They occur infrequently in children, except as a complication of shunt procedures or nonaccidental injury. Unlike acute SDH, chronic collections of blood arise as a result of the tearing of vessels rather than neural tissue. Consequently, the mass effect of the blood is more significant than the primary neural injury. 'Subacute' subdural haematoma develops between 3 and 20 days following trauma (McKissock *et al.*, 1960; Rosenorn and Gjerris, 1978). These are similar in appearance to acute collections in the early half of the period of evolution and to chronic collections in the latter half.

Blood may be present beneath the arachnoid membrane but outside the pia, namely in the subarachnoid space. The commonest cause of this is trauma. However, this thin layer of blood does not constitute a haematoma with mass effect and so for the purposes of this chapter no further reference will be made to it.

Intracerebral and intracerebellar haematoma

Deep to the pia mater is the neural tissue. Trauma may cause impaction and shearing, resulting in rupture of intraparenchymal vessels and formation of an intracerebral haematoma (ICH). Not only do these represent primary brain injury, but their mass can cause distortion, compression and subsequent secondary damage to the brain as with all haematoma.

Factors affecting outcome

Pre-injury status

Age

This is the most important parameter. Age affects outcome, independently of other factors such as level of consciousness, motor scores and pupillary changes (Hieden *et al.*, 1983). There is a linear relationship between age and mortality in adults. In severe head injury, with a GCS of 3–8, mortality increases from 28.4% in children to 47.7% in adults (Luersen *et al.*, 1988). In moderate trauma (GCS 9–12) mortality is nearly five times higher in adults than children (6.8% versus 1.4%). In minor head injuries (GCS 12–15) there is 0% mortality in children and 0.9% in adults. In children, mortality is highest at one to two years of age and reduced in adolescents. The minimum mortality is at the age of 12 years. In adults, the higher mortality is probably accounted for by extracranial factors such as ischaemic heart disease, liver disease, coagulopathies, etc. Another difference is the higher incidence of intradural haematomas in adults and the preponderance of EDHs in children. In the elderly, the higher incidence of intradural collections is probably due in part to the enlarged subdural space, as exemplified by cortical atrophy.

Associated medical factors

Pre-existing systemic disease diminishes the chances of good outcome in patients who undergo prolonged intensive care. Diabetes mellitus, ischaemic heart disease and chronic airways disease reduce tolerance to and increase the risk of infection. Pretraumatic anxiety neuroses and some personality traits mitigate against a good recovery and reintegration to society (Gilchrist and Wilkinson, 1979; Rimel *et al.*, 1981).

Radiology

Computed tomography (CT) of the brain is the gold standard for evaluating the acutely head injured patient, being technically less difficult and more sensitive and specific for acute subarachnoid blood than MRI (Gentry *et al.*, 1988a,b). CT and MRI images after head injury have been shown to improve outcome prediction (Clifton *et al.*, 1980; Cooper *et al.*, 1979; Sweet *et al.*, 1978; Tanaka *et al.*, 1988). These modalities of investigation provide information on the status of the brain parenchyma that is not possible to obtain by clinical examination or by plain radiographic films. In an analysis of 277 severe head injuries, Lobato *et al.*, (1983) identified eight consistent patterns of appearance on CT scanning that correlated with outcome measured at six months after injury. The pattern of acute hemispheric swelling following evacuation of an extracerebral haematoma was associated with a poor prognosis; 100% of the 27 patients with this CT appearance had a poor outcome. Other patterns suggesting severe diffuse injury also had a poor outcome. Where the CT scan was normal or showed only a focal lesion or a pure extracerebral haematoma, outcome was good in a high percentage of patients (68–87% depending on the radiological pattern). A recent retrospective study (Quattrocchi *et al.*, 1991) looked at the relationship to outcome of midline shift on CT scans. They found poor outcomes in 50% of cases associated with midline shift, in 14% of cases without shift and in 5% of patients with normal CT scans. Significantly, it was found that a midline shift out of proportion to the volume of intracranial haemorrhage was particularly indicative of poor outcome; and had a 75% mortality compared with 39% for patients with a haemorrhage commensurate with the degree of midline shift.

The greater sensitivity of MRI for various intraparenchymal changes may make this investigation highly useful for predicting prognosis during recovery. Most studies indicate that MRI is useful primarily in the subacute or late evaluation of head injuries where the information gained supplements that obtained by clinical examination and CT scanning (Hadley *et al.*, 1988; Snow *et al.*, 1986). In a group of 24 patients with GCS scores of 7 or less, but who had minimal or no CT abnormalities, Wilberger and colleagues (1987) found MRI abnormalities in every case. MRI was able to demonstrate white matter shear injuries, brain stem injuries and SDHs that were not seen on CT scans. None of the 19 patients who had widespread MRI abnormalities, but had normal CT scans and intracranial pressure (ICP), made a significant neurological recovery. When lesions on deferred or late MRI scans (up to 1 week post-injury) are studied in the context of neuropsychological deficits, the extent of abnormality bears a clear relationship to the degree of impairment on neuropsychological testing (Wilson *et al.*, 1988).

Intracranial mass lesions

Previously, little importance had been placed on the type of intracranial lesion as a cause of coma and subsequent outcome. However, the type of lesion is important, independent of its severity (i.e. GCS score) in determining the subsequent clinical course (Genarelli *et al.*, 1982). In a series of 124 patients with severe head injuries, those with intracranial haematomas were three times more likely to exhibit late deterioration than patients with diffuse brain injury (Clifton *et al.*, 1980). In the early 1980s, Gennarelli described outcome in patients with a GCS of 3–5 to be good in 68% of those with diffuse injury who were in coma for 6–24 hours, but good in only 8% of those in coma with acute subdural haematoma (Gennarelli *et al.*, 1982). Lobato and co-workers (1983) confirmed the correlation between a reduced GCS and poor outcome. They also noted that patients with the same severity of injury showed considerable variation in mortality and that outcome depended on the type of intracranial lesion.

Acute subdural haematoma

Subdural haematomas are associated with a higher mortality than any other mass lesion following trauma (Stone *et al.*, 1983). Reviews of outcome after acute SDHs show more than a 35% risk of death, 13 of 16 reported series had a mortality in excess of 50% (Cooper, 1993). Factors known to correlate with outcome in acute SDH include age, neurological status, timing of operation, operative findings and raised ICP.

Age

Younger patients have better outcomes. McKissock *et al.* (1960) found the average age of survivors was 36 years, compared with 51 years for the non-survivors. Hernesniemi (1979) demonstrated an increased mortality over the age of 60 years. When Fell *et al.* (1975) compared outcome in patients under and over 40 years old, they found similar mortality rates (42% compared with 49%). Outcome only differed significantly when patients less than 10 years or over 60 years old were compared. The mortalities were 33% and 69%, respectively. Stone *et al.* (1983) reported a similar overall recovery of 54% and a good functional (GOS grades 1 and 2) recovery of approximately 30% for each decade below 50 years of age. Patients over 50 years had a good functional recovery in 14%. Howard *et al.* (1989) compared clinical status and outcome in a series of adult patients aged below 40 with those over 60 years. They found that the mean volume of SDH was five times larger in the elderly, and the mean midline shift on CT scans was 1.2 cm in the elderly, but 50% less in the younger age group. Cerebral atrophy is probably the reason for the larger volume of blood demonstrated in the older age group, although this does not explain the midline shift. Although the GCS for the two groups was similar, the mortality rate was 74% in the older age group and only 18% in those aged less than 40 years. No elderly patient with a GCS of less than 13 achieved a satisfactory outcome. SDH in children also has a poor outcome. Pagni *et al.* (1975) reported an 83% mortality in children with acute SDH. Focal mass lesions and diffuse injury in the same child result in a poorer outcome.

Neurological status

Level of consciousness is an important determinant of outcome. Jamieson *et al.* (1972a) found that in patients who were unconscious at the time of surgery the mortality was 90%, but, in those who were conscious there was a mortality of 40–65%. Others have confirmed this finding (Hernesniemi, 1979; Klun and Fettich, 1984; McKissock *et al.*, 1960). The presence of pupillary abnormalities also conveys a higher associated mortality (Klun and Fettich 1984; McLaurin and Tutor, 1961; Richards and Hoff 1974). Seelig *et al.* (1981a) reported a 'functional' ('good' and 'moderate disability' on the GOS) survival of only 10% in patients with reduced or absent oculocephalic reflexes and decerebrate posturing.

Timing of surgery

Seelig *et al.* (1981b) examined the relationship between mortality and the time between the injury and evacuation of the SDH in 82 consecutive comatose patients with acute SDH. Those patients operated on within four hours of injury had a mortality of 30%, compared with 90% in those whose operation was delayed for more than 4 hours. Haselberger *et al.* (1988) analysed the interval between the onset of coma and surgery rather than the time between the injury and surgery. This study demonstrated a mortality rate of 47% in those comatose for less than 2 hours. Those waiting longer had a mortality of 80%, with only 4% making a good recovery. However, two recent studies of patients with a GCS of less than 8 have failed to reveal a relationship between outcome and timing of surgery (Wilberger *et al.*, 1990; 1991). However, it seems likely that the severity of the primary injury to the brain parenchyma sustained at the time of impact is a more important determinant of outcome than the absolute timing of the evacuation of any acute SDH (Cooper, 1993).

Operative findings

Whether the size of the SDH has any bearing on final outcome is not clear. Some authors have found an association (Howard *et al.*, 1989). Certain groups have gone further, to state that volumes of SDHs greater than 100 ml have an associated higher mortality (Howard *et al.*, 1989; Stone *et al.*, 1983; Richards and Hoff, 1974). However, the older literature does not support this (Laudig *et al.*, 1941; Mckissock *et al.*, 1960; Symonds, 1940). Bilateral SDHs have a significantly poorer prognosis with regard to mortality.

Intracranial pressure

Regardless of intracranial pathology, elevated ICP has an adverse effect on outcome in all patients with severe head injury (Becker *et al.*, 1977; Miller *et al.*, 1977). This inevitably has a deleterious effect in patients with SDH (Stone *et al.*, 1983).

Chronic subdural haematoma

Patients with chronic SDHs have a variable outcome, but this is considerably better than those with acute SDHs. The reported mortality ranges from 0 to 38% (Dronfield *et al.*, 1977; Hubschman,

1980; Markwalder *et al.*, 1981; Rashkind *et al.*, 1972). Larger series report an average mortality rate of 10% or less (Cameron, 1978; Kaste *et al.*, 1979; Luxton and Hornson, 1979). Luxton (1979) reported a 4% incidence of minor morbidity and a 17% incidence of serious disability following chronic SDH. Rashkind *et al.* (1972) reported that 75% of his patients returned to their normal state.

No consensus exists on the influence of age on outcome following chronic SDH. Hubschman (1980) reported a relatively high mortality rate of 23% in elderly and debilitated patients, whereas Munro (1942) found no association between age and outcome. The outcome of treatment of SDHs (including acute) in children is similar; 75% of infants will have normal development and 25% will show some degree of psychomotor retardation (McLaurin and Tobin 1989). It is not possible to determine if the retardation is caused by the subdural effusion or by the primary insult. Cameron (1978) stated that a patient's neurological state had no effect on outcome and reported that 13 of 15 patients who were in coma at the time of operation made a complete recovery. Seven per cent were not improved at 3 months follow-up, and 4% had died. Haematoma size does not appear to affect outcome (McKissock *et al.*, 1960). Mortality rates of patients with bilateral haematomas are approximately the same (11%) as for unilateral SDHs.

Extradural haematoma

The mortality rates reported for EDH vary from 5% to 43% (Baykaner *et al.*, 1988; Bricolo and Pasut 1984; Cook *et al.*, 1988; Jamieson and Yelland 1968; Seeling *et al.*, 1984). Factors known to affect outcome include age, concurrent intradural lesions, site of haematoma, time interval between injury and surgery, level of consciousness and neurological deficits at the time of surgery.

Age

As with all head trauma, in EDH, advancing age is associated with increasing mortality and morbidity. McLaurin and Ford (1964) reported an unsatisfactory outcome in only 18% of patients of less than 20 years of age but 52% in patients over the age of 20. Dhellemmes *et al.* (1985) reported a 9% mortality in children under 15 years. Although a difference between paediatric and adult mortality has not been universally demonstrated, the appar-

ently favourable prognosis in children may be related to a lower incidence of concurrent diffuse injury (Kalff *et al.*, 1989).

Concurrent intradural lesions

The concurrent presence of intradural blood (SDH and ICH) has been shown to be associated with a quadruple increase in mortality and morbidity in EDH (Jamieson and Yelland, 1972; Lobato *et al.*, 1988; McLaurin and Ford 1964).

Site of haematoma

There is some controversy about whether the site of an EDH affects outcome. In a series reported by Cordobes *et al.* (1981) there was little difference in outcome between frontal and temporal haematomas, although patients with parietal and occipital collections appeared to fare better. Frontal and vertex haematomas seem to have the most favourable prognosis (Jamieson and Yelland, 1968). It has been postulated that mortality is more closely related to the speed of haematoma formation than to its location. Temporal haematomas form more rapidly than do others due to arterial bleeding, usually from the middle meningeal artery (Gallagher and Browder, 1968; McLaurin and Ford 1964).

Time to surgery

Mortality is at its highest (20–60%) in patients who develop symptoms shortly after head trauma (Jamieson and Yelland, 1968; Kvarnes and Trumpy, 1978; Phonprasert *et al.*, 1980), whereas operations performed after the third day, in patients with slowly expanding lesions, are generally associated with a mortality of less than 10%

Level of consciousness

Mortality is significantly higher in comatose patients with EDHs of volumes greater than 150 ml (Rivas *et al.*, 1988), although this does not appear to be the case in patients who are conscious.

Neurological deficits

In those patients sustaining EDH, unconsciousness, pupillary abnormalities and decerebration are all associated with a less favourable outcome than when these features are absent. Seeling *et al.* (1984) reported a 41% mortality in patients who were comatose at the time of surgery. Cook *et al.* (1988) found GCS score and pupillary reactivity to be the most significant factors predicting outcome. They also noted the presence of intradural CT scan abnormalities and devised an 'extradural score' that was highly predictive (88% accuracy) of outcome. A score of zero was associated with a 3% risk of an unfavourable outcome, whereas a patient with a score of 5 had a 100% chance of a bad outcome. Overall, the mortality for EDHs was 9%.

Intracranial pressure

When raised ICP is associated with EDH, there is a higher mortality and morbidity. Lobato *et al.* (1988) reported that comatose patients with an ICP greater than 35 mmHg (normal range less than 15 mmHg) had a mortality of 73.3%; those below this had an 18% risk.

Intracerebral haematomas

In one early series, the mortality for EDH associated with traumatic ICHs was 72.4% (Browder and Turney, 1942). More recently, Jamieson and Yelland (1972) documented a 25% mortality in 63 patients. In this series, mortality was closely related to the patients' level of consciousness after injury. Those unconscious at the time of surgery had a mortality of 45%, whereas those lucid prior to operation had a mortality risk of 6%.

Posterior fossa haematomas

Posterior fossa EDHs are rare, although they are the most frequently encountered traumatic mass lesion of the posterior fossa (Wright, 1966; Zuccarello *et al.*, 1981). Children are particularly susceptible. One series reported only 17 infratentorial cases, of which 50% were children, compared with 344 cases of EDH in the supratentorial compartment (Wright, 1966). In posterior fossa EDH, outcome is related to the GCS score. In one series (Holzschuh and Schuknecht, 1989) only 20% of patients with a score of 3–7 had a good outcome, whereas in those patients with a score of 8–15, there was a 70% good outcome.

Subdural haematomas of the posterior fossa are uncommon, being less than 1% of the total number of intracranial SDHs. Traumatic ICH of the posterior fossa is even more rare. Estridge and Smith (1961) could only find 15 cases in a review of the literature. McKissock *et al.* (1960) identified only two cases in a series of 389 intracranial SDHs. Outcome is poor; at best only 50% survive (Fisher *et al.*, 1958; Wright, 1966; Young and Schmidek, 1982). In a review of the literature Raftopoulos *et al.* (1990) reported a mortality of 42–71% in patients over 12 years of age. As might be expected, those with a subacute or chronic course had a lower mortality than those presenting acutely.

Post-traumatic seizures

Seizure activity may be defined as an intermittent, stereotyped disturbance of consciousness, behaviour, emotion, motor function or sensation, that on clinical grounds is believed to result from cortical neuronal damage. The presence of an intracranial haematoma is a primary risk factor for post-traumatic seizures (PTS), with incidences of up to 25% reported (Annegers *et al.*, 1980; Jennett, 1975). PTS may be divided into two groups. 'Early' seizures are those occurring within one week of trauma. The remainder are 'late' seizures.

Early post-traumatic seizures

Fifty per cent of early PTSs are focal; they recur less often than late PTSs. Adults and children have the same incidence (except those under five years, in whom it is higher). A post-traumatic amnesia of more than 24 hours is a predisposing factor. The incidence of early PTS is related to the severity of trauma and whether or not surgery was performed. Subdural and intracerebral haematomas carry an incidence of 36% and 30% respectively (Jennett, 1975). Patients who have had chronic SDHs experience early post-operative seizures in 11% of cases (Cameron, 1978). In patients with EDH, there is an overall incidence of approximately 10%, with one-third having the their first fit after evacuation of the haematoma (Jennett, 1975).

Late post-traumatic seizures

The reported incidence of this condition varies widely. This appears to be due to differing inclusion criteria, follow-up periods and patient populations. In the most reliable reported series, 56% of cases occur within one year and 70% within two years following injury. They are more common in patients who have experienced early PTS (except children) and in those sustaining acute intracranial haematomas. After severe head injury, the risk of late PTS is 7.1% at one year and 11.5% at five years postinjury. There is an annual incidence of 3–5% thereafter (Jennett, 1975; Annegers *et al.*, 1980). Extradural haematomas are known to result in a 20–22% incidence of late PTS. Subdural and intracerebral haematomas have a 42–50% incidence (Jennett, 1974, 1975). Late epilepsy in adults is more likely to begin in the first year, although up to 20% many have their first seizure more than four years after injury. Mathematical models to predict PTS have been formulated (Feeney and Walker 1979).

Long-term sequelae

High levels of preinjury education and skilled occupation, stable personalities and good home environments are related to a better prognosis for the resumption of employment after head injury (Gilchrist and Wilkinson, 1979; Rimel *et al.*, 1981). Gains in cognitive function are the most impressive during the first 12 months after injury (Mandleberg, 1975, 1976; Mandleberg and Brooks, 1975). In theory, patients who survive an injury should reach a steady state at some point. This could be said to represent the final outcome. In practice this is difficult to ascertain. Bond and Brookes (1976) have studied the rate of recovery using the eventual GOS. They found that most patients with outcomes of 'persistent vegetative state' or 'severely disabled' had reached a 'steady state' by 3 months. In patients who ultimately make a good recovery, 68% had reached this state by 3 months and 90% by 6 months. Of patients destined to be 'moderately disabled', 67% were at their final functional state by 3 months and 95% by 6 months (Bond and Brooks, 1976). Heiden and associates (1983) reported similar findings for recovery rates using the International Data Bank figures. Thus, it appears that 90% of patients will reach their final outcome at 6 months.

Children of less than 15 years of age who survive a severe head injury rarely remain in a chronic vegetative state or are severely disabled. Ninety per cent will recover to a moderate disability or better within 3 years (Brink *et al.*, 1980; Bruce *et al.*, 1979; Carlsson *et al.*, 1968). Fifty per cent of children who have sustained coma of longer than 24 hours duration managed normal schooling (Heiskanen and Kaste, 1974). However, those in coma for longer than 2 weeks were unable to do even moderately well at school; 50% of this group were unable to continue with normal education. Even coma lasting for a few days appears to have an effect on school performance (Heiskanen and Kaste, 1974). The severity of injury is highly significant. Those more severely injured have not only higher levels of disability but reach their ultimate level of ability sooner.

When compared with adults, children have a lower incidence of traumatic mass lesions requiring surgery (Teasdale *et al.*, 1990), but outcome in the presence of a haematoma requiring surgery is the same in children and adults. Alberico *et al.* (1987) looked prospectively at 100 patients aged under 19 years with major head trauma. In this group, paediatric patients had a significantly better outcome at 1 year postinjury than adults. Children who had normal ICP measurements had a higher percentage of good outcomes (70%) than adults with normal ICP values (48%), but there was no significant difference in outcome between paediatric and adult patients who had mass lesions or raised ICP. Surgically treatable mass lesions were found in 46% of adults and in 24% of children. The importance of age cannot be overstated. Except in those under 4 years of age, mortality increases with advancing age, and good outcome decreases.

Outcome prediction will inevitably be imprecise in those patients who have intracranial haematomas, as deficits may be a consequence of the primary neural trauma. The subsequent liberation of blood would then merely reflect the severity of the underlying trauma. In contradistinction, in some patients who have sustained a relatively minor trauma, but with the liberation of significant volumes of blood, this exerts secondary effects of far greater importance than the initial primary trauma. Current methods of clinical examination and radiology are unable to discriminate between these primary and secondary insults. Consequently, outcome prediction in patients with intracranial haematomas will remain relatively inaccurate.

References

Alberico AM, Ward JD, Choi SC, *et al.* (1987) Outcome after severe head injury, relationship to mass lesions, diffuse injury, and ICP course in pediatric and adult patients. *J Neurosurg* **67**: 648–56.

Annegers JF, Grabow JD, Groover RV, *et al.* (1980) Seizures after head trauma: a population study. *Neurology* **30**: 683–89.

Baykaner K, Alp H, Ceviker N, *et al.* (1988) Observations of ninety-five patients with extradural hematoma and review of the literature. *Surg Neurol* **30**: 339–41.

Becker DP, Miller JD, Ward JD, *et al.* (1977) The outcome from severe head injury with early diagnosis and intensive management. *J Neurosurg* **47**: 491–502.

Bond MR, Brooks DN. (1976) Understanding the process of recovery as a basis for the investigation of rehabilitation for the brain injured. *Scand J Rehabil Med* **8**: 127–33.

Bricolo AP, Pasut LM. (1984) Extradural hematoma: toward zero mortality. A prospective study. *Neurosurgery* **14**: 8–12.

Brink JD, Imbus C, Woo-Sam J. (1980) Physical recovery after severe closed head trauma in children and adolescents. *J Paediatr* **97**: 721–27.

Browder J, Turney MF. (1942) Intracerebral hemorrhage of traumatic origin. Its surgical treatment. *NY State J Med* **42**: 2230–35.

Bruce DA, Raphaely RC, Goldberg AI, *et al.* (1979) The pathophysiology, treatment and outcome following severe head injury in children. *Childs Brain* **5**: 174–91.

Cameron MM. (1978) Chronic subdural haematoma: a review of 114 cases. *J Neurol Neurosurg Psychiatry* **41**: 834–39.

Carlsson CA, Von Essen C, Lofgren J. (1968) Factors affecting the clinical course of patients with severe head injury. Parts 1 and 2. *J Neurosurg* **29**: 242–51.

Clifton GL, Grossman RG, Makela M, *et al.* (1980) Neurological course and correlated computerized tomographic findings after severe closed head injury. *J. Neurosurg* **52**: 611–24.

Cook RJ, Dorsch NWC, Fearnside MR, *et al.* (1988) Outcome prediction in extradural haematomas. *Acta Neurochir (Wien)* **95**: 90–94.

Cooper PR (editor). (1993) *Head Injury.* Baltimore MD: Williams and Wilkins.

Cooper PR, Maravilla K, Moody S, *et al.* (1979) Serial computerized tomographic scanning and the prognosis of severe head injury. *Neurosurgery* **5**: 566–69.

Cordobes F, Lobato RD, Rivas JJ, *et al.* (1981) Observations on 82 patients with extradural haematoma. Comparison of results before and after the advent of computerized tomography. *J Neurosurg* **54**: 179–86.

Dhellemmes P, Lejeune J-P, Christiaens J-L, *et al.* (1985) Traumatic extradural hematomas in infancy and childhood. Experience with 144 cases. *J Neurosurg* **62**: 861–64.

Dronfield MW, Mead GM, Langman MJS. (1977) Survival and death from subdural haematoma on medical wards. *Postgrad Med J* **53**: 57–60.

Estridge MN, Smith RA. (1961) Acute subdural hemorrhage of posterior fossa. Report of a case with review of the literature. *J Neurosurg* **18**: 248–49.

Feeney DM, Walker AE. (1979) The prediction of post-traumatic epilepsy. A mathematical approach. *Arch Neurol* **36**: 8–12.

Fell DA, Fitzgerald S, Moiel RH, *et al.* (1975) Acute subdural hematomas. Review of 144 cases. *J Neurosurg* **42**: 37–42.

Fisher RG, Kim JK, Sachs E. (1958) Complications in posterior fossa due to occipital trauma – their operability. *JAMA* **167**: 176–82.

Gallagher JP, Browder EJ. (1968) Extradural hematoma. Experience with 167 patients. *J Neurosurg* **29**: 1–12.

Genarelli TA, Spielman GM, Langfitt TW, *et al.* (1982) Influence of the type of intracranial lesion on outcome from severe head injury. A multicentre study using a new classification system. *J Neurosurg* **56**: 26–32.

Gentry LR, Godersky JC, Thompson B. (1988a) Review of the distribution and radiopathologic features of traumatic lesions. *AJR* **150**: 663–72.

Gentry LR, Godersky JC, Thompson B, *et al.* (1988b) Prospective comparative study of intermediate-field MR and CT in the evalution of closed head trauma. *AJR* **150**: 673–82.

Gilchrist E, Wilkinson M. (1979) Some factors determining prognosis in young people with severe head injuries. *Arch Neurol* **36**: 355–58.

Hadley DM, Teasdale GM, Jenkins A, *et al.* (1988) Magnetic resonance imaging in acute head injury. *Clin Radiol* **39**: 131–39.

Haselberger K, Pucher R, Auer LM. (1988) Prognosis after acute subdural or epidural haemorrhage. *Acta Neurochir* **90**: 111–16.

Heiden JS, Small R, Caton W, *et al.* 1983 Severe head injury. Clinical assessment and outcome. *Phys Ther* **63**: 1946–51.

Heiskanen O, Kaste M. (1974) Late prognosis of severe brain injury in children. *Dev Med Child Neurol* **16**: 11–14.

Hernesniemi J. (1979) Outcome following acute subdural haematoma. *Acta Neurochir* **49**: 191–98.

Holzschuh M, Schuknecht B. (1989) Traumatic epidural haematomas of the posterior fossa: 20 new cases and a review of the literature since 1961. *Br J Neurosurg* **3**: 171–80.

Howard MA, Gross AS, Dacey RG, *et al.* (1989) Acute subdural hematomas: an age-dependent clinical entity. *J Neurosurg* **71**: 858–63.

Hubschman OR. (1980) Twist drill craniostomy in the treatment of chronic and subacute subdural hematoma in severely ill and elderly patients. *Neurosurgery* **6**: 233–36.

Jennett B. (1974) Epilepsy and acute traumatic intracerebral haematoma. *J Neurol Neurosurg Psychiatry* **38**: 378–81.

Jennett B. (1975) Epilepsy after non-missile head injuries. London: William Heinemann Medical.

Jennett B, Teasdale G, Braakman R, *et al.* 1979 Prognosis of patients with severe head injury. *J Neurosurg* **4**: 283–89.

Jamieson KG, Yelland JDN. (1968) Extradural hematoma. Report of 167 cases. *J Neurosurg* **29**: 13–23.

Jamieson KG, Yelland JDN. (1972) Traumatic intracerebral hematoma. Report of 63 surgically treated cases. *J Neurosurg* **37**: 528–32.

Kalff R, Kochs W, Pospiech J, *et al.* (1989) Clinical outcome after head injury in children. *Childs Nerv Syst* **5**: 156–59.

Kaste M, Waltimo O, Heiskanen O. (1979) Chronic bilateral subdural haematoma in adults. *Acta Neurochir* **48**: 231–36.

Klun B, Fettich M. (1984) Factors influencing the outcome in acute subdural haematoma. A review of 330 cases. *Acta Neurochir* **71**: 171–78.

Kvarnes TL, Trumpy JH. (1978) Extradural haematoma. Report of 132 cases. *Acta Neurochir* **41**: 223–31.

Laudig GH, Browder EJ, Watson RA. (1941) Subdural hematoma. A study of 143 cases encountered during a five year period. *Ann Surg*, **113**: 170–91.

Lobato RD, Cordobes F, Rivas JJ, *et al.* (1983) Outcome from severe head injury related to the type of intracranial lesion. *J Neurosurg* **59**: 762–74.

Lobato RD, Rivas JJ, Cordobas F, *et al.* (1988) Acute epidural hematoma: an analysis of factors influencing the outcome of patients undergoing surgery in coma. *J Neurosurg* **68**: 48–57.

Luersen TG, Melville R, Marshall LF, *et al.* (1988) Outcome from head injury related to patients age – a longitudinal study of adult and pediatric head injury. *Neurosurgery* **68**: 409–16.

Luxton LM, Harrison MJG, (1979) Chronic subdural haematoma. *Q J Med* **189**: 43–53.

Mandleberg IA. (1975) Cognitive recovery after severe head injury: 2. Wechsler Adult Intelligence Scale during post-traumatic amnesia. *J Neurol Neurosurg Psychiatry* **38**: 127–32.

Mandleberg IA. (1976) Cognitive recovery after severe head injury: 3. WAIS verbal and performance IQs as a function of post-traumatic amnesia duration and time from injury. *J Neurol Neurosurg Psychiatry* **39**: 1001–1007.

Mandleberg IA, Brooks DN. (1975) Cognitive recovery after severe head injury: 1. Serial testing on the Wechsler Adult Intelligence Scale. *J Neurol Neurosurg Psychiatry* **38**: 1121–26.

Markwalder T-M, Steinsiepe KF, Rohner M, *et al.* (1981) The course of subdural hematomas after burr-hole craniostomy and closed-system drainage. *J Neurosurg* **55**: 390–96.

McKissock W, Richardson A, Bloom WH. (1960) Subdural haematoma: a review of 389 cases. *Lancet* **i**: 1365–69.

McLaurin RL, Ford LE. (1964) Extradural hematoma. Statistical survey of 47 cases. *J Neurosurg* **21**: 364–71.

McLaurin RL, Tobin RB. (1989) Post-traumatic haematomas. In: McLaurin RL, Schut L, Venes JL, Epstein F, (editors). *Pediatric neurosurgery: Surgery of the developing nervous system*. Philadelphia: Saunders, 277–89.

McLaurin RL, Tutor FT. (1961) Acute subdural hematoma: review of ninety cases. *J Neurosurg* **18**: 61–67.

Miller JD, Becker DP, Ward JD, *et al.* (1977) Significance of intracranial hypertension in severe head injury. *J Neurosurg* **47**: 503–16.

Munro D. (1942) Cerebral subdural hematomas. A study of 310 verified cases. *N Engl J Med* **227**: 87–95.

Pagni CA. (1990) Post-traumatic epilepsy: incidence and prophylaxis. *Acta Neurochir Suppl* **50**: 38–47.

Pagni CA, Signovone G, Crotti F, *et al.* (1975) Severe traumatic coma in infancy and childhood. Results after surgery and resuscitation. *J Neurosurg Sci* **19**: 120–28.

Phonprasert C, Suwanwela C, Hongsaprabhas C, *et al.* (1980) Extradural hematoma: analysis of 138 cases. *J Trauma* **20**: 679–83.

Quattrocchi KB, Prasad P, Willets NH, *et al.* (1991) Quantification of midline shift as a predictor of poor outcome following head injury. *Surg Neurol* **35**: 183–88.

Raftopoulos C, Reuse C, Chaskis C, *et al.* (1990) Acute subdural haematoma of the posterior fossa. *Clin Neurol Neurosurg* **92**: 57–62.

Rashkind R, Glover MB, Weiss SR. (1972) Chronic subdural hematoma in the elderly: a challenge in diagnosis and treatment. *J Am Geriatr Soc* **20**: 330–34.

Richards T, Hoff J. (1974) Factors affecting survival from acute subdural hematoma. *Surgery* **75**: 253–58.

Rimel RW, Giordani B, Barth JT, *et al.* (1981) Disability caused by minor head injury. *Neurosurgery* **9**: 221–29.

Rivas JJ, Lobato RD, Sarabia R, *et al.* (1988) Extradural hematoma: analysis of factors influencing the course of 161 patients. *Neurosurgery* **23**: 44–51.

Rosenorn J, Gjerris F. (1978) Long-term follow-up review of patients with acute and subacute subdural hematomas. *J Neurosurg* **48**: 345–49.

Seelig JM, Greenberg RP, Becker DP, *et al.* (1981a) Reversible brain-stem dysfunction following acute traumatic subdural hematoma. A clinical and electrophysiological study. *J Neurosurg* **55**: 516–23.

Seelig JM, Becker DP, Miller JD, *et al.* (1981b) Traumatic acute subdural hematoma. Major mortality reduction in comatose patients treated within four hours. *N Engl J Med* **304**: 1511–18.

Seelig JM, Marshall LF, Toutant SM, *et al.* (1984) Traumatic acute epidural hematoma: unrecognised high lethality in comatose patients. *Neurosurgery* **15**: 617–20.

Snow RB, Zimmerman RD, Gandy SE, *et al.* (1986) Comparison of magnetic resonance imaging and computed tomography in the evaluation of head injury. *Neurosurgery* **18**: 45–52.

Stone JL, Rifai MHS, Sugar O, *et al.* (1983) Subdural haematomas: I. Acute subdural haematomas: progress in definition, clinical pathology, and therapy. *Surg Neurol* **19**: 216–31.

Sweet RC, Miller JD, Lipper M, *et al.* (1978) Significance of bilateral abnormalities on the CT scan in patients with severe head injury. *Neurosurgery* **3**: 16–21.

Symonds C. (1937) Mental disorders following head injury. *Proc R Soc Med* **30**: 1081–94.

Symonds CP. (1940) Delayed traumatic intracerebral haemorrhage. *Br Med J* **i**: 1048–51.

Tanaka T, Sakai T, Uemura K, *et al.* (1988) MR imaging as a predictor of delayed posttraumatic cerebral hemorrhage. *J Neurosurg* **69**: 203–209.

Teasdale G, Jennett B. (1974) Assessment of coma and impaired consciousness: a practical scale. *Lancet* **ii**: 81–84.

Teasdale GM, Murray G, Anderson E, *et al.* (1990) Risk of acute traumatic intracerebral haematoma in children and adults: implications for managing head injuries. *Br Med J* **300**: 363–67.

Wilberger JE, Deeb Z, Rothfus W. (1987) Magnetic resonance imaging in cases of severe head injury. *Neurosurgery* **20**: 571–76.

Wilberger JE, Harris M, Diamond DL. (1990) Acute subdural hematoma: morbidity and mortality related to timing of operative intervention. *J Trauma* **30**: 733–36.

Wilberger JE, Harris M, Diamond DL. (1991) Acute subdural hematoma: morbidity, mortality and operative timing. *J Neurosurg* **74**: 212–18.

Wilson JTL, Wiedmann KD, Hadley DM, *et al.* (1988) Early and late magnetic resonance imaging and neuropsychological outcome after head injury. *J Neurol Neurosurg Psychiatry* **51**: 391–96.

Wright RL. (1966) Traumatic hematomas of the posterior cranial fossa. *J Neurosurg* **25**: 402–409.

Young HA, Schmidek HH. (1982) Complications accompanying occipital skull fracture. *J Trauma* **22**: 914–20.

Zuccarello M, Pardatscher K, Andrioli GC, *et al.* (1981) Epidural hematomas of the posterior cranial fossa. *Neurosurgery* **8**: 434–37.

6

Cerebrospinal fluid fistulae

David G Hardy

Introduction

A cerebrospinal fluid fistula occurs when there is a defect in both the dural and arachnoidal coverings of the brain sufficient to allow the escape of cerebrospinal fluid (CSF). The escape of the spinal fluid can be direct, as in a penetrating wound to the head, or more commonly indirect, as cerebrospinal fluid rhinorrhoea or otorrhoea. The fistulous connection between the spinal fluid pathways and the exterior is most commonly the result of trauma, but spontaneous fistulae may also occur. Usually these are the result of a congenital defect in the skull and its coverings, or as a consequence of erosion from tumour or infection. Spontaneous fistulae are more likely to occur in the presence of raised intracranial pressure or hydrocephalus. The medicolegal significance of CSF fistulae lies in their association with craniocerebral trauma and in their tendency, not infrequently at some delay, to give rise to disabling or life-threatening conditions such as bacterial meningitis.

Traumatic cerebrospinal fluid fistulae

Introduction

The commonest cause of a CSF fistula is head trauma. A post-traumatic CSF fistula may be expected to complicate 2–3% of all patients who have been admitted to hospital following a head injury (Brawley and Kelly, 1967; Lewin, 1954). It will occur in approximately 6% of those who have sustained a severe head injury (i.e. coma lasting

more than 6 hours, or post-traumatic amnesia lasting more than 24 hours). The reported incidence of CSF fistulae in those patients who have suffered a skull fracture varies from 2% to 17% (Raaf, 1967). However, there is little direct correlation between the development of a fistula and the severity of the injury. In approximately 50% of patients in whom CSF leakage occurs there has been no, or only a transient, loss of consciousness (Mincy, 1966).

Direct leakage

When direct leakage of CSF occurs, this is usually from a penetrating wound to the head or via a compound fracture of the skull. In these patients, the site of the leakage is usually obvious and, as most compound injuries are subjected to early wound debridement and repair, long-term complications from CSF leakages of this type are rare. However, on occasion, an 'innocent' looking scalp laceration may conceal an unsuspected underlying compound fracture with penetration into the CSF pathways (Hagan, 1971). If the correct diagnosis is missed then 'unexplained' meningitis may occur, usually 6–14 days after the injury (Braakman, 1972).

Aerocoele (pneumocoele)

Although CSF otorrhoea and rhinorrhoea are the more common manifestations of a CSF fistula, the presence of air inside the head (aerocoele or pneumocoele) may also indicate the presence of a dural/arachnoidal tear and consequently the ability to develop a CSF fistula, even if no leak has yet occurred. Although the dural/arachnoidal tear may be presumed to have occurred at the same time as the injury, in about 33% of patients the air in the head only becomes evident after 48 hours. About 33% of patients who have traumatic CSF fistulae will also have air visible within the head. If air enters the head it is usually seen in the subdural or subarachnoid spaces, but, in about 20% of cases, it can also be seen within the ventricular system (Cairns, 1937). Despite the fact that intracranial air indicates a potential CSF fistula, in practice only about 50% of patients go on to develop a leak (Grant, 1923; North, 1971).

Time of onset

If CSF leakage occurs, its onset may be immediate or delayed. Fistulae of immediate onset occur at or shortly after the causative traumatic episode. Between 70% and 90% of cases will leak within the first 48 hours (Eljamel and Foy, 1990b; Laun, 1982). If the onset of the leak is delayed, it may occur weeks, months or occasionally years after the traumatic event. Although 95% of CSF fistulae of delayed onset will present within 3 months of the trauma, there are rare but nevertheless well documented reports of the leak occurring some years later (Gotham *et al.*, 1965; Okada *et al.*, 1991; Russell and Cummins, 1984). In those patients in whom considerable delay has occurred between the traumatic event and the onset of the leak, the 'cause' of the delay has usually been a plug of brain parenchyma herniating through the fracture line (Jefferson and Reilly, 1972; Lewin, 1966). At some later stage this plug may be displaced (e.g. by coughing, sneezing or straining) and CSF leakage then commences. In the more usual cases of leakage of delayed onset, the fistula is presumed to occur when post-traumatic brain swelling and any intracranial bleeding have resolved and the brain shrinks, then allowing leakage to occur (Lewin, 1966).

Although an established CSF leak may persist for weeks, in over 50% of patients the leak will last for only 2–3 days (Leech and Paterson, 1973; Lewin, 1954). When rhinorrhoea occurs, in approximately 85% of patients it will cease within 1 week. When otorrhoea occurs, in 95% of patients this will stop spontaneously within 1 week (Brawley and Kelly, 1967; Raaf, 1967; Raskind and Doria, 1966).

Site of leak

The most common type of CSF fistula to develop is in association with a fracture of the skull base. However, although up to 15.6% of all patients with head injuries may sustain fractures of the skull base, well under half of these will develop a CSF fistula (Brawley and Kelly, 1967; Calcalerra, 1980; Dagi *et al.*, 1983). The most common site for a fistula to occur is in the anterior half of the skull base, especially in the region of the cribriform plate. This is both anteriorly situated and fragile, and thus particularly vulnerable to trauma. If fracturing of the cribriform plate occurs, the fragments of bone are not infrequently driven upwards where they readily penetrate the dura (Cooper, 1987). Although the most common presentation of a CSF fistula is with rhinorrhoea, in approximately 7% of patients otorrhoea will occur (Henry and Taylor, 1978). For otorrhoea to occur, the skull fracture must involve the petrous bone and there must be an associated perforation or laceration of the tympanic membrane. In fractures of the petrous bone in which the tympanic membrane is intact the CSF drains via the eustachian tube to present as rhinorrhoea. Around 20–25% of patients with fractures of the temporal bone will have otorrhoea (Henry and Taylor, 1978). These fractures may be longitudinal or transverse. Longitudinal fractures are four to six times more common than transverse fractures and are usually associated with rupture of the tympanic membrane and ossicular dislocation; otorrhoea is common in this group. In transverse fractures, damage to the drum is less likely and therefore these are more likely to present with rhinorrhoea (Henry and Taylor, 1978). Associated facial palsy may occur in up to 50% of this group (Hicks *et al.*, 1980).

In approximately 6%, the leak will involve the sphenoid bone. Fluid may accumulate in the sphenoid sinus overnight when the patient is recumbent, to present as a profuse gush in the morning on becoming upright (the 'reservoir' sign) (Dandy, 1944).

Since the majority of CSF leaks occur through the region of the cribriform plate, anosmia is common. This is not infrequently complete and bilateral, although, if the fracture is strictly unilateral, then unilateral anosmia may occur. Unilateral rhinorrhoea is a reliable predictor of the side of the fistula in 95% of patients (Lewin, 1954). Anosmia is reported to occur in 80% of patients with rhinorrhoea. If a sense of smell is present then a fistula within the frontoethmoidal region is unlikely. CSF leakage will occur in 15–30% of those in whom the frontal sinus is involved (Ray and Bergland, 1969). Fractures of the posterior wall of the frontal sinuses are particularly likely to penetrate the dura (Wallis and Donald, 1988).

Diagnosis

If the leakage is profuse the diagnosis is usually self-evident. However, if there is major nasal or craniofacial trauma, the fluid emerging may be heavily blood-stained and therefore difficult to distinguish from traumatic serosanguinous exudate. Similarly, in those in whom onset may have been delayed, it may be necessary to distinguish spinal fluid from the profuse watery discharge of a common cold or an allergic rhinitis.

Testing the fluid for glucose may be helpful. Glucose levels of >30 mg/100 ml are usually taken to indicate the presence of CSF. However, the test is likely to be unreliable in the presence of blood, and 'false-positive' rates of 40–75% have been reported (Gadeholt, 1964; Healy, 1969). More recently the B_2 transferrin test (Tau protein) has been found to give >98% reliability, even when the CSF is diluted 1:10 by other fluids (Oberascher, 1988). The B_2 transferrin protein is a by-product of the neuroaminidase activity in the brain and is found only in CSF (Irjala *et al.*, 1979). The test relies upon the immunofixation identification of this fraction within the CSF. As the test is so reliable, it has now become the method of choice for the identification of CSF (Keir *et al.*, 1992).

If the CSF leak is intermittent or stops spontaneously then it may not be possible to obtain CSF samples. Further CSF leakage may occasionally be precipitated by the head being in the dependent position. Arranging for the collection of a specimen first thing in the morning when the patient rises may also be helpful, as this is when the leak is likely to be at its most profuse. In some patients it may be difficult to determine the side as well as the site of the leak. Unilateral anosmia, unilateral deafness and the presence of a fluid level behind the ear drum on otoscopy may all be helpful, but good radiology is essential. Plain skull radiographs may reveal the site of the fracture, and erect and supine views may identify fluid levels in the paranasal or sphenoidal air sinuses. CT scanning, especially using 'bone window' settings, may sometimes reveal fractures not visible on plain radiographs. About 20–25% of patients who have

developed a CSF fistula have no radiologically evident fracture on plain skull radiographs, or the site of the leak cannot be identified (Ray and Berglund, 1969).

Radionuclide scanning using radioisotope-labelled human serum albumin or other isotope tracers may be helpful, as may CT head scanning enhanced with intrathecal contrast (Di Chiro *et al.*, 1968; Park *et al.*, 1983). However, each of these techniques requires the presence of an active leak, and false negatives are common. MRI scanning can also be helpful. In a small proportion of patients, all such investigations fail to reveal the source, especially if the leakage is delayed or intermittent.

Treatment

Since most CSF fistulae stop spontaneously, it may appear that no specific treatment is required. However, for many years the conservative treatment of CSF fistulae has been known to be associated with a risk of meningitis (Hand and Sanford, 1970). The incidence of meningitis and the morbidity and mortality rates associated with this complication are variously reported (Brawley and Kelly, 1967; Eljamel, 1993; Leech and Paterson, 1973; Mincy, 1966; Raaf, 1967). Incidences from 3% to 50% have been reported but a recent and reliable study indicates an overall incidence of about 31% in 160 patients with traumatic CSF fistulae before surgical repair (Eljamel and Foy, 1990a). The risk appears to be somewhat greater if there is an aerocoele present and if the leak persists for more than seven days. The overall incidence of infection in the first week is about 10%. When a pneumocoele is present, this rises to about 15%. Recent research has indicated the cumulative risk at the end of the first week to be 9–11%; in the second week it rises to 18%. If no dural repair is undertaken, the cumulative risk appears to be 7% per week for the first month, and 8.1% per month for the first 6 months. After 6 months it becomes 8.4% per year. The cumulative risk at 10 years is computed to be 85% (Eljamel and Foy, 1990a). The most common infecting organism is *Pneumococcus*; this is found in 61% of patients. In fractures around the middle ear, gram-negative organisms such as *Haemophilus influenzae* may also be found (Bryan and Jernigan, 1979). Although pneumococcal meningitis is particularly virulent and lethal when it occurs spontaneously, it appears to be less so when the infection occurs as a complication of a CSF fistula (Spetzler, 1980; Dandy, 1944). The reasons for this are not clear; nevertheless mortality rates of 4–20% have been reported if this organism is implicated (Eljamel and Foy, 1990a). If meningitis occurs, there is a 4% risk that it will progress to a brain abscess and a 10% risk that the patient will develop an associated hydrocephalus (Eljamel and Foy, 1990a). If infection does occur, then aggressive treatment with appropriate antibiotics is mandatory. Recurrent attacks occur in about 31% of patients who have been treated conservatively (Eljamel and Foy, 1990a). Often these attacks are without demonstrable neurological sequelae, but the prognosis for children with meningitis secondary to CSF fistulae appears to be poorer, and more aggressive treatment of the initial attack is required (Caldicott *et al.*, 1973; Einhorn and Mizrahi, 1978).

Prophylactic antibiotic therapy

Prophylactic antibiotic therapy, usually with penicillin or a sulphonamide, has regularly been advocated for those patients with a proven CSF fistula and by some authorities for all those with skull base fractures, even when a fistula has not occurred (Brawley and Kelly, 1967). In view of the high cumulative risk of meningitis and the unfortunate outcome that may occur if this develops, it seems a not unreasonable policy. However, the evidence is mixed concerning the effectiveness of prophylactic antibiotics. In one recent study, 61% of patients with CSF fistulae who did not receive prophylaxis developed meningitis compared with only 34% of those who did (Eljamel and Foy, 1990a). In a small subgroup treated with penicillin and sulphadiazine, only 25% developed meningitis. However, when the various published studies are subjected to statistical review, the evidence suggests that antibiotic prophylaxis is probably ineffective in preventing meningitis in the long term (Dagi *et al.*, 1983; Eljamel, 1993; Hoff *et al.*, 1976; Ignelzi and Vanderark, 1975; Klastersky *et al.*, 1976). Since there is some risk of inducing antibiotic resistance it may indeed be hazardous (Bryan and Jernigan, 1979; Price and Sleigh, 1970). It has even been suggested that the exhibition of prophylactic antibiotics in comatose patients may increase the incidence of chest infection in this latter group (Klastersky *et al.*, 1976; MacGee *et al.*, 1970; Raff, 1967). Thus, the weight of current evidence does not seem to favour routine antibiotic prophylaxis in the presence of a

CSF leak or aerocoele, but the data are so far inconclusive.

Surgical repair

The justification for the surgical repair of CSF fistulae rests upon two premises: the risk of persisting or recurrent leakage, and the risk of meningitis if such a leak does occur. It is worth noting that, if a basal skull fracture occurs, there is a risk of meningitis of about 3% without any associated CSF leak (Brawley and Kelly, 1967).

Most authors recommend that surgery should be delayed until the patient's condition has stabilized and the swelling due to the initial trauma has subsided (Raaf, 1967; Westmore and Whittam, 1982). Early operation risks a complication rate of 25% (Leech and Paterson, 1973). Meningitis and failure to stop the leak are the most common of these complications. If meningitis has occurred, it should be treated before any further surgical intervention is carried out. However, if early surgical intervention is necessary for other reasons (e.g. to evacuate an intracranial haematoma) then any visible dural defect should be repaired as part of that initial surgery. Similarly, if the fistula is through a direct or possibly contaminated penetrating injury to the head or as part of a compound depressed fracture, it too should usually be repaired early, preferably within 12 hours of the injury (Lewin, 1966). Temporary packing of the nose or sinuses to reduce the volume of leakage prior to surgery is to be avoided. The requirement for surgical intervention varies with the extent, severity and location of the fistula. In fractures of the petrous bone, the fragments are rarely displaced and spontaneous healing of the dural laceration usually occurs. Surgical repair in this group is therefore rarely indicated (Hicks *et al.*, 1980; Lewin, 1966). Fractures of the facial skeleton, especially of the middle third, are not infrequently associated with CSF leakage. In one large series, 43% of patients with middle third fractures had evidence of a dural tear or CSF fistula (O'Brien and Reade, 1984). Early reduction of these fractures together with repair of the leak minimizes the risk of recurrent leakage or infection in this group (Jefferson and Reilly, 1972). Early reduction and fixation of middle third facial fractures will result in cessation of the rhinorrhoea within 3 days in 60% of patients (Steidler *et al.*, 1980). However, with manipulation or fixation alone, the leak may recur or persist. When manipulation and fixation are combined with formal repair the risk of meningitis or further leak is then negligible (Eljamel, 1994).

The surgical procedure of choice is a dural repair. In the majority of patients, this is best undertaken intradurally, but an extradural approach has also been used (Calcalerra, 1980; McCormack *et al.*, 1990). With an intradural approach, the site or sites of the leak can be more clearly visualized. Up to 14% of patients may have more than one dural defect (Laun, 1982). When identified, the dural defect or defects may be covered with a patch of pericranium, temporalis fascia or fascia lata (Ray and Berglund, 1969). Although with the intradural approach the patch is usually firmly held in position by the overlying brain, it may occasionally be necessary to use a few tacking stitches, fibrin glue, or fragments of muscle or fat to hold the patch in position. It is rarely necessary to repair the bony cranial defect except as a cosmetic procedure, but if this is done, bone paté, free bone graft, acrylic or metal may be used. If there is evidence of hydrocephalus the procedure may require to be combined with a lumbar drain or some type of shunting procedure. If the frontal paranasal sinus is involved, cranialization of the sinus and excision of the sinus mucosa are recommended (Wilson *et al.*, 1988).

In a small number of patients (1.3%) no source for the leak is identified. In these circumstances, packing of both the cribriform plate region and the sphenoid sinus with muscle or fat is recommended (Laun, 1982). Even if this is undertaken, and if no source for the leak is identified, then a high rate of recurrence of the leak is likely (Ljunggren, 1980). Despite apparently successful surgery, leakage may persist in 4–27% of patients, but if re-operation is then undertaken a seal is usually achieved (Eljamel and Foy, 1990b; Laun, 1982; Ray and Berglund, 1969; Wilson *et al.*, 1988). If the fistula has been clearly identified as coming from the sphenoid or pituitary region then an extradural transsphenoidal or transethmoidal approach may be adopted. This type of procedure is likely to be successful in 86% of patients (Wilson *et al.*, 1988). With this type of surgical approach a postoperative lumbar drain may be helpful (Von Haacke and Croft, 1983).

The success rate for the intradural repair of CSF fistulae is 98% in those with otorrhoea and 90% in others (Eljamel and Foy, 1990b). Re-exploration for persistent or recurrent leak may be required in about 10% of patients. Recurrent leak rates varying from 4–20% have been reported. The operative mortality in one recent series was reported to be 1.3% (Eljamel and Foy, 1990b). Post-traumatic meningitis following a successful operative repair has been reported as occurring in 4% in a recent series (Eljamel and Foy, 1990b).

Cerebrospinal fluid fistulae in children

Post-traumatic CSF fistula is not uncommon in older children, but is rare under the age of 2 years (Caldicott *et al.*, 1973). This is because in the neonate the skull is flexible and the paranasal sinuses have not yet developed. By the age of two years, the cribriform plate is ossified and therefore vulnerable to trauma. The extradural sinuses are pneumatized by the age of 3 years. By age 4 years the frontal sinuses have begun to develop and by age 5 years the mastoid air system has also developed. The sphenoid sinus does not appear until the age of 10 years and is therefore unlikely to be the site of the CSF leakage in children. The overall incidence of skull base fracture in children is 6–14% (Einhorn and Mizrahi, 1978). In most patients secondary infection does not occur (Einhorn and Mizrahi, 1978) but, if it does, the prognosis is poorer and aggressive treatment of the infection is necessary.

Spontaneous cerebrospinal fluid fistulae

Spontaneous CSF fistulae are less likely to be the subject of medicolegal proceedings, except when they may be considered to have occurred coincidentally with, or at some time after, an episode of head trauma.

In one series, 15% of patients considered to have developed a spontaneous CSF fistula had a history of antecedent head trauma insufficient to require medical attention (Eljamel and Foy, 1991). Thus, those providing medicolegal advice may wish to consider whether an episode of CSF leakage occurring at some time after an episode of alleged head trauma may indeed be a spontaneous CSF leak.

Spontaneous CSF fistulae are rare and constitute approximately 10% of all CSF fistulae (Eljamel and Foy, 1991; Nussey, 1966; Ommaya, 1976). They are more likely to occur in the presence of raised intracranial pressure from intracranial mass lesions or hydrocephalus (Rovit *et al.*, 1969). About 45% of those with spontaneous CSF fistulae will have raised intracranial pressure (Ommaya *et al.*, 1976). The presence of an intracranial mass or chronically raised CSF pressure may lead to erosion of the dural and arachnoidal membranes overlying especially the cribriform plate and the posterior frontal sinuses. The lamina cribrosa is often very thin and therefore vulnerable to erosion (O'Connell, 1964), but the commonest cause of CSF fistula when the CSF pressure is raised is a pituitary tumour (Ommaya, 1976). Mass lesions in the parasellar region and malignant paranasal growths may also give rise to spontaneous CSF fistulae, but these tend to occur rather late in the course of the primary disease (Locke, 1924).

Congenital defects in the skull base may also occur; 25% of spontaneous CSF fistulae will be associated with a congenital defect (Kaufman *et al.*, 1977; Ommaya *et al.*, 1976). These occur most frequently in the region of the cribriform plate and anterior skull base, but may also be found in the region of the otic cleft. A 'concealed' nasal encephalocoele or meningocoele may occur. In these patients the lamina cribrosa is deficient and the intracranial contents herniate into the upper part of the nasal cavity or the paranasal sinuses. This may be misdiagnosed by the unsuspecting ENT surgeon as a nasal polyp. Excision of this may then be followed by profuse rhinorrhoea or an episode of 'unexplained' meningitis (Nussey, 1966).

The 'empty sella' syndrome may also give rise to spontaneous CSF leakage. In this condition there is usually an elevated CSF pressure. This, it has been postulated, progressively compresses and erodes the diaphragma sellae, the pituitary gland and eventually the floor of the sella turcica (Gabriele, 1968). The arachnoidal membrane progressively herniates through the defect, eventually giving way and resulting in a (usually profuse) CSF leak (Brisman *et al.*, 1969).

Similar pulsatile erosions, often in association with congenital bony defects, may also occur in association with the middle ear (otic) cleft (Kaufman *et al.*, 1977). In these patients the leak may present as either rhinorrhoea or, if there is an associated perforation of the tympanic membrane, as otorrhoea (Kramer *et al.*, 1971). As in the case of traumatic CSF fistulae, it may on occasion prove difficult to localize the site of a spontaneous leak. In approximately 60% of patients plain skull radiographs will be abnormal, as will a similar proportion of (metrizamide enhanced) CT scans (Ahmadi *et al.*, 1985). Isotope studies, MRI scans, etc. may also prove helpful (Lantz *et al.*, 1980). If

a spontaneous CSF fistula develops, 13–33% will stop spontaneously, but in most patients the cessation is temporary (Ommaya, 1976). The treatment of choice is dural repair and in this group a shunting procedure may well be necessary (Spetzler *et al.*, 1977). If dural repair is not carried out then meningitis may develop in up to 60% of those affected (Eljamel and Foy, 1991). Even if dural repair is carried out, up to 25% will have a recurrence of the leak and about 6% will develop meningitis, despite an apparently successful dural repair (Eljamel and Foy, 1991).

References

Ahmadi J, Weiss MH, Segall HD, Shulz DH, Zee C, Giannotta SL. (1985) Evaluation of cerebrospinal fluid rhinorrhoea by metrizamide tomographic cisternography. *Neurosurgery* **16**: 54–60.

Braakman R. (1972) Depressed skull fracture: data treatment and follow up in 25 consecutive cases. *J Neurol Neurosurg Psychiatry* **35**: 395–402.

Brawley BW, Kelly WA. (1967) Treatment of basal skull fractures with and without cerebrospinal fluid fistulae. *J Neurosurg* **26**: 57–61.

Brisman R, Hughes J, Mount L. (1969) Cerebrospinal fluid and the empty sella. *J Neurosurg* **31**: 538–43.

Bryan CS, Jernigan FE. (1979) Post-traumatic meningitis due to ampicillin resistant *Hemophilus influenzae*. *J Neurosurg* **51**: 240–41.

Calcalerra TC. (1980) Extracranial surgical repair of cerebrospinal rhinorrhoea. *Ann Otol* **89**: 108–16.

Caldicott WJH, North JB, Simpson DA. (1973) Traumatic cerebrospinal fluid fistulas in children. *J Neurosurg* **38**: 1–9.

Cairns H. (1937) Injuries of the frontal and ethmoidal sinuses with special reference to cerebrospinal fluid, rhinorrhoea and aerocoeles. *J Laryngol* **52**: 589–623.

Cooper TR. (1987) *Head injury*, second edition. Baltimore: Williams & Wilkins.

Dagi TF, Meyer FB, Poletti CA. (1983) The incidence and prevention of meningitis after basilar skull fracture. *Am J Emerg Med* **1**: 295–98.

Dandy WE (1944) Treatment of rhinorrhea and otorrhea. *Arch Surg* **49**: 75–85.

Di Chiro G, Ommaya AK, Ashburn WL, Briner WH. (1968) Isotope cisternography in the diagnosis and follow up of cerebrospinal fluid rhinorrhoea. *J Neurosurg* **28**: 522–29.

Einhorn A, Mizrahi EM. (1978) Basilar skull fractures in children. The incidence of CNS infection and the use of antibiotics. *Am J Dis Child* **132**: 1121–24.

Eljamel MS. (1993) Antibiotic prophylaxis in unrepaired CSF fistulae. *Br J Neurosurg* **7**: 501–506.

Eljamel MS. (1994) Fractures of the middle third of the face and cerebrospinal fluid rhinorrhoea. *Br J Neurosurg* **8**: 289–93.

Eljamel MS, Foy PM. (1990a) Acute traumatic CSF fistulae; the risk of intracranial infection. *Br J Neurosurg* **4**: 381–85.

Eljamel MS, Foy PM. (1990b) Post-traumatic CSF fistulae: the case for surgical repair. *Br J Neurosurg* **4**: 479–83.

Eljamel MS, Foy PM. (1991) Non-traumatic CSF fistulae: clinical history and management. *Br J Neurosurg* **5**: 275–79.

Gabriele OF. (1968) The empty sella syndrome. *AJR* **104**: 168–70.

Gadeholt H. (1964) The reaction of glucose-oxidase test paper in normal nasal secretion. *Acta Otolaryngol* **58**: 271–72.

Gotham JE, Meyer JS, Gilroy J, Bauer RB. (1965) Observations on cerebrospinal fluid rhinorrhoea and pneumocephalus. *Ann Otol* **74**: 214–33.

Grant FE. (1923) Intracranial aerocoele following fracture of the skull. Report of a case with review of the literature. *Surg Gynecol Obstet* **36**: 251–55.

Hagan RE. (1971) Early complications following penetrating wounds of the brain. *J Neurosurg* **34**: 132–41.

Hand WL, Sanford JP. (1970) Post-traumatic bacterial meningitis. *Ann Intern Med* **72**: 869–74.

Healy CE. (1969) Significance of a positive reaction for glucose in rhinorrhea. *Clin Paed* **8**: 239.

Henry RC, Taylor PH. (1978) Cerebrospinal fluid otorrhoea and otorhinorrhoea following closed head injury. *J Laryngol Otol* **92**: 743–56.

Hicks GW, Wright JW, Wright JW. (1980) Cerebrospinal fluid otorrhoea. *Laryngoscope* **90**: (suppl 25): 1–25.

Hoff J, Brewin A, Hoisang U. (1976) Antibiotics for basilar skull fracture. *J Neurosurg* **44**: 649.

Ignelzi RJ, Vanderark GD. (1975) Analysis of the treatment of basilar skull fractures with and without antibiotics. *J Neurosurg* **43**: 721–26.

Irjala K, Sunopaa J, Laurent B. (1979) Identification of CSF leakage by immunofixation. *Arch Otolaryngol* **105**: 447–48.

Jefferson A, Reilly G. (1972) Fracture of the floor of the anterior cranial fossa. The selection of patients for dural repair. *Br J Surg* **59**: 585–92.

Kaufman B, Neilsen F, Weiss M, Brodkey JS, White RJ, Sykora GF. (1977) Acquired spontaneous non-traumatic normal pressure cerebrospinal fluid fistulae originating from the middle fossa. *Radiology* **122**: 379–87.

Keir G, Zeman A, Brookes G, Porter M, Thompson EJ. (1992) Immunoblotting and transferrin in the identification of cerebrospinal fluid otorrhoea and rhinorrhoea. *Ann Clin Biochem* **29**: 210–13.

Klastersky J, Sadeghi M, Brihaye J. (1976) Anti-microbial prophylaxis in patients with rhinorrhoea or otorrohea. A double blind study. *Surg Neurol* **6**: 111–14.

Kramer SA, Yanagisawa E, Smith HW. (1971) Spontaneous cerebrospinal fluid otorrhoea simulating serous otitis media. *Laryngoscope* **81**: 1083–89.

Lantz EJ, Forbes GS, Brown ML, Laws ER. (1980) Radiology of cerebrospinal fluid rhinorrhoea. *Am J Neuroradiol* **1**: 391–98.

Laun A. (1982) Traumatic cerebrospinal fluid fistulas in the anterior and middle cranial fossae. *Acta Neurochir* **60**: 215–22.

Leech PJ, Paterson A. (1973) Conservative and operative management for cerebrospinal fluid leakage after closed head injury. *Lancet* **i**: 1013–15.

Lewin W. (1954) Cerebrospinal fluid rhinorrhoea in closed head injuries. *Br J Surg* **42**: 1–18.

Lewin W. (1966) Cerebrospinal fluid rhinorrhoea with non-missile injuries. *Clin Neurosurg* **12**: 237–52.

Ljunggren K. (1980) Liquorrhoea: a review of 6 cases. *Acta Neurochir* **51**: 173–86.

Locke CE. (1924) The spontaneous escape of cerebrospinal fluid through the nose: its occurrence with brain tumour. *Arch Neurol Psychiatry* **15**: 309–24.

MacGee EE, Cauthen JC, Brackett CE. (1970) Meningitis following acute traumatic cerebrospinal fluid fistula. *J Neurosurg* **33**: 312–16.

McCormack B, Cooper PR, Perskey M, Rothstein S. (1990) Extracranial repair of cerebrospinal fluid fistula: techniques and results in 37 patients. *Neurosurgery* **27**: 412–17.

Mincy JE. (1966) Post-traumatic cerebrospinal fluid fistula of the frontal fossa. *J Trauma* **6**: 618–22.

North JB. (1971) On the importance of intracranial air. *Br J Surg* **58**: 826.

Nussey AM. (1966) Spontaneous cerebrospinal fluid rhinorrhoea. *J Neurol Neurosurg Psychiatry* **27**: 241–46.

O'Connell JEA. (1964) Primary spontaneous cerebrospinal fluid rhinorrhoea. *J Neurol Neurosurg Psychiatry* **27**: 241–46.

Oberascher G. (1988) Cerebrospinal fluid otorrhoea – new trends in diagnosis. *Am J Otol* **9**: 102–108.

O'Brien MD, Reade PC. (1984) The management of dural tear resulting from mid facial fracture. *Head Neck* **6**: 810–18.

Okada J, Tsuda T, Takasugi S, Nishikada K, Toth Z, Matsumoto K. (1991) Unusually late onset of cerebrospinal fluid rhinorrhoea after head trauma. *Surg Neurol* **35**: 213–17.

Ommaya AK. (1976) Spinal fluid fistulae. *Clin Neurosurg* **23**: 363–92.

Ommaya AK, Di Chiro G, Baldwin M, Pennybacker JB. (1976) Non-traumatic cerebrospinal fluid rhinorrhoea. *J Neurol Neurosurg Psychiatry* **31**: 214–25.

Park JHL, Strelzow VV, Friedman WH. (1983) Current management of cerebrospinal fluid rhinorrhoea. *Laryngoscope* **93**: 1294–300.

Price DJE, Sleigh JD. (1970) Control of infection due to *Klebsiella serogenes* in a neurosurgical unit by withdrawal of all antibiotics. *Lancet* **ii**: 1213–15.

Raaf J. (1967) Post-traumatic cerebrospinal fluid leaks. *Arch Surg* **95**: 648–51.

Raskind R, Doria A. (1966) Cerebrospinal fluid rhinorrhoea and otorrhoea of traumatic origin. *J Int Coll Surg* **46**: 223–36.

Ray BS, Berglund RM. (1969) Cerebrospinal fluid fistula: clinical aspects, techniques of localisation and methods of closure. *J Neurosurg* **30**: 399–405.

Rovit RL, Schecter MM, Nelson K. (1969) Spontaneous high pressure cerebrospinal rhinorrhoea due to lesions obstructing flow of cerebrospinal fluid. *J Neurosurg* **30**: 406–12.

Russell T, Cummins BH (1984) Cerebrospinal fluid rhinorrhoea 34 years after trauma: a case report and review of the literature. *Neurosurgery* **15**: 705.

Spetzler RF, Wilson CB. (1973) Dural fistulae and their repair. In: Youmans JR, editor. *Neurological Surgery*. Philadelphia: Saunders, 2209–27.

Spetzler RF, Wilson CB. (1977) Simplified percutaneous lumboperitoneal shunting. *Surg Neurol* **7**: 25–29.

Spetzler RF. (1980) Cerebrospinal fluid fistula. In: Wilson CB, Hoff JT, editors. *Current Surgical Management of Neurological Disease*. New York: Livingstone, 243–8.

Steidler NE, Cook RM Reade PC. (1980) Residual complications in patients with middle third facial fractures. *Int J Oral Surg* **9**: 259–66.

Von Haacke NP, Croft CB. (1983) Cerebrospinal fluid rhinorrhoea and otorrhoea: extracranial repair. *Clin Otolaryngol* **8**: 317–27.

Wallis A, Donald PJ. (1988) Frontal sinus fractures: a review of 72 cases. *Laryngoscope* **98**: 593–98.

Westmore GA, Whittam DE. (1982) Cerebrospinal fluid rhinorrhoea and its management. *Br J Surg* **69**: 489–92.

Wilson SG, Davidson B, Corey JP, Haydon RC. (1988) Comparison of complications following frontal sinus fractures managed with exploration, with or without obliteration over 10 years. *Laryngoscope* **98**: 516–20.

7

Cranial nerve injuries (I, V and IX–XII)

M J Davies, T T King

Introduction

Of the olfactory, trigeminal, glossopharygeal, vagus, accessory and hypoglossal nerves, the most frequently injured is the olfactory. Injuries to the other nerves in this group will rarely be seen by clinicians and may therefore go unrecognized initially, because the severity of the injury required to produce damage to these nerves makes it frequently fatal. The true incidence of these lesions is, therefore, unknown but in survivors they are clearly rare.

Olfactory nerve

Injury to the olfactory nerve is often overlooked both by patients and their doctors. It does not, as a rule, cause the patient much distress in comparison to injury of the nerves controlling vision (including ocular movement), facial movement and hearing. When damage to the olfactory nerve is unilateral the patient may be unaware of the problem unless specifically tested. Clinicians often fail to test the sense of smell unless their attention is drawn to it by the presence of CSF rhinorrhoea. Indeed, it is not uncommon to find no means available of assessing properly the sense of smell when the patient is being examined. Nevertheless, anosmia can have major implications for patients. In some it will prevent them from resuming their former occupations.

Definitions

Anosmia is the complete loss of the sense of smell. It may be unilateral or bilateral but is only of significance to the patient if it is bilateral. In unilateral anosmia the patient is unaware of the defect provided the contralateral olfactory tract is functioning normally.

Hyposmia is a condition in which the patient can detect and correctly identify some odours but not others.

Parosmia is a condition in which all odours appear the same, although they cannot be identified. The patient reports that everything smells foul and unpleasant or has a 'burning' smell. Less frequently, some odours are correctly identified but others smell foul.

Schechter and Henkin (1974) have divided abnormalities of olfaction into seven subgroups. Interested readers are referred to their paper.

Epidemiology

Although injuries to the olfactory nerves are common after head injuries, there are few large and unselected series examining the true incidence and long-term outcome of this injury. Early reports in the literature did not quantify the severity of the head injuries and tended to rely on the patients' reports of altered or absent olfaction, rather than on clinical testing. The incidence ranges from 1% to 66% in various series (Bakay and Glasauer, 1980; Glaser and Shafer, 1932; Hagan, 1967; Hughes, 1964; Jacobi *et al.*, 1986; Kitchens, 1991; Leigh, 1943; Lewin, 1954; Mock, 1950; Sumner, 1964, 1976; Lewin, 1966). Loss of smell following head injury is not always complete, several authors having described post-traumatic hyposmia and parosmia (Bakay and Glasauer, 1980; Hagan, 1967; Hughes, 1964; Jacobi *et al.*, 1986; Leigh,

1943; Lewin, 1954; Mock, 1950; Schechter and Henleiin, 1974; Sumner, 1964, 1976; Lewin, 1966). The first large and unselected series was published by Leigh in 1943. He found 72 cases of anosmia out of 1000 consecutive head injuries. Lewin (1954) found an incidence of 5% in the survivors of a series of 1000 patients (7% of these died). Mock (1950) reported an incidence of 38% in patients with basal skull fracture. Sumner (1976) found an incidence of 7.1% in his series of 1167 consecutive head injuries. He found that the incidence increases with the severity of the head injury, up to approximately 30% in the most severe injuries, or in patients in whom there has been a fracture of the anterior cranial fossa. Lewin (1954) found that the incidence of anosmia rose to 78% in those patients who had CSF rhinorrhoea.

The incidence in children appears to be considerably lower than in adults. Kitchens (1991) found only one case of anosmia in a series of 73 children with basal skull fractures (1.4%) while Jacobi *et al.*, (1986) found an incidence of 3.2% in a series of 741 paediatric head injuries, although the anosmia was permanent in only 1.2%. Other authors report an incidence of 1.4% in paediatric head injuries. Jacobi *et al.* (1986) also found that there was a predilection to anosmia in children in whom the period of post-traumatic amnesia was greater than 24 hours.

The incidence of anosmia varies according to the site of impact on the head. A commonly quoted figure is that approximately one-third of cases of anosmia follow blows to the occipital region and that most of the remaining cases are due to blows to the frontal region. Sumner (1976), in his series of 1167 consecutive head injuries, looked at the frequency of blows to different parts of the head and found that 78% of blows occurred to the frontal region and only 7.5% to the occipital region. He found that the risk of anosmia following a blow to the head was much greater in an occipital injury (21%) than in a frontal injury (3.9%). Blows to the parietal region had an intermediate risk of anosmia (10.4%).

Clinical assessment

Assessment of olfactory function often proves unsatisfactory. This is not necessarily because the patient cannot detect the odour but more often because they cannot correctly identify the particular odour. Sumner (1962) conducted a study to determine which substances were best for testing the sense of smell and found that the most common odours used were not those that were most frequently identified correctly. He found that the most suitable substances are coffee, benzaldehyde (almond), tar and oil of lemon. In his study of 200 people, all these substances had an identification rate greater than 50%.

It is important before testing olfaction in patients with recent injuries to evaluate the nasal airway, looking for blood or mucosal swelling, which may interfere with the test. The substances are then presented one at a time to each nostril whilst the opposite nostril is occluded. The examiner should be careful to avoid spilling any of the test substances on the fingers and, if a smoker, should not present the test substances with the smoking hand. Goland (1937) described the use of olfactometry in 'acute traumatic craniocerebral encephalopathies'. In this process, the odoriferous substance is presented to the patient by a process of 'blast injection' into the nostril whilst the patient stops breathing. He found that a greater concentration of the test substance was required on the side of the cerebral contusion. This method of assessing olfactory function is not commonly used.

Structural pathology

The site of the lesion producing alteration in the sense of smell is still not clearly proven. It is commonly assumed that the olfactory fibres are damaged as they pass through the cribriform plate. Cairns (1937) on reviewing a selected group of patients with frontal injuries and rhinorrhoea, commented that, although autopsy material showed frequent injury to the cribriform plate, findings at operation often showed similar lesions although the patient did not have anosmia. Leigh (1943), Lewin (1954), Hagan (1967), Russell (1942, 1960) and Jafek *et al.* (1989) all support the view that the damage occurs as the olfactory filaments pass through the cribriform plate. Jafek *et al.* (1989) postulated that as the olfactory epithelium regenerates following head trauma the receptor cells attempt to send axons centrally but that the lamina cribrosa undergoes fibrotic healing, and the axons, unable to penetrate the fibrosis, are deflected back into the peripheral tissues. Other theories have been proposed, including damage to the olfactory bulb (Lewin, 1954) or to the anteromedial temporal lobe and/or its connections (Goland, 1937).

Prognosis

Recovery from post-traumatic anosmia does occur but there are wide differences in the literature concerning the incidence. Glaser and Shafer (1932) had seven patients with anosmia in their series of 255 who were followed for between one and five years, and in whom they found no recovery. Leigh (1943) recorded recovery in six of his 72 patients (8%) and noted that it usually occured within six months of the injury. Schechter and Henkin (1974) found no recovery in any of their patients. However, they noted that patients who sustained anosmia following head injury had low total serum zinc levels and increased total serum copper levels. They also showed that a lowering of total body zinc produces hypogeusia and hyposmia and that correction of the zinc deficiency results in correction of the abnormalities of taste and smell. They suggested that correction of the lowered total zinc levels in patients with head injuries may result in some improvement in their altered olfaction. Sumner (1976) reported an overall recovery of 39% in his patients, although there appeared to be two separate subgroups amongst those who recovered. The first subgroup recovered within 10 weeks; he suggested that this was due to the disappearance of oedema and blood clot in the absence of actual destruction of neural tissue. The second subgroup recovered much more slowly, taking up to five years in some cases. Sumner (1976) found that the chance of improvement following severe head injury was only about 10%. He found no correlation between the severity of the head injury and the time taken for the anosmia to recover, although very transitory anosmia was not seen after severe head injuries. He also found that recovery, when it occurred, was usually complete but if full recovery did not occur the patient had a patchy defect, affecting a few odours only. Parosmia may occur during the recovery phase (Bakay and Glasauer, 1980; Leigh, 1943; Sumner, 1976; Lewin, 1966) and sometimes the patient is left with permanent parosmia which may affect all or only some odours.

Complications

Loss of the sense of smell results in loss of the appreciation of some of the more enjoyable aspects of life: food, flowers, perfume, a good wine (Elliott, 1974). It can, however, have more serious implications because of the inability to smell gas or smoke or to realize that something is burning. It is not possible to pursue certain occupations with an impaired sense of smell (e.g. chef, fireman, wine taster, gas-fitter, chemist).

Patients with anosmia often complain of a lack of normal taste sensation. The explanation for this is not clear. It is commonly thought that the smell of food affects our perception of its taste but the central pathways for the two sensations are not anatomically close. Sumner (1976) suggests that there are connections between the olfactory pathway and not only the ventromedial thalamic nuclei but also the taste relay in the posteromedial thalamic nuclei. Sumner (1976) found that taste recovers in most patients but Schechter and Henkin (1974) did not find this in any of their 29 patients followed for up to 23 years.

Trigeminal Nerve

Epidemiology

Peripheral injuries to the trigeminal nerve are not uncommon but intracranial injuries are rare. Hughes (1964) quoted an incidence of all types of injury to this nerve of 3.6% in traumatic head injuries, but commented that it was more commonly involved extracranially than intracranially. He quoted a 0.5% incidence of intracranial involvement and found that this was associated with multiple cranial nerve palsies, brain stem dysfunction and extensive basal fractures. Aucott, 1988, however, reports a case of 'modest' head injury, with only brief loss of consciousness, in which the patient suffered trigeminal injury affecting predominantly the first and second divisions. Jefferson and Schorstein (1955) described 66 patients with trigeminal nerve injury whom they had personally treated. These included 14 injuries related to gunshot wounds and 16 of ganglionic injury. They found that the majority of trigeminal injuries were associated with facial fractures and affected the peripheral branches of the nerve after they exited the skull base. The most common branches damaged were the supraorbital and infraorbital nerves. These injuries were usually related to fractures or lacerations around the orbital rim. Jacobi *et al.* (1986) reported trigeminal lesions in 4.2% of paediatric head injuries. The deficits were still present at six months in 2.2% of these patients.

Clinical Assessment

A full assessment of the area of supply of the trigeminal nerve must be performed. This includes both sensory and motor testing. Sensation to both light touch and pinprick must be assessed as well as the corneal reflex. The corneal reflex is tested by asking the patient to look upwards or to the side opposite to the cornea to be tested. The cornea is then touched lightly with a wisp of cotton wool. The symmetry of the response must be noted and the patient asked if the stimulus feels the same on each side. The motor component supplies the medial and lateral pterygoids, temporalis, masseter, mylohyoid and the anterior belly of digastric. This part of the nerve is tested by the patient opening and closing the mouth against resistance and moving the jaw from side to side against resistance, and by palpating the temporalis and masseter muscles whilst the patient clenches his teeth.

Structural pathology

Intracranial lesions of the trigeminal nerve may be due to penetrating injuries (particularly in wartime), but they are more commonly associated with skull base fractures and, in particular, compression injuries to the head (Bakay and Glasauer, 1980; Jefferson and Schorstein, 1955; Lewin, 1966). The most common sites of entry for penetrating injuries are in the face or the temple (Jefferson and Schorstein, 1955). High parietal and frontal penetrating injuries are rarely complicated by trigeminal injury. Intracranial injuries of the trigeminal nerve generally occur with more severe head trauma, as reported by Jacobi *et al.* (1986) in their series of 741 paediatric head injuries, in which nearly all cases of trigeminal injury occurred in patients with a period of post-traumatic amnesia of greater than 24 hours. Six of the patients with post-traumatic amnesia of more than one week had unilateral trigeminal motor involvement. This was permanent in four.

Compression injuries to the head result in fractures of the petrous bone, which can be of two types: longitudinal (80–90%) or transverse (5%). Longitudinal fractures are caused by the skull being squeezed from side to side. They tend to involve both the middle and external ear and cause damage to the facial and acoustic nerves. Transverse fractures result from anteroposterior compressive forces and can extend forward to the basal foramina in the middle fossa. These tend to affect cranial nerves V–VIII (Yadav and Khosla, 1991). The most commonly proposed mechanism of trigeminal injury is that the gasserian ganglion, or its roots or divisions, are caught, stretched or severed by fractures through the petrous bone or the exit foraminae of the skull base. Jefferson and Schorstein (1955) had one patient who came to autopsy following a closed head injury with a fracture extending across the skull base from the left to the right and involving the medial third of the right middle fossa, petrous tip and basisphenoid. The ganglion showed internal disruption and haemorrhage, with a tearing of the sensory root. Summers and Wirtshafter (1979) suggested that separation of the occipitosphenoid synchondrosis with upward displacement of the brain stem produced a traction injury of the trigeminal root around the entrance to Meckel's cave. A haematoma associated with a fracture around Meckel's cave could also produce compression of the ganglion. Russell and Schiller (1949), in experiments on crushing skulls, noted that there was a backward rotation of the petrous tip. This opened up the foramen lacerum and might cause rupture of the ganglion. Jefferson and Schorstein (1955) also commented that concurrent injury to the carotid artery and the trigeminal and other nerves in the cavernous sinus can occur with both penetrating and blunt trauma, but that such injuries would usually be fatal and therefore few come to medical attention.

The most commonly affected peripheral branches are the supraorbital, infraorbital and the inferior alveolar nerves. The supraorbital nerve is commonly damaged by lacerations or fractures involving the forehead or supraorbital margin. The resulting sensory loss involves the lateral forehead and extends back to the vertex in a tapering fashion. The infraorbital nerve is commonly damaged by fractures of the maxilla and zygoma. It results in numbness over the cheek and the lateral border of the nose, but may also result in a loss of sensation over some of the upper teeth, gum and palate, depending on where the nerve is damaged and the exact anatomical arrangement of its branches in any particular patient. The inferior alveolar nerve can be damaged by mandibular fractures and will result in an area of numbness over the lower lip and possibly the distal gum and incisor teeth.

Prognosis

Recovery following trigeminal injury is variable, but the more central the injury, the lower the prospect of recovery. Root disruption will not recover and ganglionic injuries rarely recover. Only one patient of 16 with ganglionic injury in Jefferson and Schorstein's series (1955) showed any recovery; they thought that this failure indicated severe ganglionic damage. Jacobi *et al.* (1986), however, thought that failure to recover indicated midbrain damage, but, in the absence of other signs of midbrain injury, we think this an unlikely explanation. Jefferson and Schorstein (1955) found that injuries to the divisions of the trigeminal nerve usually recovered within one year but this depends on whether the nerve is completely divided or some anatomical continuity still exists. With damage to the more peripheral branches (supraorbital, infraorbital, inferior alveolar) the area of sensory loss usually decreases with time (Lewin, 1966), either due to regeneration or axonal sprouting. There is no evidence that loss of sensation to the scalp will result in the loss of hair colour (Hughes, 1964).

Recovery from injury to the mandibular division depends upon which branches have been affected (Netterville and Civantos, 1993). Loss of the auriculotemporal and/or the meningeal branch is readily compensated. Loss of the buccal, lingual and inferior alveolar branches causes these patients to 'lose' the food bolus in the mouth. Netterville and Civantos (1993) recommend swallowing therapy to enable some compensation, but no explanation of this therapy is given. Isolated paralysis of the tensor veli palati is usually compensated for by the function of the levator veli palati with only limited dysfunction of the soft palate. Loss of the tensor tympani results in a small decrease in aural attenuation, which is compensated for by the stapedius muscle. Neither of these usually require specific therapy.

Paralysis of the temporalis, mylohyoid and pterygoids causes lateral shifting of the mandible during mastication, for which patients can usually compensate, providing contralateral function is normal. On the other hand, wasting of temporalis following denervation can lead to a significant cosmetic deformity, which may require surgical correction by placing an implant deep to the muscle. This can be fashioned from methylmethacrylate (Netterville and Civantos, 1993).

Complications

The most serious complication of trigeminal nerve injury is neuroparalytic keratitis; there is very little information in the literature about its incidence.

Jefferson and Schorstein (1955), in their series of 66 trigeminal injuries reported only one occurrence. Jacobi *et al.* (1986) reported two patients with neuroparalytic keratitis following damage to the nasociliary nerve. Extrapolating from results of procedures to section the trigeminal nerve for neuralgia, it would seem that 10–15% of these patients may develop ophthalmic complications (Hughes, 1993). Onofrio (1975) reported first division anaesthesia in nine of 135 patients following thermocoagulation for neuralgia. Of these, two developed neuroparalytic keratitis. Fraioli *et al.* (1989) had a 1.9% incidence of keratitis in 533 patients treated with thermocoagulation. Incomplete recovery of sensation following lesions of the trigeminal nerve may result in hyperpathia over the area and neuralgic pain (Bakay and Glasauer, 1980; Hughes, 1964; Jacobi *et al.*, 1986; Jefferson and Schorstein, 1955; Russell, 1942, 1960). Herpes zoster infection has been recorded following trigeminal injury (Hughes, 1964; Jacobi *et al.*, 1986).

Ninth–twelfth nerves

Injuries to the lowest four cranial nerves, either singly or in combination, are rare (Bauer, 1962; Jennett, 1974; Kitchens, 1991; Yadav and Khosla, 1991), most probably because the severity of the injury required to cause such damage to the nerves proves fatal for the patient (Bauer, 1962; Hughes, 1964; Jacobi *et al.*, 1986). Although injury to individual members of this group of nerves can occur, in most cases multiple nerves are involved. Patients with injuries to nerves IX–XII nearly always have to be ventilated in the acute phase due to the severity of their injuries. Assessment of lower cranial nerve function is frequently impossible at the time of presentation and diagnosis is therefore delayed until the patient is extubated and able to be assessed more accurately. The commonest aetiology appears to be a fall onto the back of the head resulting in a fracture of the posterior cranial fossa (Bakay and Glasauer, 1980; Massaro and Lauotte, 1993; Orbay *et al.*, 1989; Russell, 1960), but other causes are penetrating injuries (Bauer, 1962; Overholt *et al.*, 1992; Santosh *et al.*, 1973) or injuries to the cervical spine or craniocervical junction (Dukes and Bannergee, 1992; Fruin and Pirotte, 1977; Helliwell *et al.*, 1984; Maclean and Taylor, 1991; Page *et al.*, 1973; Rosa *et al.* (1984). Helliwell *et al.* (1984) have reported a case of bilateral VI and X nerve palsies following a whiplash injury. Other authors have proposed a vascular aetiology as a cause for cranial nerve palsies following cervical spine injuries, suggesting brain stem ischaemia secondary to vertebral artery spasm or compression (Grundy *et al.*, 1984; Schneider and Schemm, 1961).

We shall first look at injuries to individual nerves in this group and then progress to those involving various combinations of these four nerves.

Single nerve injuries

Glaser and Shafer (1932) had one case of injury to the glossopharyngeal nerve without involvement of nerves X–XII, but it was not stated whether this was an isolated injury or whether other cranial nerves were also affected. No comment was made about recovery in this patient.

Isolated injury to the vagus nerve has been reported in three patients by Myer and Fitton (1988); all three occurred in children and all were related to child abuse. Two of the cases required intubation and ventilation and the deficit was discovered only after several unsuccessful attempts were made to extubate the child. Chaten *et al.* (1991) described nine patients with postextubation vocal cord paralysis. Seven of these had been intubated for neurological disorders, including one case of child abuse and one of subdural effusions, both of whom had raised intracranial pressure. In both patients, the vocal cord paralysis resolved within four months. They suggested that raised intracranial pressure results in stretching, compression or ischaemia of the vagus nerve during its intracranial course. Pfenninger (1987) reported a case of failed extubation due to bilateral vocal cord paralysis following severe head injury in a patient who had dysfunction of cranial nerves VI, IX and X. He also suggested stretching or compression of these nerves in the posterior fossa as the most likely mechanism.

Isolated injury to the intracranial portion of the spinal accessory nerve has not been reported. Isolated injury to the extracranial portion of the spinal accessory nerve may follow blunt trauma to the posterior triangle of the neck, or a traction injury where the shoulder is depressed whilst the head is forced in the opposite direction. Lorei and Hershman (1993) report that such injuries may occur in football, lacrosse and hockey. Such an injury results in paralysis of the trapezius muscle but the sternomastoid muscle is spared because the injury occurs distal to its innervation.

Isolated injuries to the hypoglossal nerve appear to be associated with either hyperextension injuries to the cervical spine, in particular at the atlanto-occipital junction, or with fractures of the occipital condyles (Dukes and Bannergee, 1992; Massaro and Lanotte, 1993; Orbay *et al.*, 1989). This nerve may be damaged on one or both sides, depending on the force causing the injury. Recovery from hypoglossal nerve injury is variable, whether isolated or in association with other cranial nerve injuries. In the 20 patients we reviewed in the literature, 14 showed either partial or complete recovery, four showed no recovery; in two, no comment about recovery was made (Dukes and Bannergee, 1992; Fruin and Pirotte, 1977; Hammer, 1991; Hashimoto *et al.*, 1988; Maclean and Taylor, 1991; Massaro and Lanotte, 1993; Mock, 1950; Orbay *et al.*, 1989; Page *et al.*, 1973; Rosa *et al.*, 1984; Santosh *et al.*, 1973).

Combination injuries

Unilateral dysfunction of nerves IX and X (Avellis syndrome) was first described by George Avellis, a German laryngologist, in 1891. It results in unilateral paralysis of the larynx and soft palate, the aetiology in nearly all cases being vascular. However, the syndrome has been reported following trauma. Kitanaka *et al.* (1992) reported two cases following mild to moderate trauma to the head. In neither was there loss of consciousness at the time of injury. In both patients, the onset of the disturbance was delayed by several hours, and both had normal accessory nerve function. Neither had any demonstrable fractures around the jugular foramen on high resolution CT scanning. Both were treated with steroids and vitamin B_{12} with improvement, one patient making a complete recovery by two years, the other being lost to follow-up, at which time there was only mild hoarseness. The site of the injury was thought to be at the jugular foramen, but it was unclear why the accessory nerve was spared. Kitanaka *et al.* (1992) postulates that this nerve is less vulnerable than the ninth and the tenth.

Maclean and Taylor (1991) reported two patients with injury to the ninth, tenth and eleventh nerves unilaterally following head trauma and an associated fracture of the cervical spine or skull. One patient made a complete recovery by six weeks, whereas the other had only partial functional improvement by twelve months. Fractures of the cervical spine may be associated with vertebral artery thrombosis and subsequent lateral medullary syndrome with IX, X and XI palsies. This has also been observed in the absence of any fracture but following chiropractic manipulation (Carpenter, 1961; Tissington Tatlow and Bammer, 1957).

Unilateral paralysis of the lowest four cranial nerves is referred to as the 'Collet–Sicard' syndrome, the traumatic variety being most frequently reported in relation to war wounds or to self-inflicted injury in attempted suicide by gunshot (Bauer, 1962; Fishbone, 1976; Santosh *et al.*, 1973). Overholt *et al.* (1992) described the same constellation of findings following a penetrating injury of the jugular foramen by a piece of wood, although they attached the eponym 'Villaret's syndrome' to their case. Initially, the patient may have dyspnoea and excessive salivation with difficulty with swallowing. Occasionally the dyspnoea is so severe that urgent tracheostomy is required to enable adequate ventilation; this also minimizes the risk of aspiration pneumonitis. The dysphagia can be expected to recover with time, most patients eventually resuming a normal diet as long as the contralateral lower cranial nerves are normal (Grundy *et al.*, 1984; Maclean and Taylor, 1991; Netterville and Civantos, 1993). The affected cranial nerves, however, may not recover. Injection of the affected vocal cord may be required to improve the voice quality and the patient's ability to cough (Netteville and Civantos, 1993).

Although the matter is not related to the injuries under discussion it is of interest that Fleminger and Smith (1946) reported a patient with achalasia of the oesophagus following a depressed skull fracture of the occipital region. This only resolved after the administration of octyl nitrate more than two months following the injury, there being no recurrence after a single dose treatment.

Complications

Isolated loss of glossopharyngeal function will have some effect on the elevation of the pharynx, but little effect on swallowing overall. Loss of the parasympathetic supply to the parotid gland on the side of the injury can result in decreased salivation, which may lead to chronic parotitis. Unilateral glossopharyngeal loss does not affect the feedback loop from the carotid body and sinus, but bilateral loss may lead to marked disturbance in haemodynamic control. This may require alpha receptor blockade in the acute phase and may require long-term clonidine therapy (Netterville and Civantos, 1993; Rosa *et al.*, 1984).

Unilateral damage to the vagus nerve will result in difficulty with swallowing, with unilateral palatal and pharyngeal paralysis. With swallowing therapy, compensation for the former will usually occur with time. The latter does not cause major morbidity, but the resultant nasal regurgitation and marked nasal tonality of speech may be troublesome. Netterville and Civantos (1993) have designed a procedure in which the nasopharyngeal surface of the paralysed hemipalate is sutured to the posterior pharyngeal wall, creating a unilateral palatal adhesion, which will compensate for the paralysis. It should be performed only after adequate time for spontaneous recovery has been allowed.

The other major effect of unilateral vagal nerve damage is loss of ipsilateral vocal cord movement, which results in a hoarse voice, aspiration and an inefficient cough. In the acute phase the patient may be quite dyspnoeic and require tracheostomy. In the longer term, a silastic implant or injection of the paralysed cord may improve the symptoms.

Injury to the spinal accessory nerve results in loss of function of the sternocleidomastoid and trapezius muscles. The former is not usually noticed, but the latter results in disability from shoulder droop and shoulder pain. Exercises to strengthen the levator scapulae and rhomboids will help in supporting the shoulder (Netterville and Civantos, 1993).

Unilateral hypoglossal injury results in ipsilateral paralysis of the tongue. Whilst initially this can cause some difficulty in eating and speaking, in time, most patients compensate well. Bilateral hypoglossal palsy causes serious morbidity and patients have severe difficulty in swallowing anything, including their own secretions. In the early period they require a nasogastric tube to allow adequate nutrition. If there is no recovery, they require a feeding gastrostomy.

References

Aucott WR. (1988) Central trigeminal injury: a sign of basal skull fracture. *J R Coll Surg Edin* **33**: 161–62.

Bakay L, Glasauer FE. (1980) Cranial nerve injuries. In: *Head injury.* Boston, MA: Little, Brown, 263–76.

Bauer F. (1962) Foramen jugulare syndrome caused by bullet wound. *J Larygol Otol* **76**: 367–71.

Cairns H. (1937) Injuries of the frontal and ethmoidal sinuses with special reference to cerebrospinal rhinorrhoea and aeroceles. *J Laryngol Otol* **52**: 589–623.

Carpenter S. (1961) Injury of neck as cause of vertebral artery thrombosis. *J Neurosurg* **18**: 849–53.

Chaten FC, Lucking SE, Young ES, Mickell JJ. (1991) Stridor: intracranial pathology causing postextubation vocal cord paralysis. *Pediatrics* **87**: 39–43.

Dukes IK, Bannergee SK. (1992) Hypoglossal nerve palsy following hyperextension neck injury. *Injury* **24**: 133–34.

Elliott B. (1974) Lost bouquets. In: Potter JM, editor. *The practical management of head injuries.* London: Lloyd-Luke, 86–89.

Fishbone H. (1976) Irreversible injury of the last four cranial nerves (Collett–Sicard syndrome). *Handbook Clin Neurol* **24**: 179–81.

Fleminger JJ, Smith MC. (1946) Achalasia of oesophagus following depressed fracture of base of skull. *Lancet* **i**: 381–83.

Fraioli B, Eposito V, Guidetti B, *et al.* (1989) Treatment of trigeminal neuralgia by thermodilution, glycerolization, and percutaneous compression of the gasserian ganglion and/or retrogasserian rootlets: long-term results and therapeutic protocol. *Neurosurgery* **24**: 239–45.

Fruin AH, Pirotte TP. (1977) Traumatic atlantooccipital dislocation. Case report. *J Neurosurg* **46**: 663–66.

Glaser MA, Shafer FP. (1932) Skull and brain traumas: their sequelae. *JAMA* **98**: 271–76.

Goland PP. (1937) Olfactometry in cases of acute head injury. *Arch Surg (Lond)* **35**: 1173–82.

Grundy DJ, McSweeny T, Jones HWF. (1984) Cranial nerve palsies in cervical injuries. *Spine* **9**: 339–43.

Hagan PJ. (1967) Posttraumatic anosmia. *Arch Otolaryngal* **85**: 85–89.

Hammer AJ. (1991) Lower cranial nerve palsies. *Clin Ortho P* **266**: 64–69.

Hashimoto T, Watanabe O, Takase M, *et al.* (1988) Collett–Sicard syndrome after minor head trauma. *Neurosurgery* **23**: 367–69.

Helliwell M, Robertson JC, Todd GB, Lobb M. (1984) Bilateral vocal cord paralysis due to whiplash injury. *Br Med J* **288**: 1876–77.

Hughes B. (1964) The results of injury to special parts of the brain and skull: the cranial nerves. In: Rowbotham GF, editor. *Acute injuries to the head.* Edinburgh: Livingstone, 408–33.

Hughes RAC. (1993) Diseases of the fifth cranial nerve. In: Dyck PJ, Thomas PK, editors. *Peripheral neuropathy.* London: Saunders, 801–17.

Jacobi G, Ritz A, Emrich R. (1986) Cranial nerve damage after paediatric head trauma: a long-term follow-up study of 741 cases. *Acta Paediatr Hung* **27**: 173–87.

Jafek BW, Eller PM, Esses BA. (1989) Post-traumatic anosmia. *Arch Neurol* **46**: 300–304.

Jefferson G, Schorstein J. (1955) Injuries of the trigeminal nerve, its ganglion and its divisions. *Br J Surg* **42**: 561–82.

Jennett WB. (1974) Injury to cranial nerves and optic chiasm. In: Brock S, editor. *Injury of the brain and spinal cord and their coverings,* 5th edition. New York: Springer, 162–66.

Kitanaka C, Sugaya M, Yamada H. (1992) Avellis syndrome after minor head trauma: report of two cases. *Surg Neurol* **37**: 236–39.

Kitchens JL. (1991) Basilar skull fractures in childhood with cranial nerve involvement. *J Pediatr Surg* **26**: 992–94.

Leigh AD. (1943) Defects of smell after head injury. *Lancet* **i**: 38–40.

Lewin W. (1954) Cerebrospinal fluid rhinorrhoea in closed head injuries. *Br J Surg* **42**: 1–18.

Lewin W. (1966) Injuries to cranial nerves and visual pathways. In: *The management of head injuries.* Baltimore: Wilkins & Wilkins, 137–46.

Lorei MP, Hershman EB. (1993) Peripheral nerve injuries in athletes. *Sports Med* **16**: 130–47.

Maclean JGB, Taylor A. (1991) Combined lower cranial nerve injury: complication of upper cervical or basal skull fracture. *JR Coll Surg Edinb* **36**: 188–89.

Massaro F, Lanotte M. (1993) Fracture of the occipital condyle. *Injury* **24**: 319–20.

Mock HE. (1950) Cranial nerve injuries. In: *Skull fractures and brain injuries.* Baltimore, MD: Williams & Wilkins, 765–76.

Myer CM, Fitton GM. (1988) Vocal cord paralysis following child abuse. *Int J Pediatr Otorhinolaryngol* **15**: 217–20.

Netterville JL, Civantos FJ. (1993) Rehabilitation of cranial nerve deficits after neurotologic skull base surgery. *Laryngoscope* **103**: 45–54.

Onofrio BM. (1975) Radiofrequency percutaneous gasserian ganglion lesions. Results in 140 patients with trigeminal pain. *J Neurosurg* **42**: 132–39.

Orbay T, Aykol S, Seckin Z, Ergun R. (1989) Late hypoglossal nerve palsy following fracture of the occipital condyle. *Surg Neurol* **31**: 402–404.

Overholt EM, Dalley RW, Winn HR, Weymuller EA. (1992) Penetrating trauma of the jugular foramen. *Ann Otol Rhinol Laryngol* **101**: 452–54.

Page CP, Story JL, Wissinger JP, Branch CL. (1973) Traumatic atlantooccipital dislocation. Case report. *J Neurosurg* **39**: 394–97.

Pfenninger J. (1987) Bilateral vocal cord paralysis after severe blunt head injury – a cause of failed extubation. *Crit Care Med* **15**: 701–702.

Rosa L, Carol M, Bellagarrigue R, Ducker TB. (1984) Multiple cranial nerve palsies due to a hyperextension injury to the cervical spine. *J Neurosurg* **61**: 172–73.

Russell WR. (1942) Medical aspects of head injury. *Br Med J* **ii**: 521–23.

Russell WR, Schiller F. (1949) Crushing injuries to the skull: clinical and experimental observations. *J Neurol Neurosurg Psychiatry* **12**: 52–60.

Russell WR. (1960) Injury to cranial nerves and optic chiasm. In: Brock S, editor. *Injuries of the brain and spinal cord,* 4th edition. London: Cassell, 118–26.

Santosh KM, Barrios M, Fishbone H, Khatib R. (1973) Irreversible injury of cranial nerves 9 through 12 (Collett–Sicard syndrome). *J Neurosurg* **38**: 86–88.

Schechter PJ, Henkin RI. (1974) Abnormalities of taste and smell after head trauma. *J Neurol Neurosurg Psychiatry* **37**: 802–10.

Schneider RC, Schemm GW. (1961) Vertebral artery insufficiency in acute and chronic spinal trauma. *J Neurosurg* **18**: 348–60.

Summers CG, Wirtshafter JD. (1979) Bilateral trigeminal and abducens neuropathies following low velocity crushing head injury. *J Neurosurg* **50**: 508–11.

Sumner D. (1962) On testing the sense of smell. *Lancet* **ii**: 895–96.

Sumner D. (1964) Post-traumatic anosmia. *Brain* **87**: 107–20.

Sumner D. (1976) Disturbances of the senses of smell and taste after head injuries. *Handbook Clin Neurol* **24**: 1–25.

Tissington Tatlow WF, Bammer HG. (1957) Syndrome of vertebral artery compression. *Neurology* **7**: 331.

Yadav YR, Khosla VK. (1991) Isolated 5th to 10th cranial nerve palsy in closed head trauma. *Clin Neurol Neurosurg* **93**: 61–63.

8

Post-traumatic epilepsy

Byron Young, Robert P Rapp, Richard J Kryscio

Introduction

Post-traumatic epilepsy is divided into two types. Early post-traumatic epilepsy is characterized by one or more seizures occurring within one week of head injury and without any other obvious causes. Seizures occurring more than one week after head injury are referred to as late post-traumatic epilepsy. Temkin *et al.*, (1991) subdivided the category of early epilepsy, to distinguish seizures occurring within the first 24 hours from those occurring from day 2 to day 7; those occurring during the first 24 hours are called immediate seizures. The most common classification, however, is that used by Jennett (1975b) and adopted by most other authors (i.e. seizures are divided simply into early and late epilepsy).

A generalized seizure occurring within a few moments of injury is termed immediate epilepsy and is distinguished by most investigators from the early seizures that occur after this time. An immediate seizure follows a mild injury, is an infrequent occurrence, and, unlike early seizures, does not predispose to subsequent seizures (Jennett, 1975b).

Post-traumatic epilepsy is a not infrequent occurrence. An estimated 422 000 people are hospitalized for head injury each year in the USA (Kalsbeck *et al.*, 1980). The incidence of early epilepsy in large head injury studies ranges from 2.5% to 7% (Annegers, 1980; Jennett, 1975b). In the retrospective study by Annegers *et al.* (1980) of a civilian population during the first year after head injury, late seizures occurred in 7.1% of patients.

In the series by Jennett (1975b) of unselected head injuries, 5% of the patients admitted to hospital developed late epilepsy.

Early post-traumatic epilepsy

Risk and characteristics of early epilepsy

The risk of early post-traumatic seizures is related to the type and severity of the brain injury. Subdural and intracerebral haematomas are associated with a 30–36% incidence of early seizures (Jennett, 1975a). Epidural haematomas, frontal and parietal depressed skull fractures, and brain injuries with focal neurological signs or post-traumatic amnesia longer than 24 hours in duration are associated with an early seizure incidence of 9–13% (Caveness and Liss, 1961; Jennett, 1975a,b). Patients with missile wounds received in combat have an early seizure incidence of about 2–6% (Ascroft, 1941; Russell and Whitty, 1957). The incidence of early seizures in civilians who have suffered missile wounds has not been established in any large series. Only 1–2% of patients with minor head injuries and no neurological signs have an early seizure (Jennett, 1975b).

Age also seems to be a factor that determines the susceptibility to early seizures. In the series by Jennett (1975b), early seizures occurred more frequently in children under five years of age. Early seizures more often began in the first hour and within 24 hours in children than in adults.

Slightly less than one-third of early seizures occur within an hour of injury, one-third occur during the next 24 hours, and slightly more than one-third occur during the remaining days of the first week after injury (Jennett, 1975b). Rish and Caveness (1973) also reported that early post-traumatic seizures occur most frequently during the first five days after a combat head injury, with a peak incidence on the first day.

Focal seizures account for approximately one-half of early seizures. Most early focal seizures are focal motor seizures. Focal seizures occur more frequently after missile injuries than after blunt injuries (Jennett, 1975b).

Significance of early epilepsy

The primary significance of early epilepsy is as a predictor of an increased risk of developing late post-traumatic seizures. Approximately 25% of patients with an early seizure also have late seizures. This high frequency of late following early seizures includes even mild injuries that would, in the absence of an early seizure, have only a slight risk for late seizures. The risk for late seizures is unaffected by the number or type of early seizures, except that early focal seizures in children do not increase the risk of late seizures (Jennett, 1975b).

The occurrence of an early seizure complicates the treatment of head-injured patients. Depression of consciousness after a seizure hinders the evaluation of the patient's neurological condition. Costly computed tomographic (CT) scans may have to be repeated to rule out the possibility of a newly developed intracranial mass lesion. Occasionally, secondary complications, such as aspiration pneumonitis, are caused by post-traumatic seizures. Eleven per cent of all patients, and 22% of children under the age of five, develop status epilepticus (Jennett, 1975b). A series of 116 patients who were able to talk after a head injury, but who subsequently died, included two children, only mildly injured, whose sole cause of death was poorly controlled epilepsy (Rose et al., 1977).

Late post-traumatic epilepsy

Risk and characteristics of late epilepsy

Although researchers have developed many experimental animal models for post-traumatic epilepsy (Purpura et al., 1972), no animal model exactly reproduces the human brain injury milieu leading to post-traumatic epilepsy. Thus, the mechanisms responsible for the development of late post-traumatic epilepsy have not yet been well elucidated. Because very few late seizures occur during the first two months after head injury (Jennett, 1975b), a time period of approximately eight weeks seems to be necessary for the development of the epileptogenic focus. Some of the elements that have been suggested as causes for the development of the epileptogenic focus include:

1. Biochemical, electrical and structural changes;
2. The development of pacemaker neurones;
3. Decreased inhibitory controlling mechanisms;
4. Biochemical deficits in acetylcholine, glutamic acid and potassium;
5. Postsynaptic hypersensitivity;
6. Impairment of acid–base balance;
7. The deposition of iron salts from the haemorrhage;
8. Lipid peroxidation;
9. Genetic factors.

(Caveness, 1976; Goldensohn and Ward, 1975; Jasper, 1970; Penfield and Erickson, 1971; Pollen and Trachtenberg, 1970; Potter, 1978; Schmidt et al., 1959; Tower, 1952, 1960; Westrum et al., 1964; Willmore and Rubin, 1984; Willmore and Triggs, 1984; Willmore et al., 1978; Wyler and Ray, 1985.)

The severity of the head injury plays an important role in the development of late epilepsy. The incidence of post-traumatic seizures after traumatic intracranial haematoma is very high; one-fifth of patients who have suffered epidural haematomas and almost one-half of patients with subdural or intracerebral haematomas will develop late seizures (Jennett, 1975a). The incidence of late epilepsy after depressed skull fractures depends upon a wide range of factors and ranges from only 4% to over 60%. Other associated factors, such as focal signs, dural laceration, post-traumatic amnesia longer than 24 hours in duration, or an early seizure, greatly increase the incidence of late seizures in patients with depressed fractures. In the absence of these factors, the incidence of late epilepsy is below 10% (Jennett, 1975b). Approximately one-third of patients with combat missile wounds develop post-traumatic seizures (Caveness et al., 1979). Certain characteristics of the injury are important risk factors for subsequent seizures. The extent of focal damage, the association of focal damage and prolonged coma, and injuries adjacent to the central sulcus increase the incidence of late seizures. In the Vietnam war head injury series (Caveness *et al.*, 1979), half of the patients having early seizures also had late seizures.

Severe head injuries are not the only injuries that have a high association with late epilepsy. A patient with a mild injury, but having an early seizure, has a 25% chance of having late seizures. A mild injury alone, without significant loss of consciousness and no early epilepsy, is associated with only a 1–2% chance of late seizures. Jennett's series provides considerable data based on the features of the injury for the accurate calculation of the exact risk of the individual patient for late epilepsy (Jennett, 1975b).

Electroencephalography (EEG) performed soon after head injury is a poor predictor of the risk of late seizures (Courjon, 1970). However, after a late seizure has occurred, the presence of focal EEG abnormalities suggests an increased risk of further seizures. According to Jennett and van de Sande (1975), the early EEG findings do not provide enough additional information to be helpful to the clinician in predicting late epilepsy. Patients with severe injuries have a high incidence of EEG abnormalities and of late seizure development. Patients with early normal EEGs not infrequently develop late epilepsy. At one year after injury, there is a significant difference in EEG findings in patients with and without late seizures, but this is too late to be useful as a predicting factor. Even at one year, 55% of those patients with no late epilepsy have abnormal EEG records (Jennett and Teasdale, 1981). Caveness *et al.* (1979), Potter (1978) and others have suggested that the individual's personal or constitutional make-up, such as genetic traits, may play an important role in susceptibility to post-traumatic epilepsy. The significance of these factors remains unestablished. Schaumann *et al.* (1994) found that 'the role of genetic factors in post-traumatic epilepsy is minor, or at least not readily detectable...'.

The frequency of late seizures varies widely. There may be only a single seizure or so many that no effort is made to keep count. According to Caveness *et al.* (1979), once post-traumatic epilepsy is established, there is little change in the frequency of attacks. Caveness divided the patients in his Vietnam war series into three frequency patterns: those who had experienced one to three, four to 30, or more than 30 seizures. Each of these groups comprised approximately one-third of the seizure patients. In this series, which was based on

a 10-year follow-up, half of those patients having early seizures also developed late seizures. There was a highly significant relationship between the frequency and duration of seizures; the greater the frequency of seizures, the greater the probability of their persistence.

Mechanisms of late post-traumatic epilepsy

Surgical specimens removed to control post-traumatic epilepsy show neuronal and oligodendroglial loss, gliosis and haemosiderosis. The epileptogenic focus is adjacent to the injury site. The hyperirritable epileptogenic focus may be caused by mechanical stress or by long-standing localized ischaemia (Jasper, 1970). Tower (1960) and Tower and Elliott (1952) demonstrated that an epileptogenic focus has biochemical defects in acetylcholine, glutamic acid and potassium metabolism. Schmidt *et al.* (1959) attributed the burst of autonomous electrical activity in the epileptogenic focus to a dendritic depolarization and to the difference in potential between the cell body and the dendritic network. Westrum *et al.* (1964) proposed that the decreased synaptic endings or dendrites within the epileptogenic focus permit postsynaptic hypersensitivity. Gliotic changes may also impair the glial control of acid–base balance and allow an excessive excitability of adjacent neurones (Pollen and Trachtenberg, 1970).

Post-traumatic epilepsy is characterized by a latency period between the time of the trauma and the appearance of the first seizure. The brain injury presumably sets into motion a series of biochemical, electrical and structural changes that lead to the development of an epileptogenic focus (Rapport and Ojemann, 1975). The time taken for the development of the epileptogenic focus in humans appears to be about eight weeks. After this 'incubation' phase, late seizures make their appearance. In the series by Jennett (1975b), the seizure incidence during the first week after head injury was 30 times the incidence in any one of the seven subsequent weeks.

Post-traumatic epilepsy: prophylaxis clinical trials

Many clinical and laboratory investigations suggest that administering anticonvulsants as a prophylactic measure will reduce the incidence of post-traumatic epilepsy. Young (1990) and Temkin *et al.* (1991) provide reviews of these reports. Some early clinical trials indicated that administering a prophylactic anticonvulsant drug reduced the incidence of late seizures, but these trials were not well designed. More recent and better controlled studies do not support this conclusion.

Prophylaxis of early post-traumatic epilepsy

Young *et al.* (1983a) performed a randomized, double-blind, placebo-controlled study to determine whether administering phenytoin soon after severe head injury decreased the incidence of epilepsy in the first week. Two hundred and forty-four patients were randomized into two groups and were given either phenytoin or a placebo. The patients in the phenytoin group were given the drug within 24 hours of being admitted to the hospital. At one, three and seven days after injury, plasma concentrations of at least $10 \mu g/ml$ had been achieved in more than 78% of the phenytoin patients. No significant difference was found in the percentage of patients in either group who had early seizures ($p = 0.99$), and there was no significant difference between the treated and placebo groups in the interval from injury to first seizure ($p = 0.41$). The early administration of phenytoin was thus not effective as a prophylaxis in reducing the occurrence of seizures in the first week after head injury. The authors therefore recommended that anticonvulsant drugs should be administered as prophylaxis only after an early seizure has occurred.

Temkin *et al.* (1990) performed a double-blind, placebo-controlled study of 404 severely head-injured patients who were considered to be at high risk for the development of post-traumatic seizures; they were randomly assigned to receive either phenytoin or a placebo. The purpose of the study was to obtain and maintain high therapeutic levels of serum phenytoin in the 'treated' group of patients. These patients received an initial loading dose of phenytoin within the first 24 hours after injury. Results demonstrated that the phenytoin group had a cumulative early seizure rate of $3.6 \pm 1.3\%$, whereas $14.2 \pm 2.6\%$ of the placebo group had seizures. The authors found a significant difference between the placebo and the prophylactic phenytoin groups and concluded that phenytoin reduced the risk of early seizures by 73%. The authors did not, however, make specific recommendations about whether or not phenytoin should be administered prophylactically to prevent early seizures.

Prophylaxis of late post-traumatic epilepsy

Many patients make an excellent recovery from head injuries but retain a significant disability because of post-traumatic seizures. Late post-traumatic epilepsy has considerably more severe medical, economic, social and psychological consequences than early post-traumatic epilepsy. Late post-traumatic seizures greatly lessen the chance of gainful employment after rehabilitation.

A large body of experimental evidence suggests that anticonvulsant prophylaxis tends to prevent epilepsy induced by a variety of epileptogenic causes (Rasmussen, 1969; Young *et al.*, 1983b). However, the evidence from older clinical studies testing the efficacy of prophylaxis for late post-traumatic seizures is conflicting and, by modern standards, fraught with methodological deficiencies (Birkmayer, 1951; Caveness *et al.*, 1979; Hoff and Hoff, 1947; Murri *et al.*, 1992; Popek, 1972; Wohns and Wyler, 1979; Young *et al.*, 1979; Zervit and Musil, 1981). The rationale for prophylactic administration of anticonvulsant drugs is to prevent or arrest the progression of the development of the epileptogenic focus.

In the series by Temkin *et al.* (1990), of the patients followed for up to two years, no significant difference in the seizure rates could be demonstrated between those taking phenytoin and those given a placebo. Twenty-seven per cent of the patients treated with phenytoin and 21% of the patients given a placebo developed late post-traumatic seizures. Temkin could not demonstrate that phenytoin was effective as a prophylaxis against late post-traumatic epilepsy. Of the patients who could be followed, 70% had therapeutic phenytoin levels at their subsequent clinic visits. By the end of the first year, 21% of the phenytoin group and 15% of the control group had experienced late seizures. At the end of two years, 27% of the phenytoin group and 21% of the control group had suffered seizures.

Young *et al.* (1983b) performed a randomized, double-blind, placebo-controlled study of 179 patients to determine whether administering phenytoin soon after head injury would decrease the incidence of late post-traumatic epilepsy. Patients in the study were followed for 18 months to detect the occurrence of seizures and serially to measure concentrations of plasma phenytoin. No significant difference in the percentage of late seizures was found between the treated and placebo groups ($p = 0.75$), and there was no significant difference between the two groups in the time between injury and seizures. The results of this study demonstrated that low therapeutic ranges of phenytoin provided no prophylaxis against late post-traumatic seizures.

Because Young *et al.* (1983b) found that no patients with phenytoin plasma concentrations of 12 µg/ml or higher had a seizure, they could not conclude that higher therapeutic plasma concentrations of phenytoin and higher compliance rates would not have significantly decreased the occurrence of post-traumatic epilepsy. In the study by Temkin *et al.* (1990), seven of nine patients receiving phenytoin had therapeutic levels on the day of their first seizure. This observation provides even stronger evidence that phenytoin does not prevent the development of late post-traumatic seizures.

Murri *et al.* (1992) treated 390 severely head-injured patients with phenobarbitone for 12 months after injury; 293 patients completed the study. The study was not a randomized trial; all patients received an intramuscular dose of 1.5–3.0 mg/kg body weight per day, commencing within 24 hours of injury. Phenobarbitone plasma concentrations were maintained at between 5 µg/l and 30 µg/ml. Six patients (2.04%) had at least one seizure during the 12-month study period. The authors used historical controls to conclude that phenobarbitone, even at low doses, can have a prophylactic effect on post-traumatic epilepsy.

Temkin et al.'s combined analysis

Temkin *et al.* (1991) reviewed four studies of prophylactic administration of anticonvulsants to prevent early and late post-traumatic epilepsy. The authors concluded that the studies of Young *et al.* (1983b) and Temkin *et al.* (1990) were compatible and, when combined, showed an estimated decrease in early seizures of 64%. This analysis of late seizure studies estimated that phenytoin contributed to a 10% increase in late seizure incidence.

However, the conclusions drawn by Temkin *et al.* (1991) from their meta-analysis of the Young and Temkin studies are questionable. The study by Young *et al.* (1983b) had a negative finding for early seizures (an estimated 3.9% crude incidence in both the treatment and control groups), whereas the study by Temkin *et al.* (1990) had a positive finding for early seizures (an estimated 3.6% actuarial incidence in the treatment group, which is significantly less than the actuarial incidence of 14.2% in the control group). Temkin *et al.* (1991) combined Young's crude rates with their own actuarial rates to conclude that the combined evidence from both studies favours the active treatment. The evidence supporting this conclusion is highly questionable. Although it is reasonable to use actuarial methods, such as a stratified Cox proportional hazards model, to combine the data from the two studies, the evidence for combining these studies is marginally significant ($p = 0.08$; cf the Appendix to Temkin *et al.*, 1991).

Meta-analysis is designed to combine the evidence over several clinical studies. In this case there were only two studies; both reached disparate conclusions. The positive result in the trial by Temkin *et al.* (1990) is clearly due to an inordinately high rate of seizures in the control group, a rate not experienced in the study by Young *et al.* (1983b). Hence, on combining the studies, the evidence comes primarily from this high rate. It is doubtful that the patient populations being treated in these two studies are comparable. Had there been more than two studies with varying rates on the control groups, the conclusions reached by Temkin *et al.* (1991) would have been more convincing. The fact that there are only two studies weakens the conclusions of this analysis.

Recommendations for prophylaxis and treatment

Prophylaxis must be distinguished from treatment or suppression of an established epileptogenic focus. To be considered successful as prophylaxis, the anticonvulsant regimen must prevent the development of the epileptogenic focus and consequent seizures. Once this has been accomplished, the administration of the prophylactic agent can cease after two or three months with significantly less risk of seizure occurrence. By contrast, successful treatment suppresses the electrical activity of the developed epileptogenic focus so that seizures do not occur. Seizures are still likely in this group, however, if the anticonvulsant drug is withdrawn.

Considering the available data, we cannot recommend the prophylactic administration of phenytoin to prevent early or late seizures. If an early seizure occurs, however, phenytoin should be administered intravenously in an attempt to prevent subsequent seizures. Phenytoin should be given for approximately 10 days and then discontinued. No prophylaxis should be given to prevent late post-traumatic seizures; such prophylaxis is not justified on the basis of the evidence obtained in well controlled studies of late seizure prophylaxis. Other drugs, such as phenobarbitone or valproate, have not been tested adequately enough to justify their prophylactic administration. A trial currently being conducted at the National Institute of Neurological Disorders and Stroke is testing whether prophylactically administered valproate reduces the incidence of late post-traumatic epilepsy.

When should the administration of anticonvulsants be started? Most authors recommend starting therapy for unprovoked epilepsy only after two seizures have occurred. Others recommend beginning treatment after the first unprovoked seizure in the presence of predictors of subsequent seizures, such as focal seizures, EEG abnormalities, focal neurological signs, or structural lesions visible on brain imaging studies. Post-traumatic seizures should be considered provoked seizures, and treatment should be started after a single late seizure. When a late seizure occurs, an anticonvulsant drug (phenytoin, valproate or carbamazepine) should be administered. Treatment should be initiated after the first late post-traumatic seizure, because such seizures are likely to be multiple. The duration of treatment for patients with late post-traumatic seizures should probably follow the principles for treatment of all seizures, regardless of their cause.

Opinions, however, vary widely about when and how to discontinue anticonvulsant drugs in patients with established non-post-traumatic epilepsy. Many authors stop anticonvulsants only after two seizure-free years, whereas others wait for four years. Treiman (1993) does not stop anticonvulsants in patients with predictors of subsequent seizures. Although numerous authors suggest tapering off antiepileptic drugs over a prolonged period, presumably to lessen the risk of seizure recurrence, recent evidence does not confirm the need for this practice. Tennison *et al.* (1994) studied a group of children who had a variety of types of epilepsy and analysed the risks of and factors influencing seizure recurrence after tapering off of anticonvulsant drugs. Neither the length of the taper interval (six weeks or nine months) nor the seizure-free interval (two years or four years)

before discontinuing drugs was a significant factor in seizure recurrence. EEG spikes, however, were significantly related to seizure recurrence. Marks *et al.* (1991) found that acute withdrawal of anticonvulsant drugs did not significantly affect frequency, clinical features or electrical onset of seizures.

No well designed study has established the efficacy of any of the currently available anticonvulsant drugs as prophylactic agents. Because anticonvulsant drugs administered prophylactically do not prevent the development of the epileptogenic focus, other researchers, including Willmore (1990), have suggested the investigation of drugs that might block the epileptogenic process, such as antiperoxidants and antioxidants. Dakin and Weaver (1993) advocate the use of quantum pharmacology to model the molecular events in the developing epileptogenic focus to obtain the data necessary for designing an effective prophylactic drug. Quantum pharmacology is 'the application of the techniques of computational theoretical chemistry (molecular mechanics, molecular dynamics, *ab initio* quantum mechanics and semi-empirical quantum mechanics) to the structural analysis of biological macromolecules of pharmaceutical interest'. Dakin and Weaver (1993) illustrate this technique for analysis of iron-induced lipid peroxidation of membranes at the injury site. Application of this technique may enable the design of a new prophylactic drug on the basis of the mechanism of development of the post-traumatic epileptogenic focus rather than on the expensive conventional practice of screening several drugs in large groups of subjects to test for efficacy.

Resection of the epileptogenic focus is rarely required to control post-traumatic seizures that are intractable to medical management. Late post-traumatic seizures tend to diminish with time, and surgery should not be performed for at least two years after the injury. The general principles of the surgical treatment of post-traumatic epilepsy are the same as those for surgical treatment of other focal seizures. The classic report by Rasmussen (1969) indicated that 40% of patients become seizure-free after surgery, 26% have a significant reduction in seizure frequency, and 35% have no or only a moderate reduction in seizure frequency.

References

Annegers JF, Grabow JD, Groover RV, *et al.* (1980) Seizures after head trauma: a population study. *Neurology* **30**: 683–89.

Ascroft PB. (1941) Traumatic epilepsy after gunshot wounds of the head. *Br Med J* **1**: 739–44.

Birkmayer von W. (1951) Die Behandlung der traumatischen Epilepsie. *Wien Klin Wochenschr* **63**: 606–609.

Caveness WF. (1976) Epilepsy: a product of trauma in our time. *Epilepsia* **17**: 207–15.

Caveness WF, Liss HR. (1961) Incidence of post-traumatic epilepsy. *Epilepsia* **2**: 123–29.

Caveness WF, Meirowsky AM, Rish BL, *et al.* (1979) The nature of posttraumatic epilepsy. *J Neurosurg* **50**: 545–53.

Courjon J. (1970) A longitudinal electro-clinical study of 80 cases of post-traumatic epilepsy observed from the time of the original trauma. *Epilepsia* **11**: 29–36.

Dakin KA, Weaver DF. (1993) Mechanisms of post-traumatic seizures: a quantum pharmacological analysis of the molecular properties of an epileptogenic focus following iron-induced membrane peroxidation. *Seizure* **2**: 32.

Goldensohn ES, Ward AA Jr. (1975) Pathogenesis of epileptic seizures. In: Tower DB, editor. *The nervous system.* New York: Raven Press, 249–60.

Hoff von H, Hoff H. (1947) Fortschritte in der Behandlung der Epilepsie. *Monatsschr Psychiatrie Neuro* **114**: 105–18.

Jasper HH. (1970) Physiopathological mechanisms of post-traumatic epilepsy. *Epilepsia* **11**: 73–80.

Jennett B. (1975a) Epilepsy and acute traumatic intracranial hematoma. *J Neurol Neurosurg Psychiatry* **38**: 378–81.

Jennett B. (1975b) *Epilepsy after non-missile head injuries*, 2nd edition. Chicago: Year Book.

Jennett B, Teasdale G. (1981) *Management of head injuries* (Contemporary neurology series, vol. 20.) Philadelphia: Davis.

Jennett B, van de Sande J. (1975) EEG prediction of post-traumatic epilepsy. *Epilepsia* **16**: 251–56.

Kalsbeck WD, McLaurin RL, Harris BSH III, *et al.* (1980) The national head and spinal cord injury survey: major findings. *J Neurosurg* **53**: S19–S31.

Marks DA, Katz A, Scheyer R, *et al.* (1991) Clinical and electrographic effects of acute anticonvulsant withdrawal in epileptic patients. *Neurology* **41**: 508–12.

Murri L, Arrigo A, Bonuccelli U, *et al.* (1992) Phenobarbital in the prophylaxis of late posttraumatic seizures. *Ital J Neurol Sci* **13**: 755–60.

Penfield W, Erickson TC. (1971) *Epilepsy and cerebral localization.* Springfield, IL: Charles C Thomas, 3–7.

Pollen DA, Trachtenberg MC. (1970) Neuroglia: gliosis and focal epilepsy [abstract]. *Science* **167**: 1252–53.

Popek K. (1972) Preventive treatment of post-traumatic epilepsy following severe brain injury. *Cesk Neurol* **35**: 169–74.

Potter JM. (1978) The personal factor in the maturation of epileptogenic brain scars: review and hypothesis. *J Neurol Neurosurg Psychiatry* **41**: 265–71.

Purpura DP, Penry JK, Woodbury DM, *et al.* (1972) *Experimental models of epilepsy – a manual for the laboratory worker.* New York: Raven Press.

Rapport RL, Ojemann GA. (1975) Prophylactically administered phenytoin: effects on the development of chronic cobalt-induced epilepsy in the cat. *Arch Neurol* **32**: 539–48.

Rasmussen T. (1969) Surgical therapy of post-traumatic epilepsy. In: Walker AE, Caveness WF, editors. *The late effects of head injury.* Springfield, IL: Charles C Thomas, 277–305.

Rish BL, Caveness WF. (1973) Relation of prophylactic medication to the occurrence of early seizures following craniocerebral trauma. *J Neurosurg* **38**: 155–58.

Rose J, Valtonen S, Jennett B. (1977) Avoidable factors contributing to death after head injury. *Br Med J* **2**: 615–17.

Russell WR, Whitty CWN. (1957) Studies in traumatic epilepsy: I. Factors influencing the incidence of epilepsy after brain wounds. *J Neurol Neurosurg Psychiatry* **15**: 93–98.

Schaumann BA, Annegers JF, Johnson SB, *et al.* (1994) Family history of seizures in posttraumatic and alcohol-associated seizure disorders. *Epilepsia* **31**: 51.

Schmidt RP, Thomas LB, Ward AA Jr. (1959) The hyperexcitable neurone: micro-electrode studies of chronic epileptic foci in the monkey. *J Neurophysiol* **22**: 285–96.

Temkin NR, Dikmen SS, Wilensky AJ, *et al.* (1990) A randomized, double-blind study of phenytoin for the prevention of post-traumatic seizures. *N Engl J Med* **323**: 497–502.

Temkin NR, Dikmen SS, Winn HR. (1991) Management of Head Injury. Post-traumatic seizures. *Neurosurg Clin North Am* **2**: 425–35.

Tennison M, Greenwood R, Lewis D, *et al.* (1994) Discontinuing antiepileptic drugs in children with epilepsy. A comparison of a six-week and a nine-month taper period. *N Engl J Med* **330**: 1407–10.

Tower DB. (1960) *Neurochemistry of epilepsy: seizure mechanisms and their management.* Springfield, IL: Charles C Thomas,

Tower DB, Elliott KAC. (1952) Activity of acetylcholine system in human epileptogenic focus. *J Appl Physiol* **4**: 669–76.

Treiman DM. (1993) Current treatment strategies in selected situations in epilepsy. *Epilepsia* **34**: (suppl 5): S17–S23.

Westrum LE, White LE, Ward AA Jr. (1964) Morphology of the experimental epileptic focus. *J Neurosurg* **21**: 1033–46.

Willmore LJ. (1990) Post-traumatic epilepsy: cellular mechanisms and implications for treatment. *Epilepsia* **31**(suppl 3): S67–S73.

Willmore LJ, Sylpert GW, Munson JB. (1978) Recurrent seizures induced by cortical iron injection: a model of posttraumatic epilepsy. *Ann Neurol* **4**: 329–36.

Willmore LJ, Triggs WJ. (1984) Effect of phenytoin and corticosteroids on seizures and lipid peroxidation in experimental posttraumatic epilepsy. *J Neurosurg* **60**: 467–72.

Willmore LJ, Rubin JJ. (1984) The effect of tocopherol and dimethyl sulfoxide on focal edema and lipid peroxidation induced by isocortical injection of ferrous chloride. *Brain Res* **296**: 389–92.

Wohns RNW, Wyler AR. (1979) Prophylactic phenytoin in severe head injuries. *J Neurosurg* **51**: 507–509.

Wyler AR, Ray MW. (1985) Anticonvulsant prophylaxis against posttraumatic seizures. *Contemp Neurosurg* **7**: 1–6.

Young B. (1990) Post-traumatic epilepsy. In: Youmans JR, editor. *Neurological surgery: a comprehensive reference guide to the diagnosis and management of neurological problems*, 3rd edition. Philadelphia: Saunders, 2243–49.

Young B, Rapp R, Brooks WH, *et al.* (1979) Posttraumatic epilepsy prophylaxis. *Epilepsia* **20**: 671–81.

Young B, Rapp RP, Norton JA, *et al.* (1983a) Failure of prophylactically administered phenytoin to prevent early post-traumatic seizures. *J Neurosurg* **58**: 231–35.

Young B, Rapp RP, Norton JA, *et al.* (1983b) Failure of prophylactically administered phenytoin to prevent late posttraumatic seizures. *J Neurosurg* **58**: 236–41.

Zervit Z, Musil F. (1981) Prophylactic treatment of post-traumatic epilepsy: results of a long-term follow-up in Czechoslovakia. *Epilepsia* **22**: 315–20.

9

Motor sequelae and involuntary movement disorders

David M Frim, G Rees Cosgrove

Introduction

Movement is a fundamental property of human activity and is initiated and controlled by an intact and functioning motor system. The two basic subdivisions of this system are the pyramidal and the extrapyramidal systems. The pyramidal system comprises neurones whose cell bodies are located in cerebral cortex (upper motor neurones) and whose axons descend to synapse with other neurones whose cell bodies exist in the brain stem or spinal cord (lower motor neurones). These neurones then connect via peripheral nerves to the motor endplates of the muscles. This lower motor neurone is often called the 'final common pathway' because it is acted upon by numerous neural inputs and is the ultimate pathway through which nervous impulses reach the target muscle. The extrapyramidal system includes all other descending pathways (i.e. exclusive of the pyramidal tract), which act directly or indirectly on primary motor neurones. This, together with the cerebellar input, modulates and co-ordinates the smooth integrated functioning of the pyramidal system.

Lesions of the pyramidal system result in simple motor deficits, such as muscle weakness or complete paralysis. These simple syndromes are easily defined and are often the consequence of identifiable brain or spinal cord injury. Lesions of the extrapyramidal system may result in more complex motor disorders including hyperkinesias, dystonias and rigidity, but the exact location of the traumatic injury is often indeterminate.

The purpose of this chapter is to review the various constellations of motor sequelae and involuntary movement disorders that can be seen after central nervous system injury. These movement disorders may be found in combination, or with variable expression at different times in the same individual. Although any motor symptom is possible after central nervous system (CNS) trauma, the likely sequelae fall into five distinct clinical groups: paralysis; parkinsonism; cerebellar symptoms of ataxia or tremor; dystonia; and dyskinesias.

Although each of these types of movement disorder has a general anatomical explanation, the presence of one or several of these symptoms does not necessarily correlate with a precise anatomically identifiable lesion. For this reason it is often difficult to find objective data other than the history and clinical examination to support the connection between the head trauma and the movement disorder. All of these motor phenomena can also be caused by a variety of non-traumatic aetiologies. These include the neurodegenerative disorders, toxic exposure, cerebrovascular insult, inflammation or neoplasia. The general approach to ascribing a traumatic cause to a movement disorder is: (1) the lack of pre-existing pathology; (2) the presence of some form of demonstrable CNS injury; and (3) the development of a motor disorder at some time after the acute changes (e.g. coma) caused by the CNS injury have resolved. This time scale may be hours, days or months after injury (Hanson *et al.* 1970; Koller *et al.*, 1989; Kremer *et al.*, 1947), and may or may not be accompanied by any structural correlates (Gerstenbrand *et al.*, 1970).

Definitions

Paralysis may be defined as a loss or impairment of motor function due, in part, to disruption of normal neuromuscular initiation, conduction or execution. Complete paralysis is described as plegia and incomplete paralysis or weakness as paresis. Paralysis is also described by the specific limb or extremity affected: hemiplegia is a complete paralysis of one side of the body; quadriplegia is a paralysis of all four extremities; paraplegia is a paralysis of the lower extremities; diplegia is paralysis of any two corresponding extremities; and monoplegia is a paralysis of only one extremity. Paralysis is subdivided into flaccid, where no movement is present, and spastic, where stimulation of sensory inputs, for instance stretch reflexes, causes an exaggerated involuntary motor response. Patients who are not completely paralysed following an injury may also exhibit spasticity, in that normal movements, such as walking or lifting, cause exaggerated motor feedback after normal sensory responses. These exaggerated movements define the symptoms of spastic gait, spastic arm motion, etc. Spasms are involuntary contractions of large groups of muscles that last for several seconds or minutes and are frequently painful.

Post-traumatic parkinsonism is characterized by hypokinesia, tremor and muscular rigidity. This constellation of symptoms, when idiopathic and progressive, is described as Parkinson's disease, which is a degeneration of the dopaminergic neurones of the substantia nigra. Presumed traumatic injury to the substantia nigra or its dopaminergic outflow may cause similar symptoms without the relentless progression seen in idiopathic Parkinson's disease patients.

Tremor is an involuntary repetitive trembling or quivering, generally of the extremities. It can be coarse, of high amplitude and low frequency (3–6 cycles per second), or fine, of low amplitude and high frequency (10–20 cycles per second). Essential tremor is a fine idiopathic tremor that usually begins in the arms and can spread throughout the body. It is exacerbated by stress or anxiety and sometimes by volitional movement. Intention tremor is that which is brought on by voluntary,

co-ordinated movement. Rest tremor disappears during voluntary, co-ordinated movement, but reappears during rest periods. Almost all tremors disappear during sleep. Post-traumatic tremor presumably arises after injury to the extrapyramidal motor system, particularly the cerebellum and brain stem, as described below.

Ataxia is a failure of muscular co-ordination or an irregularity of precise motor functions. It is usually ascribed to cerebellar dysfunction where it is defined as cerebellar ataxia (a hypotonia, asynergy and muscular dysco-ordination ipsilateral to cerebellar injury). It may affect the trunk, the extremites or both. Because of the proximity of the cerebellum and the midbrain, post-traumatic ataxia is often associated with a post-traumatic intention tremor.

Dystonia is a disorder of muscular tonicity characterized by abnormal posturing and twisting movements due to involuntary tonic muscular contractions. It can affect any part of the head and neck, trunk or limbs. Dystonic movements tend to involve many muscle groups simultaneously to produce grotesque posturing and writhing movements. The abnormal posturing can be brought on by normal activities (e.g. walking) or may occur at rest. Post-traumatic dystonia may be a result of severe spasticity or may arise from an unknown aetiology.

Dyskinesias are uncontrolled involuntary movements that result in exaggerated, incomplete or abortive movement. Choreiform movements are extremely variable, coarse, quick, jerking movements that begin suddenly and show no rhythmicity. They may also continue in sleep. Athetoid movements are continuous writhing arhythmic movements that disappear with sleep. Hemiballismus is a rare condition characterized by unco-ordinated sudden activity of the axial and proximal musculature such that the limbs may flail about. Post-traumatic dyskinesias presumably arise from injury to the caudate and putamen, sustained at the time of the trauma.

Tics or habit spasms are brief recurrent stereotyped compulsive movements, usually involving a small segment of the body. They may be controlled voluntarily for a short time and are often felt to be psychogenic.

Myoclonus refers to abrupt, sudden isolated muscle contractions, which occur irregularly, especially in the limbs. They may be relatively minor and produce no appreciable movement of the muscle group or they may be extremely violent and even throw the patient to the ground.

Epidemiology

Kremer *et al.* (1947) mentioned that the proportion of head injuries causing a permanent motor disability represented about one in 700 of those patients seen at the Military Hospital for Head Injuries, Oxford, in the mid-1940s. There is no other published series, to our knowledge, which addresses the incidence of motor deficit after CNS trauma. Modern Glasgow Coma Scale outcome data do not separate motor responses from other functions; it is therefore difficult to define a given probability. In general, the more severe the head injury the more likely it is that the patient will have some associated motor deficit. In individual patients, the predictive value of CT- or MRI-documented tissue loss in the brain or spinal cord is high for expected plegia or paresis. Spasticity is almost always seen after CNS injuries causing plegia.

Involuntary movement disorders are even more difficult to quantify; controversy still exists surrounding the exact aetiology of these disorders following head trauma. The literature on involuntary post-traumatic movement disorders comprises mainly case reports and small series of patients whose motor symptoms are thought to be related to previous head trauma. This approach can only begin to define a spectrum of possible motor sequelae to central nervous system trauma. Unfortunately, the case report approach provides a numerator without a denominator for the fraction of times that CNS trauma will cause a movement disorder. Relative to idiopathic causes of involuntary movement disorders, the presumed incidence is low, in that series describing treatments of involuntary movements that collect both traumatic and nontraumatic patients usually have a preponderance of nontraumatic patients. This is an estimate based on the series described for the various subsections of this chapter and has no statistical power. Perhaps the best summary statement is that post-traumatic movement disorders occur with low frequency after head injury and that paralytic and post-paralytic syndromes are much more common than involuntary movement disorders. We must await a large series of trauma patients analysed for post-traumatic movement sequelae before we can define a quantitative incidence. Until this is done, the exact risk of motor disability after head injury will likely remain unclear.

Therefore, in the field of post-traumatic movement disorders, we are at a stage where we are unable to predict the occurrence of motor sequelae to CNS injury, unable to define the risk of motor deficits after specific CNS trauma, and have not fully defined all the possible types of motor dysfunction that can be caused by CNS injury.

Clinical assessment

Post-traumatic paralysis or paresis is easily noted on physical examination and can be assessed by standard examination techniques. The accepted rating of motor strength is based on a five-point scale: 0 for no movement; 1 for flickering movement; 2 for movement too weak to oppose gravity; 3 for movement barely opposing gravity; 4 for strength less than full; 5 for full strength. In this fashion, post-traumatic weakness can be documented and followed for recovery. Spasticity can also be followed in patients whose paralysis is not flaccid. We define spasticity on a four-point scale: 1+ for mild exaggeration of deep tendon reflexes; 2+ for moderate exaggeration of reflexes; 3+ for severe exaggeration of reflexes; and 4+ for a full range of involuntary movement in an extremity after tendon stretch. Other findings on physical examination relative to post-traumatic paralysis and spasticity include measurements of muscle bulk. As muscles are denervated and lose the neurotrophic input of the CNS, they will lose size. Lower motor neurone lesions result in early atrophy, while upper motor neurone lesions may be associated with atrophy after months or years. This can be quantitated by limb width and circumference measurements. Extremity tone can also be affected after a paralytic CNS injury. Hypertonicity is a form of spasticity that can accompany the recovery from a CNS injury. When it impedes other movements or becomes an abnormal posture, then dystonia results.

In examining tremors, the distribution, rate, rhythm and the effects of movement and rest should be noted. This allows for an accurate description of the tremor without having to resort to potentially inaccurate labels. More complex dyskinesias may be described in similar fashion or recorded on videotape.

The standard diagnostic technique for assessing head injury and the potential for permanent functional loss is the CT scan. Serial CT scanning provides excellent assessment of brain tissue loss and resolution of intracerebral haematomas or contusions. This enables a prediction of functional outcome based on loss of motor cortex or descending pathways. For both head and spinal cord injury, MRI has proven to be extremely useful and sensitive for evaluation of blunt trauma. Again, the documentation of brain tissue loss versus oedema or compression may provide some predictive value in terms of functional outcome. Electrophysiological examination for nerve conduction (in peripheral nerve injury) or denervation (in CNS injury) can also provide some prognostic support to an assessment of neurological outcome. Total peripheral denervation after a central injury is a predictor of poor recovery.

Categories of disease

The following subsections describe the major motor sequelae of CNS injury. As mentioned, it is not an exhaustive list, but rather a summary of the most common post-traumatic motor system sequelae. Issues such as pathology, prognosis, management and complications will be discussed with regard to each subsection where relevant.

Post-traumatic paralysis

Injury to the primary motor cortex, corticobulbar white matter fibres (in the corona radiata, internal capsule and brain stem), or the corticospinal tracts in the ventral spinal cord, will all result in loss of motor function. If the injury results in tissue loss and neuronal death then this loss of function will be permanent and will result in a spastic paralysis of the affected muscle groups. A variety of injuries can cause paralysis by interruption of these motor pathways. Most common are the penetrating injuries to the brain and spinal cord, which cause direct disruption of these pathways. Blunt trauma can also disrupt motor pathways and cause paralysis. The pathophysiology of this event is most likely to be cerebral contusion causing a small or moderate intraparenchymal haemorrhage in the motor cortex or descending tracts. The haemorrhage associated with an intracerebral contusion may cause permanent loss of motor function or only transient weakness, which resolves as the clot clears. However, a large clot with significant mass effect can cause vascular compromise and lead to permanent tissue loss and functional impairment (Becker *et al.*, 1990).

Blunt trauma to the head, particularly in children, can cause a syndrome of widespread oedema,

presumably from a diffuse axonal shearing injury. This syndrome is associated with prolonged coma and, in many patients, cognitive dysfunction upon awakening. There can be associated motor sequelae due to the white matter injury, most notably spastic paresis of the trunk or extremities. Any of the involuntary movement disorders described below can arise after such a diffuse injury. Direct disruption of the vascular supply to motor pathways, either by penetrating or blunt trauma, will cause syndromes identical to those reported for strokes within a vascular distribution (Gennarelli, 1990).

Significant tissue loss in the pyramidal system of the CNS will result in a spastic paralysis of the affected body part. This motor loss is generally permanent and currently without accepted direct treatment. Minor tissue loss may also result in weakness or paresis and some return of function may occur over time. Complications arising from this motor loss can be classified as early or late. In the early stage, while patients are still hospitalized, potentially comatose, and unable to move their extremities, complications such as skin breakdown and the development of decubitus ulcers can cause significant morbidity. Deep vein thrombosis and pulmonary embolism can be an additional cause of morbidity in the neurosurgical patient (Black *et al.*, 1985; Frim *et al.*, 1992). Late complications include limb atrophy, flexion contractures, spasticity and dystonia.

Physical and occupational therapies to improve the general usefulness of residual function can be very helpful. Continued passive movement of affected limbs can reduce the incidence and severity of contractures by maintaining a reasonable range of movement. Splinting devices and brace appliances may also be used to avoid the contractures that limit the range of movement in paralysed limbs. Pharmacotherapy with antispasticity drugs such as baclofen, dantrolene and diazepam can provide some relief. Local injection of long-term neuromuscular blockers, such as botulinum toxin, can interrupt the tonic muscular contraction in severely spastic patients or in those with dystonic postures. When medical therapy fails, a variety of surgical approaches can be considered in selected patients. These include myelotomy, rhizotomy, peripheral neurectomy or insertion of an intrathecal baclofen pump. Orthopaedic procedures to relieve fixed musculoskeletal deformities may also provide significant functional improvement.

Acquiring 'coping mechanisms' to overcome the loss of function is the general goal of treatment.

A multidisciplinary rehabilitation team is best suited to evaluate and treat the paralysed post-traumatic patient after the acute injuries have resolved. Rehabilitation frequently requires long-term inpatient and outpatient care before maximal functional recovery is reached. Future research towards transplantation of functional CNS tissue in the motor system, may in due course provide some hope for restorative treatment of post-traumatic motor system tissue loss (Wictorin and Bjorklund, 1992).

Post-traumatic parkinsonism

Parkinson's disease is the idiopathic 'shaking palsy' first described by Parkinson (1817) and later found to be associated with loss of substantia nigra dopaminergic neurones (Adams and Victor, 1989). Post-traumatic parkinsonism is a separate entity that shares the clinical picture of Parkinson's disease but is associated with trauma. Trauma as an aetiology for parkinsonism has been well described, even in the early case reports of Patrick and Levy (1922), where a significant proportion of their 146 cases were associated with trauma. They also noted a lengthy but variable interval between the traumatic event and the onset of parkinsonian symptoms. Epidemiological evidence has shown a positive correlation between head trauma and parkinsonism (Godwen-Austen *et al.*, 1982), and, in a twin study, Ward *et al.* (1983), demonstrated a correlation between head trauma and parkinsonism in the affected twin.

The 'punch-drunk' syndrome of boxers is a particularly well described post-traumatic parkinsonian state (Critchley, 1957; Mawdsley and Ferguson, 1963). This syndrome is characterized by diffuse brain injury, slow speech, blunted affect, akinesia and a parkinsonian resting tremor. The pathological findings in this condition are those of diffuse atrophy accompanied by specific degeneration of the substantia nigra dopaminergic neurones (Cassasa, 1924; Courville, 1945). The cause of this parkinsonian-like pathology is debated. Some have argued that direct repeated trauma to the head can cause sufficient shearing force to injure the substantia nigra or its vascular supply (Maki *et al.*, 1980; Zulch, 1969). Others have suggested that the brain stem is immune to direct injury because of its deep location and that degenerative mechanisms intrinsic to the brain are accelerated by repeated trauma (Bruetsch and DeArmond, 1935; Holbourn,

1943; Mawdsley and Ferguson 1963; Rosenblum *et al.*, 1981; Tanner *et al.*, 1987).

Anecdotal evidence suggests post-traumatic parkinsonian symptoms can be correlated with injury to the substantia nigra. There is a report of an elderly man who struck his head, developed parkinsonian features within a year, and went to autopsy soon thereafter (Bruetsch and DeArmond, 1935). His brain had evidence of petechial haemorrhage in the caudate-putamen, and nigral depigmentation. Though the haemorrhagic changes in the striatum were suggestive, there was no direct evidence that the patient's deterioration was related to underlying Parkinson's disease. Another case of post-traumatic parkinsonian symptoms in a young man one month after significant head trauma was associated with substantia nigra hypodensities on CT scan (Nayernouri, 1985). There is also a report of parkinsonian symptoms after a gunshot wound to the substantia nigra (Morsier, 1960).

Idiopathic Parkinson's disease can respond well to L-dopa treatment (Adams and Victor, 1989). Similarly, L-dopa has been used successfully to treat the parkinsonian component of a woman in her 20s with hemiatrophy–hemiparkinsonism presumably induced by birth trauma (Koller *et al.*, 1989). Stereotactic thalamotomy has also been used to treat post-traumatic parkinsonian symptoms refractory to medical therapy (Niisuma *et al.*, 1982; Scott and Brody, 1971) in a manner similar to idiopathic Parkinson's disease patients who are refractory to medical treatments.

The prognosis of post-traumatic parkinsonism is somewhat different from that of idiopathic parkinsonism and more closely resembles that of 'toxic' parkinsonism seen after acute overdoses of certain drugs. Parkinson's disease progresses as a relentless degeneration of motor function. Post-traumatic parkinsonism usually stabilizes after the initial loss in function. From this baseline, various treatment options can begin to restore function. If we accept that parkinsonian symptoms result from traumatic destruction of the nigral dopaminergic cells, then only through the restoration of dopaminergic transmission, (i.e. oral levodopa therapy) or by reduction in feedback generally inhibited by nigral dopaminergic pathways (i.e. thalamotomy) can normal function be restored. This situation is identical to any other nigral destructive process but without the progressive features. Research into transplantation techniques to restore a population of substantia nigra dopamine cells holds some promise for a permanent solution to this problem.

Post-traumatic ataxia and tremor

Injuries to the midbrain, cerebellum and the cerebellar outflow tracts can cause syndromes of tremor (the most common of which is intention tremor), cerebellar dysfunction (most commonly limb or truncal ataxia), and dysarthria (cerebellar speech) (Gerstenbrand *et al.*, 1970; Richardson, 1989). These syndromes, although rare when compared with the frequency of post-traumatic paralysis, have been well described.

The syndrome of direct cerebellar trauma causing cerebellar signs of ataxia and imbalance has been reported (Cantu, 1969). These deficits were short-lived and appeared to resolve within several weeks of the injury. A second type of post-traumatic cerebellar dysfunction has been reported as a late consequence of head injury causing coma (Gerstenbrand *et al.*, 1970). In this report, as patients regained their cortical function, a significant proportion experienced gait and truncal ataxia, some exhibited a unilateral 'wing-beating' phenomenon, and many had dysfunction of extraocular movements. A significant proportion of these patients came to autopsy, but no firm correlation of these symptoms with specific neuroanatomical loci could be made. In general, all had lesions in the upper brain stem or cerebellum. There was a general correlation of ataxia with direct cerebellar injury, particularly in the vermis, as described for short-term injury (Cantu, 1969), but the observation of ataxia also correlated with lesions of the cerebellar output pathways and the midbrain (Gerstenbrand *et al.*, 1970). Very few of the patients who exhibited post-traumatic tremors in this series had symptoms that did not improve or resolve with time. The peak incidence of the tremor appeared to be during the period of early mobilization. Very few of the patients required any sort of intervention when they had reached their full rehabilitation. Other deficits, most notably the spastic paraparesis, as described above, were permanent and represented supratentorial tissue loss.

Richardson (1989) has defined three separate post-traumatic intention tremor syndromes, based on observations made in patients presenting to his institution:

1. 'Post-traumatic cerebellar syndrome', in which intention tremor is bilateral and has no other associated symptoms except cerebellar signs;
2. 'Post-traumatic midbrain syndrome', when the tremor is unilateral and ipsilateral and associated with contralateral weakness and pyramidal tract findings;
3. 'Post-traumatic intention tremor syndrome', when the tremor is a 'pure' bilateral intention tremor in a young person, which develops several weeks to months after head trauma with no other sequelae.

The time course of these syndromes is variable, as is the functional outcome. Richardson (1989) described an eight-year-old boy with post-traumatic midbrain syndrome whose symptoms developed three months after severe head injury, which included cerebral and brain stem contusion and oedema. His weakness and tremor did not improve until he underwent cerebellar stimulating electrode implantation five years later. In a second case of severe head injury and prolonged coma, a 22-year-old man recovered to the point of being able to ambulate with a walker and feed himself. His initial recovery included severe cerebellar signs, a dysarthric, explosive speech pattern ('cerebellar dysarthria') and a mild unilateral intention tremor contralateral to a hemiparesis. His tremor was somewhat better with beta blockade. A third case illustrated the pure intention tremor syndrome in a 19-year-old girl who suffered severe head trauma and prolonged coma. She eventually awoke with a hemiparesis that progressed to disabling intention tremor in her hand and head. A contralateral cryothalamotomy provided some return of useful hand function.

Koller *et al.* (1989) reviewed several cases of post-traumatic essential tremor after severe or seemingly minor head trauma. These may respond to beta blockade, as does idiopathic essential tremor. Due to the small number of reported cases, the anatomical localization of post-traumatic essential tremor must for the present remain obscure.

Tremor syndromes can be very disabling and are generally refractory to medical therapy. For this reason, stereotactic ablative neurosurgery is often attempted in an effort to abolish the tremor and improve quality of life in such patients (Andrew *et al.*, 1982; Bullard and Nashold, 1988, 1984; Cooper, 1960; Eiras and Garcia-Cosamalon, 1980; Fox and Kurtzke, 1966; Hirai *et al.*, 1983; Iwadate *et al.*, 1989; Krauss *et al.*, 1994; Niizuma *et al.*, 1982; Ohye *et al.*, 1982; Richardson, 1989; Samra *et al.*, 1970; Spiegel *et al.*, 1963; van Manen, 1974). Surgical results are often mixed and are dependent upon the specific clinical syndrome, the functional target, and the series of patients reported. In general, the surgical results for traumatic movement disorders are less favourable than for idiopathic parkinsonism because usually there has also been injury to cortical, subcortical and cerebellar structures.

Post-traumatic dystonia

As previously defined, dystonia is a tonic contraction of the postural muscles that leaves the patient in an abnormal posture. This definition includes tonic posturing of extremities or trunk as well as the complex head, spine and extremity posture of torticollis. This tonic movement disorder is probably caused by some disruption of the extrapyramidal pathways linking the caudate, pallidum and thalamus. The corticospinal or pyramidal tracts appear to be spared in injuries causing dystonia. Observations of dystonia occurring after trauma with demonstrated contralateral striatal injury on imaging studies most strongly support this localization (Koller *et al.*, 1989; Marsden *et al.*, 1980; Pettigrew and Jankovic, 1985).

There is a variable time delay between head trauma and the presentation of dystonia. The onset of postural changes may be minutes (Perlmutter and Raichle, 1984) or years (Messimy *et al.*, 1977). The sustained trauma can be severe (Drake, 1987) or relatively minor (Maki *et al.*, 1980), yet the postural changes can be functionally significant. The incidence of head trauma as a cause of dystonia is very difficult to assess. Depending upon the series reported, the incidence ranges from 7% to 15% (Burke *et al.*, 1980; Marsden *et al.*, 1980; Pettigrew and Jankovic, 1985). The converse statement, identifying the incidence of dystonic posturing after head trauma, has, to our knowledge, not been studied.

Focal dystonia after neck or peripheral trauma has also been reported. Torticollis after neck injury is not uncommon (Sheehy and Marsden, 1980), as is the peripheral cramping seen after extremity injury (Gowers, 1893; Wilson, 1955). Oromandibular dystonic movement can also be seen after facial and mandibular trauma, or with trauma as simple as tooth extraction (Koller *et al.*, 1989).

Treatment of post-traumatic dystonia is not rewarding. Pharmacological treatment of the dystonic state with antispasmodics can provide some relief. Hypertonicity in specific muscle groups may be somewhat relieved by local injections of botulinum toxin. Surgical therapy, such as stereotactic thalamotomy or selective dorsal rhizotomy,

has been used in an attempt to improve function in a dystonic limb (Koller *et al.*, 1989).

Post-traumatic dyskinesias

Dyskinetic movements, such as hemiballismus, facial and limb tics, and myoclonic jerking, are all exceedingly rare complications of head trauma, if the paucity of case reports is any guide. Hemiballismus is generally thought to be caused by injury to the subthalamic nucleus but no convincing pathological correlations have been reported. We could find reports of four patients with complex tics after trauma; one of these was a three-year-old child who developed tics and bellowing noises after a motor vehicle accident (Erikson and Perrson, 1969). These symptoms lasted for roughly 10 years. A second case of an 18-year-old who developed facial twitching, sniffing and snorting several months after sustaining blunt trauma to the head has also been reported (Fahn, 1982). Koller *et al.* (1989) reported a man who developed tics after closed head trauma and a second patient who had an exacerbation of pre-existing Tourette's syndrome after head trauma.

Myoclonic jerking can be seen after cortical injury and may relate to post-traumatic seizure activity. Cortical injury, even when the trauma is relatively mild, can presumably cause a focal contralateral myoclonus (Watanabe *et al.*, 1984). Focal peripheral injury, such as neck trauma or spinal cord segmental trauma, can also cause a myoclonic syndrome (Jankovic and Pardo, 1986). Head trauma has been the presumed cause of both palatal (Matuso and Ajaz, 1979) and lingual (Troupin and Kamm, 1974) myoclonus.

Psychogenic movement disorders

The variety of potential post-traumatic movement disorders makes diagnosis of a primary psychogenic movement disorder particularly difficult. Clearly, a classic 'conversion reaction' can take the form of a paralytic syndrome, and psychogenic factors can lead to a variety of dystonic states, tics, ballistic movements and automatisms that can easily be mistaken for one of the above-mentioned post-traumatic syndromes. There is no clear way to separate the organic from the psychogenic other than by history, likely anatomical distribution of the abnormality, the associated neurological findings, the course of the disease, and the rarity of true post-traumatic dyskinesia. Response to treatments such as placebo and suggestion can also be valuable, as can be an analysis of secondary gain issues, such as litigation of personal injury compensation. The diagnosis of psychogenic movement disorder must always be by exclusion until more objective measures for post-traumatic movement disorder are developed.

Summary and conclusions

The complex nature of movement disorders renders difficult any attempt to assign a specific syndrome to a specific traumatic event. The majority of post-traumatic motor sequelae are paralytic or paretic and can be more easily documented, followed for improvement, and assigned an anatomical location based on radiological findings. However, all these injuries pose a host of rehabilitative difficulties that need to be addressed in order to maximize functional recovery. Presentation of the post-traumatic involuntary movement disorders as a series of case studies allows the identification and classification of the post-traumatic motor syndromes. However, we have been unable precisely to define the exact risk of developing such a syndrome after head and neck trauma. For this reason, the possibility that a specific traumatic event might have caused a post-traumatic movement disorder will always exist. If the motor disorder falls within one of the above described syndromes and has an onset temporally related to a traumatic event, then the likelihood of a causal connection is improved. One must view such a link with some caution, however, as there is still no discrete, reliable measure that relates the anatomical injury directly to any specific post-traumatic movement disorder. Only with the development of such an objective test will we be able truly to define the cause of a specific post-traumatic syndrome. Until that time, we are left only with educated speculation.

References

Adams RD, Victor M. (1989) *Principles of neurology*. New York: McGraw Hill.

Andrew J, Fowler CJ, Harrison MJG. (1982) Tremor after head injury and its treatment by stereotaxic surgery. *J Neurol Neurosurg Psychiatry* **45**: 815–19.

Becker DP, Gade GF, Miller JD. (1990) Prognosis after head injury. In: Youmans JR, editor. *Neurological surgery*. Philadelphia: Saunders, 2194–229.

Black PMcL, Baker MF, Snook CP. (1986) Experience with external pneumatic calf compression in neurology and neurosurgery. *Neurosurgery* **18**: 440–44.

Bruetsch WL, DeArmond M (1935) The parkinsonian syndrome due to trauma. A clinico-anatomical study of a case. *J Nerv Ment Dis* **81**: 531–43.

Bullard DE, Nashold BS. (1984) Stereotaxic thalamotomy for treatment of posttraumatic movement disorders. *J Neurosurg* **61**: 316–21.

Bullard DE, Nashold BS. (1988) Post-traumatic movement disorders. In: Lunsford LD, editor. *Modern stereotactic neurosurgery* Boston: Martinus Nijhoff, 341–52.

Burke RE, Fahn S, Gold AD. (1980) Delayed onset dystonia in patients with 'static' encephalopathy. *J Neurol Neurosurg Psychiatry* **43**: 489–97.

Cantu RC. (1969) Transient traumatic cerebellar dysfunction: report of a syndrome. *Int Surg* **52**: 392–94.

Cassasa CSB. (1924) Multiple traumatic cerebral hemorrhages. *Proc NY Pathol Soc* **25**: 101–106.

Cooper IS. (1960) Neurosurgical alleviation of intention tremor of multiple sclerosis and cerebellar disease. *N Engl J Med* **263**: 441–44.

Courville CB. (1945) Effects of closed cranial injuries on the midbrain and upper pons. *Res Publ Assoc Res Nerv Ment Dis* **24**: 131–50.

Critchley M. (1957) Medical aspects of boxing, particularly from a neurological standpoint. *Br Med J* **i**: 357.

Drake ME. (1987) Spasmodic torticollis after closed head injury. *J Natl Med Assoc* **79**: 561–63.

Eiras J, Garcia-Cosamalon J. (1980) Sindrome mioclonico posttraumatico. Effectividad de las lesiones talamicas sobre las mioclonias de accion. *Arch Neurobiol* **43**: 17–28.

Eriksson B, Persson T. (1969) Gilles de la Tourette's syndrome. Two cases with organic brain injury. *Br J Psychiatry* **115**: 351–53.

Fahn S. (1982) A case of post-traumatic syndrome. In: Friedhoff AJ, Chase TN, editors. *Gilles de la Tourette syndrome* New York: Raven Press, 349–50.

Fox JL, Kurtzke JF. (1966) Trauma-induced intention tremor relieved by stereotaxic thalamotomy. *Arch Neurol* **15**: 257–58.

Frim DM, Barker FG, Poletti CE, Hamilton AJ. (1992) Postoperative low-dose heparin decreases thromboembolic complications in neurosurgical patients. *Neurosurgery* **30**: 830–33.

Gennarelli TA. (1990) Mechanisms of cerebral concussion, contusion, and other effects of head injury. In: Youmans JR, editor. *Neurological surgery*. Philadelphia: Saunders, 1953–64.

Gerstenbrand F, Lucking CH, Peters G, Rothemund E. (1970) Cerebellar symptoms as sequelae of traumatic lesions of upper brainstem and cerebellum. *Int J Neurol* **7**: 271–82.

Godwin-Austin RB, Lee DN, Marmot MG, *et al.* (1982) Smoking and Parkinson's disease. *J Neurol Neurosurg Psychiatry* **45**: 577–81.

Gowers WR. (1993) Manual of disease of the nervous system, vol. II. Darien, CT: Hofner.

Hanson, RA, Bewerberg W, Byers BK. (1970) Changing motor problem in cerebral palsy. *Dev Med Child Neurol* **12**: 309–14.

Hirai T, Miyazaki M, Nakajima H. *et al.* (1983) The correlation between tremor characteristics and the predicted volume of effective lesions in stereotaxic nucleus ventralis intermedius thalamotomy. *Brain* **106**: 1001–18.

Holbourn AHS. (1943) Mechanics of head injuries. *Lancet* **ii**: 438–41.

Iwadate Y, Sacki N, Namba H, *et al.* (1989) Post-traumatic intention tremor – clinical features and CT findings. *Neurosurg Rev* **12**(suppl 1): 500–507.

Jankovic J, Pardo R. (1986) Segmental myoclonus: clinical and pharmacologic slides. *Arch Neurol* **43**: 1025–31.

Koller WC, Wong GF, Lang A. (1989) Posttraumatic movement disorders: a review. *Mov Disord* **4**: 20–36.

Kraus JK, Mohadjer M, Nobbe F, *et al.* (1994) The treatment of posttraumatic tremor by stereotactic surgery. *J Neurosurg* **80**: 810–19.

Kremer M, Russell WR, Smyth GE. (1947) A mid-brain syndrome following head injury. *J Neurol Neurosurg Psychiatry* **10**: 49–60.

Maki Y, Akimoto H, Enomoto T. (1980) Injuries of basal ganglia following head trauma in children. *Childs Brain* **7**: 113–23.

Marsden CD, Obeso JA, Zarran JJ, Lang AE. (1980) The anatomical basis of hemidystonia. *Brain* **108**: 463–83.

Matuso F, Ajaz ET. (1979) Palatal myoclonus and denervation supersensitivity in the central nervous system. *Ann Neurol* **5**: 72–78.

Mawdsley C, Ferguson FR. (1963) Neurological disease in boxers. *Lancet* **ii**: 795–801.

Messimy R, Diebler C, Metzger J. (1977) Dystonic de torsion du membre superieur gauche probablement consecutive a une traumatisme craniale. *Rev Neurol* **133**: 199–206.

Morsier GDZ. (1960) Parkinsonism consecutifia une lesione traumatique du nojau rogue et du locus niger. *Psychia Neurol* **139**: 60–64.

Nayernouri T. (1985) Posttraumatic parkinsonism. *Surg Neurol* **24**: 263–64.

Niizuma H, Kwak R, Ohyama H, *et al.* (1982) Stereotactic thalamotomy for postapoplectic and posttraumatic involuntary movements. *Appl Neurophysiol* **45**: 295–98.

Ohye C, Hirai T, Miyazaki M, *et al.* (1982) VIM thalamotomy for the treatment of various kinds of tremor. *Appl Neurophysiol* **45**: 275–80.

Parkinson J. (1817) Essay on the shaking palsy. London: Sherwood, Neely and Jones.

Patrick HT, Levy DM. (1922) Parkinson's disease. A clinical study of one hundred and forty-six cases. *Arch Neurol Psychiatry* **7**: 711–20.

Perlmutter JS, Raichle ME. (1984) Pure hemidystonia with basal ganglion abnormalities on position emission tomography. *Ann Neurol* **15**: 228–33.

Pettigrew IC, Jankovic J. (1985) Hemidystonia: a report of 22 patients and a review of the literature. *J Neurol Neurosurg Psychiatry* **48**: 650–57.

Richardson RR. (1989) Rehabilitative neurosurgery: posttraumatic syndromes. *Stereotact Funct Neurosurg* **53**: 105–12.

Rosenblum WI, Greenberg RP, Seelig JM, Becker DP. (1981) Midbrain lesions: frequent and significant prognostic features in closed head injury. *Neurosurgery* **9**: 613–20.

Samra K, Waltz JM, Riklan M. *et al.* (1970) Relief of intention tremor by thalamic surgery. *J Neurol Neurosurg Psychiatry* **33**: 7–15.

Scott MR, Brody JA. (1971) Benign early onset Parkinson's disease: a syndrome distinct from classic postencephalitic parkinsonism. *Neurology* **21**: 355–58.

Sheehy MD, Marsden CD. (1980) Trauma and pain in spasmodic torticollis. *Lancet* **i**: 777–78.

Spiegel EA, Wycis HT, Szekely EG. *et al.* (1963) Campotomy in various extrapyramidal disorders. *J Neurosurg* **20**: 871–84.

Tanner CM, Chen B, Wong WZ. *et al.* (1987) Environmental factors in the etiology of Parkinson's disease. *Can J Neurol Sci* **14**: 419–23.

Troupin AS, Kamm RF. (1974) Lingual myoclonus: case report and review. *Dis Nerv Syst* **35**: 378–80.

van Manen J. (1974) Stereotaxic operations in cases of hereditary and intention tremor. *Acta Neurochir Suppl* **21**: 49–55.

Ward CD, Duvoisin RC, Ince SE. *et al.* (1983) Parkinson's disease in 65 pairs of twins and in a set of quadruplets. *Neurology* **33**: 815–24.

Watanabe K, Kuroiwa Y, Toyokura Y. (1984) Epilepsia partialis continua: epileptogenic focus in motor cortex and its participation in transcortical reflexes. *Arch Neurol* **41**: 1040–44.

Wictorin C, Bjorklund A. (1992) Axon outgrowth from grafts of human embryonic spinal cord in the lesioned adult rat spinal cord. *NeuroReport* **3**: 1045–48.

Wilson SAK. (1955) *Neurology*, vol. 3, 2nd edition. London: Butterworth.

Zulch K. (1969) Medical causation. In: Walker AE, Caveness WF, Critchley M, editors. *The late effects of head injury*. Springfield, IL: Charles C Thomas, 464–65.

10

Sensory sequelae and cranial central pain

Mark A Young, Argye Hillis, F A Lenz

Introduction

Many individuals survive head injury and many may end up with significant neurological sequelae. In the USA alone, an estimated 50 000–75 000 people per year sustain head injuries (Frankowski et al., 1985). A significant percentage of these patients may also endure associated injury to the neck and spine. Disability resulting from these injuries has achieved near-epidemic proportions; in the USA, an associated annual cost of 12.5 billion dollars has been estimated (Ditunno, 1992). Although the aetiology, severity and outcome of injury is variable, it is well recognized that the physical and psychosocial after-effects can endure for months or even years after injury (Ruff et al., 1986). The purpose of this chapter is to outline the effects of head injury on somatosensory function, specifically hemi-inattention and central pain. There are no precise figures for the incidence of sensory impairment or pain secondary to injuries of the intracranial central nervous system (cranial central pain) in patients with head injuries.

Much of the data reviewed in this chapter will be taken from the stroke literature since there are few studies of the sensory sequelae of head injury and since the functional effects of injuries to the same part of the brain are often independent of the mechanism of injury. The discussion of sensory inattention will encompass: impact on activities of daily living and on cognitive processes; a classification of types of hemineglect; and the clinical features of hemispatial neglect, including aetiology, diagnosis, therapy and prognosis. The closing section will be devoted to a consideration of central pain syndromes.

Hemi-inattention

Functional impairments due to hemi-inattention

Sensory hemi-inattention is a term used to describe a failure to respond to stimuli on the side (of space, the body or the visual field) contralateral to brain damage. In at least some patients it seems to be a multimodality sensory manifestation of an underlying 'neglect' or failure to process mental representations of spatially-encoded information on one side. The terms hemi-inattention and hemispatial neglect will be used almost interchangeably in this chapter, although it is recognized that hemispatial neglect is a broader term that encompasses both hemi-inattention and hemidyskinesia (see below). Even though the sensory input on the affected side is encoded or 'sensed' (seen, heard or felt), the patient acts as though he or she is unaware of it. This impairment leads to substantial functional deficits. For example, patients with hemi-inattention often eat from only one side of the plate, dress only one side of the body, shave or wash only one side of the face, or use make-up only on one side. The ability to drive is also affected by failure to respond to stimuli on the left or the right (Gianotsos and Matheson, 1987). Since hemi-inattention is often accompanied by a denial of deficits (anosognosia) it may be difficult to persuade such patients of their disability.

A number of cognitive skills are disrupted by hemi-inattention. The most commonly noted disturbance is in reading. Patients may fail to read one side of the page, or even fail to read the side of the word contralateral to brain damage (Ellis *et al.*, 1987a; Kinsbourne and Warrington, 1962; Nichelli *et al.*, 1993; Riddoch, 1991). For example, accord might be read as 'record' by a patient with right brain damage and left inattention, whereas accord might be read as 'account' by a patient with left brain damage and right inattention. Similar errors in writing, such as spelling errors limited to the side of the word contralateral to the brain damage, have also been reported (Barbut and Gazzaniga, 1987; Baxter and Warrington, 1983; Caramazza and Hillis, 1990a and Hillis and Caramazza, 1989, 1991). Calculation with multidigit numbers is frequently impaired since digits are ignored on the unattended side, so that patients may have trouble with such tasks as reading phone numbers or copying addresses. Finally, patients with hemi-inattention have a tendency to get lost when on their own, because of unilaterally impaired processing of maps or internal spatial routes (Bisiach *et al.*, 1993).

On any sort of task where stimuli in the response field are spatially arranged, patients may show a response bias toward items on the side ipsilateral to the brain damage (Costa *et al.*, 1969). Furthermore, some patients have trouble in performing verbal and other tasks (listening, naming, etc.) on the unattended side of their body, even when they can perform the same tasks on the other side (Coslett *et al.*, 1993). For instance, right brain damaged patients may ignore people speaking to them from the left, but listen to those on the right. Many patients incur trauma on the unattended side (e.g. from bumping into walls, getting fingers caught on one side of the wheelchair), which is often complicated by the patient's apparent unawareness of the injury. Such trauma is particularly worrisome in patients who are anticoagulated (Fleet *et al.*, 1987). The incidence of thromboembolism may also be increased in extremities on the unattended side, as these are often used less frequently even in the absence of organic weakness or impaired function.

Clearly, hemi-inattention resulting from brain damage is a common problem which can substantially interfere with everyday functioning.

Furthermore, Denes *et al.* (1982) have studied the recovery over six months in simple motor tasks and activities of daily living in 48 patients (24 with right brain damage and 24 with left brain damage) and showed that the presence of unilateral spatial neglect was the most crucial variable in determining recovery. They concluded that patients with hemi-inattention showed least improvement in independence and social adjustment, even when confounding variables (such as extent of motor impairment) were controlled.

Types of hemispatial neglect/inattention

The most commonly reported spatially-specific deficit in processing sensory stimuli is failure to respond to visual stimuli on the side opposite to the damaged hemisphere (visual hemi-inattention or neglect) (Jackson, 1876; Jeannerod, 1987). However, unilateral tactile neglect (Villardita, 1987) and olfactory neglect (Bellas *et al.*, 1988) have also been reported. No clear dissociation between hemi-inattention in one sensory modality compared with other modalities has been reported. This is consistent with the view that the sensory defect reflects an underlying failure in a modality-independent processing mechanism. Nevertheless, a number of dissociations along lines other than sensory modality have been documented, indicating that different forms of hemispatial disorders may exist. Many authors have drawn a distinction between sensory inattention (failure to respond to sensory stimuli on the contralesional side) and motor neglect or failure to make a movement towards the contralesional side ('hemi-dyskinesia') (Bisiach *et al.*, 1985a; Watson *et al.*, 1978). These authors have suggested that patients showing sensory inattention may have more parietal damage, whereas those with hemidyskinesia may have more frontal lesions. This hypothesis is strengthened by functional brain imaging.

Positron emission tomography scans of normal subjects performing visuospatial attention tasks show that an area in the right parietal lobe is activated when subjects attend to a stimulus in the periphery whether or not they make an overt response, whereas an area of the right frontal lobe is activated when the subjects make an overt response to a stimulus in the periphery (Corbetta *et al.*, 1993). A second type of dissociation that has been described is sensory inattention or impaired scanning of half of the environment versus unilateral neglect of internal representation or failure to process an internally reconstructed image. However, when both sensory attention and processing of images are thoroughly investigated, individuals who show impaired processing of sensory stimuli also show impaired processing of images and vice versa. This finding indicates that sensory inattention may be due to impaired processing of the sensory image on one side. Along the same lines, it has been argued that sensory inattention is a reduction in directed attention to the contralateral side (Heilman and Van Den Abell, 1980), due to a unilateral impairment in the representation of the environment that guides sensory attention (Bisiach and Berti, 1987; Mesulam, 1981).

Within the visual realm, even finer dissociations have been documented. For example, some patients with right brain damage show neglect of the left side of near space, but not of far space, while others show the opposite pattern of performance when tested using comparable tasks in the two conditions. For example, Halligan and Marshall (1991) described a patient who neglected the left side of lines in line bisection tasks presented within arms' reach, but was accurate in bisecting (with a light pen) lines presented outside of arms' reach. Similarly, Guariglia and Antonucci (1992) reported a patient with right brain damage who showed left neglect of the body (personal space) but no neglect of extrapersonal space. Other authors have documented inattention or neglect of the left side of space with respect to the midline of body, contrasted with neglect of the left side of space with respect to the line of sight (Bisiach *et al.*, 1985b).

Theories of hemispatial neglect/inattention

There is no consensus about the underlying 'cause' of hemi-inattention. Contrasting theories of inattention and neglect variously account for the associations and dissociations that have been reported (Bisiach and Vallar, 1988; DeRenzi, 1982; for detailed reviews). Sensory theories, which propose that different types of hemi-inattention result from primary sensory deficits (e.g. homonymous hemianopia) combined with general intellectual deterioration (Battersby *et al.*, 1965; Lawson, 1962) can account for the fact that hemi-inattention often co-occurs with homonymous hemianopia and other sensory deficits. However, these theories fail to account for hemi-inattention

in the absence of any documented sensory deficits. Furthermore, Vallar *et al.*, (1991) have shown that the presence of homonymous hemianopia and hemianaesthesia may be overestimated in patients with hemi-inattention, since failure to respond to stimuli often mimics failure to 'see' or 'feel' the stimuli. They reported three patients with right brain damage who showed left inattention along with left homonymous hemianopia and/or left hemianaesthesia by clinical examination, who nevertheless showed preserved visual and somatosensory evoked potentials in response to left-sided stimuli. In contrast, patients with left hemisphere damage who showed right homonymous hemianopia and/or hemianaesthesia without right inattention did not have preserved evoked potentials. These data indicate that the 'hemianopia' and 'hemianaesthesia' in the patients with hemi-inattention were a manifestation of their attentional (neglect) disorder, rather than of their primary sensory deficits. Additional evidence inconsistent with 'sensory' theories of neglect comes from the numerous reports that patients show 'unconscious' processing of information on the neglected side. For example, McGlinchey-Berroth *et al.*, (1993) have reported that right brain damaged patients' decisions about words or pictures presented in the 'intact' (right) hemifield were affected by preceding stimuli presented in the 'neglected' (left) hemifield, even though the patients denied having seen the left-sided stimuli. This means that, although the patients had no overt awareness of the stimuli on the left, the stimuli nevertheless affected the speed with which they processed subsequent stimuli on the right, indicating that they must have processed the left-sided stimuli to some level.

The most widely accepted theories accounting for hemispatial neglect are attentional theories, which propose that hemispatial neglect is a failure to direct attention to the side opposite the damaged brain (Heilman and Van Den Abell, 1980; Kinsbourne, 1975, 1977) or difficulty in disengaging attention from the side ipsilateral to the brain damage (Posner *et al.*, 1984). Attentional theories account for the different types of neglect (e.g. sensory inattention versus hemidyskinesia) by assuming that they result from damage to different components of an attentional network (Heilman and Valenstein, 1979; Mesulam, 1981) or to different stages of attention (Posner *et al.*, 1984). However, they may have difficulty in explaining cases in which the patients 'attend' to the entire stimulus, but nevertheless fail further to process the contralateral side of the stimulus. To illustrate this, Hillis and Caramazza (1990) reported patients who made unilateral errors in reading words (errors on the contralesional side of the word only; e.g. house read as 'fuse' after right brain damage and as 'hound' after left brain damage), even after they read every letter of each word correctly. For example, one patient with right brain damage read shower as 's-h-o-w-e-r ... it says power', showing that he had attended to and processed the entire stimulus to some level but only the right side was incorporated into his response. Attentional theories also have trouble in explaining cases of 'dyschiria' in which stimuli on the 'neglected' (usually left) side are transposed to the unaffected right side. For instance, in copying figures, patients with left neglect often transpose elements from the left side of the figure to the right, indicating that they indeed attended to the left-sided components to some degree (Bisiach and Berti, 1987). Representational theories propose that hemispatial neglect is due to unilateral disruption of internal representations that encode sensory stimuli and guide exploration of the environment. Within such theories, different types of neglect or inattention may result from damage at different levels of representation, such as selective impairment of object-centred versus retinal-centred representations (Behrmann and Moscovitch, 1994; Caramazza and Hillis, 1990b; Driver and Halligan, 1992.

Aetiology

Although all theories of neglect/inattention can account for variations in the syndrome resulting from damage to separate regions of the brain, there has been no clear evidence linking specific 'types' of neglect with specific brain lesions. The site of lesion that most often results in severe hemispatial (left) neglect is right parietal damage (Critchley, 1953; Vallar and Perani, 1985). However, hemispatial neglect has been reported to occur after damage to right frontal regions (Heilman and Valenstein, 1972), the right thalamus (Watson *et al.*, 1981), the right basal ganglia (Ferro *et al.*, 1987; Roeltgen *et al.*, 1989), left parietal cortex and/or cingulate cortex (Coslett *et al.*, 1993; Ogden, 1985, 1987), and the left thalamus (Ferro, 1987). Although studied most frequently in patients who have sustained strokes (due to the common occurrence of strokes in the distribution of the middle cerebral artery territory, which includes the parietal lobe), hemi-inattention has also been reported as a result of tumour (Jackson,

1876), and of surgical or traumatic brain injury (Kumasegawa and Mitsuyama, 1990). Patients who have sustained traumatic brain injury may incur damage to any of the regions implicated in hemispatial neglect, although discrete lesions may not be visible on CT or MRI scans.

Diagnosis

The most commonly implemented tests for hemispatial deficits are pencil and paper tasks, such as line cancellation tasks. In these the patient is required to cross out lines scattered across both sides of a page (Albert, 1973). Other examples include line bisection, in which patients may 'neglect' the contralateral segment of the line (Bisiach *et al.*, 1983), drawing and copying (Oxbury *et al.*, 1974), and visual-search tasks, in which the patient searches for a figure on the left to match to one on the right (Gainotti *et al.*, 1972). A few tests have been published that incorporate several of these tasks as well as functional activities like reading, writing, calculation and dressing. Normative data are available for some, such as the Behavioural Inattention Test (Halligan *et al.*, 1989; Wilson *et al.*, 1987).

An important aspect of diagnosing hemispatial (visual) neglect is that of differentiating it from associated deficits that may also affect processing of visual stimuli, such as visual field loss, oculomotor dysfunction and loss of binocularity (with concomitant diplopia, loss of stereopsis, impaired fusion capability, or impaired vertical or lateral phoria/alignment). Other associated deficits that may confound performance on tasks are anosognosia for hemiplegia and anosognosia for hemianopia (Bisiach *et al.*, 1986) and extinction (Heilman and Valenstein, 1972). Extinction refers to the failure to respond to a stimulus on one side only when it is accompanied by a comparable stimulus presented simultaneously to the opposite side. This 'double simultaneous extinction' has been observed in the visual (Bender, 1977), the auditory (DeRenzi *et al.*, 1984), the tactile (Ferro *et al.*, 1987) and the olfactory (Bellas *et al.*, 1988) modalities.

Prognosis

In a longitudinal study of 20 patients, Colombo *et al.* (1982) found that most symptoms of gross hemi-inattention or neglect improve within one month and resolve completely within one year, but approximately 25% of patients show little or no improvement after one year or longer. Similarly, in a 60-month study of 41 patients with right brain damage, Heir *et al.* (1983) found that, on a test of hemi-inattention, 80% of patients showed recovery within the first 12 weeks after brain damage, but the remaining 20% failed to show subsequent recovery during the 60-month follow-up. Patients with persisting hemispatial neglect are unable to drive, often need assistance in dressing and eating, and may not be able to hold down jobs that require reading, writing, calculation or attention to any spatially arrayed material. Furthermore, the residual deficits seem to be lifelong and remarkably resistant to therapy (Halligan *et al.*, 1989).

Some factors have been identified as predictors of recovery. The most important prognostic factor for recovery from hemi-inattention seems to be the degree of recovery by a few months post insult (Colombo *et al.*, 1982; Halligan *et al.*, 1989; Sunderland *et al.*, 1987). Patients with relatively small lesions or with haemorrhagic lesions appear to improve more rapidly than those with large lesions or infarctions, whereas age and sex are not significant factors in the rate or probability of recovery (Heir *et al.*, 1983). Initial severity is also not a significant predictor of recovery (Ferro *et al.*, 1987).

Extinction is slower to recover than hemi-inattention and may represent the residual hemispatial deficit in many patients (Heir *et al.*, 1983; Karnath, 1988). Similarly, homonymous hemianopia tends to persist indefinitely, but compensation may improve over months or years. Peripheral stimulation may (Zihl, 1980; Zihl and Von Cramon, 1979) or may not improve the functional visual fields in patients with right hemisphere damage (Gianutsos and Matheson, 1987).

Rehabilitation may also accelerate recovery in patients with hemispatial neglect. Many rehabilitation programmes employ training of compensatory strategies (Pierson-Savage *et al.*, 1988). Others use computerized visuoperceptual and attention tasks (Gianutsos and Matheson, 1987). One of the most carefully designed series of studies of the effectiveness of rehabilitation for hemi-inattention has incorporated perceptual and scanning training (Diller & Gordon, 1981; Diller and Weinberg, 1977; Weinberg *et al.*, 1977, 1979). Most of these studies show significant improvement on untrained, structured tasks, such as reading as treatment progressess; however, complete resolution of neglect as a result of rehabilitation efforts has not been documented.

Medical intervention has also shown some promise in ameliorating symptoms of neglect. For example, transient resolution of hemispatial visual neglect has been achieved in individual patients with vestibular stimulation, using cold water in the contralateral ear (Cappa *et al.*, 1987; Geminiani and Bottini, 1992; Rubens, 1985). As another example, Fleet and coworkers (1987) described positive effects of dopamine agonist therapy. They reported two patients with hemi-inattention, including one with chronic deficits, who showed improved performance on cancellation tasks after the introduction of bromocriptine (15 mg daily), and who showed a decline in performance after withdrawal of the medication. Neither patient showed complete recovery, but one patient reportedly bumped into things on her left less frequently at home during the treatment period. Although the population size was limited and there was no attempt at blinding, these results warrant further investigation.

Summary

Within the broader category of hemi-spatial neglect, hemi-inattention refers to a heterogeneous group of deficits in responding to stimuli specifically on the side contralateral to the brain damage. These are relatively common and strikingly disabling deficits and can result from a variety of forms of brain damage, although they are most frequently reported after right-sided damage. Although the symptoms frequently resolve within weeks or months after injury, in approximately 25% of patients they persist for the duration of their lives. In these patients, the functional outcome is poor. Rehabilitation or medical interventions can improve performance on structured tasks, but residual functional impairments in responding to information on one side of space are the rule.

Cranial central pain

Cranial central pain syndrome (CCPS) is defined here as pain secondary to injury of the intracranial central nervous system. CCPS was first described in association with thalamic stroke by Dejerine and Roussy (1906). Later, Riddoch defined 'central pain' as 'spontaneous pain and painful overreaction to objective stimulation, resulting from lesions confined to the central nervous system, including dysaesthesias of a disagreeable kind' (Riddoch, 1938). Recent studies make it clear that lesions not only within the thalamus but throughout the central nervous system can produce central pain (Cassinari and Pagni 1969: Tasker *et al.*, 1991).

Aetiology

The clinical feature that is common to many central pain syndromes throughout the central nervous system is injury to pathways signalling pain and temperature. In a review of central pain following surgical lesions of the central nervous system, Cassinari and Pagni (1969) identified injury to the spinothalamic tract as the anatomical lesion in central pain syndromes. Boivie *et al.* (1989) have demonstrated diminished discrimination of thermal and pain sensation (classically spinothalamic tract functions), in all patients with post-stroke central pain syndromes. Similarly, Beric *et al.* (1988) demonstrated physiological evidence of spinothalamic tract injury in all patients with central pain following spinal cord injury. Eighty per cent of patients with spinal cord injury characterized by diminished spinothalamic tract function developed central pain.

A large body of evidence suggests that the principal sensory nucleus of the thalamus (ventral posterior) is involved in mechanisms of the central pain syndromes (Lenz *et al.*, 1992). Recent studies in humans have demonstrated that the ventral posterior nucleus of the human thalamus, which is involved in innocuous mechanoreception (Lenz *et al.*, 1988), is also involved in pain signalling pathways. The spinothalamic pathway terminates in and posterior to this nucleus. Cells in and posterior to this nucleus respond to painful thermal stimuli (Lenz *et al.*, 1993b) and stimulation at the sites where these cells are recorded produces the sensation of pain (Lenz *et al.*, 1993a,b). In pain following spinal cord transection the mechanism may involve 'bursting' activity produced by hyperpolarization of thalamic cells secondary to interruption of the spinothalamic tract (Lenz *et al.*, 1994).

Diagnosis

The diagnosis of CCPS rests upon clinical or radiological evidence of an injury to the brain plus clinical evidence of decreased discrimination of pain and temperature sensation. A latent period between the time of injury and the onset of pain is a common but not an invariable feature of the central pain syndromes. The onset of post-stroke central pain may occur during the immediate period after stroke (i.e. several days to several weeks delay) or after a latency of up to three years (Boivie and Leijon, 1991; Mauguiere and Desmedt, 1988; Michel *et al.*, 1990). Finally, it is critical to rule out other treatable somatic causes of pain before making a diagnosis of central pain.

The pain qualities of CCPS are variable. Central pain is classically described as burning and dysaesthetic, although this need not be the case. A wide spectrum of descriptors have been reported by patients and include: aching, lancinating, pricking, lacerating, pressing, shooting, squeezing, throbbing, cutting, crushing, splitting, stinging, icy feeling, sore stabbing, cramping, smarting and pulling. Leijon *et al.* (1989) described a population of 27 post-stroke central pain patients eight of whom reported superficial pain, eight deep pain and the remaining 11 both superficial and deep. The relationship between pain quality and lesion location is inconsistent. Despite the variation in reported central pain qualities, burning seems to be the predominant characteristic.

Hyperalgesia and allodynia are additional features of CCPS. A patient's threshold for touch, temperature and pain may be altered by injury so that, for example, an ordinarily innocuous stimulus such as a pinprick may be felt as a severe burning sensation. This pain may be produced by voluntary or passive movement of a joint (kinaesthetic allodynia). In such a case, pain and unpleasant tingling may occur during volitional activity of an extremity, rendering the patient functionally paralysed. Stimuli originating from visceral processes such as a full bladder or bowel can also affect central pain, although this is more commonly a feature of central pain following spinal cord injury rather than CCPS. Rarely, patients may develop a phantom supernumerary limb (peudopolymyelia) (Young and Buchsbaum, 1991).

Careful somatosensory testing is useful in patients with central pain. Somatosensory abnormalities include: paraesthesias, dysaesthesias, hyperpathia, spatial and temporal summation, numbness, and allodynia. The most common abnormality is loss of pain and temperature discrimination, as described above. The somatosensory pathways can be objectively assessed using neurophysiological techniques such as sensory evoked potential (SEPs) evoked by median and tibial/sural nerve electrical stimulation. Since this stimulation activates large primary afferent fibres innervating low threshold mechanoreceptors inhabiting the dorsal column area, abnormalities uncovered reflect alteration in vibration and touch modalities. Peripheral stimulation of afferents that activate the spinothalamic tract may be accomplished by the use of lasers to activate cutaneous nociceptors (Treede and Bromm, 1991).

Treatment

The large number of treatments described for the management of central pain speaks to the limited effectiveness of most therapeutic agents. Table 10.1 outlines some of the therapeutic interventions used to treat thalamic pain. Noradrenergic tricyclics (amitriptyline) are the only drugs for cranial central pain syndromes to have been proven effective in double-blinded, placebo-controlled, crossover trials (Leijon and Boivie, 1991). The antiepileptic drugs are utilized for central and peripheral neurogenic pain and include: carbamazepine, phenytoin, barbiturates, clonazepam, sodium valproate and vigabatrin. Antiepileptic drugs are considered to be most likely to relieve the paroxysmal type of central pain. Local anaesthetics such as lidocaine, tocainide and mexilitene have been used in the treatment of central pain (Leijon and Boivie, 1991) and the use of opioids has been advocated but is controversial

Table 10.1. Modalities of treatment employed in cranial central pain syndromes

Pharmacological	Adrenergics
	Analgesics
	Antiarrhythmics
	Antidepressants
	Antiepileptics
	Cholinergics
	Opioids
	Neuroleptics
Sensory stimulation	Deep brain stimulation
	Dorsal column stimulation
	TENS
Neurosurgery	Cordectomy
	Cortical and subcortical ablation
	Cordotomy
	Dorsal Root Entry Zone (DREZ) lesion
	Mesencephalic tractotomy
	Thalamotomy
Sympathetic blockade	

(Hammond, 1991). Adrenergic-acting medications such as clonidine have also been used to treat central pain (Leijon and Boivie, 1991), but the effectiveness of any of these agents for the treatment of central pain has never been demonstrated in a controlled trial.

Patients with CCPS may benefit from admission to a pain treatment centre. These centres provide a structured inpatient environment to facilitate care. Daily activities include physical and occupational therapies, vocational counselling, relaxation, recreation and individual psychotherapy, as well as continuing medical care. All of these factors have been shown to have merit in the management of pain. More specifically, the combination of aerobic exercise, relaxation techniques, physiotherapy (passive and active assisted exercises, superficial heat, ultrasound, cold and hydrotherapy), and the capacity to monitor medical treatments in a supervised environment appear to have demonstrated real benefit to these patients (Loeser and Egan, 1989).

Prognosis

There are few data regarding functional outcome of CPPS. Although CCPS may remit spontaneously in some patients, there has never been a prospective study to document this assertion (Boivie and Leijon, 1991; K.L. Casey, personal communication; R.R. Tasker, personal communication). In the majority of patients, CCPS is a chronic condition, which lasts for life. Some estimate of the chronicity of this condition can be made from the duration of the condition at the time of entry of patients into trials of medical therapy. In a study of patients with post-stroke central pain syndromes, patients had suffered with pain for between 1 and 13 years (mean 4.5 years) at the time of entry into the trial (Leijon and Boivie, 1989). Current therapy may have some influence upon the duration of CCPS since, in 50% of patients, treatment with noradrenergic tricyclics can relieve pain for periods of up to two years (Leijon and Boivie, 1989). Thus, most patients with CCPS face a lifetime of disability.

There are several sources of disability in CCPS, although in this syndrome a comprehensive assessment of disability has not been reported. As in many chronic pain syndromes, the intensity of pain is less disabling than the fact that it is chronic and continuous (Boivie, 1994). Patients with kinaesthetic allodynia have pain produced by changes in posture, ambulation or movement of the extremities (Leijon *et al.*, 1989). This can be a hindrance to rehabilitation and a significant source of disability. Coexisting depression is often a source of disability in patients with chronic pain. Although there are no studies of depression in patients with CCPS, evidence of depression was not found in any of the post-stroke central pain patients studied in a recent trial of pharmacological therapies (Leijon and Boivie, 1989). The emotional and mental state, such as anxiety or concentration on a task, can increase the intensity of central pain (Boivie, 1994). This phenomenon can interfere with work and may be a significant source of disability (FA Lenz *et al.* – unpublished observations). Finally, patients with CCPS often have neurological deficits in addition to pain, as has been shown in a study of patients with post-stroke central pain (Leijon *et al.*, 1989). These deficits, such as motor or cognitive impairment, are themselves a significant source of disability.

Acknowledgements

Some of the studies reviewed here were supported by grants to FAL from the Eli Lilly Corporation and the NIH (K08 NS01384, NS28598 and NS32386). The authors wish to thank Tibor Koreshi and Jennifer Minarcik for providing editorial assistance in the preparation of this manuscript.

References

Albert ML. (1973) A simple test of visual neglect. *Neurology* **23**: 658–64.

Barbut D, Gazzaniga M. (1987) Disturbances in conceptual space involving language and speech. *Brain* **110**: 1487–96.

Battersby WS, Bender MB, Pollack M, Kahn RL. (1965) Unilateral 'spatial agnosia' ('inattention') in patients with cerebral lesions. *Brain* **79**: 68–93.

Baxter DM, Warrington EK. (1983) Neglect dysgraphia. *J Neurol Neurosurg Psychiatry* **45**: 1073–78.

Behrmann M, Moscovitch M. (1994) Object-centered neglect in patients with unilateral neglect: effects of left-right coordinates of objects. *J Cognitive Neurosci* **6**: 1–16.

Bellas DN, Novelli RA, Eskanazi B, Wasserstein J. (1988) The nature of unilateral neglect in the olfactory system. *Neuropsychologia* **26**: 45–52.

Bender MB. (1977) Extinction and other patterns of sensory interaction. In: Weinstein EA, Friedland RP, editors. *Hemi-inattention and hemisphere specialization*. New York: Raven Press, 106–10.

Beric A, Dimitrijevic MR, Lindblom U. (1988) Central dysesthesias syndrome in spinal cord injury patients. *Pain* **34**: 109–16.

Bisiach E, Berti A. (1987) Dyschiria: an attempt at its systemic explanation. In: Jeannerod M, editor. *Neuropsychological and physiological aspects of spatial neglect*. New York: Elsevier Science, 183–201.

Bisiach E, Vallar G. (1988) Hemi-neglect in humans. In: Boller F, Graffman J, editors. *Handbook of neuropsychology*, vol. 1. North Holland: Elsevier Science, 195–222.

Bisiach E, Bulgarelli C, Sterzi R, Vallar G. (1983) Line bisection and cognitive plasticity of unilateral neglect of space. *Brain Cognition* **2**: 32–38.

Bisiach E, Berti A, Vallar G. (1985a) Analogical and logical disorders underlying unilateral neglect of space. In: Posner MI, Marin OSM, editors. *Attention and performance*, XI. Hillsdale, NJ: Lawrence Erlbaum, 239–46.

Bisiach E, Capitani E, Porta E. (1985b) Two basic properties of space representation in the brain. *J Neurol Neurosurg Psychiatry* **48**: 141–44.

Bisiach E, Vallar G, Perani D, Papagno C, Berti A. (1986) Unawareness of disease following lesions of the right hemisphere: anosognosia for hemiplegia and anosognosia for hemianopia. *Neuropsychologia* **24**: 471–82.

Bisiach E, Brouchon M, Poncet M, Rusconi ML. (1993) Unilateral neglect in route description. *Neuropsychologia* **11**: 1255–62.

Boivie J. (1994) Central pain. In: Wall P, Melzack R, editors. *Textbook of pain*. London: Churchill, 871–902.

Boivie J, Leijon G. (1991) Clinical findings in patients with central post-stroke pain. In: Casay KL. *Pain and central nervous system disease: the central pain syndromes*. New York: Raven Press, 65–75.

Boivie J, Leijon G, Johansson I. (1989) Central post-stroke pain – a study of mechanisms through analysis of sensory mechanisms. *Pain* **37**: 173–85.

Cappa S, Sterzi R, Vallar G, Bisiach E. (1987) Remission of hemi-neglect and anosognosia during vestibular stimulation. *Neuropsychologia* **25**: 775–82.

Caramazza A, Hillis AE. (1990a) Spatial representation of words in the brain implied by the studies of a unilateral neglect patient. *Nature* **346**: 267–69.

Caramazza A, Hillis A. (1990b) Levels of representation, coordinate frames, and unilateral neglect. *Cognitive Neuropsychol* **7**: 391–445.

Cassinari V, Pagni CA. (1969) *Central pain: a neurosurgical study*. Cambridge, MA: Harvard University Press.

Colombo A, DeRenzi E, Gentilini M. (1982) The time course of visual hemi-inattention. *Arch Psychiatry Neuro Sci* **231**: 539–46.

Corbetta M, Miexen FM, Shulman GL, Petersen SE. (1993) A PET study of visuospatial attention. *J Neurosci* **13**: 1202–26.

Coslett B, Schwartz M, Goldberg G, Haas D, Perkins J. (1993) Multi-modal hemi-spatial deficits after left hemisphere stroke. *Brain* **116**: 527–54.

Costa LD, Vaughn HG, Horwitz M, Ritter W. (1969) Patterns of behavioural deficit associated with visual spatial neglect. *Cortex* **5**: 242–63.

Critchley M. (1953) *The parietal lobes*. London: Hafner Press.

Denes G, Semenza C, Stoppa E, Lis A (1982) Unilateral spatial neglect and recovery from hemiplegia. *Brain* 105: 543–52.

DeRenzi E. (1982)* *Disorders of space exploration and cognition*, Chichester: Wiley.

DeRenzi E, Gentilini M, Patticini F. (1984) Auditory extinction following hemispheric damage. *Neuropsychologia* 22: 733–44.

Dejerine J, Roussy G. (1906) Le syndrome thalamique. *Rev Neuro (Paris)* 14: 521–32.

Diller L, Gordon WA. (1981) Rehabilitation and clinical neuropsychology. In: Filskov S, Bell T, editors. *Handbook of clinical neuropsychology*. New York: Wiley, 702–33.

Diller L, Weinberg J. (1977) Hemi-inattention in rehabilitation: the evolution of a rational remediation program. *Adv Neurol* 18: 63–82.

Ditunno JF. (1992) Functional assessment measures in CNS trauma. *J Neurotrauma* 9 (suppl 1): S301–5.

Driver J, Halligan PW. (1992) Can visual neglect operate in object-centered coordinates? An affirmative single case study. *Cognitive Neuropsychol* 8: 464–75.

Ellis AW, Flude BM, Young AW. (1987a) 'Neglect dyslexia' and the early visual processing of letters in words and nonwords. *Cognitive Neuropsychol* 4: 439–64.

Ellis A, Young A, Flude B. (1993) Neglect and visual language. In: Robertson I, Marshall JC, editors. *Unilateral neglect*. Hove: Lawrence Erlbaum, 233–55.

Ferro JM. (1987) Left thalamic neglect. *Acta Neurol Scand* 76: 310–11.

Ferro JM, Kertesz A, Black SE. (1987) Subcortical neglect: quantitation, anatomy, and recovery. *Neurology* 37: 1487–92.

Fleet WS, Valentein E, Watson RT, Heilman KM. (1987) Dopamine agonist therapy for neglect in humans. *Neurology* 37: 1765–70.

Frankowski RF, Annegers JF, Whitman S. (1985) The descriptive epidemiology of head trauma in the United States. In: Becker DP, Povlishock JT, editors. *Central nervous system research status report*. New York: Mary Ann Liebert, Inc, 33–43.

Gainotti G, Messerli P, Tissot R. (1972) Quantitative analysis of unilateral spatial neglect in relation to lateralization of cerebral lesions. *J Neurol Neurosurg Psychiatry* 35: 545–50.

Geminiani G, Bottini G. (1992) Mental representation and temporary recovery from unilateral neglect after vestibular stimulation. *J Neurol Neurosurg Psychiatry* 55: 332–33.

Gianutsos R, Matheson P. (1987) The rehabilitation of perceptual disorders attributable to brain injury. In: Meier MJ, Benton AL, Diller L, editors. *Neuropsychological rehabilitation*. Edinburgh: Churchill Livingstone, 202–41.

Guariglia C, Antonucci G. (1992) Personal and extrapersonal space: a case of a neglect dissociation. *Neuropsychologia* 30: 1001–1009.

Halligan PW, Marshall JC. (1991) Left neglect for near but not far space in man. *Nature* 350: 498–500.

Halligan PW, Marshall JC, Wade DT. (1989) Visuospatial neglect: underlying factors and test sensitivity. *Lancet* ii: 908–10.

Hammond D. (1991) Do opioids relieve central pain? In: Casey KL, editor. *Pain and central nervous system disease: the central pain syndromes*. New York: Raven Press, 233–42.

Heilman KM, Valenstein E. (1972) Frontal lobe neglect in man. *Arch Neurol (Minneap)* 22: 660–66.

Heilman KM, Valenstein E. (1979) Mechanisms underlying hemispatial neglect. *Ann Neurol* 5: 166–70.

Heilman KM, Van Den Abell T. (1980) Right hemisphere dominance for attention: the mechanism underlying hemispheric asymmetries of inattention (neglect). *Neurology (NY)* 30: 327–30.

Heir DB, Mondlock RA, Caplan LR. (1983) Recovery of behavioral abnormalities after right hemisphere stroke. *Neurology* 33: 345–50.

Hillis A, Caramazza A. (1989) The graphemic buffer and attentional mechanisms. *Brain Lang* 36: 208–35.

Hillis AE, Caramazza A. (1990) The effects of attentional deficits on reading and spelling. In: Caramazza A, editor. *Cognitive neuropsychology and neurolinguistics: advances in models of cognitive function and impairment*. London: Lawrence Erlbaum, 211–75.

Hillis AE, Caramazza A. (1991) Spatially-specific deficit to stimulus-centered letter shape representations in a case of 'neglect dyslexia'. *Neuropsychologia* 29: 1223–40.

Hillis A, Caramazza A. (1995) Spatially-specific deficits in processing graphemic representations in reading and writing. *Brain Lang* 48: 263–308.

Jackson JH. (1876) Case of a large cerebral tumour without optic neuritis and with left hemiplegia and imperception. In: Taylor J, editor. *Selecting writings of John Hughlings Jackson*. London: Hodder and Stoughton, 146–52.

Jeannerod M. (1987) *Neuropsychological and physiological aspects of spatial neglect*. New York: Elsevier Science.

Karnath HO. (1988) Deficits of attention in acute and recovered visual hemi-neglect. *Neuropsychologia* 26: 27–43.

Kinsbourne M. (1975) The mechanism of hemispheric control of the lateral gradient of attention. In: Rabbitt PM, Dornic S, editors. *Attention and performance*, V. London: Academic Press, 69–86.

Kinsbourne M. (1977) Hemi-neglect and hemisphere rivalry. *Adv Neurol* 18: Weinstein E, Friedland R, editors. New York: Raven Press.

Kinsbourne M, Warrington EK. (1962) A variety of reading disability associated with right hemisphere lesions. *J Neurol Neurosurg Psychiatry* 25: 334–39.

Kumasegawa T, Mitsuyama Y. (1990) A case with visual weakness, incomplete left homonymous hemianopia, visual inattention and unilateral spatial neglect after head injury. *Kyushu-Neuro-Psychiatry* 36: 109–15.

Lawson IR. (1962) Visual-spatial neglect in lesions of the right cerebral hemisphere: a study in recovery. *Neurology (Minneap)* 12: 23–33.

Leijon G, Boivie J. (1989) Central post-stroke pain – a controlled trial of amitriptyline and carbamazepine. *Pain* 36: 27–36.

Leijon G, Boivie J. (1991) Pharmacologic treatment of central pain. In: Casey KL, editor. *Pain and central nervous system disease: the central pain syndromes*. New York: Raven Press, 257–66.

Leijon G, Boivie J, Johansson I. (1989) Central post stroke pain – neurological symptoms and pain characteristics. *Pain* **36**: 13–25.

Lenz FA, Dostrovsky JO, Tasker RR, Yamashiro K, Kwan HC, Murphy JT. (1988) Single-unit analysis of the human ventral thalamic nuclear group: somatosensory responses. *J Neurophysiol* **59**: 299–316.

Lenz FA, Salt T, Jones EG, Boivie J. (1992) The ventral posterior nucleus of thalamus is involved in the generation of central pain syndromes. *Am Pain Soc J* **1**: 42–51.

Lenz FA, Seike M, Lin YC, Baker FH, Richardson RT, Gracely RH. (1993a) Thermal and pain sensations evoked by microstimulation in the area of the human ventrocaudal nucleus (Vc). *J Neurophysiol* **70**: 200–12.

Lenz FA, Seike M, Lin YC, *et al.* (1993b) Neurons in the area of human thalamic nucleus ventralis caudalis respond to painful heat stimuli. *Brain Res* **623**: 235–40.

Lenz FA, Kwan HC, Martin R, Tasker R, Richardson RT, Dostrovsky JO. (1994) Characteristics of somatotopic organization and spontaneous neuronal activity in the region of the human principal sensory nucleus in patients with spinal cord transection. *J Neurophysiol* **72**: 1570–87.

Loeser JD, Egan KJ. (1989) Inpatient pain treatment program. In: Loeser JD and Egan KJ, editors. *Managing the chronic pain patient.* New York: Raven Press, 37–49.

Mauguiere F, Desmedt JE. (1988) Thalamic pain syndrome of dejerine–roussy. Differentiation of four subtypes assisted by SEP data. *Arch Neurol* **45**: 1312–20.

McGlinchey-Berroth R, Milberg WP, Verfaellie M, Alexander M, Kilduff PT. (1993) Semantic processing in the neglected visual field: evidence from a lexical-decision task. *Cognitive Neuropsychol* **10**: 79–108.

Mesulam MM. (1981) A cortical network for directed attention and unilateral neglect. *Ann Neurol* **10**: 309–25.

Michel D, Laurent B, Convers P, *et al.* (1990). Douleurs corticales. *Rev Neurol (Paris)* **146**: 405–14.

Nichelli P, Venneri A, Pentore R, Cubelli R. (1993) Horizontal and vertical neglect dyslexia. *Brain Lang* **44**: 264–83.

Ogden J. (1985) Contralesional neglect of constructed visual images in right and left brain-damaged patients. *Neuropsychologia* **23**: 273–77.

Ogden J. (1987) The 'neglected' left hemisphere and its contribution to visuospatial neglect. In: M Jeannerod, editor. *Neuropsychology and neurophysiological aspects of spatial neglect.* New York: Elsevier Science.

Oxbury JM, Campbell DC, Oxbury SM. (1974) Unilateral spatial neglect and impairments in spatial analysis and visual perception. *Brain* **97**: 551–64.

Pierson-Savage JM, Bradshaw JL, Bradshaw JA, Nettleton NC. (1988) Vibrotactile reaction times in unilateral neglect: the effects of hand location, rehabilitation, and eyes open/closed. *Brain* **111**: 1531–45.

Posner MI, Walker JA, Freidrich FJ, Rafal RD. (1984) Effects of parietal injury on covert orienting of attention. *J Neurosci* **4**: 1863–74.

Riddoch G. (1938) The clinical features of central pain. *Lancet* **234**: 1093–98, 1150–56, 1205–209.

Riddoch MJ. (1991) *Neglect and the peripheral dyslexias.* Hove: Lawrence Erlbaum.

Rizzolatti G, Gentilucci M, Matelli M. (1985). Selective spatial attention: one center, one circuit, or many circuits? In: Posner MI, Marin OSM, editors. *Attention and performance*, XI. Hillsdale, NJ: Lawrence Erlbaum,.

Roeltgen MG, Roeltgen DP, Heilman KM. (1989) Unilateral motor impersistence and hemispatial neglect from a striatal lesion. *Neuropsychiatry Neuropsychol Behav Neurol* **2**: 125–35.

Rubens AB. (1985) Caloric stimulation and unilateral visual neglect. *Neurology* **35**: 1019–24.

Ruff RM, Levin HS, Marshall L. (1986) Neurobehavioral methods of assessment and the study of outcome in minor head injury. *J Head Trauma Rehabil* **1**: 43–52.

Sunderland A, Wade DT, Langton Hewer R. (1987) The natural history of visual neglect after stroke. *Int Disabil Stud* **9**: 60–65.

Tasker R, De Carvalho G, Dostrovsky J. (1991) History of central pain syndromes. In: Casey KL, editor. *Pain and central nervous system disease: the central pain syndromes.* New York: Raven Press, 59–64.

Treede RD, Bromm B. (1991) Neurophysiological approaches to the study of spinothalamic tract function in humans. In: Casey KL, editor. *Pain and central nervous system disease: the central pain syndromes.* New York: Raven Press, 233–42.

Vallar G, Perani D. (1985) The anatomy of spatial neglect in humans. In: Jeannerod M, editor. *Neuropsychological and physiological aspects of spatial neglect.* North-Holland: Elsevier.

Vallar G, Sandroni P, Rusconi ML, Barbieri S. (1991) Hemianopia, hemianesthesia, and spatial neglect: a study with evoked potentials. *Neurology* **41**: 1918–22.

Villardita C. (1987) Tactile exploration of space and visual neglect in brain-damaged patients. *J Neurol* **234**: 292–97.

Watson RT, Miller BD, Heilman KM. (1978) Nonsensory neglect. *Ann Neurol* **3**: 505–508.

Watson RT, Valenstein E, Heilman KM. (1981) Thalamic neglect: possible role of the medial thalamus and nucleus reticularis in behavior. *Arch Neurol* **38**: 501–506.

Weinberg J, Diller L, Gordon WA, *et al.* (1977) Visual scanning training effect on reading-related tasks in acquired right brain damage. *Arch Phys Med Rehabil* **58**: 479–86.

Weinberg J, Diller L, Gordon WA, *et al.* (1979) Training sensory awareness and spatial organization in people with right brain damage. *Arch Phys Med Rehabil* **60**: 491–96.

Wilson B, Cockburn J, Halligan PW. (1987) *Behavioural inattention test.* Titchfield, Hants: Thames Valley Test Company.

Young MA, Buchsbaum MJ. (1991) Pseudopolymelia in a stroke patient. *Arch Phys Med Rehabil*: 788.

Zihl J. (1980) 'Blindsight': improvement of visually guided movements by systematic practice in patients with cerebral blindness. *Neuropsychologia* **18**: 71–77.

Zihl J, Von Cramon D. (1979) Restitution of visual function in patients with cerebral blindness. *J Neurol Neurosurg Psychiatry* **42**: 312–22.

11

Neuropsychological indicators of psychosocial outcome

Mitchell Rosenthal, Scott R Millis

Introduction

Prediction of outcome after traumatic brain injury (TBI) has been a matter that has received close clinical and research scrutiny over the past two decades. Clinicians, confronted by distraught families, have needed certain signs that could be relied upon to counsel families on the likely pace of recovery that might be expected and what might be the end product of this recovery (i.e. how close to 'normal' will the patient get?). Likewise, researchers have tried to understand the nature of the recovery process by studying large groups of patients for months or years after injury to determine which factors (e.g. age, severity of injury, associated complications, timing or intensity of therapies) were most influential in determining the level of recovery. More recently, third-party reimbursers have been quite interested in predictors of outcome in order to determine guidelines for lengths of stay in acute and post acute rehabilitation settings.

As brain injury rehabilitation came of age in the late 1970s and early 1980s, there was an important paradigm shift in the field. The work of Bond (1975), Brooks and Aughton (1979), Mandleberg and Brooks (1975), and others was extremely influential in establishing that the most pervasive and disabling sequelae of traumatic brain injury were the cognitive and psychosocial deficits. This finding was in sharp contrast to the conventional wisdom that highlighted the physical impairments resulting from brain injury as the primary cause of burden and disability. These findings have been further substantiated in a series of publications that have provided longitudinal follow-up data for periods of 7–15 years post injury (Brooks *et al.*, 1987a; Thomsen, 1984). Thus, in most outcome studies that have been published in the past 15 years, measures of psychosocial outcome have been considered the most indicative of long-term successful outcome.

Although neuroimaging techniques such as computed tomography, magnetic resonance imaging, and single photon emission tomography have shown great promise in the identification of locus and the chronicity of a lesion, and may be correlated with measures of global outcome (Newton *et al.*, 1992), they may be less useful in defining specific patterns and the severity of impaired brain functions subserving cognition and behaviour. These critical aspects of cognition and behaviour are often directly related to the patient's ability to function in the community (Acker, 1986). Thus, neuropsychological measures have emerged as a quantitative, reliable and valid means of assessing and predicting the residual impairments that may be the greatest contributors to long-term psychosocial disability after TBI (Bond, 1990; Lezak, 1986). For example, the measurement of the duration of post-traumatic amnesia (PTA) has been widely used as a predictor of return to work, family burden and overall outcome (Brooks *et al.*, 1987a, b). Though imperfect, as will be discussed in detail later, these measures have been increasingly relied upon to counsel patients, families, the legal community and insurance companies on the eventual outcome to be expected several years post injury.

This chapter will be divided into three sections: the first will outline some of the problems inherent in defining psychosocial outcome measures; the second will present a selected review of recent literature and identify innovative ways of increasing the predictive power of neuropsychological measures; and this will be followed by a conclusion that provides recommendations for future research and clinical practice.

Elements of psychosocial outcome

The task of selecting the most relevant and quantifiable psychosocial outcome measures is not easy. Although neurosurgical studies, such as the Traumatic Coma Data Bank study (Marshall *et al.*, 1991) continue to employ the Glasgow Outcome Scale as the primary outcome measure, it is too global to accurately reflect the critical components of community reintegration as identified by rehabilitation practitioners (Bond, 1990). Even the Disability Rating Scale (Rappaport *et al.*, 1982), which is an expansion of the Glasgow Outcome Scale, is not designed to measure certain critical dimensions of psychosocial functioning (e.g. family integration, capacity for independent living, quality of interpersonal relationships etc.).

For these reasons, investigators have sought more specific measures of psychosocial outcome, which would reflect the extent to which an individual with a brain injury has returned to a reasonable level of productivity and to independent functioning in the community. Perhaps the most frequently used measure of productivity has been return to work. Investigators have used a variety of strategies to measure return to work, including simple measures of return versus nonreturn (Brooks *et al.*, 1987b), levels of employability (Ben-Yishay *et al.*, 1987), or percentage of time engaged in competitive employment activity (i.e. monthly employment ratio) (Wehman *et al.*, 1989).

Although return to work is considered an important index of psychosocial outcome, it is not so useful for many of the victims of moderate and severe brain injury who fail to return to work within one year post injury (Ben-Yishay *et al.*, 1987; Brooks *et al.*, 1987b; Rappaport *et al.*, 1982). Therefore, investigators have attempted to measure other critical aspects of psychosocial outcome and community integration. A recent effort by Willer and associates (1993, 1994) in the Traumatic Brain Injury Model Systems Project has been the development of a single measure to capture many of the salient aspects of community

re-entry. This 15-item self-report measure, known as the Community Integration Questionnaire, evaluates such diverse areas as responsibility for child care, housework, financial matters, employment status, involvement in leisure activities, shopping and social activities.

It is clear that the accuracy of prediction of psychosocial outcome from neuropsychological measures is not dependent solely on the reliability and validity of the neuropsychological data. It is just as dependent on the particular ways that researchers define psychosocial adjustment and on the specific measures that are selected for use in a particular study.

Psychometric issues

A common approach used in previous neuropsychological studies of outcome has been to correlate patient performance on standardized laboratory cognitive tests with global or specific measures of employment status, psychosocial adjustment, or functional independence. The interpretation and the practical application of these findings have been hampered by the methodological and statistical limitations of the studies: small sample sizes, lack of cross-validation, test batteries that are not comparable across studies, the use of measures available only to the author-investigator of a specific study, and samples marked by diverse or unique characteristics that limit generalization. Many studies also have had limited dissemination because they have appeared only as dissertations or poster presentations at professional conferences. Even with these limitations, some statistically significant relationships exist between neuropsychological tests and psychosocial outcome, including rehabilitation outcome and the capacity for dressing, financial management and independent living (Acker, 1986). Further discussion of specific findings will be presented in the following sections.

The issue, then, is not whether there are statistical associations between neuropsychological tests and psychosocial outcome, but what can be done to increase predictive power and validity. There are a number of possibilities. First, it may be desirable and necessary to abandon the sole reliance on traditional neuropsychological data to conceptualize and measure neuropsychological functioning for the prediction of outcome. Some neuropsychological tests that were developed in the 1940s and 1950s expressed patient test performances in single, global scores. Although providing useful information, single test scores may be insufficient adequately to describe most cognitive processes. For example, recently developed procedures that have incorporated advances from cognitive neuropsychology and information-processing theory have advanced our understanding of the complexity of memory impairment after TBI (Crosson *et al.*, 1988; Millis and Dijkers, 1993). In addition, the unidimensional quality and dissimilarity between many traditional neuropsychological measures and complex real-life situations may confound whatever positive or negative findings result from research studies. The problem, sometimes referred to as a lack of 'ecological validity', is inherent in many neuropsychological measures (Acker, 1986). A related notion is that some quasi-neuropsychological measures, such as awareness of deficits, may contribute more to prediction of outcome than do conventional measures of neuropsychological impairment (Ezrachi *et al.*, 1991; Prigatano and Altman, 1990).

Secondly, neuropsychological outcome research may need to include variables from other areas of functioning for analysis in combination with psychometric data: metabolic and biochemical, injury characteristics, patient and family behaviour in the community, and environmental factors. As an example, Schretlen (1992), in a study of 46 TBI survivors at eight years post injury, found that combining neuropsychological tests with an injury severity variable accounted for about 50% of the outcome variance. Measures of sustained, divided attention and the self-monitoring of judgement, along with the duration of hospitalization were predictive of psychosocial outcome (e.g. earned income, marital status, felony convictions, substance abuse). However, it should be stressed that not all studies have found that multivariate procedures result in increasing predictive power (Ezrachi *et al.*, 1991).

Thirdly, variables may be time-sensitive and situation-specific in their capacity to predict outcome. Some variables may have good predictive capacity within the initial acute hospitalization, the subsequent acute rehabilitation, or the first six months post injury, but account for minimal variance at later intervals. For example, in a study by Walker and associates (1992), neuropsychological test scores at about four years post injury, demographic variables, and injury characteristics, were not useful in predicting vocational or academic outcome.

Fourthly, a continued reliance on correlation analysis alone may be limiting. For example, the use of multivariate and multidimensional techniques, including confirmatory factor analysis, discriminant analysis, cluster analysis, and logistic regression, seem promising in relating neuropsychological indicators to psychosocial outcome. Chelune and Moehl (1986) have discussed the application of confirmatory factor analysis in developing and validating models of 'everyday functioning' and in clarifying what neuropsychological tests are measuring.

In the following section, a selective review of outcome studies will be presented. The studies that were selected were chosen because they addressed some of the issues presented in this section: the continued usefulness of old tests and indicators, the promise of more recent innovative techniques, the combining non-neuropsychological variables with neuropsychological tests, and the application of multivariate techniques. Other review articles of interest include Acker (1986) and Chelune and Moehl (1986).

Vocational outcome and return to employment

There appear to be associations between variables that assess injury severity, demographics and acute patient behaviour, and variables that describe return to work. At six-month follow-up, Oddy *et al.* (1978), found in their sample of 49 subjects that a length of PTA greater than seven days was associated with a low rate of work resumption. In defining coma as an 'inability to respond purposefully', Gilchrist and Wilkinson (1979) reported that 82% of subjects with coma of less than one week returned to work, compared with 11% of subjects with coma greater than seven weeks ($n = 72$).

Reyes and associates (1981) developed a five-point scale to rate the post-traumatic activity level (PTAL) of patients emerging from coma (coma, sluggish, appropriately active, restless, agitated). Patients were rated at the time of admission to inpatient rehabilitation (mean time post injury = 10.5 weeks; mean length of coma = 1.5 weeks). At four-year follow-up, there was a significant relationship between PTAL and return to work ($p < 0.01$). Patients who had been rated as sluggish or agitated on admission had low rates of returning to employment of 9% and 25%, respectively. In contrast, patients rated as active or restless showed a higher rate of job resumption of 71% and 68%, respectively. In addition to injury severity variables and early behavioural ratings, premorbid demographic variables such as age, education, employment and income have been associated with return to work in patients with moderately severe brain injury (Rimel *et al.*, 1982).

The Halstead–Reitan Neuropsychological Test Battery (HRNTB) and allied procedures have been used to predict return to work after TBI. In a study of 18 patients who had received neuropsychological rehabilitation several years post injury, Prigatano and associates (1984) found a trend for unemployed subjects to show greater impairment on some neuropsychological tests, but the differences were not statistically significant. However, employed subjects showed significantly greater improvement on follow-up assessment on the Wechsler Memory Quotient, Visual Reproduction subtest and number of difficult paired associates from the Wechsler Memory Scale and the Digit Symbol subtest of the Wechsler Adult Intelligence Scale (WAIS). In addition, employed patients performed at a significantly improved level on the general psychopathology, hyperactivity and stability scales of the Katz Adjustment Scale (KAS). Also notable in this study was the indication that traditional cognitive tests alone were insufficient for describing and predicting outcome, and that behavioural and psychosocial measures might be useful in combination. The unemployed subjects were rated as significantly more deviant on the KAS prior to testing than employed subjects.

Fraser and associates (1988) extended the application of the HRNTB to brain injury vocational outcome in their study of 97 patients with mild, moderate and severe injuries. Patients who did not return to work at one year post injury showed deficits in the following areas on neuropsychological tests at one month post injury: motor speed, cognitive flexibility, visuospatial memory, visuospatial problem solving and manipulatory skills, and the overall level of neuropsychological functioning.

More recent studies combine demographic and injury variables, neuropsychological data, and behavioural ratings to predict vocational outcome. Ezrachi and associates (1991) evaluated patients (mean time post injury = 34.65 months) prior to admission to their rehabilitation programme, at the completion of the programme, and six months later. At admission, the variables most highly related to later employment status (36% of variance) in order of importance were: community adaptation skills (Behavioral Competence Index), verbal aptitude (WAIS), duration of coma, and staff rating of patient's capacity for self-appraisal. At the conclusion of the programme, the most important variables associated with employment six months later (61% of variance) were staff ratings of the patient's acceptance of the programme, verbal aptitude, the patient's behavioural involvement with others, the duration of coma, psychomotor dexterity, and the capacity for self-appraisal.

Using survival methodology for data analysis, Dikmen and associates (1994) were able to derive multivariate models to predict the probability of returning to work after traumatic brain injury. This investigation may be a landmark study because of its prospective design, large sample (n = 366), full range of brain injury severity levels, trauma control group inclusion, long follow-up period (24 months), and low rate of attrition (8% lost to follow-up at one year and 6% of those targeted for follow-up lost between one and two years). The variables identified as important in predicting return to work were the Glasgow Coma Scale (GCS) score, Abbreviated Injury Scale extremities score, age, education, pre-injury job stability, the HRNTB Impairment Index and the Name Writing Test. For example, in a 30-year-old patient with a mild head injury and a GCS score of 13, a mild extremity injury, a bachelor's degree, and a stable pre-injury job history, there is about a 92% chance of returning to work by six months. Subjects with the highest work return rate of 96% by one year tended to obtain low Halstead Impairment Index scores at one month. Only 87% of the trauma control subjects returned to work by one year, which suggested to Dikmen and associates (1994) that, 'In some cases, it is likely that failure to resume employment has little to do with the injury and more to do with the young subject's unstable work history' (p. 184).

Other investigators have found typical neuropsychological tests less useful for predicting return to work. Walker and associates (1992), in their study of 71 patients with severe traumatic brain injury 3.9 years post injury, found that neuropsychological test scores, demographics and injury characteristics were not helpful in predicting vocational outcome. However, behavioural ratings by patients' relatives of social, emotional and physical functioning (Portland Adaptability Inventory) significantly discriminated the level of vocational outcome (77% correctly classified; 71% correct in cross-validation). Similarly, a structured behavioural assessment that involved the task of assembling a wheelbarrow correlated significantly with all work performance ratings six months later, whereas only two of the neuropsychological tests correlated with the work performance ratings (Butler *et al.*, 1988).

It is clear that neuropsychological assessment must include measures of injury severity, psychosocial functioning, and demographics to evaluate and predict vocational outcome. Traditional neuropsychological tests may be best used in the early stages post injury and supplemented with additional variables in the later stages. In addition to neuropsychological test performance, individual differences, such as vocational stability, age, education, premorbid substance abuse and adequacy of social adjustment, are likely to be important in predicting outcome after brain injury.

Social adjustment

Relating neuropsychological assessment to social adjustment after TBI faces a similar challenge to that in vocational adjustment. It appears that several types of variables may be helpful in predicting later adjustment. Measures of different aspects of injury severity have been reported to be associated with social adjustment. Oddy and Humphrey (1980) found that the length of PTA greater than seven days was related to fewer social encounters at six and 12 months post injury. Variables measured within 24 hours post injury (GCS, plasma glucose, serum potassium and leucocyte count) showed significant correlations at long-term follow-up (mean time = 3.6 years) with psychosocial functioning as measured by the KAS, Sickness Impact Profile (SIP), and Profile of Mood States (Stambrook *et al.*, 1990). For example, the combination of GCS, glucose level and leucocyte count accounted for 66% of the variance on general psychopathology on the KAS.

Tellier, and associates (1991) evaluated 50 patients with mild to severe TBI (82% with moderate and severe injuries) at 8.5 months post injury with the HRNTB. Psychosocial adjustment was assessed at 2.7 years post injury with the SIP, KAS and Prigatano's Competency Rating Form. The most significant predictors of later psychosocial outcome were neuropsychological measures of motor slowness, visuospatial functioning, memory and complex attention. However, an overall composite variable, the Average Impairment Rating, was superior to all other predictors.

Klonoff and associates (1986) combined demographic variables, injury-related data, and neuropsychological data to assess predictors and indicators of quality of life in a sample of 71 patients two to four years post injury with mild to severe TBI. Acute GCS scores were related to later social role functioning. Deficits in memory and visuoconstructional ability were associated with social withdrawal and confusion. Lower education, the presence of frontal lobe damage, and post-traumatic seizures were also related to a poorer quality of life.

Other studies have approached the prediction of social adjustment after TBI with behavioural-orientated neuropsychological measures. A procedure to evaluate memory with functional activities, the Rivermead Behavioral Memory Test, in combination with a traditional test of complex attention and organizational functioning, Trails B, accounted for 36% of the variance on a measure of social behaviour (Malec *et al.*, 1991). As important as the cognitive and behavioural repertoire of the brain-injured survivor might be in social adjustment, the quality of the environment might be equally crucial. Kaplan (1991) found that perceived social support and family cohesion were associated with psychosocial status. Patients with higher levels of cohesion and support had better outcomes.

Premorbid psychosocial stressors appear to play an important role in social adjustment after mild head injury. Fenton *et al.*, (1993) followed a group of 45 consecutively admitted patients with mild head injury (MHI group) without a history of alcohol abuse. A group of control subjects matched for age, sex and socioeconomic status was also included. The MHI group had significantly more adverse life events in the year preceding the accident than did the control group. Fenton and associates also compared MHI patients who reported psychosocial difficulties with MHI patients whose symptoms had remitted. At six weeks post injury, the symptomatic patients had four times as many chronic social difficulties as the MHI patients whose symptoms had resolved. At six months, chronic social difficulties were twice as common in the MHI patients with persistent symptoms compared with the MHI patients whose symptoms had remitted.

Independent functioning in the community

As with predicting vocational outcome and social adjustment, similar approaches have been used to relate neuropsychological assessment to functional independence. The HRNTB and allied procedures have been shown to predict late outcome of level of living independence and self-care (Chelune *et al.*, 1986; DeTurk, 1975; Goodwin, 1983; Oddy and Humphrey, 1980). Performances on specific neuropsychological procedures may predict effectiveness in activities of daily living. In a sample of 37 brain-injured adults, dressing was highly correlated ($r = 0.60$) with three visuoconstructional measures (DeTurk, 1975). Performance at five months post injury on a visual choice reaction time test was related to patients' capacities to perform activities of daily living at 12 months (Baum and Hall, 1981). In predicting motor vehicle driving capacity, performances on two WAIS subtests, Picture Completion and Picture Arrangement, were significantly correlated (0.72 and 0.46), using Pearson, with open road driving (van Zomeran, 1981). However, these WAIS subtests may be useful in assessing driving capacity only for patients who have not yet resumed driving (Sivak *et al.*, 1981).

Combining neuropsychological test data with demographics and injury-related data has also been useful in predicting levels of functional independence. In the Klonoff and associates (1986) study discussed earlier, current deficits in complex attentional/motor performances as measured by the Finger Tapping Test and Visual Choice Reaction Time, with no paralysis or peripheral nerve impairment, were associated with decreased mobility, and problems with dressing, washing, body control and ambulation. Acute GCS scores were also related to later activities of daily living performance.

Recent interest in the neuropsychological assessment of the severely disabled patient (i.e. Levels of Cognitive Functions Scale II to IV) has led to the development of a plethora of new procedures, e.g. Western Neuro Sensory Stimulation Profile (Ansell and Keenan, 1989), Sensory Stimulation Assessment Measure (Rader *et al.*, 1989), and Coma Recovery Scale (Giacino *et al.*, 1991). These measures provide a detailed analysis of basic responses and may have potential for prediction of later outcome. Giacino *et al.* (1991) found that rate of recovery (change score) on the Coma Recovery Scale during the first month of rehabilitation was significantly correlated with outcome ($p < 0.01$) at three months on a measure that assessed arousal, self-care, employability and dependence on others (i.e. the Disability Rating Scale).

Test validity and the detection of malingering

A basic prerequisite for using neuropsychological test scores for predicting outcome is that patients have given their best effort during the examination so that the test scores are valid and reliable. The presumption that the test scores represent a patient's true neuropsychological status cannot automatically be assumed in all cases, particularly in those involving litigation. There can be powerful financial and social incentives that induce exaggerated disability. Pankratz (1988) has described the problem as follows:

> Accurate assessment is dependent on patient cooperation because neuropsychological techniques mostly measure behaviors that can be consciously modified. That is, because a patient can report wrong information, respond slowly, act uncoordinated, and deny comprehension, his cooperation must be secured in order to evaluate his case satisfactorily (p. 169).

The clinical challenge of differentiating feigned impairment from bona fide neuropsychological dysfunction has resulted in the development of new tests as well as the delineation of 'malingering profiles' with conventional neuropsychological tests. Of particular importance has been the development of forced-choice procedures such as the Portland Digit Recognition Test (Binder, 1993), the Hiscock and Hiscock Forced-Choice Procedure (Guilmette *et al.*, 1993), and the Recognition Memory Test (Millis, 1992). In these forced-choice procedures, the patient is given a stimulus item to remember (e.g. a word or a number) and is then presented with a two-choice recognition task with the original stimulus item and a foil. This dichotomous format provides a known level of chance performance (i.e. 50% correct). As performances deviate below chance, the probability that the patient is deliberately choosing the wrong answer is increased.

Because not all malingerers perform below chance on forced-choice procedures, another approach to detect malingering is to use standard neuropsychological measures to determine test performance patterns and derive statistical formulae that differentiate brain-injured patients from known simulators or presumed malingerers. Among other procedures, investigators have been able to discern profiles associated with malingering using the Halstead-Reitan Neuropsychological Test Battery (Trueblood and Schmidt, 1993) and Wechsler Memory Scale Revised (Mittenberg *et al.*, 1993).

There is no single, quick and valid malingering test and it is not likely that one will be forthcoming. Instead, the detection of malingering is a multivariate process that employs a comprehensive neuropsychological assessment, determination of initial injury severity, and consideration of psychosocial influences and alternative medical and psychological diagnoses.

Conclusion

Regarding TBI, it has often been stated that 'one rule is worth a thousand exceptions'. Such a statement seems particularly relevant to the prediction of psychosocial outcome after TBI. The approach of using neuropsychological tests as a predictor of outcome has advanced our understanding of the science of prediction, but, nevertheless, much still remains to be done. As noted earlier, the research studies of the past two decades have led to some important judgements. Prediction of an individual's outcome cannot be reliable if it is based on single measures (e.g. length of PTA, duration of coma, age, estimated pre-injury IQ, presence or absence of seizures, or score on a single neuropsychological measure). A more promising approach appears to be one that combines selected neuropsychological measures with other types of data, such as metabolic, neurological, behavioural and environmental, in more sophisticated multivariate analyses. This methodology would be likely to result in more accurate predictions that will account for a greater proportion of the variance than is commonly found in current correlation studies.

Future investigators also need to consider selecting or developing neuropsychological measures that 'score high marks' on the following parameters: (1) sensitivity to change over time; (2) ecological validity or real-world relevance; and (3) high reliability and validity with a brain-injured population. Similarly, measures of psychosocial outcome need to be chosen that: (1) recognize the multidimensional nature of the outcome variable (e.g. return to work as not simply a yes–no dichotomy); (2) incorporate the broader definitions of productivity, which include maintaining independent living status; and (3) are most relevant to an individual's quality of life.

For the clinician confronted with an individual with traumatic brain injury and with a family who are concerned about the ultimate psychosocial outcome, there is reason for cautious optimism. Past research efforts have expanded our knowledge of which neuropsychological measures and variables appear to have the most predictive value. Yet, it still remains incumbent on the clinician to employ clinical judgement to provide the family with a useful opinion on which to plan their future.

Acknowledgements

The preparation of this manuscript was supported, in part, by a grant (G0087C2022) from the National Institute on Disability and Rehabilitation Research. An earlier version of this manuscript appeared in *NeuroRehabilitation* 1992; **2**(4): 1–8.

References

Acker MB. (1986) Relationships between test scores and everyday life functioning. In: Uzzell B, Gross Y, editors. *Clinical neuropsychology of intervention.* Boston: Martinus Nijhoff, 85–118.

Ansell BJ, Keenan MA. (1989) The Western Neuro Sensory Stimulation Profile: a tool for assessing slow-to-recover head-injured patients. *Arch Phys Med Rehabil* **70**: 104–108.

Baum B, Hall K. (1981) Relationship between constructional praxis and dressing in the head injured. *Am J Occup Ther* **35**: 438.

Ben-Yishay Y, Silver SM, Piasetsky E, Rattock J. (1987) Relationship between employability and vocational outcome after intensive holistic cognitive rehabilitation. *J Head Trauma Rehabil* **2**(1): 35–48.

Binder LM. (1993) Assessment of malingering after mild head trauma with the Portland Digit Recognition Test. *J Clin Exp Neuropsychol* **15**: 170–82.

Bond MR. (1975) Assessment of the psychosocial outcome after severe brain injury. In: Porter R, Fitzsimons DW, editors. *Outcome of severe damage to the central nervous system.* (CIBA Foundation Symposium 34.) Amsterdam: Elsevier, 141–57.

Bond MR. (1990) Standardized methods of assessing and predicting outcome. In: Rosenthal M, Griffith ER, Bond MR, Miller JD, editors. Rehabilitation of the adult and child with traumatic brain injury. Philadelphia: Davis, 59–74.

Brooks DN, Aughton ME. (1979) Cognitive recovery during the first year after severe brain injury. *Int Rehabil Med* **1**: 160–65.

Brooks N, Campsie L, Symington C, *et al.* (1987a) The effects of severe brain injury on patient and relative within seven years of injury. *J Head Trauma Rehabil* **2**(3): 1–13.

Brooks N, McKinlay W, Symington C, *et al.* (1987b) Return to work within the first seven years of severe head injury. *Brain Inj* **1**: 5–19.

Butler R, Namerow N, Anderson L, *et al.* (1988) Behavioral assessment in neuropsychological rehabilitation. *Clinical Neuropsychol* **3**: 325–43.

Chelune G, Moehl K. (1986) Neuropsychological assessment and everyday functioning. In: Wedding D, Horton AM, Webster J, editors. *The neuropsychology handbook.* New York: Springer, 489–525.

Crosson B, Novak T, Trenerry M, *et al.* (1988) California Verbal Learning Test (CVLT) performance in severely head-injured and neurologically normal adult males. *J Clin Exp Neuropsychol* **10**: 754–68.

DeTurk J. (1975) Neuropsychological measures in predicting rehabilitation outcome. *Dissertation Abstr Int* **36**: 437B.

Dikmen S, Temkin N, Machamer J, *et al.* (1994) Employment following traumatic brain injuries. *Arch Neurol* **51**: 177–86.

Ezrachi O, Ben-Yishay Y, Kay T, *et al.* (1991) Predicting employability in traumatic brain injury following neuropsychological rehabilitation. *J Head Trauma Rehabil* **6**(3): 71–84.

Fenton G, McClelland R, Montgomery A, MacFlynn G, Rutherford W. (1993) The postconcussional syndrome: social antecedents and psychological sequelae. *Br J Psychiatry* **162**: 493–97.

Fraser R, Dikmen S, McLean A, *et al.* (1988) Employability of head injury survivors: first year postinjury. *Rehabil Couns Bull* **31**: 276–88.

Giacino JT, Kezmarsky A, DeLuca J, Cicerone KD. (1991) Monitoring rate of recovery to predict outcome in minimally responsive patients. *Arch Phys Med Rehabil* **72**: 897–901.

Gilchrist E, Wilkinson M. (1979) Some factors determining prognosis in young people with severe head injuries. *Arch Neurol* **36**: 355–59.

Goodwin D. (1983) Cognitive and physical recovery trends in severe closed head injury. *Dissertation Abstr Int* **43**: 3066B.

Guilmette TJ, Hart KJ, Giuliano AJ. (1993) Malingering detection: the use of a forced-choice method in identifying organic versus stimulated memory impairment. *Clin Neuropsychol* **7**: 59–69.

Kaplan S. (1991) Psychosocial adjustment three years after traumatic brain injury. *Clin Neuropsychol* **5**: 360–69.

Klonoff P, Costa L, Snow W. (1986) Predictors and indicators of quality of life in patients with closed head injury. *J Clin Exp Neuropsychol* **8**: 469–85.

Lezak MD. (1986) Psychological implications of traumatic brain damage for the patient's family. *Rehabil Psychol* **31**: 241–50.

Malec J, Zweber B, DePompolo R. (1991) The Rivermead Behavioral Memory Test: laboratory neurocognitive measures, and everyday functioning. *J Head Trauma Rehabil* **5**(3): 60–68.

Mandelberg IA, Brooks DN. (1975) Cognitive recovery after severe head injury: 1. Serial testing on the Wechsler Adult Intelligence Scale. *J Neurol Neurosurg Psychiatry* **38**: 1121–26.

Marshall LF, Gautille T, Klauber M, *et al.* (1991) The outcome of severe head injury. *J Neurosurg* **75**(suppl): S28–S36.

Millis SR. (1992) The Recognition Memory Test in the detection of malingered and exaggerated memory deficits. *Clin Neuropsychol* **6**: 406–14.

Millis SR, Dijkers M. (1993) Use of the recognition memory test in traumatic brain injury: preliminary findings. *Brain Inj* **7**: 53–58.

Mittenberg W, Azrin R, Millsaps C, Heilbronner R. (1993) Identification of malingered head injury on the Wechsler Memory Scale- Revised: psychological assessment. *J Consult Clin Psychol* **5**: 34–40.

Newton MR, Greenwood RJ, Britton KE, *et al.* (1992) A study comparing SPECT with CT and MRI after closed head injury. *J Neurol Neurosurg Psychiatry* **55**: 92–94.

Oddy M, Humphrey M, Uttley D. (1978) Subjective impairment and social recovery after closed head injury. *J Neurol Neurosurg Psychiatry* **41**: 611–16.

Oddy M, Humphrey M. (1980) Social recovery during the first year following severe head injury. *J Neurol Neurosurg Psychiatry* **43**: 798–802.

Pankratz L. (1988) Malingering on intellectual and neuropsychological measures. In: Rogers R, editor. *Clinical assessment of malingering and deception.* New York: Guilford Press, 169–92.

Prigatano GP, Fordyce DJ, Zeiner HK, *et al.* (1984) Neuropsychological rehabilitation after closed head injury in young adults. *J Neurol Neurosurg Psychiatry* **47**: 505–13.

Prigatano G, Altman I. (1990) Impaired awareness of behavioral limitations after traumatic brain injury. *Arch Phys Med Rehabil* **71**: 1058–64.

Rader MA, Alston JG, Ellis DW. (1989) Sensory stimulation of severely brain-injured adults. *Brain Inj* **3**: 141–47.

Rappaport M, Hall KM, Hopkins K, *et al.* (1982) Disability rating scale for severe head trauma: coma to community. *Arch Phys Med Rehabil* **63**: 118–23.

Reyes RL, Bhattacharyya AK, Heller D. (1981) Traumatic head injury: restlessness and agitation as prognosticators of physical and psychologic improvement in patients. *Arch Phys Med Rehabil* **62**: 20–23.

Rimel R, Giordani B, Barth J, *et al.* (1982) Moderate head injury: completing the clinical spectrum of brain trauma. *Neurosurgery* **29**: 516–24.

Schretlen D. (1992) Accounting for variance in long-term recovery from traumatic brain injury with executive abilities and injury severity [abstract]. *J Clin Exp Neuropsychol* **14**: 77.

Sivak M, Olson, Kewman D, *et al.* (1981) Driving and perceptual/cognitive skills: behavioral consequences of brain damage. *Arch Phys Med Rehabil* **62**: 476.

Stambrook M, Moore A, Kowalchuck S, *et al.* (1990) Early metabolic and neurologic predictors of long-term quality of life after closed head injury. *Can J Surg* **33**: 115–18.

Tellier A, Rourke BP, Shore D, Adams KM. (1991) Predicting psychosocial outcome of traumatic brain injured adults [abstract]. *J Clin Exp Neuropsychol* **13**: 105.

Thomsen IV. (1984) Late outcome of very severe blunt head trauma: a 10–15 year second follow-up. *J Neurol Neurosurg Psychiatry* **48**: 260–68.

Trueblood W, Schmidt M. (1993) Malingering and other validity considerations in the neuropsychological evaluation of mild head injury. *J Clin Exp Neuropsychol* **15**: 578–90.

van Zomeran AH. (1981) Reaction time and attention after closed head injury. Lisse: Swets & Zeitlinger.

van Zomeran AH, Brouwer WH, Rothengatter JA, Snoek JW. (1988) Fitness to drive a car after a recovery from severe head injury. *Arch Phys Med Rehabil* **69**: 90–96.

Walker M, Hannay HJ, Davison K. (1992) PAI and the prediction of level of vocational/academic outcome post-CHI [abstract]. *J Clin Exp Neuropsychol* **14**: 29.

Wehman P, Kreutzer J, West M, *et al.* (1989) Employment outcomes of persons following traumatic brain injury: pre-injury, postinjury, and supported employment. *Brain Inj* **3**: 397–412.

Willer B, Linn R, Allen K. (1994) Community integration and barriers to integration for individuals with brain injury. In: Finlayson MAJ, Garner S, editors. *Brain injury rehabilitation: clinical considerations.* Baltimore, MD: Williams & Wilkins, 355–75.

Willer B, Rosenthal M, Gordon WA, Rempel R. (1993) Assessment of community integration following rehabilitation for traumatic brain injury. *J Head Trauma Rehabil* **8**(2): 75–87.

12

Behavioural disorders

G E Berrios

Introduction

The type and duration of the psychiatric and behavioural sequelae of head injury vary according to lesion, age, sex, genetic loading and personality. Head or brain injury is defined as damage to living brain tissue caused by an external mechanical force. It is clinically characterized by a period of altered consciousness of varied duration. In the short term, the traumatic event may rob the individual of physical and mental function (Mifka, 1976) and, in the long-term, cause neuropsychological deficit, chronic psychiatric disease and psychosocial incompetence (Bach-y-Rita, 1980; Baethmann et al., 1984; Brooks, 1984; Jennett and Teasdale, 1981; Levin et al., 1982; Lezak, 1989; Long and Ross, 1992; Richardson, 1990).

This chapter focuses on conventional forms of psychiatric disorder found in the wake of brain injury, such as neurotic symptoms, depression, schizophrenia-like states, personality disorders, delirium and traumatic dementia (for a full review of the literature, including assessment issues, see Berrios and Paykel, 1997). Reactive anxiety, dysphoria, depression and anger can also develop after neck and spinal injury without involvement of the brain. These symptoms result from personal predisposition and failures in social support rather than damage to the brain; they are not dealt with in this chapter. The conventional neuropsychological syndromes are discussed elsewhere in this volume.

Epidemiological studies tend to conflate neuropsychological and psychiatric symptoms. Hence, the specific prevalence of the latter remains unknown (Middelboe et al., 1992), as does the staging of the psychiatric sequelae and their long-term outcome (e.g. it is unclear how many patients will remain psychotic, depressed or obsessional 30 or 40 years after their injuries). One problem is that long-term studies are difficult to implement because diagnostic criteria and evaluating instruments change at regular intervals; another is that researchers deal with a changing population. The moderate industrial injury of old, affecting adults with normal premorbid personality, has now been replaced by a more severe injury occurring in younger survivors of road traffic accidents (Cohadon et al., 1991; Lee et al., 1990; Miller, 1991). This particular population is said to have a high incidence of premorbid psychiatric pathology (Parmelee et al., 1989). Lastly, the psychiatrist is also asked to see another subgroup of patients with chronic headache, fatigue, dizziness, reduced libido and irritability who show little or no detectable neurological pathology and known as the postconcussional syndrome (Bohnen and Jolles, 1992; Bruyn and Lanser, 1990; Fenton et al., 1993).

No reliable predictors are available to identify who are more likely to develop psychiatric complications following head injury, or tell for how long they might remain thus disordered. It has been suggested that the severity of future psychiatric illness correlates with the duration of post-traumatic amnesia (PTA) (Lishman, 1973; Steadman and Graham, 1970). In clinical practice, however, this predictor is not always helpful, as duration of PTA is also associated with long-term attentional, language and memory impairments, which are known to mask or obliterate long-term psychiatric illness. Furthermore, there is the reliable clinical observation (not yet empirically ascertained!) that the type of patient who presents with florid psychiatric symptomatology is likely to have exhibited a short PTA. In this group, the most useful clinical predictors remain a history of alcohol abuse (Hillbom and Holm, 1986) of abnormal pre-morbid personality or of psychiatric illness (Parmelee *et al.*, 1989).

Organic mental disorders

In the brain-injured, coma is followed by delirium. This is characterized by persistent disorientation and fluctuating confusion (Duckett and Scotto, 1992), irritability, restlessness (Brooke *et al.*, 1992) and agitation (Corrigan and Mysiw, 1988). Hyperaesthesia, over-reactivity to stimuli (Bohnen *et al.*, 1991) and inversion of sleep rhythms (Patten and Lauderdale, 1992) are commonly present. Delirium also characterizes the earlier phase of 'PTA' and may include fleeting hallucinations, and paranoid, often misidentificatory, delusions. The clinician must actively seek these symptoms, as patients often conceal their presence (fearing that they are 'going mad' and may be taken to a 'mental hospital'). This is also the time when rare neuropsychological pathologies such as reduplicative paramnesia, anosognosia and delusions of memory may be found.

As the confusional state subsides, the patient becomes more accessible to assessment. In addition to psychiatric symptoms, cortical deficits (agnosias, apraxia, aphasia), attentional disorders, and pathology of intellectual functions – ranging from mild memory problems to cognitive disintegration – can be found. The latter may on occasions be as severe as any seen in the terminal stages of the conventional dementias.

Psychotic symptoms and schizophrenia

Regardless of severity, brain-injured subjects may show isolated psychotic symptoms or recognizable psychosis. Such pathology is stressful to carers (Urbach and Culbert, 1991) and decreases treatment compliance (Salloum *et al.*, 1990). For example, hallucinations (both visual and auditory) are seen in the postinjury confusional state (Ferrey and Gagey, 1987; Muller, 1974), when their clinical meaning is uncertain. This becomes clear,

however, when subjects are fully orientated, and seizural activity must be ruled out (Morsier, 1972). For example, Varney *et al.* (1992) found that in 25 head-injured patients, the presence of olfactory hallucinations correlated with theta bursts on the EEG. Subjects who sustain brain damage in childhood are said to be more prone to develop hallucinations as adults (Albert, 1987).

Delusions, often bizarre in nature, can be found in the wake of head injury and may be an obstacle to rehabilitation (Prigatano *et al.*, 1988). Young *et al.* (1992) reported a 24-year-old man with a right temporoparietal injury who developed a Cotard's delusion (he believed he was dead). Another young man presented with a delusional reduplication of a third arm (Rogers and Franzen, 1992) and a third youngster with a left parietal lobe injury developed a somatic delusion involving his eyes (Dalby *et al.*, 1989). Kellner and Strian (1991) reported the case history of a 65-year-old man who, after a traumatic haemorrhage in the left basal ganglia, developed the bizarre delusion of having 'artificial tubes implanted into his body'. Achte *et al.* (1991) found that 28% of a sample of 3000 war veterans with moderate or severe brain injury suffered from paranoid delusions, the commonest type being jealousy. In 14 389 head-injured patients, Davison and Bagley (1969) found that 'traumatic insanity' (a concept wider than schizophrenia) had a prevalence of 2.24%. They concluded that: (1) such a figure significantly exceeded chance expectation; (2) in most of these patients there was no hard evidence for a genetic predisposition (although it is difficult to know how this conclusion was reached in view of the quality of their data); (3) there was an association with temporal lobe lesions; and (4) the commonest cause was severe closed head injury.

Recent research has tended to confirm these findings. In a follow-up study of 291 head-injured subjects, Roberts (1979) ascertained the presence of nine with 'schizophreniform psychosis'. Thomsen (1984) found eight (only one schizophreniform) in a sample of 40 severe close head injuries. Nasrallah *et al.* (1981) have reported a patient with a good premorbid history and no family history, who developed a schizophrenia-like state after head injury. Lastly, De Mol *et al.* (1982), based on the description of six patients, concluded that young men are more prone to this complication; that severity of injury does not seem to be a relevant factor in the development of traumatic psychosis; and that the clinical presentation of the latter is no different from that of conventional schizophrenia.

In a wider context, the presence of early head injury seems to be a factor in the development of schizophrenia-like states in adolescents (O'Callaghan *et al.*, 1988). Likewise, patients with schizophrenia are claimed to have a significantly higher rate of childhood head trauma than controls with mania, depression or no mental disorder (Wilcox and Nasrallah, 1987). In contrast, other authors have claimed that early brain damage may protect against schizophrenia (Lewis *et al.*, 1990). Nasrallah and Wilcox (1989) have also attempted to tease out the relative contributions of genetic and head injury components to schizophrenia, and have concluded that the latter seems more important in males. This contradicts older findings that alien tissue in the temporal lobe is more likely to cause schizophrenia-like states in the female (Taylor, 1975).

Buckley *et al.* (1993), in turn, have stated that head-injured subjects with schizophrenia, more often than those with affective symptoms, tend to bear the lesion in the dominant temporal lobe. Lastly, there have been reports of at least one case of a head-injured patient who developed a psychotic state after being treated with chlorpromazine (Sandel *et al.*, 1993), and of another who developed a similar mental state after being withdrawn from steroids (Alpert and Seigerman, 1986)

Affective disorders

Agitation and anxiety have been reported in subjects with head injuries of varying severity, and at different stages of their disease (Tuokko *et al.*, 1991). These symptoms can be present during the confusional stage or later, and may occur alone or be accompanied by other manifestations of depressive illness. It has been claimed that agitation is related to the degree of dysattention (Corrigan *et al.*, 1992), and anxiety to the severity of neuropsychological impairment (Bornstein *et al.*, 1989). Anxiety is, however, pervasive after head injury and can be found both in mild (Schoenhuber-and Gentilini, 1988) and severe (Newton and Johnson, 1985) head trauma. An interesting point is that, in a good proportion of patients, anxiety behaves as a trait (i.e. is particularly marked under stress) (Gouvier *et al.*, 1992).

The frequency and severity of depression and mania seem determined by lesion site, premorbid history, level of insight, genetic predisposition, and degree of family support. It is believed that

traumatic head injury increases the risk of depression (Fedoroff *et al.*, 1992; Silver *et al.*, 1991). This has been quantified by Gualtieri and Cox (1991) as being around a factor of 10. In a recent review, it has been claimed that 42% of subjects will suffer from depression during the first year after their injury (Fedoroff *et al.*, 1993). However, another member of this group has reported a lower incidence of depression in brain-injured than in stroke patients (subjects were matched for site of lesion) (Robinson, 1981), and also that a family history of affective disorder plays a lesser role in the development of depression than of mania (Robinson, 1988). This suggests that 'behavioural copies' of depression are common in neurological practice (Berrios *et al.*, 1987; Berrios and Dening, 1990) and that, in this patient group, depression is often difficult to distinguish from chronic hopelessness and grief (Tadir and Stern, 1985). It is also reported that neuropsychological rehabilitation may be accompanied by a reduction in 'depression' (Evans and Wilson, 1992; Ruff *et al.*, 1991). These studies do not always make clear whether 'depression' is treated as a dependent variable, although Ruff and Niemann (1990) have suggested that the latter is the case. In spite of these difficulties, Jorge *et al.* (1993a) have recently stated that the *Diagnostic and Statistical manual of mental disorders* (DSM) III-R criteria (American Psychiatric Association, 1987) remain adequate for the diagnosis of major depression in head-injured subjects. They base their claim on a comparison between head-injured patients with and without depression (however, since the groups were not matched for lesion site and type, their conclusion seems unwarranted).

Major depression can be an early (Colombel *et al.*, 1989) or a late (Burke *et al.*, 1990) complication of closed head injury. Jorge *et al.* (1993b) have suggested that the earlier form may be a direct manifestation of the lesion, and that the latter is the result of psychosocial factors. Others have used the category DSM III-R 'organic mood syndrome' to refer to the clinically similar affective disorder, which is, in general, considered as more difficult to treat than conventional depression (Barnhill and Gualtieri, 1989). Depression is also a late complication in both 'postconcussion syndrome' (Szymanski and Linn, 1992) and whiplash injury (Ettlin *et al.*, 1992). Severe depression can appear *de novo* three years after the injury (Burke *et al.*, 1990).

There have also been suggestions that the site and laterality of the head injury lesion might be of some relevance. For example, Lipsey *et al.* (1983) found that left anterior brain injuries correlated with depression, and Fedoroff *et al.* (1992) have reported an increased likelihood of major depression in left dorsolateral frontal lesions. Moehle and Fitzhugh-Bell (1988), however, did not find any relationship between laterality and depression in a sample of 186 brain-injured subjects. Likewise, on the basis of 10 brain-injured patients with a blunted prolactin response to buspirone, it has been claimed that depression is mediated in these subjects by a serotoninergic mechanism (Mobayed and Dinan, 1990). Pope *et al.* (1988) reported two patients with bipolar disorder following head injury, which proved refractory to conventional treatment but responded well to sodium valproate.

From a practical point of view, it is believed that the presence of depression predicts a bad response to rehabilitation (Ryan *et al.* 1992). Subjects who do not improve are more likely to be depressed and aggressive, to have received their injury in an assault rather than in a motor vehicle accident, and to have abused alcohol before the injury (Dunlop *et al.*, 1991). Depression is also said to correlate with fatigue, the latter being a known obstacle to rehabilitation (Walker *et al.*, 1991).

Neurotic symptoms and personality change

The incidence of obsessions is said to be increased in organic disorders in general. Clinical experience shows that this is also the case within head injuries. However, there have been few studies in this area. McKeon *et al.* (1984) have reported four subjects who developed obsessional-compulsive neurosis after a head injury, and Drummond (1988) has reported another occurrence in a 26-year-old man, starting six months after a minor head injury. The head-injury may also show less conventional symptoms. One is 'pathological affect' (i.e. intermittent and often untriggered laughing and crying) (Allman *et al.*, 1992; Robinson *et al.*, 1993; Ross and Stewart, 1987). This symptom has been reported to respond to tricyclic antidepressants, levodopa, or selective serotonic re-uptake inhibitors (Allman, 1992). Another 'symptom' is a loss of sexual drive and interest (Kreutzer and Zasler, 1989), and a reduction in the frequency of sexual intercourse. This is often related to depression (O'Carroll *et al.*, 1991)

It has been known since the nineteenth century that a change in character and personality is a manifestation of head injury, and that this seems related to lesions occurring in the frontal lobes (Stuss and Gow, 1992; Welt, 1888, quoted in Bumke, 1946). Other workers, however, have reported that premorbid traits and temporal lobe lesions may also play a role (De Mol, 1981). Personality change is apparent both to others and to the patient, and correlates well with most measurements (Dodwell, 1988; Gensemer *et al.*, 1989; Tuokko *et al.*, 1991). For reasons that are unclear, some workers assess post-traumatic personality change by means of proxy variables such as 'design fluency' and performance on the Wisconsin Card Sorting Test (Tate *et al.*, 1991). This trend is to be deprecated, for it assumes that personality change is necessarily related to the frontal lobes. Personality change is pervasive in head injury and must be assessed in detail as it has more impact on the carer than any other physical or short-term neuropsychological or psychiatric handicap (Florian *et al.*, 1991; Livingston, 1988), and is also relevant to rehabilitation (Mazaux *et al.*, 1982).

Summary

Delirium, dementia, delusions, hallucinations, occasional psychosis, affective disorders, neurotic symptoms and personality change are often found in the wake of head injury, and may be the main cause of long-term disability. Whatever the nature of the lesion, personality, sex, age and genetic vulnerability play a role in determining the severity and type of mental disorder. Undue emphasis on neuropsychology has obscured or reinterpreted psychiatric symptoms in cognitive terms. The psychiatrist must resist such reductionism. The brain-damaged patient is a person whose brain may have suffered insults seriatim, and who is struggling to readapt (Leftoff, 1983). Mental state assessments should take place at regular intervals, as psychiatric symptoms change over time. These originate as often from the lesion as from worries about the future. Much of what patients will do or say results, therefore, from a combination of limited cognition, distorted assessment of real life situations, disregulated mood, and genuine worries about problems beyond their control. The psychiatrist who can evaluate these components will have taken the first step towards the proper management of this neglected group of subjects.

References

Achte K, Jahro L, Kyykka T, Vesterinen E. (1991) Paranoid disorders following war brain damage. Preliminary report. *Psychopathology* **24**: 309–15.

Albert E. (1987) On organically based hallucinatory-delusional psychoses. *Psychopathology* **20**: 144–54.

Allman P. (1992) Drug treatment of emotionalism following brain damage. **85**: 423–24.

Allman P, Hope T, Fairburn CG. (1992) Crying following stroke: a report of 30 cases. *Gen Hosp Psychiatry* **14**: 315–21.

Alpert E, Seigerman C. (1986) Steroid withdrawal psychosis in a patient with closed head injury. *Arch Phys Med Rehabil* **67**: 766–69.

American Psychiatric Association. (1987) *Diagnostic and statistical Manual of Mental Disorders*, revised. Washington, DC: American Psychiatric Press.

Bach-y-Rita P, editor. (1980) *Recovery of function: theoretical considerations for brain injury rehabilitation.* Berne: Huber.

Baethmann A, Go KG, Unterberg A, editors. (1984) *Mechanisms of secondary brain damage.* New York: Plenum Press.

Barnhill LJ, Gualtieri CT. (1989) Two cases of late-onset psychosis after closed head injury. *Neuropsychiatry Neuropsychol Behav Neurol* **2**: 211–17.

Berrios GE, Dening T. (1990) Biological and quantitative issue in neuropsychiatry. *Behav Neurol* **3**: 247–59.

Berrios GE, Paykel ES. (1997) Psychiatric consequences of brain damage. In: Sofroniew N, Fawcett D, Dunnett S, editors *Brain damage and brain repair.* Oxford University Press, in press.

Berrios GE, Samuel C. (1987) Affective symptoms in the neurological patient. *J Nerv Ment Dis* **175**: 173–76.

Bohnen N, Jolles J. (1992) Neurobehavioural aspects of postconcussive symptoms after mild head injury. *J Nerv Ment Dis* **180**: 683–92.

Bohnen N, Twijnstra A, Kroeze J, Jolles J. (1991) A psychophysiological method for assessing visual and acoustic hyperaesthesia in patients with mild head injury. *Br J Psychiatry* **159**: 860–63.

Bornstein RA, Miller HB, Van Schoor JT. (1989) Neuropsychological deficit and emotional disturbance in head-injured patients. *J Neurosurg* **70**: 509–13.

Brooke MM, Questad KA, Patterson DR, Bashak KJ. (1992) Agitation and restlessness after closed head-injury: a prospective study of 100 consecutive admissions. *Arch Phys Med Rehabil* **73**: 320–23.

Brooks N, editor. (1984) *Closed injury: psychological, social and family consequences.* Oxford: Oxford University Press.

Bruyn GW, Lanser JBK. (1990) The post-concussion syndrome. In: Braackman R, editor. *Handbook of clinical neurology. Vol. 13. Head injury.* New York: Elsevier, 421–27.

Buckley P, Stack JP, Madigan C, *et al.* (1993) Magnetic resonance imaging of schizophrenia-like psychosis associated with cerebral trauma: clinicopathological correlates. *Am J Psychiatry* **150**: 146–48.

Burke JM, Imhoff CL, Kerrigan JM. (1990) MMPI correlates among post-acute TBI patients. *Brain Inj* **4**: 223–31.

Cohadon F, Richer E, Castel JP. (1991) Head injuries: incidence and outcome. *J Neurolog Sci* **103**: S27–S31.

Colombel JC, Bouffard V, Filipetti P, *et al.* (1989) Syndromes depressifs precoces des traumatismes craniens. *Ann Readapt Med Phys* **32**: 669–93.

Corrigan JD, Mysiw WJ. (1988) Agitation following traumatic head injury: equivocal evidence for a discrete stage of cognitive recovery. *Arch Phys Med Rehabil* **69**: 487–92.

Corrigan JD, Mysiw WJ, Gribble MW, Chock SKL. (1992) Agitation, cognition and attention during post-traumatic amnesia. *Brain Inj* **6**: 155–60.

Dalby JTh, Arboleda-Florez J, Seland TP. (1989) Somatic delusions following left parietal lobe-injury. *Neuropsychiatry Neuropsychol Behav Neurol* **2**: 306–11.

Davison K, Bagley CR. (1969) Schizophrenia-like psychoses associated with organic disorder of the central nervous system: a review of the literature. In: Herrington RN, editor. *Current problems in neuropsychiatry.* (Royal Medico-Psychological Association Publication.) Ashford, Kent: Headley, 113–84.

De Mol J. (1981) Les troubles du caractere chez les traumatises craniens adultes. *Schweizer Arch Neurol Neurochir Psychiatrie* **129**: 37–45.

De Mol J, Violon A and Brihayee J. (1982) Les decompensations schizphreniques post-traumatiques: a propos de 6 cas de schizophrenie traumatique. *Encéphale.* **8**: 17–24.

Dodwell D. (1988) Comparison of self-ratings with informant-ratings of pre-morbid personality on two personality rating scales. *Psychol Med* **18**: 495–501.

Drummond LM. (1988) Delayed emergence of obsessive-compulsive neurosis following head injury. *Br J Psychiatry* **153**: 839–42.

Duckett S, Scotto M. (1992) An unusual case of sundown syndrome subsequent to a traumatic head injury. *Brain Inj* **6**: 189–91.

Dunlop TW, Udvarhelyi GB, Stedem AFA., *et al.* (1991) Comparison of patients with and without emotional/behavioural deterioration during the first year after traumatic brain injury. *J Neuropsychiatry Clin Neurosci* **3**: 150–56.

Ettlin TM, Kischka U, Reichmann S, *et al.* (1992) Cerebral symptoms after whiplash injury of the neck: a prospective clinical and neuropsychological study of whiplash injury. *J Neurol, Neurosurg Psychiatry* **55**: 943–48.

Evans JJ, Wilson BA. (1992) A memory group for individuals with brain injury. *Clin Rehabil* **6**: 75–81.

Fedoroff JP, Starkstein SE, Forrester AW, *et al.* (1992) Depression in patients with acute traumatic brain injury. *Am J Psychiatry* **149**: 918–23.

Fedoroff JP, Jorge RE, Robinson RG. (1993). Depression in traumatic brain injury. In: Starkstein SE, Robinson RG, editors *Depression in neurologic disease*, Baltimore: Johns Hopkins University Press, 139–51.

Fenton G, McClelland R, Montgomery A, *et al.* (1993) The post-concussional syndrome: social antecedents and psychological sequelae. *Br J Psychiatry* **162**: 493–97.

Ferrey G, Gagey PM. (1987) Le syndrome subjectif et les troubles psychiques des traumatisés du crâne. *Encyclopédie Médico-Chirurgicale (Paris-France) Psychiatrie* 37520 A[10].

Florian V, Katz S, Lahav V. (1991) Impact of traumatic brain damage on family dynamics and functioning: a review. *Int Disabil Stud* **13**: 150–57.

Gensemer IB, Smith JL, Walker JC, *et al.* (1989) Psychological consequences of blunt head trauma and relation to other indices of severity of injury. *Ann Emerg Med* **18**: 9–12.

Gouvier WD, Cubic B, Jones G, *et al.* (1992) Post-concussional syndrome and daily stress in normal and head-injured college populations. *Arch Clin Neuropsychol* **7**: 192–11.

Gualtieri T, Cox DR. (1991) The delayed neurobehavioural sequelae of traumatic head injury. *Brain Inj* **5**: 219–32.

Hillbom M, Holm L. (1986) Contribution of traumatic head injury to neuropsychological deficits in alcoholics. *J Neuro Neurosurg Psychiatry* **49**: 1348–53.

Jennett B, Teasdale G. (1981) *Management of head injuries.* Philadelphia: Davis.

Jorge RE, Robinson RG, Arndt S. (1993a) Are there symptoms that are specific for depressed mood in patients with traumatic head injury? *J Nerv Ment Dis* **181**: 91–99.

Jorge RE, Robinson RG, Arndt SV, *et al.* (1993b) Comparison between acute and delayed-onset depression following traumatic brain injury. *J Neuropsychiatry Clin Neurosci* **5**: 43–49.

Kellner MB, Strian MB. (1991) Bizarre delusion and post-hemiplegic dystonia [letter]. *Br J Psychiatry* **159**: 448.

Kreutzer JS, Zasler ND. (1989) Psychosexual consequences of traumatic brain injury: methodology and preliminary findings. *Brain Inj* **3**: 177–86.

Lee ST, Lui TN, Chang CN, *et al.* (1990) Features of head injury in a developing country – Taiwan (1977–1987). *J Trauma* **30**: 194–99.

Leftoff S. (1983) Psychopathology in the light of brain injury: a case study. *J Clin Neuropsychol* **5**: 51–63.

Lewis SW, Harvey I, Ron M, *et al.* (1990) Can brain damage protect against schizophrenia? A case report of twins. *Br J Psychiatry* **157**: 600–603.

Levin HS, Benton AL, Grossman RG. (1982) *Neurobehavioral consequences of closed head injury.* New York: Oxford University Press.

Lezak MD editor. (1989) *Assessment of the behavioural consequences of head trauma.* New York: Liss.

Lipsey JR, Robinson RG, Pearlson GD, *et al.* (1983) Mood change following bilateral hemisphere brain injury. *Br J Psychiatry* **143**: 266–73.

Lishman WA. (1973) The psychiatric sequelae of head injury: a review. *Psychol Med* **3**: 304–18.

Livingston MG. (1988) The burden on families of the brain injured: a review. *J Head Trauma Rehabil* **3**: 6–15.

Long CJ, Ross LK editors (1992) *Handbook of head trauma.* New York: Plenum Press.

Mazaux JM, Barat M, Giroire JM, *et al.* (1982) Place de la reeducation des troubles des fonctions symboliques dans la prise en charge des traumatises craniens graves. *Ann Med Physique* **25**: 177–88.

McKeon J, McGuffin P, Robinson P. (1984) Obsessive-compulsive neurosis following head-injury. A report of four cases. *Br J Psychiatry* **144**: 190–92.

Middelboe T, Andersen HS, Birket-Smith M, Friis ML. (1992) Psychiatric sequelae of minor head injury. A prospective follow-up study. *Eur Psychiatry* **7**: 183–89.

Mifka P. (1976) Post-traumatic psychiatric disturbances. In: Vinken PJ, Bruyn GW, editors. *Injuries of the brain and skull, part II, vol. 24. Handbook of clinical neurology.* Amsterdam, North Holland: Elsevier, 517–74.

Miller JD. (1991) Changing patterns in acute management of head injury. *J Neurol Sci* **103** (suppl): S33–S37.

Mobayef M, Dinan TG. (1990) Buspirone/prolactin response in post-head injury depression. *J Affect Disord* **19**: 237–41.

Moehle KA, Fitzhugh-Bell KB. (1988) Laterality of brain damage and emotional disturbance in adults. *Arch Clin Neuropsychol* **3**: 137–44.

Morsier G de. (1972) Les hallucinations survenant après les traumatismes cranio-cérébraux. La schizophrenie traumatique. *Ann Med Psychol* **130**: 183–94.

Muller GE. (1974) Les syndromes post-traumatiques précoces atypiques. *Acta Neurol Belg* **74**: 163–81.

Nasrallah HA, Fowler RC, Judd LL. (1981) Schizophrenia-like illness following head injury. *Psychosomatics* **22**: 359–61.

Nasrallah HA, Wilcox JA. (1989) Gender differences in the aetiology and symptoms of schizophrenia: genetic versus brain injury factors. *Ann Clin Psychiatry* **1**: 51–52.

Newton A, Johnson DA. (1985) Social adjustment and interaction after severe head injury. *Br J Clin Psychol* **24**: 225–34.

O'Callaghan E, Larkin C, Redmond O, *et al.* (1988) 'Early-onset schizophrenia' after teenage head injury: a case report with magnetic resonance imaging. *Br J Psychiatry* **153**: 294–396.

O'Carroll RE, Woodrow J, Maroun F. (1991) Psychosexual and psychosocial sequelae of closed head injury. *Brain Inj* **5**: 303–13.

Parmelee DX, Kowatch RA, Sellman J, Davidow D. (1989) Ten cases of head-injured, suicide-surviving adolescents: challenges for rehabilitation. *Brain Inj* **3**: 295–300.

Patten SB, Lauderdale WM. (1992) Delayed sleep-phase disorder after traumatic brain injury. *J Am Acad Child Adolesc Psychiatry* **31**: 100–102

Pope HG, McElroy SL, Satlin A, *et al.* (1988) Head injury, bipolar disorder and response to valproate. *Compr Psychiatry* **29**: 34–38.

Prigatano GP, O'Brien KP, Klonoff PS. (1988) The clinical management of paranoid delusions in post-acute traumatic brain-injured patients. *J Head Trauma Rehabil* **3**: 23–32.

Richardson JTE. (1990) *Clinical and neuropsychological aspects of closed head injury.* London: Taylor and Francis.

Roberts AH. (1979) *Severe accidental injury: an assessment of long-term prognosis.* London: Macmillan.

Robinson RG. (1981) Mood change following left hemispheric brain injury. *Ann Neurol* **9**: 447–53.

Robinson RG. (1988) Comparison of mania and depression after brain injury: causal factors. *Am J Psychiatry* **145**: 172–78.

Robinson RG, Parikh RM, Lipsey JR, *et al.* (1993) Pathological laughing and crying following stroke: validation of a measurement scale and a double-blind treatment study. *Am J Psychiatry* **150**: 286–93.

Rogers MJC, Franzen MD. (1992) Delusional reduplication following closed-head injury. *Brain Inj* **6**: 469–76.

Ross ED, Stewart RS. (1987) Pathological display of affect in patients with depression and right frontal lobe damage. *J Nerv Ment Dis* **175**: 165–72.

Ruff RM, Niemann H. (1990) Cognitive rehabilitation versus day treatment in head-injured adults: is there an impact on emotional and psychosocial adjustment? *Brain Inj* **4**: 339–47.

Ruff RM, Young D, Gautille T, *et al.* (1991) Verbal learning deficits following severe head injury: heterogeneity in recovery over 1 year. *J Neurosurg* **75**(suppl): S50–S58.

Ryan TV, Sautter SW, Capps CF, *et al.* (1992) Utilizing neuropsychological measures to predict vocational outcome in a head trauma population. *Brain Inj* **6**: 175–82.

Salloum IM, Jenkins EJ, Thompson B, *et al.* (1990) Treatment compliance and hostility levels of head-injured psychiatric outpatients. *J Nat Med Assoc* **82**: 557–64.

Sandel ME, Olive DA, Raderr MA. (1993) Chlorpromazine-induced psychosis after brain injury. *Brain Inj* **7**: 77–83.

Schoenhuber M, Gentilini M. (1988) Anxiety and depression after mild head injury. *J Neurol Neurosurg Psychiatry* **51**: 722–24.

Silver JM, Yudofsky SC, Hales RE. (1991) Depression in traumatic head injury. *Neuropsychiatry Neuropsychol Behav Neurol* **4**: 12–23.

Steadman JH, Graham JG. (1970) Head injuries: an analysis and follow up study. *Proc R Soc Med* **63**: 23–28.

Stuss DT, Gow CA. (1992) 'Frontal dysfunction' after traumatic brain injury. *Neuropsychiatry Neuropsychol Behav Neurol* **5**: 272–82.

Szymanski HV, Linn R. (1992) A review of the post-concussion syndrome. *Int J Psychiatry Med* **22**: 357–75.

Tadir M, Stern JM. (1985) The mourning process with brain injured patients. *Scand J Rehabil Med* **17**(suppl): 50–52.

Tate RL, Fenelon B, Manning ML, Hunter M. (1991) Patterns of neuropsychological impairment after severe blunt head injury. *J Nerv Ment Dis* **179**: 117–26.

Taylor DC. (1975) Factors influencing the occurrence of schizophrenia-like psychosis in patients with temporal lobe epilepsy. *Psychol Med* **5**: 249–54.

Thomsen IV. (1984) Late outcome of very severe blunt head trauma: a 10–15 year second follow-up. *J Neurol Neurosurg Psychiatry* **47**: 73–77.

Tuokko H, Vernon-Wilkinson R, Robinson E. (1991) The use of the MCMI in the personality assessment of head-injured adults. *Brain Inj* **5**: 287–93.

Urbach JR, Culbert JP. (1991) Head-injured patients and their children: psychosocial consequences of a traumatic syndrome. *Psychosomatics* **32**: 24–33.

Varney NR, Hines ME, Bailey C, Roberts RJ. (1992) Neuropsychiatric correlates of theta bursts in patients with closed head injury. *Brain Inj* **6**: 499–508.

Walker GC, Cárdenas DD, Guthrie MR *et al.* (1991) Fatigue and depression in the brain-injured correlated with quadriceps strength and endurance. *Arch Phys Med Rehabil* **72**: 469–72.

Welt (1888) Cited in: Bumke O. (1946) *Nuevo tratado de enfermedades mentales.* (Spanish Translation) Barcelona: F. Seix.

Wilcox JA, Nasrallah HA. (1987) Childhood head trauma and psychosis. *Psychiatry Res* **21**: 303–306.

Young AW, Robertson IH, Hellawell DJ, *et al.* (1992) Cotard delusion after brain injury. *Psychol Med* **22**: 799–804.

13

Headache. The post-concussional syndrome

Robert Macfarlane

Post-traumatic headache

Introduction

There is a period after head injury when headache, amongst other symptoms, should be regarded as part of the normal recovery process (Jennett and Teasdale, 1981). Following concussion on the rugby field, 60% of players will experience transient head pain (Cook, 1969). Patients with minor concussion are at least as likely to suffer post-traumatic headache as those with more severe injury; the trauma need not even involve the cranium. Both Balla and Moraitis (1970) and Parker (1977) have noted that chronic headache is prevalent in trauma victims who have not sustained injury to the head.

There are many reasons why headache may persist. Organic pathology such as hydrocephalus or chronic subdural haematoma is responsible occasionally, while an element of subarachnoid haemorrhage is almost inevitable after moderate or severe head trauma (Jennett and Teasdale, 1981). Other causes include occipital neuralgia or the precipitation of migraine in sensitive subjects (Guthkelch, 1977). However, the cause of persisting headache remains obscure in the great majority of patients, and considerable debate exists about whether the cause is organic or functional. Headache is accompanied frequently by other symptoms such as impaired concentration or memory, dizziness, fatigue and irritability. The conjunction of these symptoms has been labelled the post-traumatic or postconcussional syndrome. Because headache is the most consistent and troublesome feature, it will be dealt with separately.

Definitions

Post-traumatic syndrome

Late symptoms of head injury, including headache, subjective disorders of movement (dizziness and vertigo), nervousness, irritability, inability to concentrate, impaired memory, excessive tiredness, insomnia and intolerance of alcohol (Bakay and Glasauer, 1980).

Headache

The Headache Classification Committee of the International Headache Society (1988) has characterized all types of headache; brief definitions follow.

Acute post-traumatic headache

Headache develops within 14 days of regaining consciousness (or after trauma in the absence of loss of consciousness), and disappears within eight weeks of onset.

Chronic post-traumatic headache

Headache occurs within 14 days of the injury (or after trauma if there has been no loss of consciousness), and continues for more than eight weeks.

Migraine

There are several subforms of migraine; strict criteria are applied to the definition of each. For full details see the Headache Classification Committee (1988). Brief descriptions of the two most common subtypes are as follows:

1. *Common migraine* (migraine without aura; hemicrania simplex) There are at least five attacks of headache, each lasting for between four and 72 hours, and comprising two or more of the following characteristics: unilateral, pulsating, of moderate to severe intensity (i.e. inhibiting or preventing daily activity), and aggravated by physical effort; the headache should be accompanied either by nausea/vomiting or photophobia/noise intolerance.
2. *Classical migraine* (migraine with aura) There are at least two attacks, comprising fully reversible aura symptoms, indicating a cortical or brain stem disorder. Symptoms develop generally over more than four minutes but last usually less than one hour. Headache, nausea and/or photophobia usually follow within 60 minutes, but may be absent.

Occipital neuralgia

Paroxysmal 'jabbing' pain in the distribution of the greater or lesser occipital nerves, accompanied by diminished sensation or dysaesthesia in the affected area. Commonly there is associated tenderness on palpation over the nerve.

Tension headache

Recurrent episodes of tension headache last from between 30 minutes to seven days. They are frequently described as pressing or tightening, and are usually of a mild to moderate intensity (i.e. inhibiting but not preventing daily activity). Typically the pain is bilateral and is not aggravated by physical activity. There is no nausea, but photophobia or noise intolerance may be present. Tension headache is described as episodic if the frequency averages less than 15 headaches per month or 180 per year, and chronic if it averages more than this for at least six months.

Epidemiology

Estimates of the prevalence of post-traumatic headache are very variable. They depend not only on the method by which patients are selected for study but on injury severity and the time that has elapsed from its occurrence. Another important aspect is that many patients will admit to symptoms only when asked specifically. Of 200 subjects investigated by Tubbs and Potter (1970), 11% complained spontaneously of headache, but a further 30% admitted to head pain when questioned directly. The incidence of headache in series reported between 1932 and 1970 ranged from 28% to 100% (Cartlidge and Shaw, 1981).

Injury severity

The incidence of acute post-traumatic headache appears to be relatively independent of the severity of the trauma. Russell (1932) noted that headache developed during hospital admission in 56% of patients in whom the duration of post-traumatic amnesia (PTA) was less than one hour, in 56% of those with PTA of 1–24 hours, and in 60% of those with PTA of greater than 24 hours. Guttmann (1943) reported very similar data for the first two groups, but found a 41% incidence of headache in patients with PTA of 24 hours or greater, and only 18% for those with PTA lasting seven days or longer. Others have also noted an apparently inverse relationship between length of PTA and headache (Cartlidge and Shaw, 1981; Jensen and Nielsen, 1990). Landy (1968) recorded that post-traumatic headache was almost six times more common in patients who had not suffered loss of consciousness than it was in those with PTA of more than 72 hours. Around 10% of adults and 7% of children who sustain only subconcussive trauma will still complain of headache one to two months later (Brenner *et al.*, 1944; Casey *et al.*, 1986).

Chronic headache is also more common in patients who suffer concussion than in those who sustain brain damage (Kay *et al.*, 1971). Jennett and Teasdale (1981) postulated that the relative immunity conferred by severe head injury occurs because the patient is unconscious during the period of meningism caused by traumatic subarachnoid haemorrhage, and that little is expected of these patients during their prolonged recovery period. The patient with minor concussion, however, may both remember the experience and receive little comfort from reassurance that they were fortunate to have escaped more serious injury. Premorbid personality is another important factor in determining the reaction to injury, particularly if there is a past history of depression (Cartlidge, 1978).

Duration of symptoms

The median duration of symptoms after minor head injury is one week (Lowdon *et al.*, 1989). In a prospective study of 200 patients, Russell (1932) found that 56% experienced headache during their hospital admission and 32% were still afflicted at six months. In another report of 145 minor head injuries, 74% experienced headache 24 hours after the accident, and 25% were symptomatic six weeks later (Rutherford *et al.*, 1977). Residual symptoms at this time were significantly more common in patients with neurological symptoms and signs during the first 24 hours, and were also more frequent in women, those injured in falls, and those in whom accidents had occurred at work. Similar findings have been reported by others (Brenner *et al.*, 1944). Jensen and Nielsen (1990) have also found a significantly higher incidence of chronic headache in women than men 9–12 months after trauma (49% versus 30%), as have Cartlidge and Shaw (1981) (24% versus 15% at one year).

In a prospective study of 372 survivors of head injury who were admitted to a neurosurgery unit (40% with a PTA of <1 hour; 20% with a PTA of 1–12 hours; and 40% with a PTA >12 hours), Cartlidge and Shaw (1981) found that 36% complained of headache on discharge from hospital. This symptom was still present in 27% of the group at six months, in 18% at one year, and in 24% at two years. Of patients with symptoms at discharge, 59% were asymptomatic at six months, but almost half had acquired new symptoms after leaving hospital ('late-acquired' headache). Depression and the pursuit of compensation were more common in the group who acquired new symptoms after discharge than in those who did not (39% versus 12% and 51% versus 24% respectively). Cook (1972) has also observed that patients who pursue litigation for post-traumatic symptoms are more likely to have headache than those who do not seek recompense (85% versus 70% respectively). A possible association between the persistence of symptoms and secondary financial gain is discussed in the section on 'Post-traumatic syndrome'. However, a delay in the onset of headache after injury is found also in children, few of whom are involved in compensation claims. Of 117 children studied for six years after head injury, 23% had residual headache at six months, and 25% at one year (Lanser *et al.*, 1988). A considerable number of patients in the second group had been asymptomatic at six months.

Pre-existing conditions

With the possible exception of migraine, patients with a history of head pains prior to their accident do not appear to have an increased likelihood of developing chronic post-traumatic sequelae. The relative risk of developing chronic symptoms in one recent study was 0.33 in those with and 0.42 in those without a pre-existing history of headache (Jensen and Nielsen, 1990). In addition, there was no significant difference in either the location or the nature of the symptoms experienced. Patients with a previous history of headache did, however, use significantly more analgesic medications. Alcohol ingestion at the time of injury does not correlate with headache outcome (Brenner *et al.*, 1944), but a history of chronic alcohol abuse is associated with an increase in the number of post-traumatic sequelae reported (Carlsson *et al.*, 1987).

Headache after neck injury

It has been suggested that soft tissue injury to the neck and the exacerbation of pre-existing cervical spondylosis are major factors in the genesis of post-traumatic headache (Jacobson, 1969). Balla and Karnaghan (1987) found that approximately 25% of more than 5000 patients developed head pain after whiplash injury. In those, the headache was occipital in 46%, generalized in 34%, and elsewhere in the cranium in the remaining 20%. Of 80 of the group who were the subject of a more detailed analysis, 62% developed headache within one day, and 86% within seven days. However, in some patients, headache does not develop until much later (Winston, 1987). The aetiology of headache after neck injury is thought to be injury to the ligaments and muscles at the occipito-nuchal junction, or irritation of the upper cervical dorsal roots. Experimental studies have demonstrated that subclinical apophyseal joint damage occurs after hyperextension injury to the cervical spine (La Rocca, 1978).

The head pain that follows neck injury is present most commonly either on waking, or develops during the morning (Balla and Karnaghan, 1987). The headache is usually constant and, in around 40% of patients, occurs more frequently than once per week. Personality trait, psychosocial factors, and affect are said not to predict the outcome of this type of headache (Radanov *et al.*, 1991).

Weiss *et al.* (1991) have collected seven patients with common or classic migraine, and Jacome

(1986) four of basilar migraine that developed after neck injury. Vijayan and Dreyfus (1975) have described in five patients a syndrome of intermittent severe throbbing unilateral headache associated with ipsilateral mydriasis and excessive sweating, which followed injury to the soft tissues of the neck in the region of the carotid sheath ('post-traumatic dysautonomic cephalgia'). Incomplete meiosis and ptosis developed after the headache, as well as pharmacological evidence of partial sympathetic denervation. Symptoms were ergotamine resistant, but responded promptly to propranolol.

Headache and depression

From their large prospective study, Cartlidge and Shaw (1981) have concluded that depression is an important cause of late post-traumatic headache. However, the converse is also true. Patients with minor head injury are at increased risk of developing depression when compared with controls (Merskey and Woodforde, 1972; Schoenhuber and Gentilini, 1988). It is common for patients and their families to become demoralized by both the severity of symptoms and their slow resolution. In a review of 117 patients with post-traumatic headache who were attending a headache centre at an average of 40 months after injury, 52% complained of depression, and 58% of anxiety (Barnat, 1986).

Clinical assessment

The type of pain experienced is no different whether it occurs as a solitary symptom, or as part of the post-traumatic syndrome. Tension headache is thought to account for about 85% of post-traumatic head pain, with most of the remainder being the result of neck injury, occipital neuralgia, migraine, cluster headache or injury to the temporomandibular joint (Mandel, 1989). The frequency of attacks is very variable. Jensen and Nielsen (1990) reported that around 68% experienced symptoms more than once per week, and the remainder between one and four times per month. There are few descriptions of the symptoms experienced in acute traumatic headache (Haas, 1993a). Although symptoms in the case of minor head injuries often begin either immediately or within 24 hours of injury, cluster and tension headache in particular may not develop until much later. Patients with

more severe head injury usually complain of headache as they recover (Elkind, 1989a). Headache may be generalized, polar or confined to the site of injury. Often it is exacerbated by effort, fatigue, or sudden changes in posture (Brenner *et al.*, 1944). Chronic post-traumatic headache is usually bilateral, and described as aching or throbbing. Pain is often intensified by physical or cognitive activity.

Migraine

Several papers have reported classical migraine occurring immediately after blows to the head, often in children or young adults. Such attacks may occur after very minor head trauma and at no other times (traumatic migraine) (Matthews, 1972), or more severe injury may initiate attacks of migraine, which then recur in the absence of further insults (post-traumatic migraine) (Lucas, 1972). Guthkelch (1977) studied 13 children and adolescents who suffered secondary deterioration after minor head injury, and found that 33% had a previous history of migraine and 77% a positive family history. The incidence of post-traumatic migraine in children has been estimated variously at 2–4% (Guthkelch, 1977; Snoek *et al.*, 1984). Migraine can also be precipitated by minor head trauma or whiplash injury in adults, and may occur with or without an aura. In addition, many will also suffer generalized head pain similar to that of chronic tension headache (Weiss *et al.*, 1991). Acute post-traumatic migraine usually begins within 10 minutes of impact (Haas, 1993a), whilst recurrent classical migraine may develop either within a few hours of head injury or up to 10 weeks later (Behrman, 1977). Although some authors have found an equal sex incidence for post-traumatic migraine (Behrman, 1977), others have reported a ratio of females to males of more than 3 : 1 (Weiss *et al.*, 1991).

Cluster headache

Cluster headache can also be induced by trauma (Hunter and Mayfield, 1949). The onset is often delayed until weeks or months after injury and, in the case of unilateral head trauma, the cluster is ipsilateral (Manzoni *et al.*, 1983). It is estimated that around 16% of cluster headache sufferers have a preceding history of head trauma (Turkewitz *et al.*, 1992). Like other post-traumatic sequelae, the severity of the impact does not appear to be an issue (Reik, 1987).

Other

Dysaesthesia is common over scalp lacerations, but lasts rarely for more than one year. Evans (1992) has reported patients with post-coital headache precipitated by head trauma.

Aetiology

Speed (1989) has suggested that minor diffuse axonal injury plays a role in the development of intractable headache. However, the great majority of cases occur in the absence of gross structural pathology or notable damage to the scalp or skull. Also, chronic headache does not correlate with the degree of head trauma or with CT or MRI evidence of brain injury (Haas, 1993a,b). Yamaguchi (1992) recently investigated the relationship between headache and the severity of injury in 121 patients, and found a significantly higher incidence of headache in those who sustained a mild injury than in those who suffered a more severe injury (72% versus 33%). In this series, headache also had an inverse relationship to cranial CT or EEG abnormality, but correlated positively with abnormal cervical spine radiographs. The pathological changes that are found in the brain after minor head injury are discussed later.

Kelly (1975) has argued that post-traumatic symptoms are largely iatrogenic and persist if physicians are unsympathetic or provide inadequate treatment. Another aetiological factor may be the patient's perception of the likely sequelae to injury. When 223 healthy volunteers were asked to list the symptoms that they might anticipate after head trauma, and when these were compared with those actually suffered by 100 patients who had been rendered unconscious in car accidents an average of 1.7 years previously, the features described by the two groups were remarkably similar. This prompted Mittenberg *et al.*, (1992) to conclude that the expectation of postconcussional sequelae played a significant role in their genesis.

Measurement of outcome

Many pain scoring systems have been devised to try to measure headache objectively, the best known of which are the visual analogue scale, the numeric rating scale, and the verbal descriptor scale. Other measures include the McGill Pain Questionnaire and the use of headache diaries. Further details can be found in Melzak (1983), and in Brennum and Gracely (1993).

Prognosis

There is an association between the presence of diplopia and anosmia after minor head injury and the likelihood that post-traumatic symptoms will persist for at least six weeks (Rutherford *et al.*, 1977). Brenner *et al.* (1944) have noted a similar link between headache and scalp laceration. The data from Cartlidge and Shaw (1981) suggest that, if headache is present six months after head trauma, it is likely to continue for at least one to two years. Headache was present in 27% at six months, 18% at one year, and 24% at two years. In a report of a series of 100 patients with concussion, from which cases involving litigation or compensation were excluded, Denker (1944) found that headache lasted more than two years in 22% of patients, and more than three years in 20%. Almost all patients with symptoms of more than two years' duration were over the age of 40 years.

Packard (1992) has investigated the question of the permanency of symptoms, which in some parts of the world is a prerequisite for the initiation of a claim for damages. Fifty patients were studied for an average of 23 months after legal settlements. All had been diagnosed as suffering 'permanent' post-traumatic headache on the basis of one of the following: symptoms persisting for more than one year with no evidence of further improvement; or head pain continuing for longer than six months despite adequate treatment and with no change in the pattern of symptoms for at least three months. All patients continued to report persistent symptoms one year or more after legal settlement; in only 8% had some improvement occurred.

Gender also has a bearing on the likelihood of headache chronicity. Cartlidge and Shaw (1981) found that the relative incidence of headache in women compared with men was 1.3 at discharge, 1.5 at one year, and 2.0 at two years. Jacobson (1969) concluded that the majority of minor head-injured patients lost their headaches by two months, and that all who were going to become headache-free had done so by four years. Vascular-type headaches are thought to be more likely to persist than others (Elkind, 1989a), but most instances of traumatic facial pain subside within months to one year (Elkind, 1989b).

Further management

Chronic post-traumatic headache can be difficult to manage (Haas, 1993b). Tyler *et al.* (1980) reported improvement in 21 of 23 patients treated with amitriptyline 75–250 mg daily for prolonged periods. Both Kelly (1975) and Medina (1992) concluded that supportive counselling and education were needed in addition to medication, and that unsympathetic treatment delayed recovery. Weiss *et al.* (1991) reported that post-traumatic migraine was likely to recur for months or years unless diagnosed appropriately, but that the success of therapy was similar to that for the nontraumatic variety. With the use of prophylactic antimigraine medication, they documented improvement in 78% of patients who were still involved with litigation. Post-traumatic cluster headache is said to be more resistant to treatment than its idiopathic counterpart (Evans, 1992). More recently, Medina (1992) reported that polymodal therapy, which included medication, stress education and biofeedback therapy, resulted in sufficient improvement to enable 17 of 20 patients with post-traumatic headache to return to work. Solomon and Guglielmo (1985) have reported improvements in 55% of patients treated with transcutaneous nerve stimulation. A detailed review of the treatment of post-traumatic headache can be found in Evans (1992) and in Haas (1993a,b).

Post-traumatic syndrome

Introduction

In 1866, Sir John Erichsen commented upon a series of railway workers with severe symptoms following trauma, but in whom there was little sign of external injury. He thought that molecular derangement of the spinal cord might be responsible, and the condition became known as 'railway spine'. The term post-traumatic syndrome was introduced later, at a time when it was believed that no organic brain damage was sustained in concussion. Some authors make a distinction between the 'post-traumatic' and the 'post-concussional' syndromes, reserving the latter for patients who suffer loss of consciousness. However, in the context of the medical literature this does not appear to be a useful subdivision, and the term post-traumatic syndrome will be used here throughout.

The many synonyms used to describe the symptoms of headache, dizziness, impaired concentration and memory, fatigue, diplopia, insomnia, depression, loss of libido, poor hearing, hyperacusis and tinnitus reflect the debate about its aetiology. The persistence of multiple vague symptoms after seemingly minor trauma, the lack of clinical findings or radiological abnormalities, and the fact that most patients appear normal outwardly, has led to divergent views regarding the balance between organic and psychological factors. Symonds (1940) observed that, if taken alone, these symptoms were the usual complaints of a neurotic. Post-traumatic syndrome has been described variously as traumatic neuraesthenia, traumatic psychaesthenia, post-traumatic nervous instability, and accident or compensation neurosis (Mapother, 1937; McLaurin and Titchener, 1982; Miller, 1961a; Symonds, 1940, 1962). Some authors have concluded that the consistency of these symptoms after head injury argues for a common pathophysiological basis (Binder, 1986; Kelly, 1981; Miller, 1961a,b). However, others have dismissed the existence of a single clinical entity (Lewin, 1970; Parker, 1977; Rutherford *et al.*, 1979), believing that individual symptoms are not necessarily related. Lewin (1970) has made the observation that 'when a patient with a fractured femur complains of pain in his leg and limps during the first few weeks on his feet, this is not designated as a complication, nor as a post-traumatic syndrome'.

Symptoms

Although it is often claimed that the incidence of post-traumatic syndrome is inversely proportional to the severity of the injury, both Kelly (1975) and McKinlay *et al.* (1983) have detected a significant level of symptoms in patients during the first year after major head trauma. In an evaluation of 131 patients, Rutherford *et al.* (1979) found that 8% complained of headache, 4% of anxiety, and 4% of memory loss one year after minor concussion, while lack of concentration affected 3%, and 2% suffered from insomnia or fatigue. Dizziness is second only to headache in frequency, and is rarely true vertigo. Instead it is precipitated usually by sudden changes in head position, and is associated with a feeling of faintness (Denker, 1944). The time of onset of symptoms in relation to the trauma is highly variable, as is the degree and duration of symptoms. The post-traumatic syndrome is uncommon in children (Jennett, 1972) and is generally better tolerated by younger age groups (Lundar and Nestvold, 1985).

Incidence

Because post traumatic-type symptoms are so common in the general population, Dikmen *et al.* (1986) compared their incidence in 20 mild head injuries and contrasted them against carefully matched controls. Although the study as a whole is of limited medicolegal significance because the comparison was made only one month after injury, nevertheless the high incidence of these symptoms in the general population is of interest; the data are given in Table 13.1. Similarly, behavioural problems are common in children who suffer head injury. Table 13.2 compares their incidence in 321 subconcussive head injuries with those of healthy controls.

Pathophysiology

There is now substantial evidence in the medical literature to refute the notion that minor head injury does not cause organic pathology in the brain. MRI has demonstrated clinically occult contusions and white matter lesions (Yokota *et al.*, 1991). Several experimental studies have demonstrated pathological changes in the brain stem and white matter of animals after subconcussive and minor concussive blows. Brief reviews of this literature can be found in Taylor (1967) and in

Table 13.1 Incidence of postconcussional-type symptoms one month after minor head injury, and in normal controls (adapted from Dikmen *et al.* 1986)

Symptom	Head-injured (%)	Control (%)
Irritability	68	42
Fatigue	68	41
Impaired memory	52	6
Noise intolerance	52	10
Headache	51	38
Impaired concentration	42	21

Table 13.2 Behavioural problems in the first month after subconcussive head injury in 321 children (data adapted from Casey *et al.* 1986; for each age group, the difference between the two groups is statistically significant)

Age (years)	Head injury %	Healthy controls (%)
2–4	25.0	13.1
5–14	27.1	2.7

Kelly (1981). In 1968, Oppenheimer described the histological changes in the brains of trauma victims, some of whom had sustained only mild head injury but who had died from other causes. He observed myelin destruction and retraction bulbs in the tracts between the diencephalon and the lower brain stem, indicative of diffuse axonal injury. Noseworthy and coworkers (1981), investigated auditory evoked brain stem responses (ABR) in 11 patients with the post-syndrome, and in 12 controls. They found a significant delay in wave III in the head-injured group, indicating organic changes as far rostral as the superior olivary complex. However, ABR abnormalities were not diagnostic of post-traumatic syndrome in any individual patient.

There is a high incidence of vestibular dysfunction and of asymmetrical high frequency hearing loss after head trauma; this may explain why dizziness and hyperacusis form such a prominent component of the post-traumatic syndrome. Blurred vision is reported by 14% of patients and is due most often to convergence insufficiency (Minderhoud *et al.*, 1980). Subtle intellectual disorders can be found in minor head injury victims if sought by psychological evaluation (Rimel *et al.*, 1981; Zangwill, 1966). Kelly and Smith (1981) suggest that premorbid personality has an important influence on the development of post-traumatic syndrome. This may make certain individuals, particularly those exhibiting resentment, susceptible to the effects of minor trauma, and to a poor prognosis. Kay *et al.* (1971) compared three groups discharged from a neurosurgical ward: those who had recovered fully or were suffering only a single symptom; those with more than one symptom (post-traumatic syndrome); and those with residual brain damage. They found that the 'post-traumatic' group had a higher incidence of disorders of smell, hearing and vision, or were more likely to have suffered an intracranial haematoma than the group that had recovered. They argued that the post-traumatic syndrome therefore had an organic basis. Unlike some other series, many of their 'brain-injured' group of patients also experienced a significant number of symptoms, particularly headache and dizziness.

Taylor (1967) has concluded that there is no correlation between post-traumatic sequelae and a history of previous psychiatric illness, and has argued against a predominately functional basis for persistent symptoms on the grounds that trauma affects a random sample of the population: 'Prima facie, it seems strange that 66% of the head-injured

... should be afflicted with neuroticism or excessive cupidity while most of the victims of limb, abdominal, or thoracic injury escape these stigmata.'

Symptoms and financial compensation

The existence of a relationship between the chronicity of symptoms and the prospect of secondary gain has been the subject of debate for many years. Regler (1879) was probably the first to detect a rise in the incidence of this syndrome when compensation was introduced to the USA in 1871. However, the recognition of post-traumatic symptoms predated the inauguration of compensation payment by several hundred years (for review see Evans, 1992).

From his experience of 200 head-injured patients on whom he was asked to provide medicolegal reports, Professor Henry Miller (1961a,b) wrote two very influential articles on 'accident neurosis'. He concluded that gross exaggeration of disability and malingering was common and a manifestation of the hope of financial gain rather than a result of the accident. 'The most consistent clinical feature is the subject's unshakeable conviction of unfitness to work.' He ascribed this to lack of social responsibility, and recorded that 41 of 45 patients working prior to their accident had returned to their own or similar employment within two years of financial settlement. He also observed that 'another cardinal feature is an absolute refusal to admit any degree of symptomatic improvement'. His views were supported by the results of a postal questionnaire of 63 patients conducted by Cook (1972), who found that patients seeking compensation were more likely to have symptoms of longer duration, and to return to work later, than those not seeking legal redress (88 versus 24 days). Of patients with minor head injuries who were pursuing compensation, none returned to work within one week. In contrast, 80% of patients with head injury sustained during sporting activities were working within that period. Cartlidge and Shaw (1981) have also concluded that late onset headache is unlikely to have an organic aetiology. They based this on the observation that 83% of patients with late acquired headache were seeking compensation compared with only 20% of those with early onset headache. However, these authors felt that this was largely the result of psychological factors, rather than a deliberate intention to deceive.

Some of these conclusions are, however, open to criticism. Miller followed patients referred to him by insurance companies for medicolegal reports; his series is therefore not representative of head injuries as a whole. Indeed, 50 of the patients were selected for study on the basis of gross neurotic symptoms found at the time of consultation (Miller, 1966). The major criticism of Cook's postal survey is that the response rate was less than 50%, and that patients with persisting symptoms or who were seeking compensation may have been more likely to respond than those who had recovered fully.

Kelly (1981), in contrast, noted that the post-traumatic syndrome occurred frequently when there was no question of compensation, and that the vast majority of patients returned to work before their claim was settled. Other patients remained symptomatic despite the completion of legal proceedings (Kelly and Smith, 1981). Others have concluded that organic brain damage and the psychological response to injury are responsible for the postconcussional syndrome, and that the desire for compensation is not a significant aetiological factor in the majority of cases (Alves and Jane, 1990). Symonds (1962) has been even more forthright, and states that it is questionable whether the effects of concussion, however slight, are ever fully reversible. After eliminating those involved in compensation claims, Russell (1932) found that 32% of patients still suffered chronic headache six months after injury, while dizziness was present in 24%, memory loss affected 20%, and there was 'nervousness' in 20%. McKinlay *et al.* (1983) compared two groups of 21 patients after closed head injury: those seeking and those not seeking financial reward. Although the claimants reported more symptoms than the control group, there was no significant difference in intellectual performance, behavioural changes, or in the time taken to return to work. In addition there was no suggestion that claimants made a concerted effort to appear more disabled than they were. In a study of 500 patients with post-traumatic psychoneurosis (not all the result of head injury), Thompson (1965) concluded that financial settlement had a negligible effect on the course of the illness. Occupation, a delay in settlement, or marital disharmony do not appear to determine whether or not a patient will return to work (Kelly and Smith, 1981). In Mendelson's experience (1982), around 75% of litigants failed to return to work two years after the legal case was resolved. Merskey and Woodforde (1972) compared 10 patients with post-traumatic syndrome who were not seeking compensation with 17 who had already received their settlement, and found that there was little or no difference in outcome between the two groups. Over a median follow-up of four years, 60% of the first group and 65% of the second showed either some improvement or had recovered fully. They suggested that the improvement reported by others after settlement occurred not because there was an element of pretence in the symptoms but because the uncertainty that persists until damages are agreed is harmful in itself.

However, even those who advocate staunchly that post-traumatic syndrome is a genuine illness will acknowledge that some patients malinger or simulate disability in order to enhance a claim for damages (McKinlay *et al.*, 1983). Guthkelch (1980) examined 398 consecutive head injury victims in connection with compensation claims, and labelled 6.8% as cases of 'accident neurosis'. He defined this in terms of bizarre and inconsistent complaints, exaggeration of the duration of the loss of consciousness, and attention-seeking behaviour. Kelly (1981) argues that:

> It is unreasonable to suppose that [because some patients] attempt a fraud on insurance companies, all patients who have suffered a head injury from whom a claim is outstanding and who have post-traumatic syndrome should therefore be labelled as fraudulent.

Haas (1993b) has proposed that post-traumatic headache is not related directly to trauma either to the brain or to other intracranial contents, but is caused by psychological disturbances that are created by the accident and perpetuated subsequently by other factors. These include concerns about the injury sustained or the inability to function satisfactorily at work. Mittenberg *et al.* (1992) contend that children are less likely to develop post-traumatic syndrome than adults 'because they are less able to appreciate the health risks of head trauma, and are therefore less likely to appraise any minor injury as a potential source of persistent symptoms'. Similarly, the incidence of chronic symptoms is low after sporting injuries because participants observe minor trauma repeatedly without obvious persistent ill effects, and have therefore a low expectation of experiencing long-term sequelae. In contrast, Taylor (1967) ascribed the low incidence of post-traumatic syndrome in sportsmen to motivation, and the desire to resume pleasurable activity, even if this involves suffering the inconvenience of headache.

Robertson (1988) has proposed that much of the doubt that exists in the minds of physicians, lawyers and insurance companies regarding the authenticity of post-traumatic sequelae stems from what he calls the 'three stooges model'. He argues that personal experience of the effects of head injury is very small when compared with repeated exposure to Hollywood scenes in which actors depict full recovery within moments of receiving successive violent blows to the head. He believes that, as a result of these images, the public perception of the sequelae of head trauma has been grossly distorted.

Prognosis

Comparison between different series on outcome is difficult because patient populations, definitions and the types of assessment employed vary greatly. However, the probability of suffering persistent symptoms or neuropsychological sequelae is essentially the same whether or not there is a loss of consciousness (Denker, 1944; Leininger *et al.*, 1990), and there is no correlation between the duration of PTA and the time taken to return to work (Wrightson and Gronwall, 1981). Rimel *et al.* (1981, 1982) found that 34% of minor head injuries and 66% of moderate head injuries had not resumed work three months after the event. The socioeconomic status of mild but not moderate head injury victims predicted a delay in regaining employment. By three months, 100% of executives with minor head injuries had returned to work, compared with only 68% of skilled and 57% of unskilled labourers. Older patients returned to work sooner than those in younger age groups. Neuropsychological evidence of organic brain damage and emotional stress caused by persistent symptoms were cited as explanations for the high rate of unemployment. In an unselected series of 488 paediatric head injuries (of which 93% were minor), Lundar and Nestvold (1985) found that 63% of children below the age of 10 years were symptom free three months after injury, this rising to 78% at 12 months and 81% at five years. In contrast, only 29% of children aged 10–14 years were asymptomatic at three months, 57% at 12 months, and 73% at five years. The figures for 15–19 year olds were similar to the 10–14-year age group (26%, 54% and 72% respectively). PTA was not predictive of symptoms at five years, and financial compensation was involved in only two of 28 children with persisting sequelae.

However, some caution must be exercised in making generalizations from reported series. Data are gathered almost always from attendance in emergency rooms. Beautrais *et al.* (1982) have established that families who are experiencing stressful life events are more likely to seek medical attention after accidents; this may introduce bias to the incidence of functional symptoms. A history of previous head injury is said to be a risk factor for both the number and persistence of post-traumatic symptoms (Carlsson *et al.*, 1987), as is multiple trauma (Diken *et al.*, 1986), although the significance of these factors has been disputed by others (Rimel *et al.*, 1982).

In the majority of patients, memory for new information will recover within three months, and cognitive impairment within one year (Dikmen *et al.*, 1986). In Denker's experience, dizziness had a very poor prognosis if it persisted for more than one to two years (Denker, 1944). It lasted less than two years in 82% of patients but, of the remaining 18%, it was still present in all but 2% after three years. Overall, patients of more than 40 years of age were twice as likely to have persistent sequelae as those under the age of 30 years. Although the degree of impairment for information processing speed after head injury is not related to cognitive ability, patients of higher intelligence recover more quickly than those with a lower IQ (Gronwall, 1976). This may represent greater motivation in high achievers. Memory problems affect 19% of patients at one month and 15% at six months (Minderhoud *et al.*, 1980). Other studies have reported a 19% incidence of residual memory problems at four years (Edna and Cappelen, 1987). The risk factors for persisting sequelae are given in Table 13.3. The percentage of patients with symptoms and their duration in one large series can be found in Tables 13.4 and 13.5.

Table 13.3 Risk factors for persisting sequelae after minor head injury

Predictive	Not predictive
Age >40 years	Duration of PTA
Female	Auditory-evoked brain stem responses
Low IQ	CT scan appearance
Low socioeconomic status	
Previous head injury	
Multiple trauma	
History of alcohol abuse	

Table 13.4 Distribution (percentage) of post-traumatic symptoms in adult patients at follow-up (reproduced, with permission, from Alves and Jane, 1990)

No. symptoms	Months from discharge		
	3 (*n* = 542)	6 (*n* = 485)	12 (*n* = 301)
0	33.8	50.3	53.8
1	24.7	23.7	18.3
2	16.4	12.2	12.6
3	10.5	6.0	5.6
4	6.3	4.5	3.7
5+	8.3	3.3	6.0

Conclusion

'It requires an unbiased approach on the part of the physician and a careful assessment of each

Table 13.5 Percentage of head-injured adults with post-traumatic symptoms at discharge and follow-up (reproduced, with permission, from Alves and Jane, 1990)

Symptom		Months from discharge		
	At discharge (*n* = 847)	3 (*n* = 542)	6 (*n* = 485)	12 (*n* = 301)
Headache	45.8	41.1	29.9	29.2
Dizziness	14.2	25.4	13.6	13.0
Memory problems	13.0	23.4	17.3	21.3
Weakness	10.4	15.0	7.8	8.3
Nausea	7.9	9.2	4.5	6.3
Numbness	5.8	14.7	9.1	8.6
Diplopia	4.7	9.0	3.7	5.6
Tinnitus	2.2	13.0	9.3	10.3
Hearing problems	2.0	11.2	9.3	7.0

patient's personality and his or her headache pattern to ensure that justice is done to any legal claim' (Lance, 1993). Despite Miller's treatise on accident neurosis (Miller, 1961a,b), it is difficult to disagree with the conclusion that there is no justification for a medical practitioner to state that it is well known for litigants to lose their symptoms and return to work shortly after legal settlement (Kelly, 1981).

References

Alves WM, Jane JA. (1990) Post-traumatic syndrome. In: Youmans JR, editor. *Neurological Surgery*, 3rd edition. Philadelphia: Saunders, 2230–42.

Bakay L, Glasauer FE. (1980) *Head Injury*. Boston: Little, Brown, 385–88.

Balla J, Karnaghan J. (1987) Whiplash headache. *Clin Exp Neurol* 23: 179–82.

Balla JI, Moraitis S. (1970) Knights in armour. A follow-up study of injuries after legal settlement. *Med J Aust* 2: 355–61.

Barnat MR. (1986) Post-traumatic headache patients: I. Demographics, injuries, headache and health status. *Headache* 26: 271–77.

Beautrais AL, Fergusson DM, Shannon FT. (1982) Life events and childhood morbidity: a prospective study. *Pediatrics* 70: 935–40.

Behrman S. (1977) Migraine as a sequela of blunt head injury. *Injury* 9: 74–76.

Binder LM. (1986) Persisting symptoms after mild head injury: a review of the postconcussive syndrome. *J Clin Exp Neuropsychol* 8: 323–46.

Brenner C, Friedman AP, Merritt HH, Denny-Brown DE. (1944) Post-traumatic headache. *J Neurosurg* 1: 379–91.

Brennum J, Gracely RH. (1993) Measurement of clinical and experimental head pain. In: Olesen J, Tfelt-Hansen P, Welch KMA editors. *The Headaches*. New York: Raven Press, 105–109.

Carlsson GS, Svardsudd K, Welin L. (1987) Long-term effects of head injuries sustained during life in three male populations. *J Neurosurg* 67 197–205.

Cartlidge NEF. (1978) Post-concussional syndrome. *Scott Med J* 23: 103.

Cartlidge NEF, Shaw DA. (1981) *Head Injury*. London: Saunders.

Casey R, Ludwig S, McCormick MC. (1986) Morbidity following minor head trauma in children. *Pediatrics* 78: 497–502.

Cook JB. (1969) The effects of minor head injuries sustained in sport and the postconcussional syndrome. In: Walker AE, Caveness WF, Critchley M, editors. *The late effects of head injury*. Springfield, IL: Charles C Thomas, 408–13.

Cook JB. (1972) The post-concussional syndrome and factors influencing recovery after minor head injury admitted to hospital. *Scand J Rehabil Med* 4: 27–30.

Denker PG. (1944) The postconcussion syndrome: prognosis and evaluation of the organic factors. *N Y State J Med* 44: 379–84.

Dikmen S, McLean A, Temkin N. (1986) Neuropsychological and psychosocial consequences of minor head injury. *J Neurol Neurosurg Psychiatry*, 49: 1227–32.

Edna T-H, Cappelen J. (1987) Late post-concussional symptoms in traumatic head injury. An analysis of frequency and risk factors. *Acta Neurochir (Wien)* 86: 12–17.

Elkind AH. (1989a) Headache and head trauma. *Clin J Pain* 5: 77–87.

Elkind AH. (1989b) Headache and facial pain associated with head injury. *Otolaryngol Clin North Am* 22: 1251–71.

Erichsen JE. (1866) *On railway and other injuries of the nervous system*. London: Walton and Maberly. Cited in Parker N. (1977) Accident litigants with neurotic symptoms. *Med J Aust* 2: 318–22.

Evans RW. (1992) The postconcussion syndrome and the sequelae of mild head injury. *Neurol Clin North Am* 10: 815–47.

Gronwall D. (1976) Performance changes during recovery from closed head injury. *Proc Assoc Neurol* 13: 143–47.

Guthkelch AN. (1977) Benign post-traumatic encephalopathy in young people and its relation to migraine. *Neurosurgery* 1: 101–105.

Guthkelch AN. (1980) Post-traumatic amnesia, post-concussional symptoms and accident neurosis. *Eur Neurol* 19: 91–102.

Guttmann E. (1943) Postcontusional headache. *Lancet* i: 10–12.

Haas DC. (1993a) Acute posttraumatic headache. In: Olesen J, Tfelt-Hansen P, Welch KMA, editors. *The Headaches*. New York: Raven Press, 623–27.

Haas DC. (1993b) Chronic posttraumatic headache. In: Olesen J, Tfelt-Hansen P, Welch KMA editors. *The Headaches*. New York: Raven Press, 628–37.

Headache Classification Committee of the International Headache Society. (1988) Classification and diagnostic criteria for headache disorders, cranial neuralgias and facial pain. *Cephalgia* 8(suppl 7): 1–96.

Hunter CR, Mayfield FH. (1949) Role of the upper cervical roots in the production of pain in the head. *Am J Surg* 78: 743–51.

Jacobson SA. (1969) Mechanisms of the sequelae of minor craniocervical trauma. In: Walker A, Caveness WF, Critchley M, editors. *Late effects of head injury*. Springfield, IL: Charles C Thomas, 35–45.

Jacome DE. (1986) Basilar artery migraine after uncomplicated whiplash injuries. *Headache* 26: 515–16.

Jennett B. (1972) Head injuries in children. *Dev Med Child Neurol* 14: 137–47.

Jennett B, Teadsale G. (1981) *Management of head injuries*. Philadelphia: Davis.

Jensen OK, Nielsen FF. (1990) The influence of sex and pre-traumatic headache on the incidence and severity of headache after head injury. *Cephalgia* 10: 285–93.

Kay DWK, Kerr TA, Lassman LP. (1971) Brain trauma and postconcussional syndrome. *Lancet* ii: 1052–55.

Kelly R. (1975) The post-traumatic syndrome: an iatrogenic disease. *Forensic Sci* 6: 17–24.

Kelly R. (1981) The post-traumatic syndrome. *J R Soc Med* **74**: 242–45.

Kelly R, Smith BN. (1981) Post-traumatic syndrome: another myth discredited. *J R Soc Med* **74**: 275–77.

La Rocca H. (1978) Acceleration injuries of the neck. *Clin Neurosurg* **25**: 209–17.

Lance JW. (1993) *Mechanism and management of headache*, 5th edition. Oxford: Butterworth Heinemann, 206–13.

Landy PJ. (1968) The post-traumatic syndrome in closed head injuries accident neurosis. *Proc Aust Assoc Neurol* **5**: 463–66.

Lanser JBK, Jennekens-Schinkel A, Peters ACB. (1988) Headache after closed head injury in children. *Headache* **28**: 176–79.

Leininger BE, Gramling SE, Farrel AD, Kreutzer JS, Peck EA III. (1990) Neuropsychological deficits in symptomatic minor head injury patients after concussion and mild concussion. *J Neurol Neurosurg Psychiatry* **53**: 293–96.

Lewin W. (1970) Rehabilitation needs to the brain-injured patient. *Proc R Soc Med* **63**: 28–32.

Lowdon IMR, Briggs M, Cockin J. (1989) Post-concussional symptoms following minor head injury. *Injury* **20**: 193–94.

Lucas RN. (1972) Footballer's migraine [letter]. *Br Med J* **ii**: 526.

Lundar T, Nestvold K. (1985) Pediatric head injuries caused by traffic accidents. A prospective study with 5-year follow-up. *Childs Nerv Syst* **1**: 24–28.

Mandel S. (1989) Minor head injury may not be 'minor'. *Postgrad Med* **85**: 213–25.

Manzoni GC, Terzano MG, Bono G, Micieli G, Martucci N, Nappi G. (1983) Cluster headache – clinical findings in 180 patients. *Cephalgia* **3**: 21–30.

Mapother E. (1937) Mental symptoms associated with head injury. The psychiatric aspect. *Br Med J* 1055–61.

Matthews WB. (1972) Footballer's migraine. *Br Med J* **ii**: 326–27.

McKinlay WW, Brooks DN, Bond MR. (1983) Post-concussional symptoms, financial compensation and outcome of severe blunt head injury. *J Neurol Neurosurg Psychiatry* **46**: 1084–91.

McLaurin RL, Titchener JL. (1982) Post-traumatic syndrome. In: Youmans JR, editor. *Neurological Surgery*, vol. 4, 2nd edition. Philadelphia: Saunders, 2175–87.

Medina JL. (1992) Efficacy of an individualized outpatient program in the treatment of post-traumatic headache. *Headache* **32**: 180–83.

Melzak R. (1983) *Pain measurement and assessment*. New York: Raven Press.

Mendelson G. (1982) Not 'cured by a verdict'. Effect of legal settlement on compensation claimants. *Med J Aust* **2**: 132–34.

Merskey H, Woodforde JM. (1972) Psychiatric sequelae of minor head injury. *Brain* **95**: 521–28.

Miller H. (1961a) Accident neurosis. Lecture I. *Br Med J* **i**: 919–25.

Miller H. (1961b) Accident neurosis. Lecture II. *Br Med J* **i**: 992–98.

Miller H. (1966) Mental after-effects of head injury. *Proc R Soc Med* **59**: 257–61.

Minderhoud JM, Baelens MEM, Huizenga JL, Saan RJ. (1980) Treatment of minor head injuries. *Clin Neurol Neurosurg* **82**: 127–40.

Mittenberg W, DiGiulio DV, Perrin S, Bass AE. (1992) Symptoms following mild head injury: expectation as aetiology. *J Neurol Neurosurg Psychiatry* **55**: 200–204.

Noseworthy JH, Miller J, Murray TJ, Regan D. (1981) Auditory brainstem responses in postconcussion syndrome. *Arch Neurol* **38**: 275–78.

Oppenheimer DR. (1968) Microscopic lesions in the brain following head injury. *J Neurol Neurosurg Psychiatry* **31**: 299–306.

Packard RC. (1992) Posttraumatic headache: permanency and relationship to legal settlement. *Headache* **32**: 496–500.

Parker N. (1977) Accident litigants with neurotic symptoms. *Med J Aust* **2**: 318–22.

Radanov BP, di Stefano G, Schnidrig A, Ballarini P. (1991) Role of psychosocial stress in recovery from common whiplash. *Lancet* **338**: 712–15.

Regler J. (1879) Uber die Folgen der Verletzung auf Eisenbahnen. Berlin: Reimer. Cited in: Taylor AR. (1967) Post-concussional sequelae. *Br Med J* **3**: 67–71.

Reik L. (1987) Cluster headache after head injury. *Headache* **27**; 509–10.

Rimel RW, Giordani B, Barth JT, Boll TJ, Jane JA. (1981) Disability caused by minor head injury. *Neurosurgery* **9**: 221–28.

Rimel RW, Giordani B, Barth JT, Jane JA. (1982) Moderate head injury: completing the clinical spectrum of brain trauma. *Neurosurgery* **11**: 344–51.

Robertson A. (1988) The post-concussional syndrome then and now. *Aust N Z J Psychiatry* **22**: 396–402.

Russell WR. (1932) Cerebral involvement in head injury. A study based on the examination of two hundred cases. *Brain* **55**: 549–603.

Rutherford WH, Merrett JD, McDonald JR. (1977) Sequelae of concussion caused by minor head injuries. *Lancet* **i**: 1–4.

Rutherford WH, Merrett JD, McDonald JR. (1979) Symptoms at one year following concussion from minor head injuries. *Injury* **10**: 225–30.

Schoenhuber R, Gentilini M. (1988) Anxiety and depression after mild head injury: a case control study. *J Neurol Neurosurg Psychiatry* **51**: 722–24.

Snoek JW, Minderhoud JM, Wilmink JT. (1984) Delayed deterioration following mild head injury in children. *Brain* **107**: 15–36.

Solomon S, Guglielmo KM. (1985) Treatment of headache by transcutaneous electrical stimulation. *Headache* **25**: 12–15.

Speed WG. (1989) Closed head injury sequelae: changing concepts. *Headache* **29**: 643–47.

Symonds C. (1940) Concussion and confusion of the brain and their sequelae In: Brock S, editor. *Injuries to the skull, brain and spinal cord*. Baltimore: Williams & Wilkins, 65–103.

Symonds C. (1962) Concussion and its sequelae. *Lancet* **i**: 1–5.

Taylor AR. (1967) Post-concussional sequelae. *Br Med J* **iii**: 67–71.

Thompson GN. (1965) Post-traumatic psychoneurosis: a statistical survey. *Am J Psychiatry* **121**: 1043–48.

Tubbs ON, Potter JM. (1970) Early post-concussional headache. *Lancet* **ii**: 128–29.

Turkewitz LJ, Wirth O, Dawson GA, Casaly GS. (1992) Cluster headache following head injury: a case report and review of the literature. *Headache* **32**: 504–506.

Tyler GS, McNeely HE, Dick ML. (1980) Treatment of posttraumatic headache with amitriptyline. *Headache* **20**: 213–16.

Vijayan N, Dreyfus PM. (1975) Posttraumatic dysautonomic cephalgia. Clinical observations and treatment. *Arch Neurol* **32**: 649–52.

Weiss HD, Stern BJ, Goldberg J. (1991) Post-traumatic migraine: chronic migraine precipitated by minor head or neck trauma. *Headache* **31**: 451–56.

Winston KR. (1987) Whiplash and its relationship to migraine. *Headache* **27**: 452–57.

Wrightson P, Gronwall D. (1981) Time off work and symptoms after minor head injury. *Injury* **12**: 445–54.

Yamaguchi M. (1992) Incidence of headache and severity of head injury. *Headache* **32**: 427–31.

Yokota H, Kurokawa A, Otsuka T, Kobayashi S, Nakazawa S. (1991) Significance of magnetic resonance imaging in acute head injury. *J Trauma* **31**: 351–57.

Zangwill OL. (1966) Comment on paper by Lishman WA: Psychiatric disability after head injury. The significance of brain damage. *Proc R Soc Med* **59**: 266.

14

Hypothalamic and pituitary dysfunction

O M Edwards, J D A Clark

Introduction

Documented post-traumatic hypopituitarism is rare, with only 47 cases being reported over the past 80 years, the majority occurring in the last 20 years (Edwards and Clark, 1986). However, in our study and review of the literature, we have been able to collect a further six cases over a relatively short period of time, suggesting that the complication is more frequent than had been supposed and reported. In contrast, severe injury to the hypothalamus and pituitary is a common pathological finding after fatal head injury (Ceballos, 1966; Crompton, 1971; Daniel *et al.*, 1959; Harper *et al.*, 1986; Kornblum and Fisher, 1969; Treip, 1970). Furthermore, the neuropathologist Cecil Treip, commenting on the cause of death in patients with hypothalamic and pituitary damage following head injury, suggested that in some cases 'the brain was too good to die'. These questions were addressed in a prospective study funded by the Medical Research Council into the effect of major head injury on hypothalamo–pituitary function in 60 consecutive patients admitted to our neurosurgical unit.

On admission these patients were assessed using the Glasgow Coma Scale and given sequential boluses of growth hormone release hormone, corticotrophin release hormone, thyrotrophin release hormone (TRH) and gonadotrophin release hormone. Blood was assayed for testosterone (in the male), oestradiol 17-beta (female), prolactin, thyroid stimulating hormone (TSH), leuteinizing hormone (LH), follicle stimulating hormone (FSH), growth hormone (GH) and cortisol. Fluid balance was also assessed to determine the development of diabetes insipidus (DI). These tests were performed on three occasions: on admission or as close as possible, at two weeks following admission, and at three months following the head injury. Pathological studies were carried out on the hypothalami and pituitaries of patients who died.

Definitions

Post-traumatic hypopituitarism is defined as the dysfunction of the anterior pituitary gland after an injury, usually to the head.

Post-traumatic diabetes insipidus is defined as diabetes insipidus, either transient or permanent, following head injury.

Epidemiology

The first case of hypothalamic or pituitary dysfunction following trauma was reported by a German physician, Cyran, in 1918. This was a railway worker who had sustained a skull fracture when his head was trapped between a reversing wagon and the buffers. Surprisingly, he survived the initial injury but subsequently developed loss of secondary sexual characteristics and hypothyroidism, presumed to be of pituitary origin.

Further cases were reported sporadically until an apparent recent upsurge. This may be due to several factors, including the increasing incidence of road traffic accidents, prolonged survival with improved intensive care, and an increased awareness of the condition. The six patients we identified make a total of 53 reported cases in the world literature (Table 14.1).

Table 14.1. Reported cases of post-traumatic hypopituitarism

Patient no.	Author(s)	Sex	Age at diagnosis (years)	Age at injury (years)	Trauma	Duration of coma	Skull fracture	Diabetes insipidus	Neurological sequelae
1	Cyran, 1918	M	48	32	Work injury	Unknown	Base	No	CN V
2	Reverchon and Worms, 1921	M	34	34	RTA	9 h	Base (sella)	Yes	CN V, VI, VII
3	Pascheff, 1922	M	–	–	Explosion	Unknown	Base	Temp.	CN I, II, III
4	Schereschewsky, 1927	M	28	26	Fall	2 h	No	Yes	No
5	Gross, 1940	F	27	25	Fall	3 days	No	No	CN I
6	Escamilla and Lisser, 1942	M	20	19	RTA	5 weeks	Yes	Yes	CN II, VII
7	Lerman and Means, 1945	M	46	15	Bullet	Several days	Bullet → fossa	No	Seizures
8	Lerman and Means, 1945	M	48	22	Explosion	Unknown	Unknown	No	Seizures
9	Porter and Miller, 1948	M	34	34	RTA	Several days	No	Yes	CN II
10	McCullagh and Schaffenberg, 1953	M	25	22	RTA	2 weeks	Frontotemporal	No	CN V, VI, VII
11	Lafon et al., 1955	F	33	33	Unknown	12 days	unknown	No	No
12	Witter and Tascher, 1957	M	37	37	Blunt trauma	Several days	Occipital + base	Temp.	CN I + hemianaesthesia
13	Witter and Tascher, 1957	M	43	43	Blunt trauma	Several days	Base	Temp.	CN I + hemiparesis
14	Witter and Tascher, 1957	F	48	48	Blunt trauma	Momentary	No	No	CN I
15	Goldman and Jacobs, 1960	F	22	15	RTA	Momentary	No	Yes	No
16	Werner, 1960	M	29	13	Bullet	1 week	Bullet → fossa	No	CN II
17	Altman and Pruzanski, 1961	M	68	63	RTA	No	Frontotemporal	No	CN II, VII
18	Linquette et al., 1968	M	27	26	Bullet	Unknown	Bullet → fossa	No	CN II, III
19	Klachko et al., 1968	M	39	4	RTA	11 days	Base	Yes	CN II + hemiparesis
20	Durand et al., 1969	M	62	60	Bullet	No	Bullet → fossa	No	CN II

21	Pittman et al., 1971	M	19	12	Blunt trauma	1 min	Unknown	Yes	No
22	Kanayama et al., 1972	M	46	20	Work injury	33 days	Unknown	No	No
23	Woolf and Schalch, 1973	F	21	20	RTA	Several h	Base	No	No
24	Bevilacqua and Fornaciari, 1975	M	17	15	RTA	Unknown	No	Yes	No
25	Paxson and Brown, 1976	F	14	13	RTA	5 days	Temporal	Temp.	CN III
26	Dzur and Winternitz, 1976	F	30	26	RTA	Several days	No	Temp.	No
27	Girard and Marelli, 1977	M	9	3	RTA	Several days	Yes	No	No
28	Weiss et al., 1977	F	22	20	RTA	Unknown	Facial	No	CN II, VII
29	Kanade et al., 1978	M	27	27	RTA	Unknown	Multiple (sella)	Yes	CN II, III
30	Landau et al., 1978	M	32	32	RTA	Several days	Base	Temp.	CN II, VI
31	Prosperi et al., 1978	M	12	12	Unknown	Momentary	Frontal	Yes	CN II, VI
32	Soules and Sheldon, 1979	F	23	23	Parachute	30 min	Sella	No	No
33	Salti et al., 1979	M	32	32	Bullet	2 days	Bullet → fossa	No	CN I, II, VII
34	Miller et al., 1980	F	11	4/52[a]	Child abuse	Unknown	Unknown	No	Hemiparesis
35	Miller et al., 1980	M	11	5/52[a]	Child abuse	Unknown	Parietal	No	Quadriplegia
36	Miller et al., 1980	M	7	10/52[a]	Child abuse	Unknown	Unknown	No	Hemiparesis
37	Jambart et al., 1980	M	23	18	RTA	3 h	No	No	No
38	Notman et al., 1980	M	24	24	Blunt trauma	No	Temporal + base	Yes	CN V, VII, VIII, IX, X
39	Valenta and DeFeo, 1980	F	16	15	RTA	Unknown	Yes	No	No
40	Valenta and Defeo, 1980	M	21	20	RTA	Unknown	Yes	No	CN II, VII
41	Pere et al., 1980	M	43	43	Work injury	Several h	Base (sella)	Temp.	No
42	Pere et al., 1980	M	49	27	Fall	Several days	Unknown	No	CN VI, VII
43	Bistritzer et al., 1966	M	18	16	Fall	Several days	Base	No	CN II + Hemiparesis
44	Jambart et al., 1981	M	45	45	RTA	Several h	No	No	CN II

Table 14.1. (Continued)

Patient no.	Author(s)	Sex	Age at diagnosis (years)	Age at injury (years)	Trauma	Duration of coma	Skull fracture	Diabetes insipidus	Neurological sequelae
45	Kaufman, 1981	M	20	20	RTA	1 week	Frontal	Yes	No
46	Fernandez-Castener et al., 1982	M	20	18	RTA	Unknown	No	Temp.	No
47	Gomez-Saez et al. 1982	M	27	27	RTA	13 days	Multiple (sella)	No	No
48	Edwards and Clark, 1986	F	16	16	RTA	3 weeks	No	Yes	CN II
49	Edwards and Clark, 1986	M	35	35	RTA	4 weeks	Frontal	Yes	No
50	Edwards and Clark, 1986	M	19	19	RTA	4 weeks	Frontal	No	CN II
51	Edwards and Clark, 1986	M	48	47	RTA	24 h	Base (sella)	No	CN I, IV, VI + quadriplegia
52	Edwards and Clark, 1986	M	21	18	RTA	No	Temporofrontal	No	No
53	Edwards and Clark, 1986	F	58	14	Shrapnel	Unknown	Shrapnel → fossa	Temp.	No

RTA, road traffic accident; CN, cranial nerve.
[a] Age in weeks.

Examination of these cases reveals that post-traumatic hypopituitarism occurs mainly in young males, reflecting the high prevalence of death due to trauma in this age group. The most frequent cause of the head injury was a road traffic accident. These were responsible for 27 of the 53 injuries (Table 14.1). Occasional cases have been reported after falls (Bistritzer *et al.*, 1966; Gross, 1940; Pere *et al.*, 1980; Schereschewsky, 1927) work accidents (Cyran, 1918; Kanayama *et al.*, 1972; Pere *et al.*, 1980), direct bullet and shrapnel injury to the pituitary region (Durand *et al.*, 1969; Lerman and Means, 1945; Linquette *et al.*, 1968; Salti *et al.*, 1979; Werner, 1960; and our patient 6), blunt trauma (Notman *et al.*, 1980; Pittman *et al.*, 1971; Witter and Tascher, 1957), bomb and blast injuries (Lerman and Means, 1945; Pascheff, 1922) and child abuse (Miller *et al.*, 1980). The injury is usually to the head, the only exception to this being a patient who landed feet first on soft earth, after her parachute failed to open (Soules and Sheldon, 1979). A postal survey of British endocrinologists has revealed that there is considerable under-reporting of these patients in the literature and indicated that many were identified only after the development of DI.

DI has long been recognized as a complication of head injury (Rowntree, 1924). It is said to be the most common hypothalamic disorder following trauma (Porter and Miller, 1948). However, the two largest studies have reported a low incidence, with four cases out of 2500 head-injured subjects in Pickles' (1947) series and 13 out of 5000 nonfatal closed head injuries in the study of Porter and Miller (1948). The incidence in our study of 60 subjects was two of 48 survivors, which is 15–25 times greater than that reported previously. This substantial apparent increase in reported incidence may have occurred because, since the two large studies were reported 40 years ago, there have been considerable advances in intensive care therapy, and hence in the number of severely head-injured subjects, who are more likely to develop DI (Porter and Miller, 1948; Verbalis *et al.*, 1985). It may also be due to a better recognition of the complication because of an increased awareness. There have been no previous studies of DI complicating fatal head injury. The high incidence in our study (five of 12 patients, confirms its association with severe injury.

The onset of DI in our subjects varied between 12 hours and five days after injury. This is similar to previous studies. The onset was abrupt in each subject and none had the rare triphasic pattern (Verbalis *et al.*, 1985) in which an initial phase of DI is followed by a transient antidiuretic phase before the eventual return of DI.

Anterior pituitary dysfunction has been reported in association with DI but its frequency is uncertain. Barreca *et al.* (1980) reported defective anterior pituitary hormone secretion in eight of 10 subjects; GH and TSH were the most commonly involved. Verbalis *et al.* (1985) observed deficient TSH and ACTH secretion in 40% and 36% of subjects respectively. However, neither study states how the hormone response was deemed to be deficient and the number of patients that actually required replacement therapy is not recorded. In contrast, Porter and Miller (1948) observed 1 patient with anterior pituitary insufficiency out of 18 subjects with DI, and Notman *et al.* (1980) reported one subject with hypopituitarism out of 10 cases. Neither of our survivors with DI had evidence of anterior pituitary dysfunction, although both had an elevated prolactin (PRL) level. This occurred shortly after injury and was probably due to the stress response rather than to hypothalamic damage, as their PRL levels were subsequently normal. However, subnormal hormone responses to stimulation with hypothalamic releasing factors were found in four of five patients with DI who subsequently died. The abnormal response was presumably a consequence of their more severe injuries. Thus, DI was a relatively frequent occurrence in patients who subsequently died, but was infrequent in the survivors.

Structural pathology

Pathological changes in the hypothalamus and pituitary are commonly found in patients dying of head injury. Classically, there is massive infarction of the anterior pituitary with survival of a rim of cells one to two deep, and survival of a thicker layer contiguous with the posterior pituitary. Haemorrhage is commonly found in the posterior pituitary. Daniel *et al.* (1959) suggested that these findings were due to the interruption of the blood supply to the anterior pituitary and warned that pituitary infarction should be borne in mind in patients who remain in prolonged coma. As one can see from Figure 14.1, the unique blood supply to the anterior pituitary renders it susceptible to hypotension and trauma. The anterior lobe has no direct blood supply, receiving its circulation only through the hypophyseal portal vessels. Blood

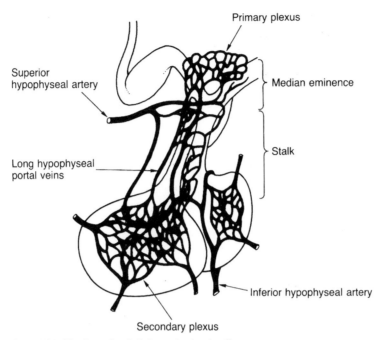

Primary plexus

Superior
hypophyseal artery

Median eminence

Stalk

Long hypophyseal
portal veins

Inferior hypophyseal artery

Secondary plexus

Figure 14.1. Blood supply of pituitary gland and stalk.

from the superior hypophyseal artery breaks up into a primary capillary plexus lying in the median eminence and pituitary stalk, from which the long and the short portal vessels supply blood to the anterior lobe. They are both derived from the primary capillary bed but the short portal vessels emerge from the lower part of the pituitary stalk below the level of the diaphragma sellae. The long portal vessels supply up to 90% of the anterior lobe, and the short portal vessels supply a variable layer of anterior lobe cells adjacent to the posterior lobe. The capsular vessels supply the surface of the pituitary. The inferior hypophyseal arteries supply the posterior lobe, entering below the diaphragma sellae. It is this unique blood supply, which can be interrupted by stalk transection or compression in intracerebral oedema, which probably accounts for the findings of massive infarction in the anterior lobe due to interruption of the portal supply, whilst a variable layer of cells contiguous with the posterior lobe survive due to a continuing supply from the short portal vessels. The rim of the pituitary survives because of the capsular vessels.

In our studies, pituitary function was assessed in 12 patients who died as a consequence of head injury; subsequently their endocrine tests were related to the post-mortem histological findings in the hypothalamus and pituitary. The histological changes observed in the anterior pituitary were similar to those previously described (Ceballos, 1966; Daniel *et al.*, 1959; Daniel and Treip, 1961; Harper *et al.*, 1986; Kornblum and Fisher, 1969) and included large centrally – situated infarcts with a small surviving rim of variable thickness (Figure 14.2). The incidence of large anterior pituitary infarctions, in nine of the 10 pituitary glands available for histological examination, was considerably greater than the incidence in the above studies. This difference may have arisen because our subjects had more severe head injuries, as all 12 died within one week of injury, whereas other studies have included less severely injured patients who died several months after injury. Hypothalamic damage was also frequently observed in our subjects, with petechial haemorrhages or small infarcts located in the paraventricular and supraoptic nuclei, median eminence and upper stalk. These findings are similar to those in previous studies (Crompton, 1971; Treip, 1970). Only one of our subjects had a stalk transection; this is in keeping with the low incidence reported by Ceballos (1966) and Harper *et al.* (1986).

Anterior pituitary necrosis develops because of an interruption of blood flow in the hypothalamo–hypophyseal portal vessels in the pituitary stalk. Although it was initially suggested by Daniel and

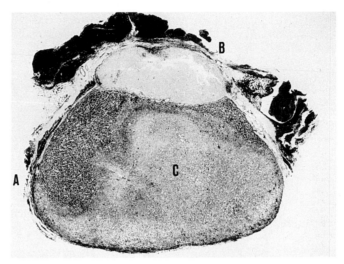

Figure 14.2. Histological section of pituitary gland showing a large area of anterior pituitary infarction. A, anterior pituitary gland; B, posterior pituitary gland; C, area of extensive necrosis.

Treip (1961) that stalk transection was the responsible mechanism, it is apparent from our study and other recent papers that this injury is infrequent. It is more likely that compression of stalk portal vessels on the diaphragma sellae due to post-injury pituitary swelling and intracerebral oedema is responsible (Harper *et al.*, 1986; Kornblum and Fisher, 1969). All 12 of our subjects had evidence of gross cerebral oedema on their CT scans, with obliteration of the lateral ventricles and perimesencephalic cisterns, and flattening of the cortical sulci. At postmortem, their brains were described as swollen and oedematous, with cerebellar coning frequently present. In these circumstances, compression of the stalk vessels seems likely.

Harper *et al.* (1986) reported a high incidence of fracture of the base of the skull in subjects with infarction of the anterior lobe, and Daniel and Treip (1966) stated that a basal fracture was one of the two consistent clinical findings in such patients, the other being prolonged coma disproportionate to the severity of the head injury. However, in our study, there was no relationship between the histological changes and the site of the skull fracture, as large pituitary infarcts were present in subjects with frontal, parietal and basal fractures and in one subject with no fracture. In addition, the direction of the injuring force did not appear important, as similar pituitary damage was observed in the six subjects whose impact was predominantly in the anteroposterior plane when compared with the other six injured by a lateral force.

It has also been suggested that hypotension and anoxia after injury may be responsible for the massive anterior pituitary infarction (Orthner and Mayer, 1967). However, all our subjects were maintained on a ventilator with their gas exchange being monitored and their blood pressure being carefully controlled.

Thus, in our patients, massive pituitary infarction was not due to hypotension or hypoxia and was independent of the direction of the injuring force or the presence of a skull fracture. It seems more likely that the severity of the injury and the consequent intracerebral oedema are, by producing stalk compression, the determinants of the resulting pituitary necrosis.

It has been suggested that the lesion responsible for the development of DI is most commonly in the pituitary stalk and occurs as a result of stretching of the relatively fixed stalk by the displaced brain at the time of injury (Porter and Miller, 1948). Animal experiments (Magoun *et al.*, 1939; Pickford and Ritchie, 1945) and studies in humans who have had their pituitary stalk sectioned (Lipsett *et al.*, 1956) have demonstrated that the development of permanent DI is dependent on the number of surviving antidiuretic hormone-secreting neurones. If less than 10–20% remain viable then permanent DI will occur (Verbalis *et al.*, 1985).

The direction of the injuring force that is most likely to produce the stalk lesion appears to be in the anteroposterior plane, as 15 of Porter and Miller's 18 subjects and six of our seven patients had frontal or occipital injuries (Porter and Miller, 1948).

Clinical assessment

Fluid balance should be carefully monitored in all head-injured subjects. If a negative balance develops then the presence of DI should be considered. Paired urine and plasma osmolality should be measured. If the urine osmolality is dilute (<300 mmol/kg) in the presence of concentrated serum (>290 mmol/kg) then treatment for DI should be commenced. In such patients, anterior pituitary function should be assessed promptly.

Because our study showed a high incidence of large anterior pituitary infarcts in fatally injured patients, it is important to exclude hypopituitarism in those who were the most severely injured. Both thyroxine and the sex hormones are initially suppressed in response to major injury and therefore cannot be used to determine if replacement therapy is required within the first week of injury. However, cortisol levels should be considerably elevated within 48 hours of injury; if a random cortisol level is less than 400 nmol/l, glucocorticoid replacement therapy should be started (100 mg hydrocortisone intravenous bolus and 50 mg thrice daily thereafter).

In addition, any apparently stable patient who becomes hypotensive should be treated as above, with a serum sample taken for cortisol immediately prior to commencing replacement treatment.

Anterior pituitary dysfunction should be considered in patients who develop unexplained hyponatraemia. Both cortisol and thyroxine levels should be checked and it should be borne in mind that a low plasma cortisol is abnormal in the stressed patient.

Clinical comparisons

Previous histological studies have not been able to compare their findings with the premortem endocrine results. Our findings of multiple hormone deficiencies in six of the patients with large pituitary infarcts is not surprising, but a further three patients had virtually normal dynamic tests. This may have arisen because these three subjects survived for four to five days after their endocrine tests were performed and thus may have developed pituitary infarction (possibly with endocrine abnormalities) at this late stage, during the period when their intracranial pressure was rising. The subject with pituitary stalk transection had no hormone response to stimulation, presumably because the blood supply to the anterior pituitary must have been severed completely.

The finding of most clinical relevance was that five subjects were glucocorticoid deficient. This occurred in three subjects with large pituitary infarcts, the subject with stalk transection and one subject in whom the pituitary was unavailable but the hypothalamus had infarction of the median eminence. Apart from the specimen with stalk transection, similar histology was observed in other subjects but was not accompanied by glucocorticoid deficiency.

Prognosis

The prognosis is dependent on the severity of the injury.

Our study identified several endocrine changes associated with a poor prognosis. Glucocorticoid insufficiency was not demonstrated in any survivors during the first week after injury, but occurred in five who were fatally injured. Similarly, a deficient PRL response was present in six of those who died but it was not observed in any survivors.

There were several other endocrine changes suggestive of a poor prognosis. A reduced TSH response to TRH was the most frequent abnormality in the nine who were fatally injured, but was also present in some survivors. The analysis of mean levels demonstrated that T_4 was lower in fatalities (T_3 just failed to achieve statistical significance), whereas FSH, LH and testosterone levels were significantly higher in those who died.

Complications

Permanent neurological sequelae are common, ranging from persistent vegetative state with quadriparesis to a single cranial nerve palsy.

The most important endocrine complication is anterior pituitary failure and, from the published reports, it is apparent that this may take many months or even years to develop. Subjects presenting with hypopituitarism should be asked about a past history of serious head injury.

Further management

Patients found to have anterior pituitary failure will require full hormone replacement therapy with glucocorticoid (hydrocortisone 10–30 mg daily), and thyroxine 50–200 μg daily. The actual amount will depend upon clinical and biochemical assessment, and must aim to keep the free thyroxine in the upper end of the normal range. Testosterone is given either as an implant every six months or as Sustanon or Primoteston depot 250 mg every two to three weeks intramuscularly or oestrogen and progestogen replacement is given. If posterior pituitary failure is present, then desmopressin may be administered, either intranasally by rhinule Desmospray or Desmopresis tablets.

References

Altman R, Pruzanski W. (1961) Post-traumatic hypopituitarism. Anterior pituitary insufficiency following skullfracture. *Ann Intern Med* **55**: 149–54.

Barreca T, Perria C, Sannia A, *et al.* (1980) Evaluation of anterior pituitary function in patients with post-traumatic diabetes insipidus. *J Clin Endocrinol Metab* **51**: 1279–82.

Bevilacqua G, Fornaciari G. (1975) Clinicopathological correlations in a case of post-traumatic pan-hypopituitarism. *Acta Neuropathol (Berl)* **31**: 171–77.

Bistritzer T, Theodor R, Inbar D, *et al.* (1966) Anterior hypopituitarism due to fracture of the sella turcica. *Am J Dis Child* **135**: 966–67.

Ceballos R. (1966) Pituitary changes in head trauma. *Ala J Med Sci* **3**: 185–98.

Crompton MR. (1971) Hypothalamic lesions following closed head injury. *Brain* **94**: 165–72.

Cyran E. (1918) Hypopoysenschadigung durch schadelbasis-fracktur. *Dtsch Med Wochenschr* **44**: 1261.

Daniel PM, Pritchard MML, Treip CS. (1959) Traumatic infarction of the anterior lobe of the pituitary gland. *Lancet* **ii**: 927–30.

Daniel PM, Treip CS. (1961) Acute massive traumatic infarction of the anterior lobe. In: Gardiner-Hill H, editor. *Modern trends in endocrinology*, 2nd series. Guildford: Butterworths, 55–68.

Daniel PM, Treip CS. (1966) Lesions of the pituitary gland associated with head injuries. In: Harris GW, Donavan BT, editors. *The pituitary gland*, vol 2. Guildford: Butterworths, 519–34.

Durand L, Maugery J, Noel G. (1969) Insuffisance ante-hypophysaire et plomb de chasses dans la selle turcique. *Bull Soc Ophtalmol Fr* **69**: 578–81.

Dzur J, Winternitz W. (1976) Post-traumatic hypopituitarism: Anterior pituitary insufficiency secondary to head trauma. *South Med J* **69**: 1377–79.

Edwards OM, Clark JDA. (1986) Post-traumatic hypopituitarism: 6 cases and a review of the literature. *Medicine (Baltimore)* **65**: 281–90.

Escamilla RF, Lisser H. (1942) Simmonds disease. *J Clin Endocrinol* **2**: 65–96.

Fernandez-Castanerr M, Martinez De Osaba MJ, Vilardell E. (1982) Insuffisance hypophysaire post-traumatique. *Ann d'Endocrinol* (Paris) **43**: 213–18.

Girard J, Marelli R. (1977) Post-traumatic hypothalamo-pituitary insufficiency. *J Pediatr* **90**: 241–42.

Goldman KP, Jacobs A. (1960) Anterior and posterior pituitary failure after head injury. *Br Med J* **2**: 1924–26.

Gomez-Saez JM, Mendez SJ, Ramon JS. (1982) Panhipopituitarismo anterior tras fractura de la silla turca. *Med Clin* (Barcelona) **78**: 159–61.

Gross D. (1940) Hypophyseunder schadeltrauma. *Arch Psychiatr Nervenkrankheiten* **111**: 619.

Harper CG, Doyle D, Hume Adams J, *et al.* (1986) Analysis of abnormalities in pituitary gland in non-missile head injury: study of 100 consecutive cases. *J Clin Pathol* **39**: 769–73.

Jambart S, Turpin G, de Genness JL. (1980) Panhypopituitarism secondary to head trauma: evidence for a hypothalamic origin of the deficit. *Acta Endocrinol* **93**: 264–70.

Jambart S, Turpin G, de Gennes JL. (1981) Panhypopituitarismes acquis post-traumatiques, idiopathiques et d'origine hypothalamique de l'adulte. *Nouv Presse Med* **10**: 975–77.

Kanade A, Ruiz AE, Tornyos K, *et al.* (1978) Panhypopituitarism and anemia secondary to traumatic fracture of the sella turcica. *J Endocrinol Invest* **1**: 263–68.

Kanayama Y, Kubo K, Furukawa Y, *et al.* (1972) A case of post-traumatic hypopituitarism. *Endocrinol Jpn* **19**: 517–23.

Kaufman JM. (1981) Panhypopituitarisme na schedeltrauma. *Tijdschir Geneeskd* **37**: 292–95.

Klachko DM, Winerr N, Burns TW, *et al.* (1968) Traumatic hypopituitarism occuring before puberty: Survival 35 years untreated. *J Clin Endocrinol* **28**: 1768–72.

Kornblum RN, Fisher RS. (1969) Pituitary lesions in craniocerebral injuries. *Arch Pathol* **88**: 242–48.

Lafon R, Passouant P, Labauge R, *et al.* (1955) Syndrome myotoniquie au cours d'un myxoedema hypophysaire post-traumqtique de l'adulte. *Rev Neurol* **93**: 759–60.

Landau H, Adin I, Spitz IM. (1978) Pituitary insufficiency following head injury. *Isr J Med Sci* **14**: 785–89.

Lerman J, Means JH. (1945) Hypopituitarism associated with epilepsy following head injury. *J Clin Endocrinol* **5**: 119–31.

Linquette M, Fossati P, Lefebvre J, *et al.* (1968) Hypopituitarisme anterieur lie a un anevrysme carotido-caverneux post-traumatique. *Rev Fr Endocrinol Clin Nutr Metab* **9**: 61–67.

Lipsett MB, MacLean JP, West CD, *et al.* (1956) An analysis of the polyuria induced by hypophysectomy in man. *J Clin Endocrinol* **16**: 183–95.

McCullagh EP, Schaffenburg CA. (1953) Anterior pituitary insufficiency following skull fracture. *J Clin Endocrinol* **13**: 1283–90.

Magoun HW, Fisher C, Ranson SW. (1939) The neurohypophysis and water exchange in the monkey. *Endocrinology* **25**: 161–74.

Miller WL, Kaplan SL, Grumbach MM. (1980) Child abuse as a cause of post-traumatic hypopituitarism. *N Engl J Med* **302**: 724–28.

Notman DD, Mortex MA, Moses AM. (1980) Permanent diabetes insipidus following head trauma: observations on ten patients and an approach to diagnosis. *J Trauma* **20**: 599–602.

Orthner H, Meyer E. (1967) Der posttraumatische diabetes insipidus. *Acta Neurol (Wein)* **30**: 216–50.

Pascheff C. (1922) Preliminary communication on injuries as a cause of diabetes insipidus with bitemporal hemianopia. *Br J Ophthalmol* **6**: 549–54.

Paxson CL, Brown DR. (1976) Post-traumatic anterior hypopituitarism. *Pediatrics* **57**: 893–96.

Pere P, Fontaine B, Mizrahi R, *et al.* (1980) L'hypopituitarisme post-traumatique. *Rev Fr Endocrinol Clin Nutr Metab* **21**: 341–47.

Pickford M, Ritchie AE. (1945) Experiments on the hypothalamo-pituitary control of water excretion in dogs. *J Physiol* **104**: 105–28.

Pickles W. (1947) Disturbances of metabolism associated with head injuries. *N Engl J Med* **236**: 858–62.

Pittman JA, Haigler ED, Hershman JM, *et al.* (1971) Hypothalamic hypothyroidism. New Eng. J. of Med., 285, 844–45.

Porter RJ, Miller RA. (1948) Diabetes insipidus following closed head injury. *J Neurol Neurosurg Psychiatry* **11**: 258–62.

Prosperi L, Bernasconi S, Cantarelli A, *et al.* (1978) Traumatic hypopituitarism associated with bitemporal hemianopia in a prepubertal child. *J Pediatr Ophthalmol Strabismus* **15**: 376–81.

Reverchon L, Worms G. (1921) Lesions traumatiques de l'hypophysee dans les fractures de la base du crane. *Bull Mem Soc Chirurg Paris* **47**: 685–89.

Rowntree LG. (1924) Studies of diabetes insipidus. JAMA **83**: 399–405.

Salti IS, Haddad FS, Amiri ZN, *et al.* (1979) Bullet injury to the pituitary gland: a rare cause of panhypopituitarism. *J Neurol Neurosurg Psychiatry* **42**: 955–59.

Schereschewsky NA. (1927) La symptomatologie et le diagnostic de la maladie de Simmonds (cachexie hypophysaire). Rev *Fr Endocrinol Clin Nutr Metab* **5**: 275–81.

Soules MR, Sheldon GW. (1979) Traumatic hypopituitarism: anterior hypophyseal insufficiency from indirect cranial trauma. *South Med J* **72**: 1592–96.

Treip CS. (1970) Hypothalamic and pituitary injury. *J Clin Pathol* **23**(suppl 4): 178–85.

Valenta LJ, De Feo DR. (1980) Post-traumatic hypopituitarism due to a hypothalamic lesion. *Am J Med* **68**: 614–17.

Valenta LJ, Sostrin RD, Eisenburg H, *et al.* (1982) Diagnosis of pituitary tumors by hormone assays and computerized tomography. *Am J Med* **72**: 861–73.

Verbalis JG, Robinson AG, Moses AM. (1985) Post-operative and post-traumatic diabetes insipidus. *Front Horm Res* **13**: 247–65.

Weiss SR, Jacobi JD, Fishman LM, Lemaire WJ. (1977) Hypopituitarism following head trauma. *Am J Obstet Gynecol* **127**: 678–79.

Werner W. (1960) Traumatischer hypopituitarismus. *Endokrinologia* **39**: 172–85.

Witter H, Tascher R. (1957) Hypophysar hypothalamische Krankheitsbilder nach stumpfem Schadeltrauma. *Fortschr Neurol Psychiatr* **25**: 523–46.

Woolf PD, Schalch DS. (1973) Hypopituitarism secondary to hypothalamic insufficiency. *Ann Intern Med* **78**: 88–90.

15

Post-traumatic hydrocephalus

J D Pickard

Introduction and definitions

Dilatation of the cerebral ventricles (ventriculomegaly) is relatively common after severe head injury and may reflect either cerebral atrophy or true hydrocephalus (see Gean, 1994; Pickard, 1982; for reviews). Hydrocephalus may be defined as an excessive accumulation of cerebrospinal fluid (CSF) within the head due to a disturbance of its secretion, flow or absorption. This definition avoids any confusion with hydrocephalus *ex vacuo*, in which the excess CSF fills the space left by cerebral atrophy. Cerebral atrophy is the result of parenchymal tissue loss that becomes manifest as swelling resolves and necrotic tissue becomes gliotic.

The deposition of blood and debris into the cerebral ventricles and subarachnoid spaces or the presence of meningitis, followed by the usual inflammatory reaction, might be expected frequently to lead to disturbances of the circulation and absorption of CSF. Hydrocephalus results when CSF production exceeds CSF reabsorption and may be either communicating (obstruction to CSF flow/reabsorption distal to the IVth ventricle) or noncommunicating (obstruction to CSF flow within the ventricular system). Surprisingly, perhaps, symptomatic hydrocephalus that necessitates a CSF diversion procedure is relatively uncommon, although its more chronic form is often underdiagnosed. There is no difficulty in defining acute hydrocephalus with sequential CT scanning in the first weeks after head injury. The distinction between atrophy and obstruction in CSF flow/ absorption becomes a problem in the succeeding months and years. The two processes may coexist.

Epidemiology

The incidence of post-traumatic hydrocephalus has been reported to vary between 8% and 72%, depending on the definition and technique (Beyerl and Black, 1984; Cardoso and Galbraith, 1985; Gudeman *et al.*, 1981; Kishore *et al.*, 1978; Levin *et al.*, 1981). Symptomatic hydrocephalus that requires a shunt is much less common, with the incidence ranging from 1% to 4% after head injury, but this may underestimate the true incidence of the condition. As discussed later, many cases of late onset symptomatic communicating hydrocephalus have no apparent cause; patients may not always remember significant past health problems such as head injury. Furthermore, there has been no long term follow-up of a cohort of head-injured patients of different severities for 25 years to see how many develop symptomatic ventricular dilatation and what are the predictive factors. Some studies are flawed by selection bias and give an estimate of the lowest incidence. For example, in the catchment population, served only by the regional neurosurgical unit in Glasgow, scrutiny of all cases of acquired hydrocephalus admitted over five years revealed 17 cases of post-traumatic hydrocephalus, which represented 0.7% of 2374 cases of severe head injury (Cardoso and Galbraith, 1985). Sixteen of the 17 patients became symptomatic within one year from the time of injury. What is not clear is how many of the 2374 patients with severe head injuries had ventriculomegaly to which symptoms had not been attributed. Some neurologists and neurosurgeons are sceptical of the existence of normal pressure hydrocephalus.

Clinical assessment

Hydrocephalus may present in different ways after head injury.

Pre-existing hydrocephalus

Patients with pre-existing but 'arrested' hydrocephalus, as, for example, with aqueduct stenosis, may be at greater risk from a head injury in general and of decompensation of their hydrocephalus in particular. Arrested hydrocephalus is a treacherous condition that may become symptomatic after quite mild trauma. Twenty four hour intracranial pressure (ICP) monitoring will often reveal periods of raised pressure and wave activity, particularly during dream sleep.

Acute hydrocephalus

Acute hydrocephalus may result from a supratentorial clot causing a midline shift and contralateral ventricular dilatation. Brain herniation at the tentorium or foramen magnum, or a posterior fossa haematoma, may present as acute hydrocephalus. Meningitis, traumatic subarachnoid haemorrhage or extensive craniotomies (anterior fossa repair) may be followed by hydrocephalus. In such patients, the presenting symptoms are those of raised ICP:- if the patient is conscious, there are headaches and/or blurring of vision (papilloedema), a deteriorating consciousness level and, finally, coning with fixed dilated pupils and apnoea. Traumatic intraventricular haemorrhage rarely causes hydrocephalus (LeRoux *et al.*, 1992).

Failure to improve

In patients in prolonged coma or in whom clinical progress has arrested, a CT scan should be performed to exclude hydrocephalus (Grosswasser

et al., 1988). It is unusual for patients not to continue to improve after head injury – if they plateau, a cause should be sought.

Normal pressure hydrocephalus (symptomatic; chronic; communicating hydrocephalus)

Hakim first described this condition after head injury in 1972 in patients with progressive 'dementia', gait disturbance and urinary incontinence who often improved with CSF diversion (Hakim and Adams, 1965). Although these symptoms may overlap clinically with other conditions, careful clinical analysis in the majority of patients will reveal a distinctive syndrome (Fisher, 1977). Typically, gait becomes disturbed first and is a symptom most likely to be improved by shunting. Patients can move their limbs perfectly normally on a couch but are unable to initiate walking ('magnet gait'). They are unstable and may eventually become bedridden and unable even to turn over. The term 'dementia' disguises the reality that patients with normal pressure hydrocephalus who respond to a shunt have mental slowing, loss of executive function and recent memory loss, which is a combination typical of the subcortical type of dementia (Vanneste, 1994). Urinary incontinence occurs late and initially presents as urgency of micturition associated with instability of the bladder detrusor muscle. The frontal lobe type of incontinence, with lack of appropriate concern and even complete lack of awareness of urinary incontinence, occurs very late.

Pathophysiology and structural pathology

There is a paucity of postmortem reports of patients with normal pressure hydrocephalus in the literature but the presumption is that subarachnoid haemorrhage or meningitis result in obliteration of the cortical subarachnoid space and the arachnoid granulations by fibrosis. These changes are not rendered visible by current *in vivo* scanning techniques.

The conventional description of the development of hydrocephalus supposes that, with acute obstruction to CSF flow, the cerebral ventricles rapidly dilate and the cerebral sulci, fissures and basal cisterns are obliterated. CSF flows into the periventricular white matter through either an intact or a disrupted ependymal lining, causing CSF oedema around the ventricles. Alternative pathways of CSF absorption become established but the details in different age groups remain ill-defined. Unconventional 'lymphatic' pathways may play a role in addition to utilization of spinal arachnoid villi in communicating hydrocephalus and less plausibly through the blood vessels in the oedematous periventricular white matter. During the stage of periventricular CSF oedema, there is destruction of nerve fibres within the oedematous zone and, over succeeding weeks and months, the periventricular white matter becomes gliotic, at which stage the changes tend to be irreversible. CSF oedema can be demonstrated by CT scanning during the acute stages of hydrocephalus in humans, but periventricular low density may be seen in the elderly population and should not be confused with the more straightforward periventricular oedema of the young (Gean, 1994). Age changes can include white matter ischaemia and infarction, and demyelination and gliosis, in a distribution that may mimic hydrocephalic periventricular oedema.

Investigations

Typically, CT scanning is sufficient to detect acute hydrocephalus by revealing ventricular dilatation and the absence of sulcal atrophy, but this is an over-simplistic approach to normal pressure hydrocephalus. Sulcal atrophy may be present in patients with normal pressure hydrocephalus who respond to shunting. Periventricular lucency in the elderly may be misleading. MRI is superior to CT scanning in resolving the nature of the periventricular changes, but a functional quantitative test of CSF absorption (computerized CSF infusion study ± 24-hour ICP monitoring) (Pickard *et al.*, 1980; Borgesen and Gjerris, 1982) is required in borderline patients before embarking on shunt procedures, which are not without risk, particularly in those patients with a low probability of improvement. A CSF tap test does not reveal all patients who might improve with a shunt (Wikkelsö *et al.*, 1986; Vanneste, 1994).

Measurement of outcome

At present, outcome in most clinics is usually assessed by interviewing the patient and the relatives, with no attempt at quantification. Ideally,

the patient should have been assessed by a neuropsychologist pre- and postoperatively, and the time to walk 10 metres recorded. The ability to cope at home may require a home visit by an occupational therapist or nurse. A diary is useful for recording the frequency of incontinence. A CT or MR scan should be performed at one week and at two to three months to assess ventricular size and exclude asymptomatic subdural collections. If patients have not improved and the ventricles have not reduced in size, valve function should be checked by a CSF infusion study. Some patients improve without shrinkage of the ventricles.

Diagnosis and complications

Acute hydrocephalus

Where acute hydrocephalus is the cause of a patient's deterioration, that patient will improve after insertion of a competent shunt but may be left with transient or long-term problems with memory, fits (from ventricular puncture: frontal > parietal), hemianopia (occipital infarction from posterior cerebral artery herniation), hemiplegia (ventricular puncture, intracranial haematoma, coning), and disorders of higher mental function, including executive dysfunction. It is unknown how many of these patients require a shunt system in the long term, but it is not safe to assume that 'they will grow out of it'. Within 12 years, 81% of shunts fail (Sainte-Rose, 1989).

Normal pressure hydrocephalus

These patients are generally more fragile and worse surgical risks than the younger age group with acute hydrocephalus. Historical series painted such a grim picture that the risks appeared sometimes to outweigh the benefits. Attention to preoperative assessment is essential. Most complications occur in those patients with a low probability of improving with a shunt.

New valves have probably improved matters. In a recent audit of 138 patients one year after insertion of a Medos programmable valve for hydrocephalus, who were considered to be at high risk of complications, the incidence of subdural collections was 16%, infection 12%, and shunt revisions 9% (UK Shunt Audit Group, 1994). In general, the consensus in the literature is that 70% of patients with normal pressure hydrocephalus improve when a cause such as trauma is known. It is too soon to know how long the benefit will last.

Further management

Long-term follow-up is not required, except by annual letter, once it has been established whether a patient will respond to a shunt and provided that the patient has a reliable general practitioner.

References

Beyerl B, Black PMcL. (1984) Post-traumatic hydrocephalus. *Neurosurgery* 15: 257–61.

Borgesen SE, Gjerris F. (1982) The predictive value of conductance to outflow of CSF in normal pressure hydrocephalus. *Brain* 105: 65–86.

Cardoso ER, Galbraith S. (1985) Post-traumatic hydrocephalus – a retrospective review. *Surg Neurol* 23: 261–64.

Fisher CM. (1977) The clinical picture in occult hydrocephalus. *Clin Neurosurg* 24: 270–84.

Gean AD. (1994) Imaging of head trauma. New York: Raven Press, 577.

Grosswasser Z, Cohen M, Reider-Grosswasser I, Stern MJ. (1988) Incidence, CT findings and rehabilitation outcome of patients with communicative hydrocephalus following severe head injury. *Brain Inj* 2: 267–72.

Gudeman SK, Kishore PRS, Becker DP, *et al.* (1981) Computed tomography in the evaluation of incidence and significance of post-traumatic hydrocephalus. *Radiology* 141: 397–402.

Hakim S, Adams RD. (1965) The special clinical problem of symptomatic hydrocephalus with normal CSF pressure: observation on CSF hydrocephalus. *J Neurol Sci* 2: 307–27.

Kishore PRS, Lippen MH, Miller JD, *et al.* (1978) Post-traumatic hydrocephalus in patients with severe head injury. *Neuroradiology* 16: 261–65.

LeRoux PD, Haglund MM, Newell DW, *et al.* (1992) Intraventricular haemorrhage in blunt head trauma: an analysis of 43 cases. *Neurosurgery* 31: 678–85.

Levin HS, Meyers CA, Grossman RG, *et al.* (1981) Ventricular enlargement after closed head injury. *Arch Neurol* 38: 623–29.

Pickard JD, Newton H, Greene A. (1992) A prospective study of idiopathic normal pressure hydrocephalus – guidelines for outpatient assessment. *J Neurol Neurosurg Psychiatry* 55: 517–18.

Pickard JD, Teasdale G, Matheson M, *et al.* (1980) Intraventricular pressure waves – the best predictive test for shunting in normal pressure hydrocephalus. In: Shulman K, Marmarou A, Miller JD, *et al.* editors. *Intracranial pressure IV*. Berlin: Springer Verlag, 498–500.

Pickard JD. (1982) Adult communicating hydrocephalus. *Br J Hosp Med* 27: 35–44.

Sainte-Rose C, Hoffman HJ, Hirsch JF. (1989) Shunt failure. *Concepts Pediatr Neurosurg* 9: 7–20.

UK Shunt Audit Group. (1994) Audit of the Medos programmable shunt – a preliminary analysis. *J Neurol Neurosurg Psychiatry* 57: 1150–51.

Vanneste J. (1994) Three decades of normal pressure hydrocephalus: are we wiser now? *J Neurol Neurosurg Psychiatry* 57: 1021–25.

Wikkelsö C, Anderson H, Blomstrand C, Lindquist G, Svendsen P. (1986) Normal pressure hydrocephalus. Predictive value of the cerebrospinal fluid tap-test. *Acta Neurol Scand* 73: 566–73.

16

Vascular pathology

O C E Sparrow

Introduction

Most injuries, however trivial, involve blood vessels, causing oedema and often bruising. The purpose of this chapter is to review injuries to significant vessels, where the vascular trauma is serious in its own right, influencing prognosis beyond the immediate risk of local haemorrhage. Whilst most such injuries affect major arteries, veins and, particularly, intracranial venous sinuses, smaller arteries can also be affected, with consequences that may be no less devastating.

Definitions

Vessel wall injury may be partial or full thickness. The terms partial disruption and full thickness tear or full thickness laceration will be used for clarity. If a full thickness tear affects all of the circumference of the vessel, transection or avulsion results.

Aneurysms following trauma are sometimes separated into 'true' and 'false', on the basis of whether they follow partial disruption or a full thickness tear of the vessel wall (Jackson *et al.*, 1976). This determines whether the wall of the aneurysm comprises damaged artery or surrounding tissue only. Although this distinction may have implications for treatment, none the less the term traumatic aneurysm will be used here for both types.

Defining what constitutes trauma may seem pedantic, but trivial injuries may be followed by potentially catastrophic dissection or occlusion of,

in particular, cervical carotid or vertebral arteries. 'Minimal trauma' will therefore be used to denote such trivial injuries and distinguish them from the significant injuries typically associated with arterial damage. This will be discussed further in the section on structural pathology.

Epidemiology

By implication, the frequency with which vascular injuries are encountered will vary with the overall incidence of trauma in the community concerned. It will also vary to a lesser extent with the demography of the population (as trauma in general affects young males disproportionately) and with the pattern of trauma. Penetrating neck injury (mostly from assault) is a major cause of vascular injury, so if stab and gunshot wounds are common, major vessel injuries will also be common.

Cervical vessels

In a Swiss study of nearly 3000 cases, Laske *et al.* (1990) found that 0.58% of subjects had supra-aortic major arterial injury, whilst Rao *et al.* (1993) found major vessel injuries in 14% of over 500 penetrating neck wounds in a New York level 1 trauma centre. From Beirut, Khoury *et al.* (1990) reported over 500 penetrating neck injuries. Carotid arteries were involved in 9% (a tenth of these involved more than one carotid injury). In the USA, blunt injury was believed to account for

3–10% of cervical vessel injuries by Fakhry *et al.* (1988), but, of 54 carotid injuries, only 2% were blunt, with 18% having a major associated venous injury (Fry and Fry, 1980). Hoang-The-Dan *et al.* (1984) described a 4% incidence of blunt carotid injury in France, while in a South African series of 124 carotid injuries, 84% affected the common carotid and the internal jugular vein was also injured in 26% (Demetriades *et al.* 1989). Davis *et al.* (1990) felt that less than 1/1000 blunt neck injuries is followed by carotid dissection, which is not the only vascular lesion to complicate blunt neck trauma.

Autopsy figures are loaded in favour of severe injuries, although the vessel injury is not necessarily responsible for death. Moar (1987) examined 200 consecutive victims of fatal road traffic accidents. Detailed examination of the common carotids and their bifurcations yielded some disruption in 29%. Of those with arterial injury, nearly 40% had dual vessel involvement, and combined intimomedial tears were present in 63%. Complete tears were present in 26% and adventitial contusions were present in 70%. Vanezis (1986) reported a similar study of 32 fatal road traffic accident victims with evidence of posterior neck injury, in whom detailed vertebral artery examination was undertaken, showing injury in 31%.

Vertebral artery injuries are less frequent than those involving the carotids. Nevertheless, they have been associated with cervical fracture-dislocations (Louw *et al.* 1990). In a further variation, Willis *et al.* (1994) looked at cervical spinal injuries adjacent to the vertebral arteries (unstable fractures, facet joint and foramen transversarium fractures), and showed that 46% had vertebral artery lesions (mostly occlusions, but also pseudo-aneurysms dissections and intimal flaps).

Intracranial vessels

As far as intracranial arteries are concerned, Mirvis *et al.* (1990) reviewed over 1300 consecutive computed tomographic (CT) head scans for trauma; 1.9% of these demonstrated clear evidence of infarction in at least one defined arterial territory. Of the 53 infarcts, 41 were in major arterial territories. Some were proved at autopsy to be, and others were believed to be, due to vessel compression by oedema or contusion, so the vessel walls may have been structurally intact. Intracranial vessel wall injury is believed to be rare, with little over 100 post-traumatic aneurysms

recorded in the literature (Soria, 1988), although another report from the same year (Buckingham *et al.*, 1988) found 67 in children alone, and added two more. However, these included extradural skull base aneurysms of the petrous and cavernous carotid. Approximately 50% of intracranial traumatic aneurysms arise from the cavernous segment of the internal carotid artery (Ferguson, 1989). Missile and penetrating injuries more commonly cause aneurysms. In 74 angiographic examinations for deeply penetrating transcranial or transorbital stab wounds, 11 (15%) aneurysms were found (Kieck and de Villiers, 1984).

A more obvious consequence of carotid arterial injury at cavernous sinus level is the formation of a carotico-cavernous fistula. After trauma, these are mostly high flow (direct) fistulae. The incidence among patients with head injuries who require admission to a neurosurgical unit has been estimated at 0.4%, rising to 2.2% for severe head injuries (Stern, 1976). Kieck and de Villiers (1984) found five (7%) carotico-cavernous fistulae amongst their 74 angiograms carried out following deep transcranial or transorbital stab wounds. A further three arteriovenous fistulae were identified at other sites.

Dural venous sinus repair constitutes approximately 10% of neurosurgical operations for war wounds, but far fewer in civilian trauma practice (Roy and Cooper, 1990).

Traumatic middle meningeal arteriovenous fistula has been reported in 1.8% of nearly 450 angiographic examinations for head injury, although the incidence of all discernable injuries of the vessel was 4% (Freckmann *et al.*, 1981).

Vessels of the scalp and face

Peick *et al.* (1988) concluded that scalp vessel traumatic aneurysms constitute less than 1% of reported aneurysms. The isolated reports of injuries to these and arteries of the face do not allow the calculation of reliable incidences.

Clinical assessment

Cervical vessels

Penetrating injury is usually obvious because of brisk arterial (or venous) haemorrhage, haematoma (which may be pulsatile), or bruit. Less frequently there may be neurological deficit appropriate to the territory of the carotid or vertebral artery, although such deficit may evolve only after arrival in hospital. Entirely separately, cervical root deficits may be present, as may spinal cord injury. This may occur after penetrating injury involving either the vertebral artery or the carotid (Lipschitz, 1976). Of particular note are ipsilateral loss of vision after carotid injury (which can precede hemispheral neurological signs) and ipsilateral Horner's syndrome (Culebras *et al.*, 1989), although these are less important in diagnosing penetrating than blunt injuries.

Blunt arterial injury is far more challenging to diagnose in time for effective treatment. When head injuries coexist, neurological deficits from the arterial injury may be difficult to interpret. Bok *et al.* (1984) and Hellner *et al.* (1993) found that 50% of internal carotid dissections associated with head or facial injuries were bilateral, although the symptoms were the same as for the unilateral cases. The onset of neurological deficits without impaired consciousness, and deficits not explained by CT scan evidence of brain injury or spinal cord or brachial plexus trauma are highly suggestive, as radiological signs of cerebral ischaemia and infarction evolve slowly (Fakhry *et al.*, 1988). Monocular blindness is an important early sign of carotid occlusion. The combination of head, facial and cervical spine injuries predisposed to blunt dissection in the case control study reported by Davis *et al.* (1990). Intraoral trauma may also cause carotid injury (Hengerer *et al.*, 1984).

Cervical subluxation or dislocation predisposes to vertebral artery injuries (Louw *et al.*, 1990), as do fractures in the vicinity of the artery, especially those involving facet joint and foramen transversarium (Willis *et al.*, 1994). The atlantoaxial segment of the artery may be particularly susceptible to blunt injury in children (Garg *et al.*, 1993). Simeone and Lyness (1976) described one and analysed 11 additional cases of posterior circulation ischaemia following cervical manipulation.

The cervical carotid and vertebral arteries are prone to spontaneous dissection, the carotids more than the vertebrals (Meyer *et al.*, 1988). Minor trauma has been implicated in many cases. The importance of minor injuries, even those that might be termed 'physiological', should not be overlooked, but, in this context, the trauma is not of sufficient magnitude to consider in its own right, and the patient presents with 'spontaneous' symptoms of dissection or occlusion (see below).

Appropriate investigations include combinations of duplex Doppler sonography, CT scan, magnetic resonance imaging (MRI), and angiography, depending on the clinical circumstances.

Intracranial vessels

Injury to intracranial vessels occurs from both penetrating and blunt injuries. A special example of the former is surgical injury, which has been responsible for some traumatic aneurysms (Jackson *et al.*, 1976). Most intradural traumatic aneurysms follow depressed fractures or penetrating injury. Knife and gunshot wounds in particular may cause vessel injury, which may not be disclosed by early angiography (Kieck and de Villiers, 1984; Nov and Cromwell, 1984). There is a major propensity for rupture. Jackson *et al.* (1976) found more than half of all such aneurysms reported in the literature had bled within 15 days of injury, with a 50% mortality. The pericallosal artery in particular seems vulnerable to injury against the falx in blunt trauma (Nov and Cromwell, 1984).

The internal carotid too is vulnerable at the skull base, and either blunt or penetrating injury can lead to a false aneurysm, or, more frequently, a carotico–cavernous fistula. Although most are high flow direct fistulae, low flow fistulae may also occur from rupture of intracavernous branches of the internal carotid artery. Narrowing and thrombosis of the artery may also occur, although occlusion is more common in the petrous segment (Bonafé and Manelfe, 1990). Carotico-cavernous fistula can follow the introduction of a needle percutaneously into Meckel's cave; the author has seen an internal maxillary artery fistula to the pterygoid venous plexus from radiofrequency thermocoagulation by this route. Although traumatic aneurysms of the carotid artery in the skull base may present with expansion causing pain or with cranial nerve palsy (typically third or sixth nerves), haemorrhage may be the first sign. Torrential epistaxis may be difficult to control. The diagnosis of carotico-cavernous fistula is usually straightforward. Pulsatile tinnitus and bruit, an injected eye with chemosis, exophthalmos (often pulsatile), ophthalmoplegia, deteriorating vision and trigeminal nerve involvement are the commonest features of the condition (Bonafé and Manelfe, 1990). Ocular involvement may be bilateral, or even contralateral. Rarely, bilateral fistulae may occur. Carotid injury in the petrous or cavernous segments is frequently associated with skull base fractures, usually involving the sphenoid bone (Bonafé and Manelfe, 1990).

Middle meningeal injury can produce either an arteriovenous fistula or a traumatic aneurysm, or both. Aneurysms can rupture causing a delayed, or 'spontaneous', extradural haematoma (Odake, 1981), but if dura has been torn, subdural (Aoki *et al.*, 1991) or even intracerebral haemorrhage may occur.

Dural venous sinus injury does not usually result in early occlusion, and although open wounds may bleed heavily, typically bleeding begins during surgical exposure. Air embolism can occur with an open sinus if the head has been elevated. Occlusion, particularly of the dominant transverse sinus or posterior two-thirds of the superior sagittal sinus, is poorly tolerated, resulting in venous engorgement and intracranial hypertension, which is frequently fatal (Roy and Cooper, 1990).

Investigation of these patients includes CT scan, MRI, transcranial Doppler sonography and angiography, depending on the clinical assessment.

Vessels of the scalp and face

Injury to scalp vessels may produce traumatic aneurysms of the occipital or superficial temporal arteries. These present with local pain, headache or a pulsatile mass (Peick *et al.*, 1988). If neglected, rupture can produce an extremely painful, huge scalp haematoma. A fistula between the occipital artery and the mastoid emissary vein may occur and is easily diagnosed clinically.

Arteries in the face can also be injured. Severe epistaxis early after facial and skull fractures is generally due to injury of the internal maxillary artery (Bonafé and Manelfe, 1990). The author has also seen a traumatic aneurysm involving this vessel after trans-sphenoidal surgery.

Some scalp aneurysms are obvious on clinical examination alone, although angiography may be necessary, sometimes as a prelude to endovascular occlusion of aneurysms or fistulae.

Spinal cord arteries

These can be affected by dissection of the aorta, due to any cause, including trauma, with onset of paraplegia. The neurological level is variable and, depends on the anatomical distribution of radicular arterial feeders (Fosburg and Brewer, 1976). Surgical injury of the major radicular vessel, or artery of Adamkiewicz, can be responsible for paraplegia during aortic aneurysm surgery or thoracotomy for other pathology.

Special investigation in relation to the spinal cord is only required if doubt about compression exists. For this purpose, MRI is the technique of choice, although CT myelography is effective in its absence.

Structural pathology

Penetrating injury

These injuries are self-explanatory. Assuming haemorrhage is controlled and flow is preserved in arteries, a full thickness laceration results in a false aneurysm, with the surrounding tissues forming the aneurysm wall (Jackson *et al.*, 1976). The exception to this is when there is a combined arterial and venous full thickness laceration. In this case, an arteriovenous fistula results. Partial thickness lacerations will weaken the wall in proportion to their depth and a true aneurysm may form. Whilst a false aneurysm will, by definition, be weaker than a true aneurysm, in other respects there is little more than histological appearance to separate them.

Blunt injury

The spectrum of blunt trauma is much wider, varying from minor self-limiting injuries, such as adventitial contusions, to complete thrombosis and rupture.

Intimal disruption can result in a flap causing occlusion and thrombosis, or dissection. The plane of the latter is usually in the outer part of the tunica media in major systemic arteries, the same as for the extracranial carotids and vertebrals. However, in cerebral arteries, it occurs immediately deep to the internal elastic lamina, usually causing acute occlusion, although rupture outwards to cause subarachnoid haemorrhage can occur. Cerebral arterial dissections are more often detected after mild than major trauma (Ferguson, 1989). In this context, Mizutani *et al.* (1982) have proposed that excessive intimal fibroelastic thickening may predispose to cerebral dissection after mild trauma. It is interesting to note that fibrointimal proliferation has been described in association with a common carotid traumatic aneurysm (Hebra *et al.*, 1993).

At autopsy, Moar (1987) found some degree of disruption in 29% of common carotid arteries from 200 consecutive fatal road traffic accident victims. Of those with abnormalities, 40% were bilateral and 63% had combined intimomedial tears. Polla-nen *et al.* (1992) demonstrated the importance of heat-labile cytosol enzymes released from dam-aged smooth muscle cells following vertebral artery injury and conceivably predisposing to vessel rupture.

Cervical dissections may progress intracranially, where rupture will cause subarachnoid haemor-rhage, but the internal carotid may rupture in the cavernous sinus, causing a carotico-cavernous fistula (Bonafé and Manelfe, 1990). Although it has been proposed that cervical carotid vessel injury may permit traumatic subarachnoid haemor-rhage because of blood tracking intradurally (Har-land *et al.*, 1983), Deck and Jagadha (1986) have described six instances in which intracranial verte-bral artery rupture would appear to have been more likely to be responsible. Similarly, ruptures of the posterior inferior cerebellar artery with associated traumatic subarachnoid haemorrhage have also been reported (Dolman, 1986; Harland *et al.*, 1983). A careful clinical description of a traumatic vertebral artery aneurysm rupturing into the cervi-cal subarachnoid space round the C6 nerve root has been reported (Kaplan *et al.*, 1993), suggesting that this proposed mechanism does occur.

Minimal trauma

Dissection of cervical vessels is known to occur spontaneously, and has frequently been described after mild injury, including physiological events such as vigorous coughing or sneezing. Neck movement can also be the precipitating factor; many cases have been reported followed cervical manipulation. Even endotracheal intubation has been implicated. In such circumstances, an under-lying vascular pathology is not necessarily demon-strated, and, in its absence, the trauma, although minimal, has been blamed. The progress of this condition, and its prognosis, are similar to the spontaneous type of dissection (Culebras *et al.*, 1989). Occlusion of vessels after minimal trauma also occurs, but whether this is on the basis of an intimal flap is not clear.

Prognosis

Neurological recovery

As many vascular injuries will lead to brain ischaemia and stroke the outcome from this condition is important. Early (one month) mortal-ity is the most appropriate measure, as later mortality in the (frequently older) spontaneous stroke victim is likely to be unduly high. One-month case fatality rates are age-related, being higher for the elderly. In the 1970s and 1980s, one-month case fatality for stroke varied from 17% to 34%, with an average of 21% (Terént, 1993). A comparable figure for patients with cerebral infarc-tion only (i.e. no haemorrhage) is only 17%, at least half of whom are still alive five years later. However, at one year, about one-third are still partially or completely dependent. This figure is similar at five years (Dombovy, 1993). For the younger victim of a post-traumatic stroke, the figures may be expected to be somewhat better, in the absence of associated traumatic central nervous system injury.

Wade and Langton Hewer (1989) found func-tionally useful recovery following stroke rarely continued beyond six months. This is similar to recovery following head injury. Separately, only activities of daily living and aphasia have been studied sufficiently in stroke, but in these the final (usually six-month) function correlates well with the initial function.

Cervical arterial injury

Specific vessel occlusions vary in their effects. Unger *et al.* (1980) reviewed over 700 reported carotid injuries. The mean age of the subjects was 28 years, and mortality was 21%. Of 186 with severe neurological deficits, 34% improved with carotid repair, while only 14% did so if the carotid was ligated. The outcome of blunt carotid injuries reported in the literature was reviewed by Pretre *et al.* (1994), who concluded that good results mostly applied to those patients who were asymptomatic, and that, for the others, the morbidity and mortality were very significant. Perry *et al.* (1980) found an overall mortality of 23%, which dropped to 14% if the carotid was repaired. There were no deaths after successful repair, although there were mild neurological deficits. Krajewski and Hertzer (1980) reviewed the literature on 96 cases of blunt carotid injury, finding a 30% mortality and 42% permanent neurological deficits. They recommen-ded surgical repair in patients who present with transient ischaemic symptoms, stroke in evolution, or mild completed strokes.

At the aortic arch level, Rosenberg *et al.* (1989) reported a series of 30 patients with 33 blunt injuries to the major branches; 27 of these survived and 18 of 20 reconstructions were patent at follow-up.

Penetrating injuries of the vertebral arteries seem safer than those involving the carotids, perhaps because the usually intact contralateral artery prevents ischaemia. Reid and Weigelt (1988) reported 43 patients with vertebral artery injury who had only 5% mortality. The 17% figure reported by Golueke *et al.* (1987) was ascribed to the fact that trauma occurred as part of a missile injury of the central nervous system in every subject. Vertebral artery dissection (mostly non-traumatic) was relatively benign in the 13 patients reported by Mas *et al.* (1987). There were no recurrences and 63% had normal vessels, 11% were occluded and the rest were much improved at follow-up. Unilateral occlusion from blunt injury probably mostly remains undiagnosed, judging from the study of Willis *et al.* (1994) on cervical bony injuries.

Intracranial vessel injury

For the major arteries, the consequences of occlusion are similar to those at cervical level, although the opportunities for successful collateral supply are reduced. In principle, the prognosis is essentially that of ischaemic stroke affecting the appropriate territory. Basilar occlusion had a particularly grave outlook, with an 86% mortality in spontaneous cases reported by Labauge *et al.* (1981). However, traumatic aneurysms are particularly dangerous. Jackson *et al.* (1976) found that half the reported patients had bled within 15 days of injury, and half of these haemorrhages proved fatal.

Major vessel patency

Patency of major arteries is important in the context of the risk of occlusive disease in later life. Carotid bifurcation disease affects significant numbers of elderly people. Thus, reliance on a single patent carotid artery will put the patient at an increased risk of ischaemic symptoms, greater than would occur if both vessels were patent. Furthermore, carotid endarterectomy is more hazardous when the contralateral carotid artery is occluded. Similar arguments apply to the vertebral arteries, but surgery is performed only infrequently.

Cervical veins are not important in the long term, as alternative venous channels open up if an internal jugular vein is occluded. However dural venous sinus occlusion is more serious, predisposing to the development of the syndrome of benign intracranial hypertension, and sometimes to hydrocephalus (Kalbag, 1976). Occasionally an acquired arteriovenous fistula involving the thrombosed sinus may form (Mohr *et al.*, 1989). If intradural veins are involved, there is a risk of intradural haemorrhage. Typically, the lateral sinus is affected.

Complications

Late complications are due mostly to unrecognized vessel injury, but incomplete follow-up of trauma patients may be partly to blame. Perry (1993) reported delayed diagnosis of 31 major vessel injuries, including 12 carotid arteries and leading to three strokes. Of the 31, over half had aneurysms; arteriovenous fistulae, dissections, thromboemboli and stenoses were less frequent. Sharma *et al.* (1991) reported eight traumatic carotid aneurysms diagnosed at various times over a 10-year period, and Pozzati *et al.* (1989) reported delays of between two weeks to six months in the presentation of blunt carotid dissection. Such aneurysms can present with lower cranial nerve compression at the skull base (Waespe *et al.*, 1988).

Intracranial arteries many also be affected. A carotico-cavernous fistula can follow internal carotid dissection (Tucci *et al.*, 1984). Nine examples of occlusion, including most major intracranial and extracranial vessels, have been reported after intervals of between 20 minutes (which can scarcely be called delayed) and 24 days (Krueger *et al.*, 1982). Kieck and de Villiers (1984) reported delayed intracranial haemorrhage in four of 11 patients. In these, the onset of neurological signs occurred from one week to several months after stab wounds to the head. Scalp vessels may also be affected, with superficial temporal and occipital aneurysms, and, rarely, arteriovenous fistulae (particularly occipital to mastoid emissary vein) often presenting late (Peick *et al.*, 1988). Arteries within the face may also form false aneurysms.

Haemorrhage may be intracranial, into the tissues of the scalp or neck, or into the paranasal air sinuses, pharynx or middle ear cleft. Life-threatening bleeding is well described, including ferocious epistaxis and otorrhagia.

Venous sinus thrombosis can also lead to delayed arteriovenous fistula formation, with pulsatile tinnitus. The lateral sinus is particularly likely to be involved. If preferential drainage is via intradural veins, intracranial haemorrhage (subdural or into the brain substance) can occur (Mohr *et al.*, 1989).

Further management

The initial management of the complications mentioned above is emergency control of any bleeding by local pressure. Packing of the ear, or nose and post-nasal space may temporarily control internal carotid haemorrhage. If this fails, digital compression of the ipsilateral carotid artery in the neck is required while arrangements are made for other types of intervention.

Definitive treatment of major vessel bleeding requires preliminary angiographic assessment, if feasible and if time permits. This may allow endovascular control of the lesion once it has been identified. For life-threatening epistaxis, emergency trapping may be necessary of the internal carotid artery between the dural penetration intracranially (if possible proximal to the ophthalmic artery origin) and its origin in the neck. If interventional radiology is readily available, this is usually unnecessary. Such heroic measures may be followed by cerebral ischaemia, and the option of revascularization by superficial temporal to middle cerebral artery bypass should be considered.

Treatment of an arteriovenous fistula is usually undertaken by the endovascular route. The most recent reports indicate that 80% of internal carotid arteries can be spared if endovascular obliteration of direct carotico-cavernous fistulae is carried out by an expert (Bonafé and Manelfe, 1990). Dural (e.g. lateral sinus) arteriovenous fistulae are more difficult to deal with by embolization, and excision is usually employed (Sundt and Piepgras, 1983). Radiosurgery (focused radiation) can also be used for these fistulae, but the very shallow volume is difficult to irradiate satisfactorily.

Aneurysms in the cervical vessels are best repaired, where possible by reconstruction. If this is not possible, then prevention or treatment of cerebral ischaemia by some form of bypass may be appropriate. For extracranial vessels, dissection is most often managed by anticoagulation or surgical reconstruction. Intracranial arterial dissection is usually diagnosed after vessel occlusion has occurred, but, if it affects the intradural vertebral artery, it is mostly diagnosed after subarachnoid haemorrhage, when ligation has been reported to be effective and safe.

References

Aoki N, Sakai T, Kaneko M. (1991) Traumatic aneurysm of the middle meningeal artery presenting as delayed onset of acute subdural haematoma. *Surg Neurol* **37**: 59–62.

Bok APL, Kieck CF, de Villiers JC. (1984) Head injury associated with carotid occlusion due to blunt cervical trauma. *S Afr J Surg* **22**: 43–50.

Bonafé A, Manelfe C. (1990) Traumatic carotid–cavernous sinus fistulas. In: Braakman R, editor. *Handbook of clinical neurology, vol. 57: Head injury.* Amsterdam: Elsevier Science 345–66.

Buckingham MJ, Crone KR, Ball WS, *et al.* (1988) Traumatic intracranial aneurysms in childhood: two cases and a review of the literature. *Neurosurgery* **22**: 398–408.

Culebras A, Hodge CJ, Petro GR. (1989) Carotid and vertebral dissecting haematomas. In: Toole JF, editor. *Handbook of clinical neurology, vol. 54: Vascular diseases. Part* II. Amsterdam: Elsevier Science, 271–85.

Davis JW, Holbrook TL, Hoyt DB, *et al.* (1990) Blunt carotid artery dissection: incidence, associated injuries, screening, and treatment. *J Trauma* **30**: 1514–17.

Deck JHN, Jagadha V. (1986) Fatal subarachnoid haemorrhage due to traumatic rupture of the vertebral artery. *Arch Pathol Lab Med* **110**: 489–93.

Demetriades D, Skalkides J, Sofianos C, *et al.* (1989) Carotid artery injuries: experience with 124 cases. *J Trauma* **29**: 91–94.

Dolman CL. (1986) Rupture of posterior inferior cerebellar artery by single blow to head. *Arch Pathol Lab Med* **110**: 494–96.

Dombovy ML. (1993) Rehabilitation and the course of recovery after stroke. In: Whisnant JP, editor. *Stroke: populations, cohorts and clinical trials.* Oxford: Butterworth-Heinemann, 218–37.

Fakhry SM, Jaques PF, Proctor HJ. (1988) Cervical vessel injury after blunt trauma. *J Vasc Surg* **8**: 501–508.

Ferguson GG. (1989) Intracranial artery aneurysms – a surgical perspective. In: Toole JF, editor. *Handbook of clinical neurology, vol. 55: Vascular diseases. Part* III. Amsterdam: Elsevier Science, 41–87.

Fosburg RG, Brewer LA. (1976) Arterial vascular injury to the spinal cord. In: Vinken PJ, Bruyn GW, editors. *Handbook of clinical neurology, vol. 26: Injuries of the spine and spinal cord. Part* II Amsterdam: Elsevier Science, 63–79.

Freckmann N, Sartor K, Herrmann HD. (1981) Traumatic arteriovenous fistulae of the middle meningeal artery and neighbouring veins or dural sinuses. *Acta Neurochir* **55**: 273–81.

Fry RE, Fry WJ. (1980) Extracranial carotid artery injuries. *Surgery* **88**: 581–87.

Garg BP, Ottinger CJ, Smith RR, *et al.* (1993) Strokes in children due to vertebral artery trauma. *Neurology* **43**: 2555–58.

Golueke P, Sclafani S, Phillips T, *et al.* (1987) Vertebral artery injury – diagnosis and management. *J Trauma* **27**: 856–65.

Harland WA, Pitts JF, Watson AA. (1983) Subarachnoid haemorrhage due to upper cervical trauma. *J Clin Pathol* **36**: 1335–41.

Hebra A, Robison JG, Elliott BM. (1993) Traumatic aneurysm associated with fibrointimal proliferation of the common carotid artery following blunt trauma: case report. *J Trauma* **34**: 297–99.

Hellner D, Thie A, Lachenmayer L, *et al.* (1993) Blunt trauma lesions of the extracranial internal carotid artery in patients with head injury. *J Craniomaxillofac Surg* **21**: 234–38.

Hengerer AS, DeGroot TR, Rivers RJ, *et al.* (1984) Internal carotid artery thrombosis following soft palate injuries: a case report and review of 16 cases. *Laryngoscope* **94**: 1571–75.

Hoang-The-Dan P, Pourriat JL, Lapandry C, *et al.* (1984) Internal carotid artery dissection. *Ann Fr Anesth Reanim* **3**: 388–91.

Jackson FE, Gleave JRW Janon E. (1976) The traumatic cranial and intracranial aneurysms. In: *Handbook of clinical neurology, vol. 24: Injuries of the brain and skull. Part* II. Amsterdam: North-Holland, 381–98.

Kalbag RM. (1976) Dural venous sinus thrombosis and head injury. Braakman R, editor. In: *Handbook of clinical neurology, vol. 24: Injuries of the brain and skull. Part* II. Amsterdam: North-Holland, 369–80.

Kaplan SS, Ogilvy CS, Gonzalez R, *et al.* (1993) Extracranial vertebral artery pseudoaneurysm presenting as subarachnoid hemorrhage. *Stroke* **24**: 1397–99.

Khoury G, Hajj H, Khoury SJ, *et al.* (1990) Penetrating trauma to the carotid vessels. *Eur J Vasc Surg*, **4**: 607–10.

Kieck CF, de Villiers JC. (1984) Vascular lesions due to transcranial stab wounds. *J Neurosurg* **60**: 42–46.

Krajewski LP, Hertzer NR, (1980) Blunt carotid artery trauma: report of two cases and review of the literature. *Ann Surg* **191**: 341–46.

Krueger H, Wodarz R, Werry WD. (1982) Cerebral arterial occlusions following blunt trauma of head and neck. *Nervenarzt* **53**: 83–90.

Labauge R, Pages M, MartyDouble C, *et al.* (1981) Occlusion of the basilar artery. A review with 17 personal cases. *Rev Neurol* **137**: 545–71.

Laske A, Bauer E, Von Segesser L, *et al.* (1990) Injuries of the large supraaortic arteries. *Schweiz Med Wochenschr* **120**: 1050–55.

Lipschitz R. (1976) Stab wounds of the spinal cord. In: Braakman R, editor. *Handbook of clinical neurology, vol. 25: Injuries of the spine and spinal cord. Part* I. Amsterdam: North-Holland, 197–207.

Louw JA, Mafoyane NA, Small B, *et al.* (1990) Occlusion of the vertebral artery in cervical spine dislocations. *J Bone Joint Surg Br* **72**: 679–81.

Mas JL, Bousser MG, Hasboun D, *et al.* (1987) Extracranial vertebral artery dissections: a review of 13 cases. *Stroke* **18**: 1037–47.

Meyer JS, Imai A, Shinohara T. (1988) Causes of cerebral ischaemia and infarction. In Toole JF, editor. *Handbook of clinical neurology, vol. 53: Vascular diseases. Part* I. Amsterdam: Elsevier Science, 155–73.

Mirvis SE, Wolf AL, Numaguchi Y, *et al.* (1990) Post-traumatic cerebral infarction diagnosed by CT: prevalence, origin and outcome. *AJR* **154**: 1293–98.

Mizutani T, Goldberg HI, Parr J, *et al.* (1982) Cerebral dissecting aneurysm and intimal fibroelastic thickening of cerebral arteries. Case report. *J Neurosurg* **56**: 571–76.

Moar JJ. (1987) Traumatic rupture of the cervical carotid arteries: an autopsy and histopathological study of 200 cases. *Forensic Sci Int* **34**: 227–44.

Mohr JP, Stein BM, Hilal SK. (1989) Arteriovenous malformations. Toole JF, editor. In: *Handbook of clinical neurology, vol. 54: Vascular diseases. Part* II. Amsterdam: Elsevier Science, 361–93.

Nov AA, Cromwell LD. (1984) Traumatic pericallosal artery aneurysm. *J Neuroradiol* **11**: 3–8.

Odake G. (1981) Spontaneous closure of a traumatic middle meningeal arteriovenous fistula accompanied by a sagittal epidural haematoma. *Neurol Med Chir* **21**: 1267–73.

Peick AL, Nichols WK, Curtis JJ, *et al.* (1988) Aneurysms and pseudoaneurysms of the superficial temporal artery caused by trauma. *J Vasc Surg* **8**: 606–10.

Perry MO, Snyder WH, Thal ER. (1980) Carotid artery injuries caused by blunt trauma. *Ann Surg* **192**: 74–77.

Perry MO. (1993) Complications of missed arterial injuries. *J Vasc Surg* **17**: 399–407.

Pollanen MS, Deck JHN, Boutilier L, *et al.* (1992) Lesions of the tunica media in traumatic rupture of vertebral arteries: histologic and biochemical studies. *Can J Neurol Sci* **19**: 53–56.

Pozzati E, Giuliani G, Poppi M, *et al.* (1989) Blunt traumatic carotid dissection with delayed symptoms. *Stroke* **20**: 412–16.

Pretre R, Reverdin A, Kalonji T, *et al.* (1994) Blunt carotid artery injury: difficult therapeutic approaches for an under-recognized entity. *Surgery* **115**: 375–81.

Rao PM, Ivatury RR, Sharma P, *et al.* (1993) Cervical vascular injuries: a trauma centre experience. *Surgery* **114**: 527–31.

Reid JDS, Weigelt JA. (1988) Forty-three cases of vertebral artery trauma. *J Trauma* **28**: 1007–12.

Rosenberg JM, Bredenberg CE, Marvasti MA, *et al.* (1989) Blunt injuries to the aortic arch vessels. *Ann Thorac Surg* **48**: 508–13.

Roy R, Cooper PR. (1990) Penetrating injuries of the skull and brain. In Braakman R, editor. *Handbook of Clinical Neurology, vol. 57: Head injury.* Amsterdam: Elsevier Science, 299–315.

Sharma S, Rajani M, Mishra N, *et al.* (1991) Extracranial carotid artery aneurysms following accidental injury: ten years' experience. *Clin Radiol* **43**: 162–65.

Simeone FA, Lyness SS. (1976) Vertebral artery thrombosis in injuries of the spine. In: Vinken PJ, Bruyn GW, editors. *Handbook of clinical neurology, vol. 26: Injuries of the spine and spinal Cord. Part* II. Amsterdam: North-Holland, 57–62.

Soria ED. (1988) Traumatic aneurysms of cerebral vessels: a case study and review of the literature. *Angiology* **39**: 609–15.

Stern WE. (1976) Carotid–cavernous fistula. In: Vinken PJ, Bruyn GW, editors. *Handbook of clinical neurology, vol. 24: Injuries of the brain and skull Part* II. Amsterdam: North-Holland, 399–439.

Sundt TM, Piepgras DG. (1983) The surgical approach to arteriovenous malformations of the lateral and sigmoid dural sinuses. *J Neurosurg* **59**: 32–39.

Terént A. (1993) Stroke morbidity. In: Whisnant JP, editor. *Stroke: populations cohorts and clinical trials*. Oxford: Butterworth-Heinemann, 37–58.

Tucci JM, Maitland CG, Pcsolyar DW, *et al.* (1984) Carotid – cavernous fistula due to traumatic dissection of the extracranial internal carotid artery. *Am J Neuroradiol* **5**: 828–29.

Unger SW, Tucker WS, Mrdeza MA, *et al.* (1980) Carotid arterial trauma. *Surgery* **87**: 477–87.

Vanezis P. (1986) Vertebral artery injuries in road traffic accidents: a post-mortem study. *J Forensic Sci Soc* **26**: 281–91.

Wade DT, Langton Hewer R. (1989) Rehabilitation after stroke. In: Toole JF, editor. *Handbook of clinical neurology, vol. 55: Vascular diseases. Part* III. Amsterdam: Elsevier Science, 233–54.

Waespe W, Niesper J, Imhof HG, *et al.* (1988) Lower cranial nerve palsies due to internal carotid dissection. *Stroke* **19**: 1561–64.

Willis BK, Greiner F, Orrison WW, *et al.* (1994) The incidence of vertebral artery injury after midcervical spine fracture or subluxation. *Neurosurgery* **34**: 435–42.

17

Neuroradiological considerations

B E Kendall

Introduction

In western society, head trauma is the most common cause of death and disablement in young persons. Overall, road traffic accidents and falls account for most severe injuries and 50% of deaths, but in young children nonaccidental injury is responsible for 25% of head injuries (HI) and it is responsible for over 80% of HI deaths in infants. Many head injuries have medicolegal implications and radiology may play an important part by demonstrating the extent and pathophysiology of the damage; this may aid in determination of the cause and prognosis.

Many patients with severe head injuries are unstable when admitted to hospital and the early management is often crucial to the prognosis. Clinical responsibility for such patients undergoing imaging studies is shared between the radiologist and the referring clinician. It is the responsibility of the latter to be sure that:

1. An accurate clinical assessment has been made and imaging is indicated.
2. Any serial observations of the patient's condition are available and are maintained in the imaging department
3. The patient is in a satisfactory condition for transfer to the imaging department and that nursing attention is maintained, when necessary, during the imaging studies.

Perfect images can be produced only on motionless patients. Head-injured patients may be unable to co-operate due to confusion, intoxication, fear or claustrophobia. When appropriate, rapidly revers-

ible sedation or, very occasionally, general anaesthesia may be indicated in order to obtain diagnostic studies.

Head injury is often only one component of the damage resulting from major trauma. Life-threatening thoracic and/or abdominal injuries with ruptured viscera and/or internal bleeding may require preliminary elucidation in which ultrasound or portable radiographic facilities may play a significant part. Any hypovolaemia must be corrected simultaneously. Priority in management should be given to the prevention of secondary hypoxic and/or ischaemic brain damage or the elevation of intracranial pressure. The establishment of adequate ventilation is a particularly important consideration in head injury, because of the secondary effects of CO_2 retention in raising intracranial pressure.

In severe cases, radiological examination designed to show intracranial bleeding and mass lesions is a high priority and must be conducted rapidly in a fashion that ensures the production of adequate films. In patients with clinical signs and/or symptoms suggesting neck injury, or in patients with reduced levels of consciousness following a head injury, a preliminary lateral radiograph, or even a CT scout view of the cervical spine, is advisable in order to exclude an unstable fracture or fracture-dislocation in which damage to the cervical spinal cord could occur with even the gentle movement necessary for the positioning of the head for imaging or during recovery when mobilization is commenced.

It is the responsibility of the radiologist to perform the correct studies for the facilitation of treatment and to produce images that document adequately any significant abnormalities that are detected. It is also the responsibility of the radiologist to comment on the diagnostic quality of the images produced and to recognize any artefacts. The significance of a negative study in the clinical context should be clearly stated.

The decisions regarding the investigations to be performed are made in consultation with the referring specialist after consideration of the history, the current disabilities and the possible underlying pathophysiologies to be elucidated. Consultation in the majority of cases is by written request. Equally it is an important duty of the radiologist to limit the use of studies that will not provide the information that the clinician requires, particularly if they are invasive or involve ionizing radiation. In particular transarterial angiography is necessary only as a pretherapeutic measure to be used prior to intervention, having been replaced by MR angiography or spiral CT for diagnostic purposes.

Brain death is a clinical diagnosis. It may be documented by electrophysiological tests but imaging is not indicated in dead or moribund subjects.

Scalp injury

Radiology makes a relatively small, but sometimes important contribution to this diagnosis. An abnormality of the soft tissues of the scalp or face is often apparent, frequently noted as an incidental feature on imaging studies of head-injured patients. Oedema, haematoma, blood breakdown products, and/or loss of tissue may be apparent. Foreign bodies, particularly metallic objects, that are evident on plain radiographs may cause artefacts on CT scans; ferromagentic foreign bodies induce phase shift and susceptibility artefacts on MRI.

An irregularity shown on imaging of the cortex of a bone underlying a scalp injury may give the first indication of osteomyelitis or bone necrosis.

Cephalhaematoma is the presence of a blood clot between a single bone of the skull vault (usually the parietal, occasionally the occipital) and the pericranium. It is limited by the connection of the pericranium to the sutures. It occurs in 2.5% of newborns and, in forceps deliveries, is not uncommonly associated with a fracture. Periosteal bone may be shown by two days of age but a prominent peripheral rim of bone is generally

evident by 10 days. Resolution is usual by 6–10 weeks, but it may persist and fill in with trabeculated bone to form a permanent, localized thickening of the vault with widening of the diploe.

Chronic subgaleal haematoma or effusion is a complication of recurrent haematoma, particularly affecting poorly controlled epileptics. The subgaleal fluid may form a thick layer within a partly calcified membrane.

Scalp injury may also occur as the result of embolization procedures, in which intentional or inadvertent blockage of scalp vessels occurs during occlusion procedures for a post-traumatic fistula or severe bleeding. Radio-opaque material may or may not be evident in the occluded vessels.

Skull fractures and cranial defects

A skull fracture is present in about 75% of severe head injuries and there is no doubt that the presence of even a simple linear vault fracture in a conscious patient is associated with a considerable increase in the incidence of intracranial damage, increasing the probability of intracranial haematoma by a factor of 400 and of craniotomy by a factor of 20. (Dacey *et al.*, 1986; Jennett and Teasdale, 1981). However, intracranial bleeding not infrequently occurs in the absence of a fracture; a fracture was absent in 44% of cases requiring craniotomy in one large series (Masters *et al.*, 1987). Fractures are not excluded by normal skull radiography and the mere demonstration of a fracture provides inadequate information about the presence and degree of intracranial damage. If there is reason to suspect intracranial haemorrhage, or when clinical assessment is complicated by alcohol or drug abuse, or a clinical feature suggests the possibility of a skull base fracture, a CT scan should be performed and/or the patient should be observed for 48 hours. Skull radiographs are not a routine requirement in the management of head trauma (Rosenorn *et al.*, 1991).

Even when in retrospect skull radiographs would have shown a fracture, failure to have taken them is not negligent if a clinical indication was lacking at the time. With one notable exception, radiographs or other studies should not be performed solely for medicolegal purposes. Only when nonaccidental injury is suspected are skeletal, including skull, radiographs indicated for the potential medicolegal benefit of a child.

Skull radiography may be indicated for elucidation of the complications of fractures for example to show a depressed fragment, which, because of overlap, appears as a relatively dense area on routine projections. The degree of any depression is more conveniently shown by a CT scan than by tangential view skull radiographs. Skull radiographs are indicated in patients who have had cerebrospinal fluid diverting procedures in order to verify the possibility of a post-traumatic shunt disconnection. When CT imaging is not available, skull radiographic studies, limited by the guidelines in the report of the Royal College of Radiologists (Clarke and Adams, 1990), are advisable.

However, skull radiographs have often been done prior to referral; correct radiological interpretation is essential for assessment of the severity of the injury and its potential complications. Failure to diagnose a skull fracture on a radiograph or a CT scan in time to avoid an intracranial complication may be a major factor in mediolegal proceedings. Failure to emphasize the inadequacy of imaging studies for diagnosis or exclusion may also assume importance.

Particular attention should be paid to any sign that may be indicative of:

1. A compound fracture and the danger of intracranial sepsis;
2. An intraorbital foreign body, particularly if metallic, which maybe a contraindication to MRI;
3. A fracture of the maxilla or mandible, which may be associated with airway obstruction or cause cosmetic disfiguration.

Skull fractures, when present, are often evident on CT scan; bone windowing should be used if necessary, and they should then be documented on film. High resolution CT scanning is the optimum procedure for the diagnosis of skull base fractures.

A fracture line is recognized by an extension through both tables of the skull, which causes it to appear darker than vascular grooves and diploic channels. When the radiograph beam used is oblique to the fracture line, the break in the inner and outer tables may be shown as overlapping lines. In a recent fracture, the margins are parallel and clearly defined, particularly when the fracture is on the side of the skull adjacent to the film, but they are not corticated. This feature is helpful in the differential diagnosis from unusual sutures and congenital cranial defects which commonly occur in neurofibromatosis type I, but which are occasionally seen as isolated anomalies. Fractures usually extend into, and frequently cross, sutures. In children in particular they may be accompanied by diastasis of the suture. As healing commences, the edges of the fracture become eroded and by about two weeks after the injury the fracture line tends to become more ill-defined. Fractures usually heal completely within six months in adults and within a much shorter period of time (as little as eight weeks) in young children.

Failure of a fracture to heal is usually associated with tearing of the underlying meninges. This results in either a pseudomeningocoele or interposition of brain substance, so that the normal brain pulsation causes erosion of the edges of the bone, resulting in a 'growing fracture' (Tandon *et al.*, 1987). This condition, which is relatively much more common in children, is associated with a soft tissue mass, which gradually increases in size and is underlying the scalp. A more clinically significant feature is damage caused to the adjacent cortex by the margins of the bone defect. This usually produces progressive loss of brain substance, resulting in an encephalomalacic cyst, which is commonly associated with neurological deficit and/or of epilepsy. Such damage may be prevented by early treatment of the dural rent and reconstitution of the skull defect.

Compound fractures are of particular importance because they provide a potential pathway for infection, which may precipitate meningitis or abscess formation. Many are evident clinically from the presence of a depressed vault fracture with overlying laceration of the scalp, or of cerebrospinal fluid leakage or bleeding.

Radiological features

The Radiological features of compound fractures include:

1. Air related to the fracture line or within the cranium. Its recognition may be subtle and require window manipulation to distinguish it from fat, which is less lucent. Gas may be:
   a. Extradural, usually extending from a sinus or mastoid and lifting dural attachments;
   b. Subdural, extending along the side of the falx or tentorium.
   c. Subarachnoid or intraventricular, with fluid levels on appropriate studies;
   d. Within brain substance.
   Air under tension (aerocoele) may be recognized from the displacement of intracranial

structures. This may be sufficient to require urgent surgical drainage to avoid brain damage from vascular compression secondary to trans-falcine or tentorial herniation.

2. Extension of a fracture into air-containing structures, such as paranasal sinuses, nasal cavity, middle ear or mastoid should be carefully sought.

3. Any intracranial foreign body.

4. Intracranial abscess: intracranial sepsis is usually suspected clinically from evidence of systemic upset and intracranial mass signs. Intraparenchymal abscess usually shows on imaging as a thin-walled ring-enhancing structure with surrounding oedema. Extracerebral abscesses, particularly extradural pus, may be much more difficult to detect; a thin layer of fluid can be associated with considerable clinical disturbance and, even if a plain scan is negative, in appropriate clinical situations a postcontrast medium study should be performed to seek an enhancing membrane.

Accidental injury

Accidental injuries may be unsuspected from the history.

In birth injury, fractures are usually associated with use of forceps and may or may not be accompanied by obvious bruising, a cephalhaematoma, or a clinically evident depression. Their significance lies in the possibility of underlying intracranial haemorrhages, especially sub- and extradural haematomas, which may involve the posterior fossa and/or require evacuation. Rarely, fractures may be caused by a narrow pelvis, usually due to pressure by the sacral promontory, on by a benign tumour such as an osteochondroma. If such fractures are not recognized, they may later cause confusion in patients in whom there is a possibility of nonaccidental injury.

Nonaccidental injury

Nonaccidental injury is suspected when there is evidence of trauma on physical examination without an appropriate history. Head injury is frequent in these circumstances and it may be suggested by craniofacial bruising or haematoma formation, swelling of the scalp, enlargement of the vault, epilepsy, diminished consciousness, or neurological deficit. Evidence of systemic trauma with meta-

physeal (Kleinman, 1990) and rib fractures, soft tissue injury such as tearing of the frenulum, burns and features of social neglect may also be evident.

Radiology plays an important role in the diagnosis and documentation of nonaccidental injury. Experimental evidence indicates that a simple linear fracture of a parietal bone may be caused by a force equivalent to a fall from a distance of one-and-a-half feet striking the vertex directly onto an unyielding surface (Taylor, 1856). Features of skull fractures indicating violence greater than can be accounted for by a fall from a height of under three feet on to a hard surface (Weber, 1985) include:

1. Fractures of the occipital bone;
2. Fracture lines with separation greater than 5 mm;
3. Multiple fractures;
4. Fractures that are complex with multiple rami;
5. Fractures associated with splaying of sutures.

It is often of importance in such subjects to attempt from the appearance of the fractures and the reaction in the adjacent bone to assess within fairly wide limits the dates between which the causative trauma could have occurred. This may be used as one indicator of the time of the injury and of whether there has been more than one incident. The presence of visible soft tissue swelling over a fracture suggests a recent injury. Generally speaking, the margins of a skull fracture remain well defined and parallel for about one to two weeks, and then tend to become progressively more ill defined as healing commences. A fracture in which the margins are not parallel will be over two weeks in age. Fractures are usually healed by eight weeks, particularly in young children. Skull fractures do not develop callus during healing and this is an important feature in deciding the age of a long bone fracture. A skeletal survey is of importance in this respect and should always be obtained (Kleinman, 1990). Consideration of the intracranial injuries in relation to the fractures may be helpful for more accurate timing (Zimmerman *et al.*, 1979).

Cranial nerve palsies may be due to compression by haematoma, aneurysm, fibrous or granulation tissue, or to tearing of the nerve at the time of injury. The latter mechanism is likely if the fracture transgresses a neural foramen or end organ. Division of a cranial nerve may be recognized if it can be visualized on high resolution MRI, particularly in the case of the second, seventh and eighth nerves. The extension of a fracture into the optic canal, internal auditory canal or otic labyrinth is easily shown with high resolution CT scanning, which may also reveal the extension of basal fractures into other cranial nerve canals.

Penetrating craniocerebral injury

Metallic fragments from a high velocity gun shot injury may pass through the skull, leaving a larger exit than entry wound; low velocity missiles tend to be retained within the cranium. When examined by CT scanning they tend to cause a considerable artefact, which may mask the degree of adjacent damage. Metallic fragments are potentially mobile and ferromagnetic fragments are a contraindication to MRI. Other metallic objects, such as knives and arrows, may be extracted following the injury, but the possibility of retained fragments should always be considered; MRI is contraindicated until these have been excluded. The metallic fragments may lie within a fluid filled cavity and may move under the influence of gravity. Many metallic foreign bodies and bone fragments are sterile, but the particles of skin and clothing carried with them are not, so that superimposed infection may occur. This may be suggested by increasing oedema adjacent to the foreign body and is confirmed by thin walled ring enhancement with surrounding oedema if an abscess forms. Erosion into the cerebrospinal fluid or damage to an adjacent blood vessel may be precipitated. For these reasons, carefully planned extraction of the metal through a nonevocative region of the brain may be considered, often using stereotactic methods.

Although penetrating trauma is usually associated with an obvious entry wound, this is not always the case. Particularly in children, self-inflicted accidental damage by a sharp object entering the eye or mouth may be associated with only superficial trauma or with asymptomatic deep penetration into brain substance. The object may be radio-opaque, but wooden skewers and pencils may be involved. These are usually of low density on CT scans and reflect little signal on MRI, where they are visible as linear, low intensity structures.

As well as infection, penetrating trauma may be associated with direct damage to blood vessels and may cause haematoma, aneurysm, dissection or arteriovenous fistula. Percutaneous needling for the treatment of trigeminal neuralgia (carotico-cavernous fistula), percutaneous transjugular catheterization (vertebro-vertebral fistula) and direct puncture of cervical vessels for angiography (vertebro-vertebral and carotid-jugular fistula) are well

recorded. These are uncommon complications and should not lead to successful litigation provided the procedure was clinically indicated and informed consent was obtained. Treatment is by interventional neuroradiology.

A rare form of penetrating trauma may occur to the foetal head during amniocentesis. This may cause brain damage either directly from intracranial haemorrhage (which may also result in hydrocephalus) or indirectly due to arterial damage causing infarction. A history of difficulty with the amniocentesis, foetal distress and/or the presence of a scar in the superficial tissues overlying the brain damage may be helpful in diagnosis. (Chong *et al.*, 1989; Naylor *et al.*, 1990; Youroukos *et al.*, 1980).

Brain damage and intracranial haematoma

Currently, cranial CT scanning is the diagnostic procedure of choice in management of head injury although MRI is playing an increasing role. Patients with a minor or moderate head injury with a negative CT scan and clinical improvement to virtual normality are generally discharged under the care of a reliable companion after a period of 12 hours' observation. If there is failure to improve, or deterioration occurs, the CT scan is repeated. A negative CT scan in a patient with a depressed conscious level may occur with:

1. Diffuse axonal injury, which may be revealed by MRI;
2. Early contusions and hypoxic ischaemic lesions, which will become evident on delayed CT scanning or on MRI;
3. Epilepsy;
4. Intoxication by drugs;
5. Metabolic disturbances.

On the combined basis of CT scanning (or MRI) and clinical observation, medical management may be supplemented by surgical intervention. Imaging may show:

1. Diffuse lesions, which, in a comatose patient may require immediate intensive care management in order to prevent secondary brain damage due to hypoxia, hypercarbia, hypotension, brain swelling with herniation, seizures or metabolic imbalance, all of which may have medicolegal implications.

2. Focal lesions, which are potentially correctable by surgery aimed at relief of raised intracranial pressure. Generally speaking focal intracerebral haemorrhages or haemorrhagic contusions causing mass effect and sited in nonevocative regions are considered for surgery in appropriate clinical circumstances if their volume exceeds about 25 ml in the supratentorial compartment, but less if they are infratentorial.

The biochemical changes that occur in a haematoma with the passage of time not only give characteristic appearances on imaging but also have constituents that can be recognized, particularly on MRI. These may allow some estimation of the time of the bleeding. This is not of particular significance when the history is reliable but there are cases, such as in nonaccidental injury, in which the timing of an incident may have important implications.

The density of blood and blood clot on CT scans is proportional mainly to the protein concentration. This is at its highest in recent, fully contracted clot and reduces as the clot is denatured.

Anaemia, admixture with cerebrospinal fluid and poor clot contraction may reduce the initial density of blood and/or clot. Blood that fails to clot may precipitate as in an haematocrit, showing a 'fluid level' with the denser part dependent.

The time to denaturation varies with the size of the clot, but isodensity generally occurs at between 14 and 28 days and hypodensity after these periods.

A diminished or increased MRI signal (depending on the sequence) may be caused by flowing protons. This phenomenon is used to show blood vessels by MR angiography. In recent haematomas, a communication between an artery and a vein may persist and circulation of blood may be shown within part of the haematoma. Oxyhaemoglobin, being diamagnetic, returns a signal similar to that of brain substance, whereas, in high field images, deoxyhaemoglobin and the other compounds of haemoglobin are paramagnetic and return a reduced signal on T2 (particularly on T2*) and gradient echo sequences when intracellular. The time taken by the haemoglobin to become reduced varies with the environment and is slower within the cerebrospinal fluid than within an enclosed cavity or within brain substance.

Intracellular methaemoglobin is formed as the haemoglobin within red blood corpuscles is oxidized. This has a short T1 and is bright; it returns low signal on T2. As lysis of the cells takes place, methaemoglobin is released and returns high signal on both T1 and T2-weighted sequences. Macrophages invade the haematoma from the periphery, engulfing the remains of the haemoglobin breakdown products, which are converted into haemosiderin particles. This causes susceptibility effects, reflecting low signal on T2-weighted sequences. Haemosiderin formation occurs in intracerebral haematomas but is unusual in extracerebral haematomas unless recurrent bleeding takes place.

Haemosiderin, by persisting for long periods, provides a useful indicator of the previous haemorrhage within the brain substance. In particular, it can help to distinguish haemorrhage and haemorrhagic contusion from infarction and nonhaemorrhagic contusion. Often, haemoglobin breakdown is at various stages in different parts of a haematoma, providing a more complex, but easily analysed, image.

Extradural bleeding is usually arterial, classically from the middle meningeal artery and often associated with skull fractures crossing arterial grooves. Binding of the dura to the skull tends to restrict the haematoma and accounts for its biconvex configuration. Rapid accumulation of the haematoma is associated with progressive neurological deficit, responding to early recognition and surgery. Basal and vertex haematomas are best shown on coronal sections and therefore by MRI, being more easily overlooked on axial CT scans. The latter usually originate from a torn venous sinus, which is displaced from the vault by a haematoma crossing the midline. Similarly, other dural attachments, including the tentorium, tend to be separated from the bone if the haematoma is both above and below it.

With all extracerebral bleeding, urgent drainage may be life saving and, since it is not usually associated with any primary brain injury, the prognosis for full recovery is good. When the clinical diagnosis is evident, delay in order to perform confirmatory radiological studies in a rapidly deteriorating patient should be avoided.

Chronic extradural haematoma is unusual. It is most frequent as a complication of shunt procedures in children and may be found incidentally, often with a calcified rim, during routine checking of hydrocephalus control.

Acute subdural haemorrhage is usually due to bleeding from brain substance and is one component of severe intracranial damage in primary brain injury. The extracerebral clot frequently extends over the surface of the damaged lobe or hemisphere and conforms in shape to the convexity. The damaged brain adds to the swelling and displacement and may be the predominant factor in patients with only a shallow but diffuse subdural haemorrhage. The radiologist should assess and record the relative contribution of each of these components, since unnecessary or too aggressive surgery may have medicolegal implications. Contralateral or, in the case of posterior fossa subdural haemorrhage, 3 ventricular hydrocephalus is a poor prognostic sign requiring urgent surgical relief of the swelling. In general, the prognosis for a good recovery is poor.

As haematomas become subacute 7–21 days after bleeding, they tend to isodensity with grey matter and may be difficult to visualize directly with CT scans. Medial deviation of the cerebral white matter and compression of the ventricle(s) usually allow a diagnosis with CT scanning, even in bilateral cases in which a midline shift is absent. With MRI, altered signal in the haematoma is always evident.

Chronic haematomas are of lower density than grey matter and are biconvex in configuration. Post-traumatic headaches, other symptoms of raised intracranial pressure, or recurrent subdural bleeding may be present.

Chronic subdural haematoma in infants includes many cases of so-called external hydrocephalus. This is mostly seen between two and six months of age, more often in boys. It is usually bilateral with fluid extending into the interhemispheric fissure. It may follow known head injury with previously documented high density subdural haematoma; more often there is no history of trauma and the aetiology is uncertain, but nonaccidental injury may be strongly suspected. Encephalomalacia and/or focal atrophy more frequent in the parieto-occipital region(s), or evidence of systemic trauma may support this premise. Presentation is usually with an enlarging or large head; focal signs are unusual, although retinal haemorrhages or cerebrospinal fluid xanthochromia may be present.

The extracerebral fluid is usually of a slightly higher density and of a T2 higher signal than cerebrospinal fluid. The underlying subarachnoid space may be visible and even dilated, and the brain may appear compressed away from the vault.

Haemosiderin tends to be present in subdural membranes only if haemorrhage is recurrent. It may also occur following haemorrhage into the subarachnoid space, being produced in Bergmann glia and resulting in meningeal haemosiderosis, which is usually restricted to cases of chronic and recurrent subarachnoid haemorrhage.

Cerebrospinal fluid fistula: meningitis

Most cerebrospinal fluid leaks cease spontaneously soon after trauma, but some persist and are an underlying cause of recurrent meningitis. The site of a fistula may be suggested by the demonstration of fluid localized, for example, to one middle ear or a paranasal sinus, or of a fracture extending through the wall of an air cavity, particularly if herniation of intracranial contents into the fracture line is evident.

In patients in whom the precise site of the leak is not evident (as, for example, with complex basal fractures or in the absence of a visible fracture line), in the presence of active cerebrospinal fluid leakage, the fistula may be shown by intrathecal injection of nonionic contrast medium. This is manipulated along the cranial base to outline the cerebrospinal fluid-filled track, followed by CT scanning. If the leakage ceases during the procedure it may be induced again by causing an increase of cerebrospinal fluid secretion by jugular compression or by raising cerebrospinal fluid pressure using a Valsalva manoeuvre.

Post-traumatic epilepsy

This occurs much more frequently with depressed fractures with an underlying cerebral laceration than with a simple contusion. Lesions are usually well shown by routine MRI, by which the degree and extent of the brain damage is defined. If no scar is evident on routine MRI, high resolution T1-weighted volume imaging using an MP RAGE or spoilt GRASS-type of sequence will reveal the cerebral cortex in greater detail.

Motor sequelae: involuntary movements; sensory sequelae: thalamic pain; impairment of memory and intelligence or of emotional control

The phase of recovery of physiological processes following head injury is generally defined as extending to the end of the period of post-traumatic amnesia (Symonds, 1962). The patient may be left with one or more of these post-traumatic symptoms.

These symptoms may occur in the presence of major brain destruction, causing postencephalomalacic cystic changes ('porencephalic cysts'), gliosis and atrophy. They are often associated with diffuse axonal injury following shear stress lesions or small brain stem haemorrhages caused by tearing of basal perforating arteries. In such patients, end stage damage may be shown on high resolution T2-weighted MRI (Gentry *et al.*, 1988a,b) as small high intensity gliotic lesions with low intensity components due to the presence of haemosiderin. These are not infrequently demonstrated in the corpus callosum and fornices as well as in the cerebral white matter. It should be noted that even with high field high resolution MRI, carried out to assess the degree of residual brain damage, only a minority of axonal shearing injuries are shown. Some of these correspond to larger lesions visible in the acute phase, particularly if these lesions are haemorrhagic. In the acute phase of major shearing injuries, CT scans may be normal but haematoma in the septum pellucidum, corpus callosum, fornix or upper brain stem, and blood within the lateral ventricles are often present on CT scans (Kido *et al.*, 1992). Such subjects often remain unconscious from the moment of impact until death.

After minor head trauma, post-traumatic behaviour disorders and the postconcussional syndrome have been shown on high field MRI to be associated with similar residua of axonal shearing in the white matter of the cerebral hemispheres (Mittl *et al.*, 1994).

Hypothalamic and pituitary lesions

If diabetes insipidus or the effects of inappropriate antidiuretic hormone secretion are recognized clinically, damage to the infundibulum or, less frequently, to the hypothalamus, may be evident. Diabetes insipidus is usually transient but, in those patients in whom it persists, MRI, and, less often CT scanning, may show disruption of the pituitary stalk associated with an enhancing T1 high signal nodule in the region of the tuber cinerium. The normal T1 high signal from a normally sited posterior pituitary is absent and, if the hypophyseal portal system is completely disrupted, the anterior pituitary gland may be small with extension of the chiasmatic cistern into the sella turcica.

Congenital disruption of the pituitary stalk may be associated with growth hormone deficiency or, less frequently, with clinical evidence of deficiency of other anterior pituitary hormones. The MRI features of stalk disruption with T1 high signal in the tuber cinerium and stalk, and hypoplasia of the pituitary gland and sella, are

usual. The condition is more frequent following breech extraction, which may also be associated with damage to the cervical spinal cord and a posterior fossa subdural haematoma.

Hydrocephalus/atrophy

Hydrocephalus is usually of the communicating type and related to bleeding into the cerebrospinal fluid and blockage of pacchionian corpuscles. Intraventricular clot may occlude the aqueduct or other narrow parts of the ventricular system, but this is generally transient.

Unilateral hydrocephalus in the acute phase of head injury may occur on the side opposite to a cerebral hemisphere mass lesion causing compression of the third ventricle. Many such cases are fatal unless surgical relief of the mass lesion is possible.

Hydrocephalus may also be related to obstruction to cerebrospinal fluid pathways or pacchionian granulations by exudate or fibrosis, especially in cases of compound injury complicated by infection.

Hypertensive hydrocephalus can generally be recognized both clinically and on imaging, and can be distinguished from brain damage with atrophy. It usually occurs within a month of head injury, but occasionally as late as three months; it may be suspected if there is failure clinically to improve to the expected degree.

All parts of the ventricular system above the obstructed region are distended, with a tendency to rounding of their contours. The restraining effect of the septum pellucidum and/or falx cerebri results in a diminished angle between the ventricular roofs; enlargement of the temporal horn(s) tends to be relatively pronounced. In early hydrocephalus, the temporal horns alone may be distended and are an important diagnostic feature. The ventricular distension tends to be more marked in regions where the brain is damaged and its compliance diminished. Communicating intracerebral cysts may also become distended. Regions of the ventricular system supported by only a thin layer of nervous tissue are particularly prone to becoming distended during hydrocephalus. These regions, which are not affected in atrophic conditions, include the anterior and posterior recesses of the IIIrd ventricle and the roof of the IVth ventricle.

Fluid distension of interstitial spaces, most marked in those close to the lateral ventricles, may be present in the acute phase. The hydrocephalus may resolve spontaneously or become balanced to a state of 'normal pressure hydrocephalus', or may persist at high pressure. If the hydrocephalus is not relieved, the distension may persist and be associated with chronic periventricular gliosis and central atrophy.

Focal and/or generalized atrophy causing ventricular and sulcal dilatation may be present within three months of head injury and may progress. It may be accompanied by wallerian degeneration of descending tracts, which return T2 high signal and show loss of volume.

Vascular lesions

These may occur soon after trauma or they may be delayed. They are diagnosed clinically and confirmed by imaging. Vascular occlusion may be precipitated by direct trauma to arterial walls causing secondary thrombosis, or by dissection with or without secondary thrombosis or distal embolism. Subarachnoid bleeding may precipitate arterial spasm sufficient to cause infarction.

Herniation of brain substance through the tentorial hiatus or under the falx cerebri may cause arterial compression and result in infarction in the distribution of the affected vessel. The extent of infarction and the nature of the occlusive process may be resolved by MRI and MR angiography or by regular or spiral CT scanning.

Arterial damage by penetrating trauma, or in relation to a fracture or dissection, may result in true or pseudoaneurysm formation. Careful assessment, prior to surgery or embolization, unless spontaneous regression or thrombosis is clearly demonstrated, is of particular importance with aneurysms within the subarachnoid space.

Arteriovenous fistulae

Large vessel fistulae are most frequent between an internal carotid artery and the cavernous sinus, and may be due to direct penetrating trauma or, more frequently, to shearing of the artery. Clinical signs of a fistula may be evident immediately after trauma but they more usually occur during the succeeding few days.

A vertebro-vertebral fistula usually accompanies damage to the cervical spine, but it may be associated with vertebral arterial dissection and is frequently not diagnosed until after the acute phase. Other fistulae may occur between external

carotid branches and adjacent veins, most frequently between the occipital or superficial temporal arteries and veins. Maxillo-maxillary fistulae are usually congenital but may also be post-traumatic. The large vessel fistulae may close spontaneously in the acute phase; this may be encouraged by intermittent arterial compression. Once a fistula has become established, spontaneous closure is rare and interventional radiology should be considered, particularly if the vascular anatomy is favourable and suggests that closure can be accomplished with preservation of the feeding artery.

Small vessel fistulae are usually between branches of dural arteries and adjacent veins or sinuses. They may be due to a persisting communication through a pseudoaneurysm or to dilatation of physiological arteriovenous connections, sometimes related to venous sinus thrombosis. These fistulae may also require occlusion by interventional neuroradiology if they are symptomatic. Increased venous pressure is associated with dysfunction of neural tissues, which may result in motor or sensory disability, epilepsy, confusion or dementia. It may also cause cranial nerve dysfunction as well as congestion of orbital muscles with ocular movement disorders and/or proptosis. Unacceptable or progressive neural dysfunction may cause the demand for interventional treatment. Interventional radiology may also be indicated if occlusion is required because drainage is through cortical vessels, since this has been shown to increase the risk of intracerebral haemorrhage.

Closure of large fistulae may be achieved by transarterial or transvenous placement of balloons or coils immediately adjacent to the venous side of the fistula to induce thrombosis within the fistula itself. Smaller arteriovenous connections may be occluded using liquid embolic material.

The success rate of embolization is well above 90%, but it does carry significant risks. These should be emphasized and discussed although in practice the incidence of permanent neurological disability is under 5%. This may be due to:

1. Loss of embolic material into the cerebral circulation.
2. Occlusion of the major feeding vessel to the fistula. Unless accidental, this is not performed without tests for the adequacy of collateral circulation. However, despite all precautions, some evidence of vascular insufficiency affecting the ipsilateral hemisphere occurs in about 10% of such occlusions.

3. Occlusion of ophthalmic artery branches, with optic nerve or retinal ischaemia.
4. Occlusion of superficial arterial branches resulting in muscular or dermal ischaemia. Consequences are muscle spasm with trismus, which is usually only transiently painful, facial hemiatrophy and refractory healing of the scalp following surgery.
5. Distended balloons may cause neural compression, particularly of the cranial nerves passing through the cavernous sinus.
6. Occlusion of part of the venous outflow may increase the flow and/or pressure in other parts of the outflow. This may change the nature of symptoms and/or be a factor in precipitating haemorrhage.

References

Chong SKF, Levitt GA, Lawson J, *et al.* (1989) Subarachnoid cysts with hydrocephalus: a complication of mid-trimester amniocentesis. *Prenatal Diagn* **9**: 677–79.

Clarke JA, Adams JE. (1990) The application of clinical guidelines for skull radiography in accident and emergency departments: theory and practice. *Clin Radiol* **41**: 152–55.

Dacey RG, Alves WM, Rimel RW, *et al.* (1986) Neurosurgical complications after apparently minor head injury – assessment of risk in a series of 610 patients. *J Neurosurg* **65**: 203–10.

Gentry LR, Godersky JC, Thompson B. (1988a) MR imaging of head trauma: review of the distribution of radiopathologic features of traumatic lesions. *Am J Neuroradiol* **150**: 663–72.

Gentry LR, Godersky GC, Thompson B, Dunn VD. (1988b) Prospective comparative study of intermediate-field MR and CT in the evaluation of closed head trauma. *Am J Neuroradiol* **150**: 673–82.

Jennet B, Teasdale G. (1981) *Management of head injury.* Philadelphia: Davis, 77–93.

Kido DK, Cox C, Hamill RW, Rothenberg BM, Woolf PD. (1992) Traumatic brain injuries: predictive usefulness of CT. *Radiology* **182**: 777–81.

Kleinman PK. (1990) Diagnostic imaging in infant abuse. *AJR* **155**: 703–12.

Masters SJ, McClean PM, Arcarese JS, *et al.* (1987) Skull X-ray examinations after head trauma. *N Engl J Med* **316**: 84–91.

Mittl RL, Grossman RI, Hiehle JF, *et al.* (1994) Prevalence of MR evidence of diffuse axonal injury in patients with mild head injury and normal head CT findings. *Am J Neuroradiol* **15**: 1583–89.

Naylor G, Roper JP, Willshaw HE. (1990) Ophthalmic complications of amniocentesis. *Eye* **4**: 845–49.

Rosenorn J, Duus B, Nielson K, *et al.* (1991) Is a skull X-ray necessary after milder head trauma? *Br J Neurosurg* **5**: 135–39.

Symonds C. (1962) Concussion and its sequelae. *Lancet* **i**: 1–5.

Tandon DN, Banerji AK *et al.* (1987) Craniocerebral erosion (growing fracture of the skull in children): Part II. Clinical and radiological observations. *Acta Neurochir* **88**: 1–9.

Taylor AS. (1856) *Medical jurisprudence.* Philadelphia: Blanchard and Lee, 368.

Weber W. (1985) Biomechanical fragility of skull fractures in infants. *Z Rechtsmed* **94**: 93–101.

Youroukos S, Papdelis F, Matsanoitis N. (1980) Porencephalic cyst after amniocentesis. *Arch Dis Child* **55**: 814–15.

Zimmerman RA, Bilaniuk LT, Bruce D, *et al.* (1979) Computed tomography of craniocerebral injury in the abused child. *Radiology* **130**: 687–90.

18

Recurrent cranial trauma

Bhupal P Chitnavis, Peter J Hamlyn

Introduction

Recurrent head injuries may be divided into two groups: those involving a second major insult, and multiple minor insults.

The factors determining outcome from a second head injury are likely to be similar to those that are relevant in an initial injury, these are:

Mechanism

Some studies (Alberico et al., 1987), though not all (Jennett et al., 1979), show that head injuries consequent upon a fall, an assault or a domestic incident carry a higher proportion of mass lesions and, in turn, are associated with a higher mortality than road traffic accidents. Motor-cyclists not wearing helmets are 15 times more likely to die than passengers in a motor car (Kraus, 1987).

Premorbid factors

Increasing age (Alberico et al., 1987; Berger et al. (1985); Carlsson et al., 1968; Luerssen et al., 1988), smoking (Carlson et al., 1987) and malnutrition (Clifton et al., 1984) all worsen outcome.

Pathology

Acute subdurals are not only the commonest (Gennarelli et al., 1982) intracranial haematomas but also carry the worst prognosis, followed by intracerebral haematomas, although site and size also influence outcome (Andrews et al., 1988).

Clinical state

The depth and length of coma correlate with outcome (Braakman et al., 1980; Choi et al., 1988; Gennarelli et al., 1982; Jennett et al., 1979; Teasdale and Jennett, 1974), as do length of post-traumatic amnesia (PTA) and preservation of brain stem reflexes (Braakman et al., 1980; Russell and Smith, 1961; Unterharnscheidt et al., 1971).

Physiological measurements

Raised intracranial pressure (Miller et al., 1981), pressure volume index (Maset et al., 1987), cerebral perfusion pressure (Changaris et al., 1987), cerebral blood flow (Overgaard et al., 1981), multimodality evoked potentials (Greenberg et al., 1977, 1981), and the electroencephalogram (EEG) (Synek, 1990) have all been shown to be predictors of outcome.

Neurochemical indices

Blood levels of catecholamines (Clifton et al., 1981, 1984) the enzyme CKBB (Bakay and Ward, 1983), and the concentration of fibrin degradation products (Crone et al., 1987) and cerebrospinal fluid lactate levels (De Salles et al., 1986) all predict outcome.

Secondary brain injury

Cerebral ischaemia as a secondary insult has been shown to increase mortality and morbidity. The control of factors leading to cerebral ischaemia mitigate this effect (Langfitt and Gennarelli, 1982).

Treatment

Early management of intracranial haematomas has been shown to improve outcome (Seelig *et al.*, 1981).

Rehabilitation

It has been shown that those entering rehabilitation programmes following head injury reintegrate into society faster (Hook *et al.*, 1976).

Outcome after a second major insult

The majority of factors given above are independent of the number of occasions on which injury occurs. Two studies have addressed the issue of prior head injury in influencing outcome. They have taken as their starting point a closed head injury severe enough to cause impaired consciousness (Carlson *et al.*, 1987; Gronwall and Wrightson, 1987).

The study by Gronwall and Wrightson (1987) matched 20 adults between 16 and 26 years of age, who had incurred a previous head injury but in whom there had been no residual disability and who went on after periods of five months to eight years to suffer a further concussive head injury, with a similar noninjured group. Both groups were then subjected to a Phased Auditory Serial Addition Test (PASAT) at weekly intervals, commencing at 48 hours until their scores were within one standard deviation of the mean score for a group of nonconcussed subjects of comparable age. There was a greater and longer lasting impairment in the second insult group, although information processing rates eventually returned to normal. However, they concluded that concussion may have both permanent and temporary components, both of which initially limit information processing, but that the test they used may not have been sensitive enough to pick up the residual permanent damage. They concluded that the effects of concussion are cumulative and that this

has an implication in those sports where concussion is commonplace.

The possibility that head injury resulting in unconsciousness, no matter how short, is capable of causing permanent sequelae was addressed in a study from Sweden, which looked at the effect of head injury sustained during life in three male populations (Carlson *et al.*, 1987). They found that the two factors most likely to predict the development of a postconcussional syndrome were the numbers of reported accidents with impaired consciousness and the duration of the longest episode of unconsciousness or PTA. The authors agreed that smoking and alcohol were important confounding variables but that even when these were taken into account there was still a significant relationship with previous head injury. They concluded that repeated mild head injury has a cumulative effect.

Recurrent trauma encephalopathy

The clearest example of recurrent head trauma in humans is provided by boxing. The literature contains different and confused terminologies: dementia pugilistica, punch drunk syndrome, boxer's encephalopathy, traumatic encephalopathy, encephalopathia traumatica boxistica and pugilistic disease. We wish to introduce a new term: 'recurrent trauma encephalopathy' (RTE), which more closely addresses the underlying pathological mechanism and broadens its applicability.

Recurrent head injury has been a feature of many sports (association football, rugby, wrestling and national hunt racing) in which it has been suggested that RTE may occur (Editorial, 1976; Foster *et al.*, 1976). Recent studies on amateur boxers have taken variously as their control groups: soccer players (Murelius and Huglund, 1991), track and field athletes (Murelius and Huglund, 1991), prospective boxers (Brooks *et al.*, 1987), rugby and water polo players (Butler *et al.*, 1993). No evidence of significantly impaired consciousness was found in the boxers over and above these groups, some of whom (track and field, prospective boxers, water polo players) are not obviously exposed to recurrent head injury.

Even in boxing, the incidence of RTE remains unclear. The populations of boxers that have been studied this century may be divided broadly into two groups. The old group (Corsellis *et al.*, 1973; Roberts, 1969) had their boxing careers prior to 1940. This group comprises largely older retired professionals who fought many bouts in contests of longer duration (15 rounds or more). The new group comprises young professionals and amateur boxers who have had relatively fewer bouts in fights of shorter duration (three to 12 rounds) on sprung floors designed to lessen the impact suffered by the head when falling (Brooks *et al.*, 1987; Butler *et al.*, 1993; Murelius and Huglund, 1991; Stewart *et al.*, 1994; Thomassen *et al.*, 1979). These studies suggest that the two groups are very different and the likelihood of finding evidence of an encephalopathy is greater in the older group.

Some studies have suggested that the occurrence of neurological signs and symptoms in former boxers is a function of the number of bouts fought and the length of boxing career. In addition, boxers in heavyweight classes appear to be more at risk (Corsellis *et al.*, 1973; Jedlinski *et al.*, 1971; Roberts, 1969). It is not clear whether this is due to the slow accumulation of relatively minor trauma or to a greater number of knockouts. Some work in animals points to the former (Unterharnscheidt *et al.*, 1971). Part of the confusion derives from the lack of a clear definition of cerebral concussion. Some have defined it as a transient loss of neuronal functioning without permanent neuronal damage (Denny-Brown and Russell, 1941).

The occurrence of neurological sequelae in older studies has ranged from 17% to 55% (Jedlinski *et al.*, 1971; Roberts, 1969). The latter figure occurs in a study in which many of the signs were subjective and mild (Jedlinski *et al.*, 1971). Whilst 21.7% of boxers in this study showed 'pronounced organic symptoms', these were not satisfactorily defined. A more recent study noted neurological abnormalities in 35% of a series of amateur boxers, although there was no control group (McLatchie *et al.*, 1987). When the same team rectified this problem, no consistent pattern of cognitive deficits was found (Brooks *et al.*, 1987). Robert's study (1969) examined 224 boxers (of 250 who had been identified as a 1.5% random sample of 16 781) who had boxed professionally in the UK between 1929 and 1955. In this series, 37 (17%) had chronic neurological sequelae. Of these, 13 demonstrated a characteristic RTE and two suffered frank dementia. Age, number of bouts and being in a heavyweight class were factors associated with an increased frequency of neurological sequelae. An earlier study by Carroll (1936) stated that about 5% of boxers suffered pugilistic disease after five years in the ring.

The most recent studies have failed to show any deleterious effects from amateur boxing (Brooks *et al.*, 1987; Butler *et al.*, 1993; Murelius and Huglund, 1991; Stewart *et al.*, 1994; Thomasson *et al.*, 1979). The participants in these studies were often in their teens and relatively inexperienced, in contrast with the case studies described by Corsellis *et al.* (1973) in their classic work (where the mean age was 69 and where more than 50% had fought over 300 contests). The International Boxing Federation, in an attempt to promote safety, has therefore limited the number of rounds. It has encouraged the early termination of ill-matched bouts and better medical supervision of concussed fighters before a return to the ring.

Thus, the consequences of modern boxing may be very different from those described in older papers.

Clinical features

RTE was first described by Martland in 1928 under the term 'punch drunk syndrome'. He described the early symptoms as usually appearing in the extremities,

> with only a very occasional and slight flopping of the foot or leg in walking or a slight unsteadiness. . . . This may not hinder fighting. . . . Then there were periods of slight mental confusion as well as distinct slowing of muscular action.

He felt that many cases did not progress. However, if they did, then,

> a distinct dragging of the leg may develop along with generalised muscular slowness along with hesitancy of movement, tremors of the hand, nodding movements of the head. . . . In severe cases there may be a staggering propulsive gait with facial characteristics of the parkinsonian syndrome. . . . Marked mental deterioration may set in.

He stated that up to half the fighters eventually developed this condition.

Pathology

The classic study by Corsellis *et al.* (1973) of 15 brains from retired boxers defined the pathology of the RTE. Macroscopically, there was atrophy of the brain, with thickened leptomeninges. On section, they found abnormalities of the septum pellucidum, in particular a cavum septum pellucidum, in 12 specimens, whilst in a study by Schwidde (1952), a cavum was found in only 20% of an unselected postmortem series of 1032 human brains. Corsellis also showed that a septal cavum was not a feature of other neurodegenerative disorders. In the cerebellum there were distinct histological differences from Alzheimer's disease and other neurodegenerative disorders. There was cortical scarring on the interior surface of the lateral lobes of the cerebellum, with Purkinje cell loss, glial fibrosis, thinning of the granular layer and nigrostriatal degeneration. Furthermore, unlike Alzheimer's disease, there was an almost total absence of senile plaques and an abundance of neurofibrillary tangles. More recent studies (using antibodies to detect the beta protein present in the plaques of Alzheimer's disease) and which utilized the same specimens as Corsellis *et al.*, showed beta protein immunoreactive deposits to be present in abundance (Roberts *et al.*, 1990). Although in most patients with Alzheimer's disease, head trauma is not an obvious factor, there are examples of isolated head injury giving rise to a dementia pathologically indistinguishable from this condition (Ruddelli *et al.*, 1982). Furthermore, in a large series of brain-damaged patients an insidious dementia occurring some years after the initial trauma was noted in 11–25% of cases, a rate more than double that of the normal population (Lewin *et al.*, 1979). This suggests a progressive problem despite the absence of continuing trauma.

Animal studies

Denny-Brown and Russell (1941) pointed out in their account on cerebral concussion that acceleration forces, similar to those in boxing (Johnson *et al.*, 1975), were a more consistent method of concussing animals than applying direct pressure to the brain. In acceleration/deceleration injuries of the head, shearing forces are applied to the brain tissue, resulting in tearing and stretching of the neural elements, particularly axons. When shearing strains are large, there is extensive destruction of axons in the white matter of the cerebral hemispheres. These lesions, recently studied by MRI, have been suggested as being the prime event in traumatic unconsciousness, and, unless associated with haemorrhage or gross disruption of fibre tracks, axonal injury is readily missed at postmortem examination (Adams *et al.*, 1982; Jenkins *et al.*, 1986). Lesser degrees of shearing injury almost certainly occur in the brains of patients exposed to less severe neurological stress. Some have found degeneration of axons in the white

matter of monkeys subjected to quite minor head injury (Jane *et al.*, 1981). These changes were not found by other workers using a different model (rat and frog) (Parkinson, 1992). However even though gross pathology may not be encountered, shearing, acceleration/deceleration injuries may still render many axons nonfunctional (Langfitt and Gennarelli, 1982). Relatively minor trauma is sufficient to cause axoplasmic stasis, which at a later stage leads to axonal disruption (Povlishok *et al.*, 1983).

Prevention

Several studies have attempted to diagnose RTE early. However, there is no evidence that early detection will influence the ultimate outcome.

EEG

Disorganized or pathological EEG recordings have been found in a number of studies on boxers (Jedlinski *et al.*, 1971; Johnson, 1969; Kaplan and Browder, 1954; Kaste *et al.*, 1982; Ross *et al.*, 1983). Some studies have suggested lower ranked boxers (Kaplan and Browder, 1954), and those with longer careers as judged by number of bouts (Ross *et al.*, 1983), showed more disorganized EEGs.

Imaging

Using MRI and CT scanning, a number of studies (Jordan *et al.*, 1992; Ross *et al.*, 1983; Kaste *et al.*, 1982) have tried to pick up the changes demonstrated by Corsellis *et al.* (1973). Jordan *et al.* (1992) performed CT scans in 338 active professional boxers and found abnormalities in 25 (7%). The most common abnormality was brain atrophy. They found no differences in boxers with abnormal CT scans compared with those with normal or borderline CT scans with regard to age, win/loss record, number of bouts, or abnormal EEG. This is at variance with other studies (Ross *et al.*, 1983). Seventeen (68%) of the 25 with abnormal CT scans reported a previous knock-out or stoppage compared with only 89 (37%) of boxers with normal CT scans. Atrophy was more frequent in those with a large cavum septum pellucidum, as in 13% of this series. However, in this study, 92% of boxers with abnormal CT scans had normal EEGs. The background prevalence of cavum septum pellucidum has been variously estimated from as high as 5.4% (MacPherson and Teasdale, 1988) to lower than 1% (Bogdanoff and Natter, 1989).

Neuropsychometry

A number of neuropsychological studies have been undertaken on boxers (Brooks *et al.*, 1987; Butler *et al.*, 1993; Cason *et al.*, 1984; Kaste *et al.*, 1982; McLatchie *et al.*, 1987; Murelius and Huglund, 1991; Roberts, 1969; Ross *et al.*, 1983, 1987; Stewart *et al.*, 1994; Thomasson *et al.*, 1979). None of these has shown neuropsychological abnormalities in amateur boxers. Others have shown that professional boxers score abnormally, though none of these studies had controls (Cason *et al.*, 1984; McLatchie *et al.*, 1987; Roberts, 1969; Ross *et al.*, 1983). Some have shown boxers to perform better after bouts (Butler *et al.*, 1993).

Conclusions

There is clear evidence that recurrent head injury carries a cumulative burden. The outcome after a second insult is likely to be worse than when that same insult is suffered *de novo*, although hard evidence has yet to emerge.

There is also clear evidence that some boxers manifest the neurological changes of RTE, both functionally and anatomically. The pathological changes described share features with other neuro-degenerative disorders and may be progressive once initiated. At present there is no established method of detecting an at-risk individual, and it is not possible to establish that early detection will ameliorate the eventual consequences.

References

Adams FJ, Gannarelli TA, Graham DI. (1982) Brain damage in non missile head injury: observations in man and subhuman primates. In: Smith WT, Cavanagh JB, editors. *Recent advances in neuropathology*, No. 2. New York: Churchill Livingstone, 165–96.

Alberico AM, Ward JD, Choi SC, Marmarou A, Young HF. (1987) Outcome after severe head injury: relationship to mass lesions, diffuse injury, and ICP course in paediatric and adult patients. *J Neurosurg* 67: 648–56.

Andrews BT, Chiles BW, Olsen WL, Pitts LH. (1988) The effects of intracerebral haematoma location on the risk of brain stem compression and on clinical outcome. *J Neurosurg* 69: 518–22.

Bakay RAE, Ward AA. (1983) Enzymatic changes in serum and cerebrospinal fluid in neurological injury. *J Neurosurg* 58: 27–37.

Berger MS, Pitts LH, Lovely M, Edwards MSB, Bartkowski HM. (1985) Outcome from severe head injury in children and adolescents. *J Neurosurg* 62: 194–99.

Bogdanoff B, Natter HM. (1989) Incidence of cavum septum pellucidum in adults: a sign of boxer's encephalopathy. *Neurology* 39: 991–92.

Braakman R, Gelpke GJ, Habbema JDF, Mass AIR, Minderhoud JM. (1980) Systemic selections of prognostic features in patients with severe head injury. *Neurosurgery* 6: 362–70.

Brooks N, Kupshik G, Wilson L, Galbraith S, Ward R. (1987) A neuropsychological study of active amateur boxers. *J Neurol Neurosurg Psychiatry* 50: 997–1000.

Butler RJ, Forsythe WI, Beverly DW, Adams LM. (1993) A prospective controlled investigation of the cognitive effects of amateur boxing. *J Neurol Neurosurg Psychiatry* 56: 1055–61.

Carroll EJ Jr. (1936) Punch-drunk. *Am J Med Sci* 191: 706–12.

Carlson GS, Svardsudd K, Welin L. (1987) Long term effects of head injuries sustained during life and in three male populations. *J Neurosurg* 67: 197–205.

Carlsson C-A, Von Essen C, Lofgren J. (1968) Factors affecting the clinical course of patients with severe head injuries. *J Neurosurg* 29: 242–51.

Cason IR, Seigel O, Shaw R, Campbell EA, Tarlau M, Didomenico A. (1984) Brain damage in modern boxers. *JAMA* 251: 2663–67.

Changaris DG, McGraw CS, Richardson JD, Garretson, HD Arpin HD, Shields CB. (1987) Correlation of cerebral perfusion pressure and Glasgow Coma Scale to outcome. *J Trauma* 27: 1007–13.

Choi SC, Narayan RK, Anderson RL, Ward JD. (1988) Enhanced specificity of prognosis in severe head injury. *J Neurosurg* 69: 381–85.

Clifton GL, Ziegher MG, Grossman RG. (1981) Circulating catecholamines and sympathetic activity after head injury. *Neurosurgery* 8: 10–14.

Clifton GL, Robertson CS, Grossman RG, Hodge S, Foltz R, Garza C. (1984) The metabolic response to severe head injury. *J Neurosurg* 60: 687–96.

Corsellis JAN, Bruton CJ, Freeman-Browne D. (1973) The aftermath of boxing. *Psychol Med* 3: 270–303.

Crone KR, Lee KS, Kelly DL. (1987) Correlation of admissions fibrin degradation products with outcome and respiratory failure in patients with severe head injury. *Neurosurgery* 21: 532–36.

Denny-Brown D, Russell WR. (1941) Experimental cerebral concussion: *Brain* 64: 93–164.

De Salles AAF, Kontos HA, Becker DP, *et al.* (1986) Prognostic significance of ventricular CSF lactic acidosis in severe head injury. *J Neurosurg* 65: 615–24.

Editorial. (1976) Brain damage in sport. *Lancet* i: 401–402.

Foster JB, Leiguarda R, Tiley PJB. (1976) Brain damage in national hunt jockeys. *Lancet* i: 981–87.

Gennarelli TA, Spielman GM, Langfitt TW, *et al.* (1982) Influence of the type of intracranial lesion on outcome from severe head injury: a multicentre study using a new classification system. *J Neurosurg* **56**: 26–32.

Greenberg RP, Becker DP, Miller JD, Mayer DJ. (1977) Evaluation of brain function in severe human head trauma with multimodality evoked potentials: II. Localisation of brain dysfunction and correlation with post traumatic neurological conditions. *J Neurosurg* **47**: 163–77.

Greenberg RP, Newton PG, Hyatt MS, Narayan RK, Becker DP. (1981) Prognostic implications of early multimodality evoked potentials in severely head injured patients: a prospective study. *J Neurosurg* **55**: 227–36.

Gronwall D, Wrightson P. (1975) Cumulative effect of concussion. *Lancet* **ii**: 995–96.

Hook O. (1976) Rehabilitation. In: Vinken PJ, Bruyn GW, editors. *Handbook of clinical neurology, vol. 24. Injuries of the brain and skull. part II.* Amsterdam: North-Holland, 683–97.

Jane JA, Steward O, Gennarelli TA, *et al.* (1981) Pathology of minor head injury. Presented at the Annual Meeting of the American Association of Neurological Surgeons, Boston, April 1981.

Jedlinski J, Gatarski J, Szymusik A. (1971) Encephalopathia pugilistical (punch drunkenness). *Acta Med Pol* X 11 3.31

Jenkins A, Teasdale G, Hadley MD, MacPherson P. (1986) Brain lesions detected by magnetic resonance imaging in mild and severe head injuries. *Lancet* **ii**: 445–47.

Jennett B, Teasdale G, Braakman R, Minderhoud J, Heiden J, Kurze T. (1979) Prognosis of patients with severe head injury. Neurosurgery **4**: 283–89.

Johnson J. (1969) Organic psychosyndromes due to boxing. *Br J Psychiatry* **115**: 45–53.

Johnson J, Skorecki J, Wells RP. (1975) Peak accelerations of the head experienced in boxing. *Med Biol Eng* **13**: 396–404.

Jordan BD, Zimmerman RD. (1990) CT and MRI in boxers. *JAMA* **263**:

Jordan BD, *et al.* (1992) CT of 338 active professional boxers. *Neuroradiology*: 509–12.

Kaplan HA, Browder J. (1954) Observations on the clinical and brain wave patterns of professional boxers *JAMA* 156: 1138–44.

Kaste M, Vilkkij, Sainio K, *et al.* (1982) Is chronic brain damage in boxing a hazard of the past? *Lancet* **ii**: 1186–87.

Kraus JF. (1987) Epidemiology of head injury. In: Cooper PR, editor. *Head injury,* 2nd edition. Baltimore, MA: Williams and Wilkins, 1–19.

Langfitt TW, Gennarelli TA. (1982) Can the outcome from head injury be improved? *J Neurosurg* **56**: 19–25.

Lewin W, Marshall TFde C, Roberts AJ. (1979) Long term outcome after severe head injury. *Br Med J* **ii**: 1533–38.

Lewin HS, Lippold SC, Goldman A, *et al.* (1987) Neurobehavioural functioning and magnetic resonance imaging findings in young boxers. *J Neurosurg* **67**: 657–67.

Luerssen TG, Klauber MR, Marshall LF. (1988) Outcome from head injury related to patients age. A longitudinal prospective study of adult and paediatric head injury. *J Neurosurg* **68**: 409–16.

Martland HS. (1928) Punch drunk. *JAMA* **91**: 1103–107.

Maset AL, Marmarou A, Ward JD, *et al.* (1987) Pressure-volume index in head injury. *J Neurosurg* **67**: 832–40.

McLatchie G, Brooks N, Galbraith S, *et al.* (1987) Clinical neurological examination, neuropsychology, electroencephalography and computed tomographic head scanning in active amateur boxers. *J Neurol Neurosurg Psychiatry* **50**: 96–99.

MacPherson D, Teasale F. (1988) CT Demonstration of a 5th ventricle – a finding to KO boxers? *Neuroradiology* **30**: 506–10.

Miller JD, Butterworth JF, Gudeman SK, *et al.* (1981) Further experience in the management of severe head injury. *J Neurosurg* **54**: 289–99.

Murelius O, Huglund Y. (1991) Does Swedish amateur boxing lead to chronic brain damage? 4. A retrospective neuropsychological study. *Acta Neurol Scand* **83**: 9–73.

Overgaard J, Mosdal C, Tweed WA. (1981) Cerebral circulation after head injury: III. Does reduced regional cerebral blood flow determine recovery of brain function after blunt head injury? *J Neurosurg* **55**: 63–74.

Parkinson D. (1992) Concussion is completely reversible: an hypothesis. *Med Hypotheses* **37**: 37–39.

Povlishok JT, Becker DP, Cheng CL, *et al.* (1983) Axonal change in minor head injury. *J Neuropathol Exp Neurol* **42**: 225–42.

Roberts AH. (1969) *Brain damage in boxers. A study of prevalence of traumatic encephalopathy among ex-professional boxers.* London: Pitman.

Roberts GW, Allsop D, Bruton E. (1990) The occult aftermath of boxing. *J Neurol Neurosurg Psychiatry* **53**: 373–78.

Ross RJ, Cole M, Thompson JS, Kyung HK. (1983) Boxers – computed tomography EEG and neurological evaluation. *JAMA* **249**: 211–13.

Ross RJ, Casson IR, Siegel O, Cole, M. (1987) Boxing injuries: neurologic, radiologic and neuropsychologic evaluation. Head and neck injuries. *Clin Sports Med* **6**: 41–51.

Ruddelli R, Strom JO, Welch RT, *et al.* (1982) Post traumatic premature Alzheimer's disease: neuropathologic findings and pathogenetic considerations. *Arch Neurol* **39**: 570–75.

Russell WR, Smith A. (1961) Post traumatic amnesia in closed head injury. *Arch Neurol* **5**: 4–17.

Saija A, Hayes RL, Lyeth BG, *et al.* (1988) The effect of concussive head injury on central cholinergic neurons. *Brain Res* **452**: 303–11.

Schwidde JT. (1952) Incidence of cavum septum pellucidum and cavum vegae in 1032 human brains. *Arch Neurol Psychiatry* **67**: 625–32.

Seelig JM, Becker DP, Miller JD, Greenberg RP, Ward JD, Choi SC. (1981) Traumatic acute subdural haematoma: major mortality reduction in comatose patients treated within four hours. *N Engl J Med* **304**: 1511–18.

Stewart WF, Gordon B, Selnes O, *et al.* (1994) Prospective study of central nervous system function in amateur boxers in the United States. *Am J Epidemiol* **139**: 573–88.

Synek VM. (1990) Revised EEG Coma Scale in diffuse acute head injuries in adults. *Clin Exp Neurol* **27**: 99–111.

Teasdale G, Jennett B. (1974) Assessment of coma and impaired consciousness: a practical scale. *Lancet* **ii**: 81–84.

Thomassen A, Juul Jensen P, DeFine OB, Braemer J, Christensen AL. (1979) Neurological, electroencephalographic and neuropsychological examination of 53 former amateur boxers. *Act Neurol Scand* **60**: 352–62.

Unterharnscheidt F, Sellier K. (1971) Von Boxen Mechanic Pathomolophogie und Klinik der Traumatischen Schaden des ZNS bei Boxern. *Fortschr Neurol Psychiatr* **39**: 109–51.

Section II

Ophthalmology

19

Neuro-ophthalmological aspects of head injury

N J C Sarkies

Introduction

Forty per cent of the brain volume is devoted to the sensation of vision. The brain captures the visual world with a sensory apparatus that refines and organizes the incoming data, and a motor apparatus that maintains stability of the visual image. Normally we are entirely unconscious of the perfect integration of these complex processes. Head injury frequently causes an alteration in the quality of the visual sensation, sometimes producing a gross disturbance, sometimes a subtle change. Many patients who suffer from head injury experience great difficulty in describing the visual disturbances they suffer. In attempting to characterize and explain the disturbance of visual function suffered by a head-injured patient, the physician requires knowledge of the normal anatomy and physiology of the visual pathway and eye movement control systems, as well as a full understanding of the structural basis of the patient's injury.

Definitions

Visual acuity

Visual acuity is defined as the resolving power of the eye, which represents the smallest angle subtended at the nodal point of the eye by two points, still allowing them to be appreciated as distinct. The visual acuity is measured clinically with the Snellen chart or Landolt rings and recorded as a fraction of unity (the latter being represented by those letters whose limbs each subtend one minute). In the UK, this percentage is recorded as a fraction of the normal testing distance of six metres. Thus unity corresponds to 6/6 and the largest letter to 6/60. In the USA, the distance is 20 feet and these acuities are recorded as 20/20 and 20/200 respectively; in Europe, acuity is generally expressed as a decimal (1.0 and 0.1). The normal person has a visual acuity that is better than unity. If the vision is so poor that even the largest letter on the chart cannot be recognized, then it is measured clinically by reducing the distance (e.g. 3/60). Still worse vision is noted by the ability to count fingers, appreciate hand movements, and perceive light, or, when this is absent, no perception of light.

Visual field

Visual field is defined as 'that portion of space in which objects are visible at the same moment during steady fixation of gaze in one direction' (Traquair, 1949).

Charts of peripheral visual fields show that the normal field extends to about 60° nasally and above, to about 70° below, and to 90° temporally. The peripheral field becomes constricted gradually with age (Fisher, 1968).

The automated static perimeters that have become widely used in clinical practice incorporate in the statistical programme a correction for the age of the subject. Many alternative methods for visual field examination are available (e.g. confrontation techniques, the Amsler grid, the Tangent screen, bowl perimeters e.g. Goldmann) (Anderson, 1981; Harrington, 1976).

Colour vision

Following lesions of the optic nerve, there is more pronounced loss of the field for red than for white. It is unknown whether this phenomenon is due to the fact that the coloured stimuli are of lower intensity or whether there is a true wavelength selectivity. Impaired colour vision tested with the pseudoisochromatic Ishihara plates or the Farnsworth–Munsell 100-Hue Test is frequently found in optic neuropathies of any cause (Glaser, 1978).

Visual agnosia

The term visual agnosia refers to a specific syndrome in which a brain-damaged patient has sufficient visual acuity and field to see an object but cannot appreciate its meaning or character. According to many observers, visual agnosia comprises a spectrum of disorders in which primary visual deficits are combined with intellectual dysfunction. Specific agnosias for colour, body parts, spatial recognition, objects, familiar faces (proposagnosia) and words (aiexia) have been described (Miller, 1982a).

Blindness

Legal blindness is defined as impairment of sight resulting in the inability to undertake an occupation for which eyesight is essential. The definition is not strictly dependent upon the absolute level of visual acuity or visual field. A useful distinction may be drawn between occupational vision and navigational vision.

Accommodation

Accommodation is the process by which the refractive power of the lens of the eye is altered to diminish retinal blur and obtain clear vision of a near object. Accommodation is measured in dioptres; one dioptre is the accommodation that occurs

when the fixation distance is one metre. The near reflex comprises accommodation, convergence and pupillary constriction.

Diplopia

Misalignment of the visual axes produced by a squint causes the images of an object to fall on noncorresponding areas of the two retinas. A patient interprets these two images as diplopia. If the patient has had a squint since early childhood, then a suppression scotoma develops so that diplopia does not occur. Early onset squints may decompensate later in life as a result of injury or intercurrent illness, and, in these circumstances, diplopia may result. Binocular diplopia must be distinguished from uniocular diplopia, which is due to an abnormality within the media of the eye (e.g. cataract).

Stereopsis or depth perception

Local stereopsis is the point-by-point matching of disparate stimulus elements in the two half-images. There is evidence from clinical studies that the maintenance of normal stereopsis requires both cerebral hemispheres and an interhemispheric link (Blakemore, 1970; Mitchell and Blakemore, 1970).

Oscillopsia

Oscillopsia is an illusory movement of the seen world that occurs when images of stationary objects move across the retina. It may be caused by abnormal eye movements or disorders of eye–head co-ordination.

Epidemiology

Estimates of the the frequency of optic nerve injury with head trauma vary according to patient selection and follow-up (e.g. 1.6% (Turner, 1943), 4.0% (Hughes, 1964), 2.7% (Roberts, 1979)).

Orbital injury commonly accompanies midfacial trauma. In a prospective series of 363 midfacial fractures, only 34 patients were without ocular injury (Dutton *et al.*, 1992). Nine patients with optic neuropathy were included in this series.

Trauma to the optic chiasm is much less common than trauma to the optic nerves. Since its recognition approximately 100 cases have been reported (Heinz *et al.*, 1994). In a series of 231 optic nerve and chiasmal injuries reported from Los Angeles, chiasmal injuries comprised only 9% of blunt optic nerve injuries and 2% of penetrating injuries (Keane and Baloh, 1992).

Trauma to the postchiasmal visual pathways may be associated with extensive brain injury.

Clinical assessment

The assessment of visual function in patients after head injury requires considerable skill and patience. Frequently, the extent of ocular injury is not recognized initially in patients who have sustained severe, perhaps life-threatening, head injury, and only becomes apparent when the patient recovers consciousness or begins rehabilitation. Tests of visual function may not be possible in patients with cognitive deficits; the examiner must tailor the tests performed to each patient's ability. The testing of visual acuity and field is subjective; therefore particular attention should be given to the objective findings on examination, especially the pupil reactions (including the swinging flashlight test), and the appearance of the optic disc. Optic atrophy does not appear until at least one month after the injury. Patients with head injury also require a thorough ocular examination to exclude ocular contusion or penetrating injury. Examination of the eye movements should include

charting of the fields of diplopia (e.g. Hess screen). In significant head injury, a computed tomography (CT) scan is now automatic.

Structural pathology

Retina and optic nerve

The patterns of visual loss from retinal or optic nerve damage may be indistinguishable. When there is a retinal lesion affecting the rods and cones, the resulting field defect corresponds to the retinal defect in size, shape, extent and intensity (Traquair 1949). When there is a retinal lesion involving the ganglion cell layer and the nerve fibre layer, the field defect conforms to the field represented by the ganglion cells whose fibres are damaged. Three patterns of visual field loss occur in patients with retinal or optic nerve damage: (1) peripheral field loss; (2) a: arcuate field loss; b: altitudinal hemianopia; and (3) central field loss.

Direct injury to the retina usually causes ophthalmoscopically visible changes within it. Indirect injury to the retina may result from local or systemic interference with its blood supply. Subtle retinal and optic nerve abnormalities may not be visible without the aid of slit-lamp biomicroscopy, red-free fundus photography, or fluorescein angiography.

All types of monocular visual field defects may be produced by trauma to the optic nerve. The finding of optic atrophy (Figure 19.1) provides objective evidence of permanent damage to the

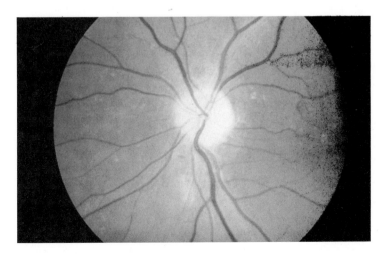

Figure 19.1. Fundus photograph showing optic atrophy.

optic nerve. Optic atrophy may develop as a result of: (1) disease within the eye affecting the nerve fibre layer or optic disc; (2) disease affecting any portion of the optic nerve; (3) intracranial disease involving the chiasm, tract or lateral geniculate body; and, rarely, (4) disease of retrogeniculate pathways (trans-synaptic degeneration).

Ophthalmoscopic features of optic atrophy comprise pallor, loss of the peripapillary nerve fibre layer, and pathological disc cupping. Confounding features include enlarged physiological cups, myopia, opacities in the media, as well as the brightness of the light source in the examiner's ophthalmoscope. Fundus photography, especially with red-free light may help in defining equivocal cases.

There is a good correlation between the degree of optic atrophy and the reduction in visual function, but the absence of optic atrophy does not preclude the possibility of optic nerve damage. Estimates based upon quantitative nerve fibre counts have emphasized that normal visual acuity and field requires only about half the normal complement of nerve fibres (Frisen and Frisen, 1976; Quigley *et al.*, 1989).

Pathological studies have demonstrated that there is a delay of up to six weeks before optic atrophy develops after injury (Kupfer, 1973; Lundstrom and Frisen, 1975; Quigley and Anderson, 1977). When a visual axon is cut, the ascending segment disintegrates and disappears because it is separated from its nutrient ganglion cell body. The rate of degeneration is proportional to the thickness of the nerve fibre. Large axons begin to show

changes within 30 hours, but small fibres may not show changes for 10 days. Ascending degeneration of the axon occurs within a few days, but the portion of the axon still connected to the cell body remains normal for three to four weeks. Then the entire remaining cell body and axon degenerates from the point of injury so that no affected ganglion cells remain viable. Injuries of the orbital optic nerve, optic chiasm and optic tract cause degeneration of the ganglion cell bodies at about six to eight weeks.

Regeneration of axons does not occur in the optic nerve of humans (Wolter, 1960), but some degree of remyelination may occur. Therefore, damage to axons in the optic nerve is permanent. Trans-synaptic degeneration of neurones occurs only *in utero* or in early infancy, when the brain is immature (Haddock and Berlin, 1950; Miller and Newman, 1981).

The mechanism of damage to the optic nerve by head injury

Though occasionally a trivial blow to the head may cause significant optic nerve injury, usually it results when the insult is severe enough to cause prolonged unconsciousness. The optic nerve may be injured directly or indirectly. Direct injury occurs with penetrating trauma, such as gunshot wounds through the temple (Keane, 1986), or orbital and frontal bone fractures. Indirect injuries are more common. Trauma to the ipsilateral outer eyebrow is transmitted to the optic nerve within the

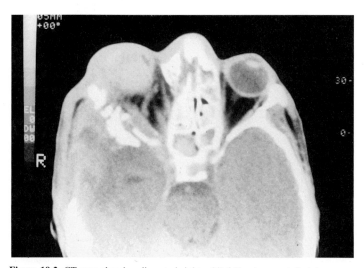

Figure 19.2. CT scan showing disrupted right orbit following craniofacial trauma. There is an intraocular haemorrhage and optic canal fracture.

canal (Anderson *et al.*, 1982). Occasionally, temporoparietal blows will damage the optic nerve. The syndromes of optic nerve avulsion, optic nerve sheath haemorrhage, orbital haemorrhage and optic canal fracture (Figures 19.2 and 19.3) may be recognized with the aid of appropriate radiographic studies.

Secondary ischaemic injury to the optic nerve may occur with head injury as a result of local or systemic vascular changes (e.g. ophthalmic artery occlusion, ipsilateral carotid artery occlusion, caroticocavernous fistula). Systemic hypoperfusion (shock) may cause bilateral optic nerve infarction (Hollenhorst and Wagener, 1950.) Delayed visual

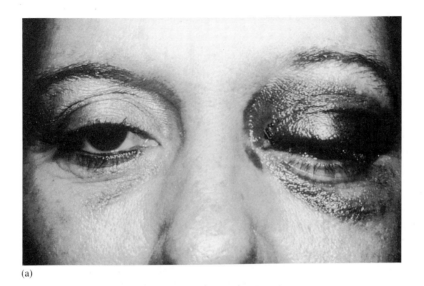

(a)

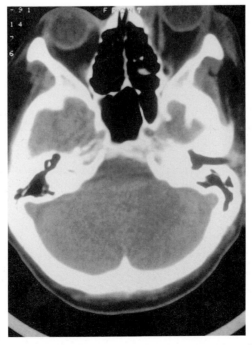

(b)

Figure 19.3. (**a**) Orbital haematomas of patient who sustained an injury with a billiard cue to the left orbit. (**b**) The CT scan shows a left proptosis with evidence of a haematoma within the optic nerve sheath.

loss following injury is usually due to evolving oedema or ischaemia within the optic canal, or compression from an orbital haematoma. Rarely, delayed visual loss may be caused by post-traumatic aneurysms (Keane, 1972), caroticocavernous fistulae (Sanders and Hoyt, 1969), or traumatic mucocoeles (Larson *et al.*, 1983). The pathophysiology of traumatic optic neuropathy is discussed in a recent review (Steinsapir and Goldberg, 1994).

The following case report illustrates the multi-factorial nature of visual loss after severe head injury.

Case report

MC was working on the repair of an articulated lorry when the vehicle jumped out of control and rolled back crushing his head. He lost consciousness for about 10 minutes, and was found bleeding from his nose and forehead.

Initial examination showed that he had no external ocular movements of the right eye, the right pupil was fixed and dilated and there was a right sided hemiparesis. Both optic discs were swollen. Radiological investigations revealed a right sided posterior fossa extradural haematoma and traumatic subdural blood, contusions in the region of the orbital gyri, intracranial air, and a maxillary facial fracture, as well as left sided rib fractures. His level of consciousness deteriorated, and he began to develop a left sided weakness and respiratory difficulties. He was treated by intubation, ventilation and posterior fossa craniectomy to evacuate the haematoma. After the operation, his level of consciousness improved and he was extubated the following day. However, the orbits became progressively more swollen; he developed bilateral external ophthalmoplegia and his vision became severely compromised. The diagnosis of traumatic bilateral caroticocavernous fistulae was confirmed by angiogram. He was treated by balloon angioplasty, closure of the fistula, and lumboperitoneal shunting.

Follow-up examination five years later showed that the visual acuities were right 6/60, left 6/12, with corrective lenses. He was unable to identify any of the Ishihara colour plates with the right eye, but he identified 9/14 plates with the left eye. He read N8 print slowly. Visual field examination showed a central scotoma on the right with a tunnel field on the left. The right eye movements were absent, and the right eye was adducted and fixed in position. The left eye movements were full. Both

pupils were 3 mm diameter and fixed to light. He had gross bilateral optic atrophy.

The mechanism of optic nerve injury in this patient was a combination of indirect optic nerve trauma due to the head injury, venous congestion from the caroticocavernous fistula, arterial occlusion due to ophthalmic artery insufficiency, and the compressive effects of raised intracranial pressure. Despite prompt and appropriate treatment of these complications of a severe crush injury to the head, he was rendered legally blind by the accident.

Treatment of optic nerve injury

The treatment of immediate visual loss due to indirect optic nerve injury is controversial. Some authors advocate high dose intravenous steroids and optic canal decompression if there is no early improvement, but any claims for the benefits of treatment must be compared with the rate of spontaneous recovery, which occurs in at least one-third of patients (Hooper, 1951; King and Walsh 1949; Turner, 1943).

There have been reports of dramatic improvement of vision in patients treated with steroids. Some authors have employed regimens of high dose dexamethasone or methylprednisolone (Seiff, 1990; Spoor *et al.*, 1990), based on the treatment of acute spinal cord injury (Bracken *et al.*, 1990).

In a study of 23 patients with traumatic optic neuropathy, high doses of intravenous steroids were given to the whole group. If significant improvement did not occur between 24 and 48 hours, decompression of an optic nerve sheath haematoma by medial orbitotomy and decompression of the optic canal by frontal craniotomy were considered on the basis of CT findings (Mauriello *et al.*, 1992). Nine of 16 patients improved after intravenous steroids alone, whereas one of three improved after optic nerve sheath decompression, and three of four improved after combined optic nerve sheath decompression and optic canal decompression. A similar nonrandomized study reported that 11 of 14 patients gained improved visual acuity after undergoing an external ethmoid approach to decompress the optic canal (Joseph *et al.*, 1990). A review of transethmoid and sphenoid decompression in 11 patients with indirect optic nerve injury showed visual improvement in eight, including four with initial total blindness (Girard *et al.*, 1992).

When visual loss is delayed the arguments for high dose steroids and surgical decompression of the optic canal are more persuasive. Yet the extreme variation in reported success rates for optic nerve decompression is perplexing (Lessell, 1989). Except for the Japanese series (Fukado, 1975), the numbers of cases reported (from the USA and Europe) are small. Many patients treated with surgery have also received steroids, which may have a delayed effect. Until more information is available from prospective randomized controlled clinical trials, the hazards of high dose steroids and transethmoidal decompression should be weighed against the possible benefits in each individual patient.

Optic chiasm

The finding of a bitemporal hemianopia is the cardinal sign of chiasmal pathology. Most compressive causes of bitemporal hemianopia produce a relative rather than an absolute loss of field. In contrast, reports of traumatic chiasmal injury have emphasized that the bitemporal field defect is absolute. The mechanism of chiasmal injury is probably tearing or stretching of the crossing fibres. Chiasmal injury may occur more commonly than has been recognized because of the associated high mortality in these patients. Specific treatment is not available (Heinz *et al.*, 1994; Savino *et al.*, 1980; Traquair *et al.*, 1935).

Optic tract

The finding of a complete homonymous hemianopia, bilateral optic atrophy (band atrophy in the contralateral eye with the temporal field loss and more generalized loss in the ipsilateral eye), and an afferent pupillary defect in the eye with the temporal field loss, indicates an optic tract lesion. Trauma causing an optic tract injury is rare (Bell and Thompson, 1978).

Lateral geniculate body and optic radiation

Lesions causing lateral geniculate body or optic radiation damage to the visual pathway are characteristically seen with vascular disease, tumours, or abscesses, rather than as a result of trauma. Parietal cortex damage occurs with head injury. Features suggesting parietal lobe involvement include a relatively congruous homonymous hemianopia, (denser below than above), conjugate movements of the eyes to the side opposite the lesion on forced eye closure (Cogan's sign), and an abnormal optokinetic response consisting of abnormal slow and fast phase eye movements when targets are moved towards the side of the lesion (Miller, 1982b). Often, parietal lesions are characterized by a lack of awareness of the field defect.

Occipital cortex

Traumatic lesions of the occipital cortex cause congruous homonymous field defects. Bilateral homonymous hemianopia of varying degree, ring scotomas, 'key-hole' fields, and altitudinal defects have been reported (Miller, 1982c). (Figures 19.4–19.6) In his studies of war casualties, Holmes observed that bullet wounds interrupting both occipital lobes were usually fatal if the lower portions were damaged, because death occurred from intracranial bleeding as a result of laceration of the venous sinuses. If the upper portions of the occipital lobes were affected, inferior field loss from both eyes resulted (Holmes, 1918). Cortical blindness may also occur as a complication of tentorial herniation from subdural and intracranial haematomas (Keane, 1980). Transient cortical blindness after head trauma in adults is usually immediate and often has a protracted course with variable outcome (Greenblatt, 1973).

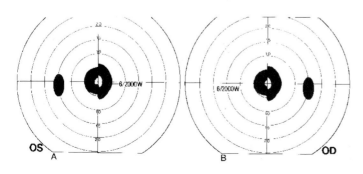

Figure 19.4. Field chart showing ring scotomas (courtesy Walsh and Hoyt).

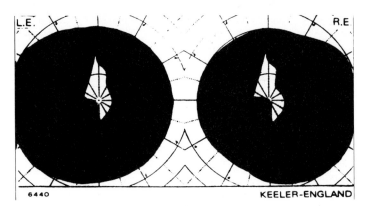

Figure 19.5. Field chart showing key-hole fields.

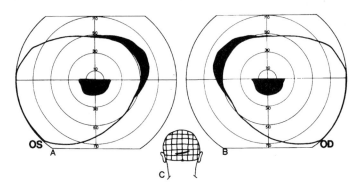

Figure 19.6. Field chart showing altitudinal scotomas (courtesy Walsh and Hoyt).

The use of visual evoked responses to light flashes is not helpful in establishing either diagnosis or prognosis in cases of cerebral blindness (Bodis-Wollner *et al.*, 1977; Spehlmann *et al.*, 1977).

Disorders of colour perception, unilateral visual inattention, and dissociation of kinetic from static perception, have been recognized in patients with occipital injuries (Riddoch, 1917).

Treatment

Apart from general measures to support recovery, there is no specific treatment known to improve prognosis after severe cerebral injury affecting the visual pathways.

Eye movement disorders

Accommodation paralysis

Symptoms of difficulty with near vision are often reported by patients who have suffered cerebral concussion or craniocervical injuries. When slit-lamp examination reveals the signs of tears in the iris sphincter, tears at the root of the iris, or recession of the anterior chamber, then the accommodation paralysis may be attributed to ocular contusion. Accommodation paralysis may also be observed in the dorsal midbrain syndrome, comprising impaired vertical eye movements, eyelid retraction, abnormal vergence movements, skew deviation and pupillary light: near dissociation, but, in most patients, the accommodation paralysis is apparently isolated and difficult to explain on an organic basis (Westcott, 1936).

III, IV and VI palsy

In most large series of acquired palsies of the oculo-motor, trochlear and abducens nerves, head injury is second only to 'idiopathic' as the most common cause (Rucker, 1958, 1976; Richards *et al.*, 1992; Keane and Baloh, 1992).

Oculomotor palsy

The oculomotor nerve is particularly vulnerable in head injury, which causes a contusion or stretching injury to the nerve where it is firmly attached to the dura beside the posterior clinoid process before it enters the cavernous sinus (Heinze, 1969). Supratentorial intracranial pressure from expanding haematoma may also compress the third nerve at this site (Hutchinson, 1867). Herniation of the hippocampal gyrus (Figure 19.7) may compress the oculomotor nerve where it passes over the ridge of dura associated with the attachment of the free edge of the tentorium to the clivus. As the pressure increases, the oculomotor nerve then becomes compressed against the posterior cerebral artery. The first sign of oculomotor compression is often a dilated pupil. Experiments have demonstrated that the most potent stimulus for pupillary dilatation is lateral displacement of the intracranial contents, rather than a marked increase in the intracranial pressure (Kerr and Hollowell, 1964). As the pressure increases, additional signs of oculomotor nerve compression occur. Although the sequence is not consistent, usually ptosis and medial rectus muscle weakness are the most apparent, especially in the obtunded patient (Miller, 1985). In 130 patients with isolated third nerve palsy studied by Green *et al.* (1964), 10.8% were caused by trauma. Of this group, 36% showed incomplete recovery, while the remaining 64% remained unchanged.

It may not be possible to distinguish between a third nerve palsy and ocular muscle contusion in orbital injuries until the orbital swelling has resolved. A fixed dilated pupil due to a third nerve palsy must be distinguished from a traumatic mydriasis due to orbital trauma. The finding of infraorbital numbness favours an inferior blow out fracture of the orbit.

Aberrant regeneration of the oculomotor nerve

Evidence of aberrant regeneration first appears about nine weeks after injury in the adult. For example, on attempted vertical gaze, the eye does not move or it retracts because both superior and inferior rectus muscles contract. Alternatively, any attempt to move the eye vertically results in elevation of the upper eyelid because fibres originally destined for other muscles innervate the levator palpebrae superioris. Anomalous reinnervation may result in a pupil that constricts on attempted adduction of the eye, yet does not constrict to light. This is sometimes called pseudo-Argyll Robertson pupils (Forster *et al.*, 1969).

Management of oculomotor palsy

Spontaneous recovery of oculomotor nerve function occurs over a period of at least 12 months. In the first few months, patients may learn to ignore the diplopia or patch the affected eye. If recovery is incomplete, then a variety of squint procedures and

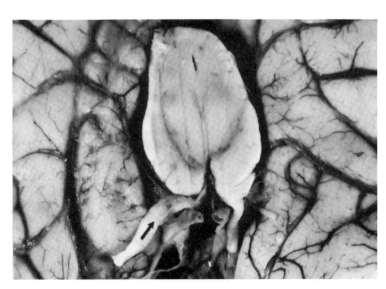

Figure 19.7. Postmortem specimen showing tentorial herniation causing compression of the third nerve (courtesy Walsh and Hoyt).

ptosis operations may be employed. When no recovery occurs, the results of squint surgery are disappointing (Saunders and Rogers, 1982).

Trochlear nerve palsy

Trochlear palsies are rarely diagnosed acutely after head injury. As the patient awakens from coma, he or she closes one eye to focus. Later, difficulty in downgaze and reading become apparent. Examination shows one eye is slightly higher, especially on gaze inwards and downwards. Contralateral head tilt will improve diplopia, whereas ipsilateral head tilting increases the separation of the images. The patient usually learns to adopt a head posture to minimize the diplopia. The differential diagnosis includes orbital muscle injury, a partial third nerve paresis, and skew deviation. Skew deviation is a vertical misalignment of the eyes, which is usually but not always comitant. According to Trobe (1984), patients with skew deviation do not suffer from torsional diplopia. Skew deviation is usually recognized by its association with other signs of brain stem or cerebellar disease.

Pathological studies by Heinze (1969) have shown that closed head trauma causes trochlear injury by avulsion of the rootlets of the nerve as it emerges from the brain stem. When damage occurs at this site, both nerves are often involved, although this may be masked until the patient undergoes surgical correction of an apparent unilateral palsy. Minor head trauma may occasionally cause an isolated trochlear palsy. Orbital trauma may also cause a trochlear nerve palsy, but the trochlea itself or the superior oblique may be directly injured. Approximately 40–50% of unilateral palsies will recover spontaneously (Rush and Younge, 1981; Sydnor *et al.*, 1982), usually within eight months, although only 25% of bilateral palsies resolve (Sydnor *et al.*, 1982).

Management of trochlear palsy

Spontaneous recovery of the trochlear nerve after head injury occurs over a period of up to 12 months. The patient may manage with a compensatory head posture, or patch the affected eye. Occasionally, a vertical prism is helpful, but this does not correct the torsional diplopia. Squint surgery for trochlear palsy has proved very beneficial, and involves: (1) weakening the antagonist inferior oblique muscle; (2) strengthening the superior oblique tendon; and (3) weakening the

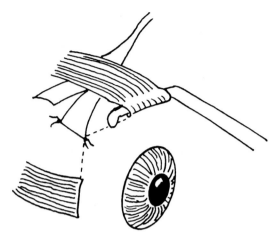

Figure 19.8. Diagram to show advancement of anterior third of superior oblique muscle for bilateral superior oblique palsy.

contralateral inferior rectus muscle (Knapp, 1981). Advancing the anterior part of the superior oblique tendon has proved most effective in bilateral trochlear palsies (Figure 19.8) (Mitchell and Parks, 1982; Price *et al.*, 1987).

Abducens palsy

The site of damage to the abducens nerve in head injury may be in the nucleus (Klingele *et al.*, 1980), the subarachnoid space, where it is stretched at its attachment to the pons or the clivus dura (Heinze, 1969), at the petrous apex (Roberts, 1976), cavernous sinus or orbit. Changes in intracranial pressure occurring spontaneously or after neurosurgical procedures are often associated with unilateral or bilateral abducens palsies. Rush and Younge (1981) reported that approximately 40% of traumatic sixth nerve palsies improve within 6–12 months, although all 15 isolated abducens palsies in another series resolved spontaneously, 33% within weeks (Falbe-Hansen and Gregersen, 1959).

Management of abducens palsies

Patients with abducens palsies should be followed for at least 6–12 months before surgical correction is considered, unless it is known that the abducens nerve is no longer intact. During this period, patients may prefer to patch one eye, and children should undergo alternate patching to discourage amblyopia. Prisms may help some patients to achieve binocular single vision in the primary position. Botulinum toxin injections of the ipsilateral medial rectus muscle may prevent contracture (Lee, 1992). When squint surgery is undertaken, vertical transposition of superior and inferior rectus muscles, combined with medial rectus weakening procedures, have proved most effective.

Complex eye movement disorders

Internuclear ophthalmoplegia

Traumatic unilateral (Beck and Meckler, 1981) and bilateral (Rich *et al.*, 1974) internuclear ophthalmoplegias have been reported. The pathology is probably ischaemia. Skew deviation commonly occurs in association with a unilateral internuclear opthalmoplegia, but rarely with a bilateral internuclear ophthalmoplegia. Skew deviation after trauma must be distinguished from a blow-out fracture of the orbit causing tethering of the inferior rectus muscle.

Vertical ophthalmoplegia

Survival after head trauma severe enough to produce the dorsal midbrain syndrome is unusual, but occasionally patients with multiple neurological damage also show the signs of damage to the mesencephalon (see above).

Cerebellar eye movement disorders

Disorders of gaze-holding and nystagmus characteristically occur with cerebellar lesions, although often these patients also have brain stem damage. The abnormalities seen include: (1) inaccurate saccades; (2) fixation instability; (3) impaired pursuit movements; (4) nystagmus (gaze-evoked, rebound, downbeat, positional); and (5) skew deviation (Leigh and Zee, 1985).

Oscillopsia

Nystagmus acquired after head trauma causes a most disabling oscillopsia, which is associated with grossly reduced visual acuity. Acquired pendular nystagmus occurs as a consequence of brain stem infarction (Gresty *et al.*, 1982). See-saw nystagmus is an uncommon disorder occasionally caused by head trauma (Leigh and Zee, 1983). It is characterized by elevation and intorsion of one eye and synchronous depression and extorsion of the other eye. Bitemporal hemianopia often coexists.

References

Anderson DR. (1981) *Testing the field of vision*. St. Louis: Mosby.

Anderson RL, Panje WR, Gross CE. (1982) Optic nerve blindness following blunt forehead trauma. *Ophthalmology* **89**: 445–655.

Beck RW, Meckler RJ. (1981) Internuclear ophthalmoplegia after head trauma. *Ann Ophthalmol* **13**: 671–75.

Bell RA, Thompson HS. (1978) Relative afferent pupillary defect in optic tract hemianopias. *Am J Ophthalmol* **85**: 538–40.

Blakemore C. (1970) Binocular depth perception and the optic chiasm. *Vision Res* **10**: 43–47.

Bodis-Wollner I, Atkin A, Raab E, *et al.* (1977) Visual association cortex and vision in man: pattern evoked occipital potentials in a blind boy. *Science* **198**: 629–30.

Bracken MB, Shephard MJ, Collins WF, *et al.* (1990) A randomised controlled trial of methylprednisolone or naloxone in the treatment of acute spinal cord injury. *N Eng J Med* **322**: 1405–11.

Dutton GN, Al-Qurainy I, Stassen LFA, Titterington DM. (1992) Ophthalmic consequences of mid-facial trauma. *Eye* **6**: 86–89.

Falbe-Hansen I, Gregersen E. (1959) The prognosis for disturbances of ocular motility following trauma to the head. *Acta Ophthalmol* **37**: 359–70.

Fisher RF. (1968) The variations of the peripheral visual fields with age. *Doc Ophthalmol* **24**: 41–67.

Forster RK, Schatz NJ, Smith JL. (1969) A subtle eyelid sign in aberrant regeneration of the third nerve. *Am J Ophthalmol* **67**: 696–98.

Fukado Y. (1975) Results in 400 cases of surgical decompression in the optic nerve. *Mod Prob Ophthalmol* **14**: 474–481.

Frisen L, Frisen M. (1976) A simple relationship between the probability distribution of visual acuity and the density of retinal output channels. *Acta Ophthalmol* **54**: 437–44.

Girard BC, Bouzas EA, Lamas G, Soudant J. (1992) Visual improvement after transethmoid-sphenoid decompression in optic nerve injuries. *J Clin Neuro-ophthalmol* **12**: 142–48.

Glaser JS. (1978) *Neuro-ophthalmology*. Hagerstown: Harper and Row, 11.

Green WR, Hackett ER, Schlezinger NS. (1964) Neuro-ophthalmologic evaluation of oculomotor nerve paralysis. *Arch Ophthalmol*, **72**: 154–67.

Greenblatt SH. (1973) Posttraumatic transient cerebral blindness: association with migraine and seizure diatheses. *JAMA* **225**: 1073–76.

Gresty MA, EII JJ, Findley LJ. (1982) Acquired pendular nystagmus: its characteristics, localising value and pathophysiology. *J Neurol Neurosurg Psychiatry* **45**: 431–39.

Haddock JN, Berlin L. (1950) Trans-synaptic degeneration in the visual system: report of a case. *Arch Neurol Psychiatr* **64**: 66–73.

Harrington DO. (1976) *The visual fields*. St. Louis: Mosby.

Heinz GW, Nunery MD, Grossman CB. (1994) Traumatic chiasmal syndrome associated with midline basilar skull fractures. *Am J Ophthalmol* **117**: 90–96.

Heinze J. (1969) Cranial nerve avulsion and other neural injuries in road accidents. *Med J Aust* **2**: 1246–49.

Hollenhorst RW, Wagener HP. (1950) Loss of vision after distant haemorrhage. *Am J Med Sci* **219**: 209–18.

Holmes G. (1918) Disturbances of vision by cerebral lesions. *Br J Ophthalmol* **2**: 353–84.

Hooper RS. (1951) Orbital complication of head injury. *Br J Surg* **39**: 126–38.

Hughes B. (1964) The results of injury to special parts of the brain and skull: the cranial nerves. In: Rowbottham GR, editor. *Acute injuries of the head*. Edinburgh: Livingston, 410.

Hutchinson J. (1867) Four lectures on compression of the brain. *Clin Lect Rep Lond Hosp* **4**: 10–55.

Joseph MP, Lessell S, Rizzo J, Momose J. (1990) Extracranial optic nerve decompression for traumatic optic neuropathy. *Arch Ophthalmol* **108**: 1091–93.

Keane JR. (1972) Posttraumatic intracavernous aneurysm: epistaxis with monocular blindness preceded by chromatopsia. *Arch Ophthalmol* **87**: 701.

Keane JR. (1980) Blindness following tentorial herniation. *Ann Neurol* **8**: 186–90.

Keane JR. (1986) Blindness from self-inflicted gunshot wounds. *J Clin Neuroophthalmol* **6**: 247.

Keane JR, Baloh RW. (1992) Posttraumatic cranial neuropathies. *Neurol Clin North Am* **10**: 849–67.

Kerr FWL, Hollowel OW. (1964) Location of pupillomotor and accommodation fibres in the oculomotor nerve: experimental observations on paralytic mydriasis. *J Neurol Neurosurg Psychiatry* **27**: 473–81.

King AB, Walsh FB. (1949) Trauma to the head with particular reference to the ocular signs. Part 1: Injuries involving the cranial nerves. *Am J Ophthalmol* **32**: 191.

Klingele TG, Schultz R, Murphy MG. (1980) Pontine gaze paresis due to traumatic craniocervical hyperextension: report of 2 cases. *J Neurosurg*, **53**: 249–51.

Knapp P. (1981) Treatment of unilateral fourth nerve paralysis. *Trans Ophthalmol Soc UK* **101**: 273–75.

Kupfer C. (1973) Retinal ganglion cell degeneration following chiasmal lesions in man. *Arch Ophthalmol* **70**: 256–60.

Landstrom M, Frisen L. (1975) Evolution of descending optic atrophy: a case report. *Acta Ophthalmol* **53**: 738–46.

Larson CH, Adkins WY, Osguthorpe JD. (1983) Posttraumatic frontal and frontoethmoid mucoceles causing reversible visual loss. *Otolaryngol Head Neck Surg* **91**: 691.

Lee JP. (1992) Modern management of sixth nerve palsy. *Aust N Z J Ophthalmol* **20**: 41–46.

Leigh RJ, Zee DS. (1983) The neurology of eye movements. Philadelphia: Davis. 205

Lessell S. (1989) Indirect Optic Nerve Injury: *Arch Ophthalmol* **107**: 382–86.

Mauriello JA, Deluca J, Krieger A, Schulder M, Frohman L. (1992) Management of traumatic optic neuropathy: a study of 23 patients. *Br J Ophthalmol* **76**: 349–53.

Miller NM. (1982a) Central disorders of visual integration. In: *Walsh and Hoyt's clinical neuro-ophthalmology*, 4th edition Baltimore: Williams & Wilkins, 153–60.

Miller NM. (1982b) Topical diagnosis of lesions in the visual sensory pathway. In: *Walsh and Hoyt's clinical neuro-*

ophthalmology, 4th edition. Baltimore: Williams & Wilkins 136–37.

Miller NM. (1982c) Topical diagnosis of lesions in the visual sensory pathway. In: *Walsh and Hoyt's Clinical Neuro-ophthalmogy*, 4th edition. Baltimore: Williams & Wilkins.

Miller NM. (1985) Topical diagnosis of neuropathic motility disorders. In: *Walsh and Hoyt's clinical neuro-ophthalmology*, 4th edition. Baltimore: Williams & Wilkins.

Miller NM, Newman SA. (1981) Transsynaptic degeneration. *Arch Ophthalmol* **99**: 1654.

Mitchell DE, Blakemore C. (1970) Binocular depth perception and the corpus callosum. *Vision Res* **10**: 49–54.

Mitchell PR, Parks MM. (1982) Surgery for bilateral superior oblique palsy. *Ophthalmology* **89**: 484–88.

Price NC, Vickers S, Lee JP, Fells P. (1987) The diagnosis and surgical management of acquired bilateral superior oblique palsy. *Eye* **1**: 78–85.

Quigley HA, Anderson DR. (1977) The histological basis of optic disc pallor. *Am J Ophthalmol* **83**: 709–17.

Quigley HA, Dunkelberg, Green WR. (1989) Retinal ganglion cell atrophy correlated with automated perimetry in human eyes with glaucoma. *Am J Ophthalmol* **107**: 453–64.

Rich JR, Gregorius FK, Hepler RS. (1974) Bilateral internuclear ophthalmoplegia after trauma. *Arch Ophthalmol* **92**: 66–68.

Richards BW, Jones FR, Younge BR. (1992) Causes and prognosis in 4278 cases of paralysis of the oculo-motor, trochlear and abducens cranial nerves. *Am J Ophthalmol* **113**: 489–96.

Riddoch G. (1917) Dissociation in visual perceptions due to occipital injuries, with especial references to appreciation of movement. *Brain* **40**: 15–57.

Roberts AH. (1979) Severe accidental head injury. London: Macmillan.

Roberts M. (1976) Lesions of the ocular motor nerves (III, IV and VI). In: Vinkin PJ, Bruyn GW, editors. *Handbook of clinical neurology*, vol. 24, part II. Amsterdam: North-Holland, 59–72.

Rucker CW. (1958) Paralysis of the third, fourth and sixth cranial nerves. *Am J Ophthalmol* **61**: 1293–98.

Rucker CW. (1966) The causes of paralysis of the third, fourth and sixth cranial nerves. *Am J Opthalmol* **61**: 1293–98.

Rush JA, Younge BR. (1981) Paralysis of cranial nerves III, IV and VI: cause and prognosis in 1000 cases. *Arch Ophthalmol* **99**: 76–79.

Sanders MD, Hoyt WF. (1969) Hypoxic ocular sequelae of carotid-cavernous fistualae. *Br J Ophthalmol* **53**: 82–97.

Saunders RA, Rogers GL. (1982) Superior oblique transposition for third nerve palsy. *Ophthalmology* **89**: 310–16.

Savino PJ, Glaser JS, Schatz NJ. (1980) Traumatic chiasmal syndrome. *Neurology* **30**: 963–170.

Seiff SR. (1990) High dose corticosteroids for the treatment of visual loss due to indirect injury to the optic nerve. *Ophthalmic Surg* **21**: 389–95.

Spehlmann R, Gross RA, Ho SU, *et al.* (1977) Visual evoked potentials and postmortem findings in a case of cortical blindness. *Ann Neurol* **2**: 531–34.

Spoor TC, Hartel WC, Lensink DB, Wilkinson MJ. (1990) Treatment of traumatic optic neuropathy with corticosteroids. *Am J Ophthalmol* **110**: 665–69.

Steinsapir KD, Goldberg RA. (1994) Traumatic optic neuropathy. *Surv Ophthalmol* **38**: 487–518.

Sydnor CF, Seaber JH, Buckley EG. (1982) Traumatic superior oblique palsies. *Ophthalmology* **89**: 134–38.

Traquair HM. (1949) An introduction to clinical perimetry. London: Kimpton.

Traquair HM, Dott NM, Russell WR. (1935) Traumatic lesions of the optic chiasma. *Brain* **58**: 398–411.

Trobe JD. (1984) Cyclodeviation in acquired vertical strabismus. *Arch Ophthalmol*, **102**: 717–20.

Turner JWA. (1943) Indirect injuries of the optic nerve. *Brain* **66**: 140–51.

Westcott V. (1936) Concerning accommodative asthenopia following head injury. *Am J Ophthalmol* **19**: 385–91.

Wolter JR. (1960) Regenerative potentialities of the centrifugal fibres in the human optic nerve. *Arch Ophthalmol* **64**: 697–707.

20

Ocular trauma

Graham R Kirkby

Epidemiology

Despite many advances in medical and surgical management, severe ocular injury remains a significant cause of permanent visual impairment. In addition, large numbers of patients with minor ocular injuries suffer considerable pain, inconvenience and time lost from work. The National Society to Prevent Blindness (1980) reported than in the USA 2.4 million eye injuries may be occurring annually of which 20 000–68 000 are serious and vision-threatening. In a national hospitalization survey in the USA between 1984 and 1987, Klopfer *et al.* (1992) found ocular trauma was the principal cause of 13.2 per 100 000 admissions and the principal or secondary diagnosis in 29.1 per 100 000. Shein *et al.* (1988) reported on 3184 patients presenting to an urban eye casualty unit in Massachusetts over a six-month period. Severe injuries totalled 5.1%; 94.9% of these were superficial injuries or contusions, and 19.1% of those affected were less than 15 years of age. Accidents in the workplace accounted for 48% of injuries and 3.4% were sporting. In a prospective survey of eye injuries over a one-year period in Glasgow, MacEwen (1989) analysed 5671 patients. Of these, 69.9% were work-related, 18.3% occurred during leisure and domestic activities, 2.3% were sporting accidents and 1.9% were assaults. Contact lenses caused 2.3% of injuries. In 5.3% the cause was unknown. Young males were

the most commonly injured and children were injured most severely.

Accidents at work have always been an important cause of eye injuries. In the USA, the *Morbidity and Mortality Weekly Report* (MMWR) in 1984 (Leads from the MMWR, 1984) estimated that there were 900 000 such injuries in 1982. The severity of these injuries seems to be reducing, however, since industrial eye injuries accounted for 71% of hospital admissions in 1923 but were only 14% in 1989 (MacEwen, 1989). By this time, sport was the commonest cause (42.2%) followed by leisure and domestic (22.6%) and assault (18.6%). The recognition of sports as a major cause of eye injury has led to calls for increased protection. In a one-year survey of severe eye injuries in sport, Jones (1988) found soccer to be the single most common cause of injury (32.7%), with the racquet sports accounting collectively for 52%. In the USA, Shein *et al.* (1988) found baseball and softball to be the commonest causes (30%) followed by racquet sports (22%).

In the USA, the National Eye Trauma System (NETS) Registry has, since 1985, collated data from participating regional centres concerning penetrating eye injuries. Dannenberg *et al.* (1992a), presenting collective experience of penetrating eye injuries in the workplace, suggested that 75% were males younger than 40 years, and this supported the observations of MacEwen (1989). Dannenberg *et al.* (1992b), reporting on penetrating injuries due to assault, found a similar preponderance of young males. It is interesting to note that an association between these injuries and alcohol consumption was discovered in 2% of workplace and in 48% of assault cases.

Assessment of the patient

History

Ophthalmic injuries at work, in sport, and due to assault, often result in a claim for compensation. The medical examiner preparing a medicolegal report will, therefore, take a careful history. Of particular importance will be the exact circumstances of the incident, the availability and wearing of ocular protection, the presence or otherwise of appropriate guards on machinery, the length of stay in hospital, the time spent off work, and the effect on the victim's occupational capabilities, on personal hobbies and on the ability to drive. A history of past ocular problems should be sought, including the wearing of spectacles. A family history should be taken, since the presence of inherited ocular diseases may be important in predicting the long-term ocular health of the examinee. General health problems, such as diabetes and hypertension, may also have a long-term capability for ocular damage and should be included in the history.

Medical records

In almost every case, it will be essential for the examiner to scrutinize the patient's medical records. Casualty cards or notes and inpatient records should all be requested. The general practitioner's records should also be seen, as they may provide evidence of past ocular complaints and of time off work following an injury. The records of the patient's optometrist may be helpful in determining the preincident visual acuity and need, or not, for spectacles.

In most instances, the clinical examination will provide objective evidence to support the subjective symptoms. However, occasionally, an individual will be encountered who is hysterical or is malingering. Details of the many tests that can be employed to detect such an individual are outwith the scope of this chapter but the examiner should be conversant with their application. The examiner can do little better than read the appropriate chapter on malingering in Duke-Elders

System of Ophthalmology (Duke-Elder and Abrams, 1970).

The examiner may be asked to express the visual loss in percentage terms. A table has been published (Duke-Elder and Abrams, 1978), but the usefulness of such figures is doubtful, since they do not take into account such other factors as visual field defects, loss of colour vision or contrast sensitivity.

In serious injuries, where treatment is ongoing, the examiner may have to prepare interim reports until a steady state is reached, when a final report can be made.

Examination

The examination should comprise a full ophthalmic examination of both eyes, including refraction if necessary. Of particular importance in blunt injuries is gonioscopy for detection of angle recession. This should be carried out in both eyes for comparison. Subsequent to the examination, supplementary tests may be required such as visual fields, orthoptic investigations and visually evoked responses.

Effect of ophthalmic trauma on stereopsis

Many victims of ocular trauma later complain of difficulty in performing fine tasks. This may be especially troublesome in those whose livelihood depends on such manipulations, for example, a skilled worker or artisan. Presumably, the reason for this difficulty is, at least in part, due to degradation in stereoscopic vision.

Levy and Glick (1974) investigated the effect of degradation of stereopsis by reducing Snellen acuity in one eye. They found that, using the Titnus Stereo Test, monocular cues provided sufficient information to distinguish the differences in circles at 200 seconds of image disparity. Acuity less than 6/60 (20/200) gave similar uniocular and binocular results. Goodwin and Romano (1985) confirmed that visual acuity and stereo acuity are related. Monocular degradation of visual acuity affected stereo acuity more between 6/7.5 (20/25) and 6/15 (20/50) than binocular degradation of visual acuity.

These studies do not, of course, take into account the gradual learning and adaptive process that an injured patient necessarily undergoes, and the clinician preparing a medicolegal report could not necessarily know the precise level of stereopsis required in any given occupation. However, they do indicate that an assessment of stereopsis in an injured individual may be necessary and they do provide some numerical back-up to the report.

Eye Injuries

Indirect

Whiplash

Whiplash injuries typically occur in rear end motor vehicle accidents. Oculomotor abnormalities represent the commonest effects (Burke *et al.*, 1992; Duke-Elder and MacFaul, 1972a) Daily (1970a, 1973, 1979) first described a splinter of retinal tissue projecting from the foveal surface and a wisp-like appearance of the inner retinal surface in several clinical situations. These included one patient with whiplash neck injury in a car accident and two others with head trauma; in one other patient, there was direct eye trauma. He attributed these changes to elevation of the posterior hyaloid in the macular region. Kelly *et al.* (1978) described a whiplash maculopathy in which there was an immediate unilateral or bilateral reduction in visual acuity. A transient greyish swelling in the foveal zone resolved eventually to leave a small foveal pit with a prominent whitish border; the vision returned to normal. Complete posterior vitreous detachment (PVD) has been described by Burke *et al.* (1992) in one patient following whiplash injury, whereas Daily (1970a,b) and Kelly *et al.* (1978) described localized premacular PVD. The writer can find no reference to retinal detachment being caused by whiplash, but the patient of PVD in Burke *et al.* (1992) may indicate this as a theoretical possibility.

Traumatic retinal angiopathy due to remote trauma

Traumatic retinal angiopathy may be predominantly arterial, venous or a mixture of the two. The whole subject is elegantly reviewed by Archer (1986). Purtscher (1910) first described a retinal angiopathy consisting of oval white spots and intravitreal haemorrhages in patients with head injuries. Subsequently, a similar mixed arterial/venous picture, with generalized retinal oedema, intraretinal haemorrhages and cotton wool spots has been reported in various situations after trauma.

Compressive chest injuries may produce a severe retinopathy, which is often unilateral, although the other eye may be subtly affected. The retinopathy resolves between six weeks and six months and most patients achieve 6/12 vision or better, although a permanent scotomata, colour vision defects and a loss of contrast sensitivity may persist. These same parameters should be assessed in patients suffering from chest compression due to seatbelts (Archer *et al.*, 1988; Beckinsale and Rosenthal, 1983; Hoare, 1970; Kelly, 1972). Archer (1988) also carried out fluorescein angiography in his patients and found vascular abnormalities present years after the event. They also had abnormal pattern reversal visually evoked responses.

Multiple long bone fractures with fat embolism syndrome (FES) may cause an ischaemic vasculopathy (Adams, 1971; Chuang *et al.*, 1985; Thomas and Ayyar, 1972). In her paper, Chuang (1985), seeking to establish the incidence of subclinical FES as judged by retinal lesions, examined 100 consecutive patients with long bone or pelvic fractures but no other major injury. She found retinopathy in four patients, three of whom were symptomatic. The symptomatic patient retained a paracentral scotoma two years after injury.

A predominantly venous angiopathy, with perivenous, preretinal and, occasionally, vitreous haemorrhage, is seen following a sudden increase of intrathoracic pressure, as in the Valsalva manoeuvre, and has recently been reported following bungee jumping (Habib and Malik, 1994). Permanent sequelae are rare, but preretinal haemorrhage has been known to result in permanent visual impairment (Duane, 1973).

Electrical injury

Electrocution by lightning or industrial accident can cause abnormalities in every part of the eye. Corneal scarring, iritis, Horner's syndrome, cataract, retinal and choroidal abnormalities, and optic nerve damage have all been reported; they were reviewed recently by van Johnson *et al.* (1987) and previously by Duke-Elder and MacFaul (1972b). Cataracts may occur immediately or be of delayed onset up to three years. They typically affect the capsule and subcapsular region, and are not invariably progressive. Visual rehabilitation following their removal depends on whether other structures, especially the retina or the optic nerve, have been damaged.

Chemical burns

Chemical burns remain common and may be sustained at home, in accidental spillage in shops and elsewhere, and in industrial accidents. Some cases result from the deliberate spraying of a chemical into the eyes by an assailant. Jones and Griffith (1992) carried out a prospective population-based survey within the chemical industry and found that an eye injury occurred once every 75 000 man hours of work (injury incidence 23 : 1000 per year). In this study, no patient required hospital admission. In many instances, ocular protection was either not worn or it failed to protect adequately. In some instances, the protector provided was incorrect for the task. Employers should provide adequate facilities adjacent to the working areas for emergency irrigation of chemical injuries, since time is of the essence in removing the substance from the eye (Duke-Elder and MacFaul, 1972c). Alkali injuries to the eye are more serious than acids because they penetrate more readily.

Roper-Hall (1965) proposed a grading system based on the work of Ballen (1963) (Table 20.1). This is still widely used and is often recorded or can be gleaned from the hospital notes. This grading is important since it can be used to determine the likely ultimate prognosis.

After a severe chemical injury, recovery may be very protracted due to defective tear film, delayed epithelialization, symblepharon formation, lid margin scarring and, sometimes, eyelash misdirection, all of which may require further treatment or surgery. Glaucoma may be present due to trabecular meshwork damage. Cataract may occur. Corneal scarring and vascularization may limit the final visual acuity and is extremely difficult to deal with surgically, since conventional corneal grafting frequently fails (Buxton and Norden, 1986). In severe bilateral chemical scarring, keratoprosthesis may be considered, although there are likely to be complications such as glaucoma, retinal detachment and retroprosthetic membranes, as well as extrusion of the prosthesis itself (Aquavella *et al.*, 1982; Cardona, 1983). It is unlikely, in a severe chemical burn, that a final report could be prepared earlier than one year after the injury.

Radiation injuries

Ultraviolet light

The commonest injury sustained due to ultraviolet light is the welder's flash. The delayed onset of pain, photophobia and reduced vision being familiar to all ophthalmologists. Repeated exposure in the industrial setting, where there is often also an excessively dusty atmosphere, may lead to chronic conjunctivitis and blepharitis (Narda *et al.*, 1990). Norn and Franch (1991) examined 217 male welders and found conjunctival spheroid degeneration in 24%, pingueculae in 57%, and pterygium in only one person, but pseudopterygium in 5%. Half the subjects had corneal scars.

Chronic exposure to ultraviolet light also occurs in those living or working in snow-bound or waterside environments. Taylor *et al.* (1989) examined 838 watermen on Chesapeake Bay; pterygium was found in 140, climatic droplet keratopathy in 162 and pingueculae in 642. The association between cataract and ordinary daylight exposure is not proven. However, 8-methoxypsoralen (8-MOP) and exposure to psoralen ultraviolet A (PUVA) is used in dermatological practice and has been shown to cause corneal opacity and cataract in animals. Boukes and Bruynzeel (1985) examined 398 patients on PUVA therapy. It was found that, in three patients, lens opacities were at least partly due to the therapy. Retinal damage

Table 20.1. Classification of severity of ocular injury in chemical burns: Roper-Hall (1965) after Ballen (1963). (Reprinted with permission of the Royal College of Ophthalmology.)

Grade	Cornea	Conjunctiva	Prognosis
I	Epithelial damage	No ischaemia	Good
II	Hazy but iris detail seen	Ischaemia less than 1/3 at limbus	Doubtful
III	Total epithelial loss Stromal haze Iris details obscured	Ischaemia affects 1/3 to 1/2 at limbus	Vision reduced Perforation rare
IV	Opaque No view of pupil or iris	Ischaemia affects more than 1/2 at limbus	Poor Prolonged convalescence Symblepharon common

from ultraviolet light is possible and is more likely in aphakic patients. For a useful summary see Kirkness and Weale (1985).

Visible light

Light can cause damage to the retina in three ways: thermally, as in laser photocoagulation; mechanically, as in Q switched lasers, and photochemically. Photochemical injury occurs environmentally in eclipse burns or solar retinopathy but may also occur in an occupational setting. Photofloods in television studios cause considerable discomfort glare due. to their high luminance. The light contains considerable blue light and ultraviolet irradiation, which may be harmful (Hietanen and Hoikkala, 1990).

Welding flash can cause macular damage. Metal arc inert gas (MIG) welders may be especially dangerous (Brittain, 1988).

McDonald and Irvine (1983) showed that prolonged exposure in ophthalmic surgery while using operating microscopes caused retinal damage as predicted by Mainster *et al.* (1983).

Infrared radiation

A characteristic posterior cortical cataract, accompanied by dehiscence of the anterior zonular lamellar, is seen in those chronically exposed to infrared irradiation, glass workers and furnacemen being particularly prone. A thermal model of the human eye has been constructed to determine changes in the intraocular temperature distribution resulting from exposure to infrared radiation (Scott, 1988).

Wainwright and Whillock (1990) used data from measurements by the Health and Safety Executive in various industrial processes. They determined, using a mathematical model of heat flow in the eye, that large temperature rises could be expected at the anterior lens surface.

Infrared radiation also contributes to photic light damage in the retina.

Microwaves

Since their introduction into many homes, there has been much discussion in the lay press of the danger of microwave ovens. There is as yet no evidence that these are dangerous or cause cataracts. Microwaves are used industrially in radar and communications equipment and their effects on the lens have been investigated *in vitro* by

Creighton *et al.* (1987) and *in vivo* in rabbit eyes by Emery *et al.* (1975). An interesting discussion on the relative merits of this and other research is presented by Joyner (1989) in his paper on 'Microwave cataract and litigation'. Since the leakage of radiation from radar cabinets and generating devices varies as the inverse square of the distance from the source (Joyner and Bangay, 1986) the power levels to which an individual is exposed rapidly reduce as they move away from the source.

Minor nonperforating injuries

Corneal Foreign Bodies

Corneal foreign bodies are some of the commonest industrial injuries. Usually there is a small corneal leucoma but visual disability is slight or absent unless there is involvement of the optic axis or complications such as infection. Few patients take more than half a day off work (Alexander *et al.*, 1991).

Corneal abrasion

Traumatic corneal abrasion usually resolves rapidly but may be subject to recurrence. Weene (1985) found a 7.69% recurrence rate in 377 consecutive patients. The size of the original abrasion did not correlate with recurrence. Sixty per cent of recurrences occurred within six months of injury. Hykin *et al.* (1994), on reviewing the natural history and management of recurrent erosion, found that of 117 such patients, 75 had a history of trauma and 23 had epithelial basement membrane dystrophy; eight had both and 11 had neither. This study found that only five of 117 patients required more than simple lubricant ointment at night to control symptoms.

Blunt trauma to the globe

General considerations

Blunt trauma is common and can damage every structure in the eye. A blow at a given point on the globe may cause an injury there (coup) or at a distant point (contrecoup) by the transmission of a shockwave through the ocular media. In addition, Delori *et al.* (1969) found that a severe blow at the front of the eye causes posterior displacement of the cornea and lens iris diaphragm, with consequent pre-equatorial expansion. At that time, the distance between the vitreous base and the posterior pole of the lens is increased. The intraocular pressure at the vitreous base in increased, countering the tractional force. As the zonule and lens capsule are distensible, traction on the suspensory ligament and the lens itself causes less damage than traction acting directly on the vitreous base, which is less distensible. The greatest shearing forces in the retina are located along the posterior border of the vitreous base, explaining the commonly found damage at that point.

Cornea

The cornea is not usually severely damaged by blunt trauma; however, the corneal endothelial cell count (ECD) may be reduced. Slingsby and Forstot (1981) found a 6.4% decrease in ECD in patients with hyphaema, but a 12.2% decrease in those with angle recession. This may mean an increased likelihood of corneal decompensation if the patient required cataract surgery in the future.

Iris and ciliary body

Damage to the iris may take the form of iris sphincter ruptures with pupil deformity. Traumatic mydriasis and iridodialysis may cause photophobia and, in the latter, uniocular diplopia. Iris pigment may be deposited on the anterior lens capsule in Vossius' ring.

Mild iritis frequently occurs in these circumstances but prolonged iritis and the precipitation of iritis in susceptible individuals has been reported by Rosenbaum *et al.* (1991).

Hyphaema occurs due to tearing of tissue in the iris or the ciliary body. Most resolve rapidly, but rebleeding may occur within a few days of injury. An incidence of 16% for this complication seems a typical figure (Thomas *et al.* 1986). Corneal blood staining occurs in the same eye, particularly in association with rebleeding, larger hyphaemas and raised intraocular pressure. Corneal blood staining does clear but may take months or years. In a child, the development of amblyopia in such circumstances may necessitate keratoplasty.

Glaucoma

Glaucoma may occur acutely after blunt trauma, either with or without hyphaema, but it may also occur months or many years later. Apart from cases of ghost cell glaucoma, in which depigmented red cells migrate into the anterior chamber from the vitreous, blocking the trabecular meshwork, the majority of post-traumatic glaucoma is due to damage to the anterior chamber angle. Clinical examination should, therefore, include gonioscopy in both eyes for comparison. In angle recession, the ciliary body is torn with displacement posteriorly of the iris root (Alper, 1963; Wolf and Zimmerman, 1962). Gonioscopic examination in the early stages after injury has shown marked variation in the amount and appearance of the recessed areas over a few days (Herschler, 1977). Tears and abnormalities of the trabecular meshwork itself are also seen. In patients with hyphaema, angle recession has been seen in 71% (Blanton, 1964), 94% (Kaufman and Tolpin, 1974; Tönjun, 1966) or even 100% (Spaeth, 1967). Attempts have been made to correlate the likelihood of glaucoma developing with the extent of angle recession. Kaufman and Tolpin (1974) found the majority of patients with 240° or even 360° of angle recession did not develop glaucoma in a 10-year follow-up study, although most had an increased coefficient of outflow. In their study, three patients (9%) had glaucoma at the end of 10 years; only two of these had late onset glaucoma (6%). Tönjun (1968) found no glaucoma in 80 patients after eight years. Blanton (1964) found 7% glaucoma after 10 years. Both of these were retrospective studies. Although late onset glaucoma with less than 180° of angle recession has been seen (Blanton, 1964), more than 240° confers higher risk (Alper, 1963; Tesluk and Spaeth, 1985). Some patients with angle recession glaucoma develop glaucoma in their uninjured eye (Herschler, 1977; Tesluk and Spaeth, 1985). This may indicate that post-traumatic angle recession glaucoma is more likely to occur in those who would develop glaucoma anyway. This, and the possibility of visual loss from glaucoma in the good eye, obviously has important medicolegal implications.

Hypotony

Hypotony may occur after blunt injury and is due to cyclodialysis. This will be revealed on gonioscopy. Profound hypotony may be corrected by surgical refixation of the detached ciliary body (Demeler, 1988).

Lens

Cataract

Traumatic contact between the cornea and the lens (or a shockwave) causes an anterior subcapsular 'rosette' cataract, which may be transient. Sectoral and other opacities may occur and may be symptomatic (visual deterioration, photophobia, etc.) or not. Progression is not inevitable unless there is capsule rupture.

Dislocation

Trauma was the commonest cause of lens subluxation or dislocation in a hospitalization study by Jarrett (1967). However, other causes such as Marfan's syndrome or syphilis (amongst others) should be excluded. Subluxation may be asymptomatic or may have refractive effects such as myopia, astigmatism or monocular diplopia. Dislocation may cause pupil block glaucoma. A posteriorly dislocated lens may cause chronic uveitis and, occasionally, phacolytic glaucoma (Rodman, 1963).

Cataract extraction in traumatic cases may be more complicated and less successful than normally because of the presence of other traumatic sequelae.

Retina and vitreous

Commotio retinae

Commotio retinae results either from a coup or a contrecoup injury. If peripheral, there is usually no permanent visual disturbance, although there may be late pigmentary changes in the retina. However, severe commotio at the macula causes a hole in 3–4% of patients, resulting in poor central vision (Archer and Canavan, 1983).

Retinal pigment epithelium

Friberg (1979) has reported traumatic retinal pigment epithelial RPE oedema consisting of a cream-coloured discoloration followed by patchy depigmentation and pigment clumping. Gass (1987) described accompanying serous retinal detachment. Gitter et al. (1968) described traumatic haemorrhagic RPE detachment in general due to underlying choroidal rupture. Visual acuity is unaffected unless there is foveal involvement. Levin et al. (1991) described two cases of retinal epithelial tears after trauma. In one patient, the trauma was directly to the eye, in the other the trauma was indirect and there was a mild Purtscher retinopathy. The clinical findings were as for other cases of RPE tears, with late depigmentation and

large window defects on fluorescein angiography. One patient had a paracentral scotoma.

Choroid

Rupture of the choroid and Bruch's membrane, manifesting as deep subretinal haemorrhage in the acute period, leads ultimately to the appearance of scarring and pigment epithelial changes in the area of the tear. These lesions characteristically occur directly at the site of injury as circumferential lesions parallel to the ora, or indirectly as peripapillary crescents. Lesions may, however, be of irregular shape (Wood and Richardson, 1990) or radial to the disc (Pruett et al., 1987).

In Wood and Richardson's (1990) series, injuries from punches tended to cause diffuse impact on the globe with indirect peripapillary ruptures only, whilst impact from projectiles, weapons and kicks caused more widespread ruptures. Choroidal ruptures in or near the macula may result in reduced visual acuity either immediately, due to haemorrhage and scarring, or later due to the development of choroidal neovascular membranes (Fuller and Gitter, 1973; Gass 1973; Smith et al., 1974). Maberley and Carvounis (1977) performed static and kinetic perimetry in nine eyes with indirect traumatic choroidal rupture and found no characteristic field defect apart from central or paracentral scotoma due to retinal involvement. Nerve fibre bundle defects were found in four patients. Nerve fibre bundle defects were also found by Wood and Richardson (1990), who suggested that these represented optic nerve injury rather than being directly attributable to the rupture.

Macular changes

Grey (1978) described macular changes similar to those seen in solar retinopathy following ocular trauma in three patients, in two of whom the vision remained impaired. Gross and Freeman (1990) described patients with post-traumatic yellow maculopathy, which was due to the alteration in colour of subretinal blood. Both cases resulted in reduced acuity when the material had dispersed.

Traumatic retinal tears and detachment

Lamellar macular holes after commotio retinae have already been mentioned above. Cooling (1986) has suggested that vitreous avulsion may account for the full thickness macular hole that, in some instances, occurs acutely after blunt trauma, and also the rare radial tears described by Carter and Park (1987). These authors described both eyes of an amateur boxer in whom there were giant tears and huge radial tears, in one eye extending through the macula.

Retinal tears appearing at the site of severe concussion do so as a result of retinal ischaemia (Archer, 1986). These tears may be large and sometimes flatten spontaneously. Most respond to conventional surgery. Nevertheless, field defects persist, corresponding to the area of retinal ischaemia.

Retinal dialysis is traditionally associated with ocular trauma. Zyon and Burton (1980), on reviewing 211 cases of retinal dialysis, concluded that most could be ascribed to trauma, a proposition supported by Ross (1981). A genetic cause for retinal dialysis was considered unlikely by Hagler (1980) and Ross (1991).

Goffstein and Burton (1982) found dialyses and giant retinal tears were the most common cause of retinal detachment after trauma, but pointed out that bilateral inferotemporal retinal dialyses were not found in their trauma group. This finding emphasizes the importance of meticulous examination of the uninjured eye using indirect ophthalmoscopy and scleral depression in such patients.

Differentiation of traumatic from nontraumatic retinal detachment

The differentiation of traumatic from nontraumatic retinal detachments may be difficult. Cox *et al.* (1966), in an important paper, examined 166 patients with retinal detachment due to ocular contusion. For inclusion in the study, all patients had to have at least one other sign of ocular contusion. Those affected were predominantly young (85% less than 40 years) and male (86.7%). The incidence of myopia was 21%, which is a little higher than in the general population. The latent interval between the trauma and the detachment was less than two years in 80%.

In 59.4%, retinal detachment was due to breaks at the ora. These detachments were of a slowly progressive type and had signs such as demarcation lines. They were not bullous. The breaks found were vitreous base tears and vitreous base avulsion tears. Retinal dialyses were accompanied by chorioretinal atrophy and pigmentation.

In 35.7% of eyes, breaks developed in areas with no vitreous attachment, and, in 26.6%, tears developed at the site of vitreoretinal attachment. These were tears similar to those seen in non-traumatic detachment, but they were frequently accompanied by typical traumatic tears. This study identified as being exclusively due to trauma bucket handle vitreous base avulsion tears and large irregular tears occurring due to ischaemia at the point of impact.

Goffstein and Burton (1982) reported on 586 detachments, of which 111 were traumatic. They presented similar data to that of Cox *et al.* (1966) on age, sex and latent interval, although more patients (28%) were myopic. They found that giant retinal tears and retinal dialyses formed 69% of the traumatic detachments, but they represented only 7% of the nontraumatic group. Their important conclusions, which are helpful in the medicolegal context, are that traumatic detachments are characterized by:

1. Unilateral vitreoretinal pathology.
2. Giant tears and dialyses (especially superior and nasal).
3. Age of onset under 40 years.
4. Latent interval between trauma and detachment less than two years.
5. Objective evidence of trauma.

Even with a history of ocular injury, trauma is unlikely to produce a detachment characterized by:

1. Bilateral vitreoretinal pathology.
2. Simple retinal tears or lattice degeneration.
3. Age over 40 years.
4. Latent interval exceeding 2 years.
5. No supporting objective evidence of trauma.

Of course, exceptions do occur, and each case must be judged on its merits and decided on the balance of probabilities.

Prognosis after surgery for traumatic retinal detachment

Retinal detachment after blunt trauma requires surgical intervention in the majority of instances. Retinal dialysis and impaction ischaemic tears may be managed with conventional scleral buckling surgery. The results of retinal dialysis surgery (Hagler, 1980) are generally anatomically excellent (98% success). Visual acuity may not be good if there was macular involvement by detachment or some other pathology; Hagler (1980) found only 40% had an acuity of 6/12 or better. Giant retinal tears can be repositioned in up to about 80% of patients (Leaver *et al.*, 1984), the visual acuity being 6/60 or better in 57% of patients at 18 months (Billington and Leaver, 1986).

Penetrating ocular trauma

General considerations

Penetrating trauma has always stimulated interest and debate in ophthamology, and ocular trauma surgery has benefited greatly from improved techniques and better understanding of the pathological processes involved. A great deal of work has been done in trying to predict the ultimate visual outcome from the situation obtaining at presentation. Of relatively recent surveys, the following are of interest.

Barr (1983) reported on 122 patients with corneoscleral lacerations. The average age was 25 years; 99 were males, and 17% of the eyes were enucleated. The best predictors of a good visual result were: good initial visual acuity; the absence of posterior uveal prolapse; the absence of lens damage; and a small laceration.

Sternberg *et al.* (1984) reported on 281 eyes and found that an initial visual acuity of 1.5/60 (20/800) or better was the most important factor. In this group, being aged less than 18 years improved prognosis. In those with vision worse than 1.5/60 (20/800), a laceration of the cornea only conferred a better outcome. A better visual outcome also occurred when the lens was not displaced and when lacerations were anterior to the rectus muscle insertions.

Hutton and Fuller (1984) reviewed 194 patients undergoing pars plana vitrectomy for severe eye injuries involving the posterior segment. They found, as had Sternberg *et al.* (1984), that an initial visual acuity of 1.5/60 (5/200) was predictive of a better final acuity, as were smaller (<12 mm) lacerations. They did not find that the position of the laceration influenced the outcome. They found the best predictor of poor outcome was the absence of the visually evoked potential (VEP), reflecting the importance for a good outcome of the structural integrity of the macula and optic nerve.

De Juan *et al.* (1993) reviewed 453 patients. The mean age 26 years; 86% of patients were male; 23% of eyes were enucleated. They also found that an initial visual acuity of 1.5/60 (5/200) was predictive of a better outcome, with 64% of eyes with poorer initial vision eventually requiring enucleation or attaining a final vision of worse than 1.5/60 (5/200). Further observations were that the presence of an afferent pupil defect signified a poorer outcome. Corneal wounds did better than corneoscleral or scleral wounds. Loss of, or subluxation of, the lens was predictive of poor outcome; the presence of a cataract was not. They

also concluded that injuries sustained with a blunt force did worse than those caused by sharp objects or projectiles. They added that double perforating injuries were likely to have a poor prognosis. De Juan (1983) found only three of 18 double perforating wounds had a final visual acuity of 1.5/60 (5/200) or better (this group contained no patients with an intraocular foreign body (IOFB)).

In conclusion, a perforating injury is likely to have a poor visual outcome if, at presentation, there is:

1. Poor visual acuity.
2. A relative afferent pupil defect.
3. A large laceration of the corneosclera or sclera, especially extending behind the recti.
4. Loss or subluxation of the lens.
5. Severe intraocular (especially vitreous) haemorrhage.
6. Retinal detachment.
7. An absent VEP.

Some of these prognostic factors are corroborated by experimental studies of the pathology of serious injury such as those of Cleary and Ryan (1979a,b,c) and Gregor and Ryan (1982a,b). The writer of a medicolegal report will, however, be more concerned with an analysis of a clinical situation that is relatively stable several months after the injury, probably after the patient has undergone one or more surgical procedures.

Corneal perforating injury and laceration

Corneal perforating injuries and lacerations without other injury have the best prognosis of all perforating eye injuries (Barr, 1983; Eagling, 1976). However, in addition to symptoms such as photophobia, visual acuity may be reduced by scarring on the optic axis or by astigmatism from a more peripheral wound. Corneal wounds of less than one-third of the corneal diameter or less than 4 mm in length are known to cause less astigmatism. The presence of iris tissue in the wound does not correlate with astigmatism, but may lead to vascularization of the scar, especially since iris incarceration is more likely in the more peripheral wound.

Patients with severe regular astigmatism who are intolerant of spectacles may undergo refractive surgery. Alternatively, contact lenses may be helpful, especially in those with irregular astigmatism. Smiddy *et al.* (1989), reporting on 26 patients, 22 of whom were also aphakic, found good results in the younger patients, and in those in whom scarring was peripheral. The average follow-up was only 10 months. Contact lenses have, of course, their own complications, but they are a cheaper and simpler alternative to penetrating keratoplasty. In scarred corneas, a rotational autograft may be helpful.

Lens injury

Damage to the crystalline lens in a perforating injury is usually manifested as cataract. The cataract may be progressive or static. If progressive, cataract extraction can be performed by a variety of methods and an intraocular lens (IOL) may or may not be implanted. If no IOL is implanted, the patient may need a contact lens. Epikeratophakia may be considered when there is contact lens intolerance. Children are a particular problem. In the USA, a nationwide study of epikeratophakia in children included 87 traumatic cases, 89% of which were successful. Of six patients able to co-operate verbally in visual acuity testing, four had vision 6/30 (20/100) or better (Morgan, 1987). Rarely, phacoanaphylactic endophthalmitis occurs. This condition must be distinguished from sympathetic ophthalmitis, although the two conditions may occur simultaneously. Easam and Zimmerman (1964) suggested that, clinically, the exciting eye is likely to be uninflamed when phacoanaphylactic endophthalmitis starts in the other eye, whereas, in sympathetic ophthalmitis, the exciting eye is usually intensely inflamed.

Iris damage

Severe perforating injuries may result in the loss of considerable iris tissue, causing photophobia, or possibly monocular diplopia, if there is peripheral iridectomy or iridodialysis. The cosmetic defect should also be considered. A contact lens with a painted iris may need to be worn.

Posterior segment perforating injury

These are the most serious type of perforating injury. The major risk is of retinal detachment. This occurs due to fibrocellular proliferation in the vitreous base region, which causes retinal breaks in this area, particularly small retinal dialyses. Vitrectomy surgery is commonly used, but results are difficult to compare because of the many variations in injuries sustained.

Intraocular foreign bodies

General considerations

The National Eye Trauma System Registry (Dannenberg *et al.*, 1992a), on reviewing 635 penetrating injuries found 35% involved an IOFB. These serious injuries therefore remain relatively common. Many injuries are sustained at work. Young males aged 20–40 years are most commonly affected (Roper-Hall, 1954).

The Management of IOFB has changed greatly over the years, as has much of ocular surgery. Before the advent of the operating microscope, Roper-Hall (1954) presented 555 IOFBs. They were extracted, if magnetic, via the anterior route (corneal), via the pars plana or via the posterior route (i.e. through the retina). Forty-nine per cent of patients secured a visual acuity of 6/18 (20/60) or better. After the introduction of the operating microscope, Percival (1972) presented a series of 245 eyes, 61% of which obtained 6/12 (20/40) vision or better. Williams *et al.* (1988) reported on 105 IOFBs, 60% of which obtained 6/12 (20/40) or better, despite the introduction by this time of vitreoretinal surgical techniques. Although the rate of enucleation is now less, these figures do not seem to indicate impressive progress over such a long period.

Magnetic extraction of IOFB, the mainstay of surgical management till the 1970s, is now reserved by most surgeons for those foreign bodies that are small, can be seen clearly and that are not stuck in the retina. Good results have been obtained, however, in other circumstances by some authors (Shock and Adams, 1985).

The prognosis in IOFB injury depends on a number of factors. Williams *et al.* (1988) found that, at presentation, predictors of a good visual outcome were an initial visual acuity of 6/12 (20/40) or better, and the need for two or less operations. The predictors of a poor visual outcome were an initial visual acuity of 6/12 (20/40) or worse and a wound length of 4 mm or greater, independent of localization. The size of the IOFB is important, with airgun and BB pellets having a particularly dismal prognosis. De Juan *et al.* (1983) found that all patients in their series had visual acuity of less than 1.5/60 (5/200). In Moore *et al.*'s (1987) series, of 16 intraocular airgun pellets, 11 eyes were enucleated, two were blind and no other eye had a vision better than counting fingers. Presumably these poor results reflect the large amount of force applied to the globe by these relatively blunt but heavy projectiles.

Anterior chamber

Most of these are easily removed. Small foreign bodies may fall into the anterior chamber angle under the influence of gravity. They may declare themselves by causing recurrent uveitis or localized corneal oedema. Gonioscopy is advised in the clinical examination of IOFB patients for medicolegal reports.

Lens

Foreign bodies in the crystalline lens may cause cataract necessitating their removal. They may, however, remain incarcerated there for many years without progressing.

Posterior segment

An IOFB in the ciliary body may be difficult to identify during surgery to remove it. An electric foreign body locator can be invaluable in this situation. IOFBs entering the vitreous may either stop there, where they are suspended in the gel, or may sink under the influence of gravity to lie on or about the inferior retina or pars plana. Those with more momentum strike the posterior pole, occasionally passing out of the eye, as in a double perforating injury. Double perforating injuries have a poorer prognosis.

Other IOFBs strike the posterior pole and then either drop down on to the inferior retina or ricochet across the eye. In general terms, the initial point of impact on the retina causes a break, but the amount of reaction renders detachment due to that break very unusual indeed. Field defects due to disruption of the nerve fibre layer at this point of impact can be charted and may be extensive. In these patients, this parameter of visual performance should always be presented in a medicolegal report.

Most retinal detachments in IOFB injuries result from anterior tractional breaks, as seen in penetrating injuries without IOFB.

Siderosis

An iron-containing foreign body within the eye is slowly absorbed, causing deposition of iron around the foreign body (direct siderosis), or the iron is disseminated through the eye (indirect siderosis) (Duke-Elder and McFaul, 1972d). Siderosis has been reported to occur within 18 days of injury (Davidson, 1933) but may not appear for several years (Duke-Elder and McFaul, 1972d). The pathological changes involved in the generalized condition consist of the deposition of ferritin throughout the cytoplasm of cells, with accumulations in siderosomes. This damages the lysosomes, enzymes leak and cells degenerate (Tawara, 1986). There is a tendency for there to be more ferritin in the posterior segment in posterior segment IOFBs. Likewise, there is more ferritin in the anterior chamber structures in anterior IOFBs. Clinically, generalized siderosis is manifested by iris heterochromia and mydriasis, glaucoma, cataract and retinal degeneration. Some cases, in which the IOFB is very small, resolve spontaneously (Duke-Elder and McFaul, 1972a).

The electroretinogram was first shown to be a sensitive indicator of siderosis by Karpe (1948). The first change is an increase in the size of the 'a' wave. The 'b' wave then diminishes. Knave (1969), using Karpe's division of the 'b' wave into three stages, identified that, once stage II has been reached, the prognosis becomes very poor (for further information on electrodiagnostic tests in ocular metallosis, see Galloway, 1981). If an IOFB is left in the eye, serial electroretinography is necessary to detect the onset of siderosis. Knave (1969) found that the onset of electroretinographic evidence of siderosis, in the presence of an iron-containing particle, averaged one month.

Sneed and Weingeist (1990) reported the management of 14 patients with an IOFB with siderosis. The foreign body was extracted in 12 patients and cataract was extracted in 11. The final acuity was better than 6/12 (20/40) in all these patients, indicating that excellent visual results can be attained with modern management, even in established siderosis bulbi.

Sympathetic ophthalmitis

General considerations

Sympathetic ophthalmitis is a granulomatous uveitis occurring in both eyes following an accidental or surgical insult to one eye. It is said to occur in 2 of 1000 perforating injuries and after 1 in 100 000 intraocular operations (Liddy and Stuart, 1972). The insult is almost always a perforating injury (eyes with blunt trauma have been found to have a globe rupture), or intraocular operation, although one case following cyclocryotherapy has been reported by Sabates (1988). In the overwhelming majority of accidental or surgical injuries there has been incarceration of, or injury to, uveal tissue.

The condition is characterized clinically by the onset of granulomatous uveitis in the injured (exciting) eye with 'mutton fat' keratic precipitates, to be followed not long after by uveitis in the uninjured (sympathizing) eye. In the posterior segment, this takes the form of whitish retinal pigment epithelial lesions (Dalen–Fuchs nodules). There may be disc oedema.

Treatment

At this stage, treatment commences to save the sympathizing eye, usually with topical and systemic steroids. Hakin *et al.* (1992) reported on 18 patients treated with steroids, and, in some instances, other immunosuppressant agents such as azathioprine or cyclosporin. The results in their series were good, with 10 of 18 patients retaining 6/9 acuity or better, and only one patient having less than 6/60. The use of topical and systemic steroids and the inflammation itself leads to complications such as glaucoma and cataract. In Hakin's series, seven patients required cataract extraction and six developed a raised intraocular pressure. Mackley and Azar (1978), in a study of 17 patients whose follow-up averaged 10.6 years, found that 47% developed cataract and 43% glaucoma. Cataract extraction may be successful (Hakin *et al.*, 1992). Reynard and Minkler (1983) described six patients with sympathetic ophthalmitis who underwent cataract surgery and found that all the eyes developed mild or severe postoperative uveitis and that three patients retained perception of light vision only.

Prevention

The onset of sympathetic ophthalmitis has been observed to occur between five days and 66 years after injury (Lubin *et al.*, 1980). The same authors observed that the onset in 65% of patients was between two weeks and three months, and 90% occured within one year. It is generally stated that enucleation of the injured eye within two weeks of injury confers protection from sympathetic ophthalmitis.

McClellan *et al.* (1987) described patients with very late onset sympathetic ophthalmitis (11 years, 38 years and 62 years). In the first two patients, further surgery had been carried out on the exciting eye respectively seven years and five days earlier. The authors pointed out the possible dangers of

secondary surgical intervention in injured eyes many years after the injury. The risks of surgical intervention had been noted previously by Lewis *et al.* (1978) with reference to vitrectomy surgery, which is now commonly employed in attempts to salvage eyes that previously may have been enucleated or at least have had only one operation to effect an initial repair.

There is considerable controversy about whether enucleation of the exciting eye should be performed once sympathetic ophthalmitis is established. Lubin *et al.* (1980) found that enucleation of the exciting eye within two weeks of the onset of sympathetic ophthalmia was beneficial to the clinical course of the sympathizing eye. A much earlier study by Winter (1955) found enucleation conferred no such advantage.

Prevention and protection

The decrease in hospital admissions due to industrial ocular accidents has probably resulted from safer processes and the introduction of ocular protection. In the United Kingdom, the Factories Act 1961, the Health and Safety at Work Act 1974, and the Protection of Eyes Regulations 1974, require employers to provide eye protectors, shields or fixed shields which conform to all the requirements of the certificates of approval. A useful booklet on the law and ocular protection is published by the Royal Society for the Prevention of Accidents (Rousell, 1979) and the British Standards Institution (1988) has published a guide for selection, use and maintenance of eye protection for industrial and other uses. Despite the regulations, companies do not necessarily supply protective eyeware or may supply the wrong type for the industrial process being undertaken.

Watts (1988) found that, despite workers wearing protection of the correct type, it may nevertheless be ineffective. Alternatively, the operative may fail to wear the protection provided by the employer (Dannenberg *et al.*, 1992a; MacEwen, 1989). Clearly, a detailed history of the provision and wearing of eye protection must be taken in every industrial accident. It is often helpful to obtain for inspection the protection supplied or worn at the time of the accident.

Jones (1988) found that, despite calls for increased eye protection in sports, many sportsmen decline to wear it, or state that they know nothing of its availability. It seems that mandatory facial protection, such as for ice hockey players in some regions of the USA, may be the best way forward (Shein *et al.*, 1988). Certainly, the compulsory wearing of seatbelts in the United Kingdom has dramatically reduced the number of serious eye injuries in motor accidents (Cole *et al.*, 1987; Vernon and Yorston, 1984). Careful enquiry should be made in such accidents about whether seatbelts were worn at the time. Similarly, in sporting accidents, the history should elicit whether the individual knew of the existence of protective eyeware, since such knowledge could reduce the liability of the injuring party if none was worn.

Suggested further reading

Duke-Elder S, editor. (1972) *System of ophthalmology.* Injuries: vol 14, parts I, II. London: Kimpton.

Eagling EM, Roper-Hall MJ. (1986) *Eye injuries.* London: Butterworth.

Shingleton BS, Hersch PS, Kenyon KR. (1991) *Eye trauma.* St Louis: Mosby.

References

Adams CBT. (1971) The retinal manifestations of fat embolism. *Injury* 2: 221–24.

Alexander MM, MacLeod JDA, Hall NF, Elkington AR. (1991) More than meets the eye: a study of the time lost from work by patients who incurred injuries from corneal foreign bodies. *Br J Ophthalmol* 75: 740–42.

Alper MG. (1963) Contusion angle deformity and glaucoma: gonioscopic observations and clinical course. *Arch Ophthalmol* 69: 455–67.

Aquavella JV, Rao GN, Brown AC, Harris JK. (1982) Keratoprosthesis: results, complications and management. *Ophthalmology* 89: 655–60.

Archer DB. (1986) Traumatic retinal vasculopathy. *Trans Ophthalmol Soc UK* 105: 361–84.

Archer DB, Canavan YM. (1983) Contusional Injuries of the Eye: Retinal and Choroidal Lesions. *Aust J Ophthalmol* 11: 251–64.

Archer DB, Earley OE, Page AB, Johnston PB. (1988) Traumatic retinal angiopathy – associated with wearing of car seat belts. *Eye* 2: 650–59.

Ballen PH. (1963) Mucous membrane grafts in chemical (lye) burns. *Am J Ophthalmol* 55: 302–12.

Barr CC. (1983) Prognostic factors in corneoscleral lacerations. *Arch Ophthalmol* 101: 919–24.

Beckinsale AB, Rosenthal AR. (1983) Early fundus fluorescein angiographic findings and sequelae in traumatic retionpathy: case report. *Br J Ophthalmol* 67: 119–23.

Billington BM, Leaver PK. (1986) Vitrectomy and fluid/silicone oil exchange for giant retinal tears: results at 18 months. *Graefes Arch Clin Exp Ophthalmol* 224: 7–10.

Blanton FM. (1964) Anterior chamber angle recession and secondary glaucoma. *Arch Ophthalmol* 72: 39–43.

Boukes RJ, Bruynzeel DP. (1985) Ocular findings in 340 long-term treated PUVA patients. *Photodermatology* 2: 178–80.

British Standard 7028. (1988) Guide for selection, use and maintenance of eye protection for industrial and other uses.: British Standards Institution.

Brittain GPH. (1988) Retinal burns caused by exposure to MIG-welding arcs: report of two cases. *Br J Ophthalmol* 72: 570–75.

Burke JP, Orton HP, West J, *et al.* (1992) Whiplash and its effect on the visual system. *Graefes Arch Clin Exp Ophthalmol* 230: 335–39.

Buxton JN, Norden RA, (1986) Adult penetrating keratoplasty: indications and contra-indications. In: Brightbill FS, editor. Corneal surgery, theory technique and tissue. St Louis: Mosby, 129.

Cardona H. (1983) Prosthokeratoplasty. *Cornea* 2: 179.

Carter JB, Park DW. (1987) Unusual retinal tears in an amateur boxer. *Arch Ophthalmol* 105: 1138.

Chuang EL, Miller FS, Kalina RE. (1985) Retinal lesions following long bone fractures. *Ophthalmology* 92: 370–74.

Cleary PE, Ryan SJ. (1979a) Experimental posterior penetrating eye injury in the rabbit. I: Method of production and natural history. *Br J Ophthalmol* 63: 306–11.

Cleary PE, Ryan SJ. (1979b) Experimental posterior penetrating eye injury in the rabbit. II: Histology of wound, vitreous and retina. *Br J Ophthalmol* 63: 312–21.

Cleary PE, Ryan SJ. (1979c) Method of production and natural history of experimental posterior penetrating eye injury in the rhesus monkey. *Am J Ophthalmol* 88: 210–20.

Cole MD, Clearkin L, Dabbs T, Smerdon D. (1987) The seatbelt law and after. *Br J Ophthalmol* 71: 436–40.

Cooling RJ. (1986) Traumatic retinal detachment: mechanisms and management. *Trans Ophthalmol Soc UK* 105: 575–79.

Cox MS, Schepens CL, Freeman HM. (1966) Retinal detachment due to ocular contusion. *Arch Ophthalmol* 76: 678–85.

Creighton MO, Larsen LE, Stewart-Dehaan PJ, *et al.* (1987) *In vitro* studies of microwave induced cataract II. Comparisons of damage observed for continuous wave and pulsed microwaves. *Exp Eye Res* 45: 357–73.

Daily L. (1970a) Macular and vitreal disturbances produced by traumatic vitreous rebound. *South Med J* 63: 1192–98.

Daily L. (1970b) Foveolar splinter and macular wisps. *Arch Ophthalmol* 83: 406–11.

Daily L. (1973) Further observations on foveolar splinter and macular wisps. *Arch Ophthalmol* 90: 102–103.

Daily L. (1979) Whiplash injury as one cause of the foveolar splinter and macular wisp. *Arch Ophthalmol* 97: 360.

Dannenberg AL, Parver LM, Brechner RJ, Khoo L. (1992a) Penetrating eye injuries in the workplace. The National Eye Trauma System Registry. *Ophthalmology* 110: 843–48.

Dannenberg AL, Parver LM, Fowler CJ, (1992b) Penetrating eye injuries related to assault. The National Eye Trauma System Registry. *Arch Ophthalmol* 110: 849–52.

Davidson M. (1933) Siderosis bulbi. *Am J Ophthalmol* 16: 331–35.

De Juan E, Sternberg P, Michaels RG. (1983) Penetrating ocular injuries. Types of injury and visual results. *Ophthalmology* 90: 1318–22.

Delori F, Pomerantzeff O, Cox MS. (1969) Deformation of the globe under high speed impact: its relation to contusion injuries. *Invest Ophthalmol* **8**: 290–301.

Demeler U. (1988) Surgical management of ocular hypotony. *Eye* **2**: 77–79.

Duane TD. (1973) Valsalva haemorrhagic retinopathy. *Am J Ophthalmol* **75**: 637–42.

Duke-Elder S, Abrams D. (1970) Ophthalmic optics and refraction. In: Duke-Elder S, editor. *System of ophthalmology*, vol. 5. London: Kimpton, 487–501.

Duke-Elder S, Abrams D. (1978) *Duke-Elder's practice of refraction*, 9th edition. Edinburgh: Churchill Livingstone, 105.

Duke-Elder S, MacFaul PA. (1972a) The indirect ocular effects of remote injuries. In: Duke-Elder S, editor. *System of ophthalmology*, vol. 14, part 1. London: Kimpton, 716.

Duke-Elder S, MacFaul PA. (1972b) Electrical injuries. In: Duke-Elder S, editor. *System of ophthalmology*, vol. 14, part 2. London: Kimpton, 813–35.

Duke-Elder S, MacFaul PA. (1972c) Chemical injuries. In: Duke-Elder S, editor. *System of ophthalmology*, vol. 14, part 2. London: Kimpton, 1043.

Duke-Elder S, MacFaul P. (1972d) Retained foreign bodies. In: Duke-Elder S, editor. *System of ophthalmology*, vol. 14, part 1. London: Kimpton, 525–44.

Eagling EM. (1976) Perforating injuries of the eye. *Br J Ophthalmol* **60**: 732–36.

Easam HA, Zimmerman LE. (1964) Sympathetic ophthalmia and bilateral phacoanaphylaxis. *Arch Ophthalmol* **72**: 9–15.

Emery AF, Kramar P, Guy A, Lin JC. (1975) Microwave induced temperature rises in rabbit eyes in cataract research. *Trans ASME J Heat Transfer* **97**: 123–28.

Friberg TR. (1979) Traumatic retinal pigment epithelial oedema. *Am J Ophthalmol* **88**: 18–21.

Fuller B, Gitter KA. (1973) Traumatic choroidal rupture with late serous detachment of the macula. *Arch Ophthalmol* **89**: 354–55.

Galloway NR. (1981) Ophthalmic electrodiagnosis, 2nd edition. London: Lloyd-Luke, 171–73.

Gass JDM. (1973) Choroidal neovascular membranes. Their visualisation and treatment. *Trans Am Acad Ophthalmol Otolaryngol* **77**: 310.

Gass JDM. (1987) *Stereoscopic atlas of macular diseases: diagnosis and treatment*, 3rd edition. St Louis: Mosby, 170.

Gitter KA, Slusher M, Justice J. (1968) Traumatic haemorrhagic detachment of retinal pigment epithelium. *Arch Ophthalmol* **79**: 729–32.

Goffstein R, Burton TC. (1982) Differentiating traumatic from non-traumatic retinal detachment. *Ophthalmology* **89**: 361–68.

Goodwin RT, Romano PE. (1985) Stereoacuity degradation by experimental and real monocular and binocular amblyopia. *Invest Ophthalmol Vis Sci* **26**: 917–23.

Gregor Z, Ryan SJ. (1982a). Combined posterior contusion and penetrating injury in the pig eye. I: A natural history study. *Br J Ophthalmol* **66**: 793–98.

Gregor Z, Ryan SJ. (1982b) Combined posterior contusion and penetrating injury in the pig eye. II: Histological features. *Br J Ophthalmol* **66**: 799–804.

Grey RHB. (1978) Foveo-macular retinitis, solar retinopathy and trauma. *Br J Ophthalmol* **62**: 543–46.

Gross JG, Freeman WR. (1990) Post traumatic yellow maculopathy. *Retina* **10**: 37–41.

Habib NE, Malik TY. (1994) Visual loss from bungee jumping. Lancet **343**: 487.

Hagler WS. (1980) Retinal dialysis: statistical and genetic study to determine pathogenic factors. *Trans Am Ophthalmol Soc* **78**: 686–733.

Hakin KN, Pearson RV, Lightman SL. (1992) Sympathetic ophthalmia: visual results with modern immunosupressive therapy. *Eye* **6**: 453–55.

Herschler J. (1977) Trabecular damage due to blunt anterior segment injury and its relationship to traumatic glaucoma. *Trans Am Acad Ophthalmol Otolaryngol* **83**: 239–48.

Hietanen MTK, Hoikkala MJ. (1990) Ultraviolet radiation and blue light from photofloods in television studios and theatres. *Health Phys* **59**: 193–98.

Hoare GW. (1970) Traumatic retinal angiopathy resulting from chest compression by safety belt. *Br J Ophthalmol* **54**: 667–69.

Hutton WL, Fuller DG. (1984) Factors influencing final visual outcome in severely injured eyes. *Am J Ophthalmol* **97**: 715–22.

Hykin PG, Foss AE, Pavesio C, Dart JKG. (1994) The national history and management of recurrent corneal erosion: a prospective randomised trial. *Eye* **8**: 35–40.

Jarrett WH. (1967) Dislocation of the lens: a study of 166 hospitalised cases. *Arch Ophthalmol* **78**: 289–96.

Jones NP. (1988) One year of severe eye injuries in sport. *Eye* **2**: 484–87.

Jones NP, Griffith GAP. (1992) Eye injuries at work: a prospective population based survey within the chemical industry. *Eye* **6**: 381–85.

Joyner KH. (1989) Microwave cataract litigation: a case study. *Health Phys* **57**: 545–49.

Joyner KH, Bangay MJ. (1986) Exposure survey of civilian airport radar workers in Australia. *J Microwave Power* **21**: 209–19.

Karpe G. (1948) Early diagnosis of siderosis retinae by the use of electroretinography. *Doc Ophthalmol* **2**: 277–96.

Kaufman JH, Tolpin DW. (1974) Glaucoma after traumatic angle recession: a ten year prospective study. *Am J Ophthalmol* **78**: 648–54.

Kelly JS. (1972) Purtscher's retinopathy related to chest compression by safety belts. Fluorescein angiographic findings. *Am J Ophthalmol* **74**: 278–83.

Kelly JS, Hoover RE, George T. (1978) Whiplash maculopathy. *Arch Ophthalmol* **96**: 834–35.

Kirkness CM, Weale RA. (1985) Does light pose a hazard to the macula in aphakia? *Trans Ophthalmol Soc UK* **104**: 699–702.

Klopfer J, Tielsch JM, Vitale S, See LC, Canner JK. (1992) Ocular trauma in the United States. Eye injuries resulting in hospitalisation, 1984 through 1987. *Arch Ophthalmol* **110**: 838–42.

Knave B. (1969) Electroretinography in eyes with retained intraocular metallic foreign bodies. A clinical study. *Acta Ophthalmol Suppl* **100**: 1–66.

Leads from the MMWR. (1984) Leading work related diseases and injuries: United States. *JAMA* **251**: 2503–504.

Leaver PK, Cooling RJ, Feretis EB, Lean JS, McLeod D. (1984) Vitrectomy and fluid/silicone oil exchange for giant retinal tears: results at 6 months. *Br J Ophthalmol* **68**: 432–38.

Levin LA, Seddon JM, Topping T. (1991) Retinal pigment epithelial tears associated with trauma. *Am J Ophthalmol* **112**: 396–400.

Levy NS, Glick EB. (1974) Stereoscopic perception and Snellen visual acuity. *Am J Ophthalmol* **78**: 722–24.

Lewis ML, Gass JDM, Spencer WH. (1978) Sympathetic uveitis after trauma and vitrectomy. *Arch Ophthalmol* **96**: 263–67.

Liddy MB, Stuart J. (1972) Sympathetic ophthalmia in Canada. *Can J Ophthalmol* **7**: 157–59.

Lubin JR, Albert DM, Weinstein M. (1980) Sixty five years of sympathetic ophthalmia: a clinicopathologic review of 105 cases (1913–1978). *Ophthalmology* **87**: 109–21.

Maberley AL, Carvounis EP. (1977) The visual field in indirect traumatic rupture of the choroid. *Can J Ophthalmol* **12**: 147–52.

MacEwen CJ. (1989) Eye injuries: a prospective survey of 5671 cases. *Br J Ophthalmol* **73**: 888–94.

Mackley TA, Azar A. (1978) Sympathetic ophthalmia: a long term follow-up. *Arch Ophthalmol* **96**: 257–62.

Mainster MA, Ham WT, Delori FC. (1983) Potential retinal hazards. Instrument and environmental light sources. *Ophthalmology* **90**: 927–32.

McClellan KA, Billson FA, Filipic M. (1987) Delayed onset sympathetic ophthalmia. *Med J Aust* **147**: 451–54.

McDonald HR, Irvine AR. (1983) Light induced maculopathy from the operating microscope in extracapsular cataract extraction and intraocular lens implantation. *Ophthalmology* **90**: 945–51.

Moore AT, McCartney A, Cooling RJ. (1987) Ocular injuries associated with the use of airguns. *Eye* **1**: 422–29.

Morgan KS, McDonald MB, Hiles DA, *et al.* (1987) The nationwide study of epikeratophakia for aphakia in children. *Am J Ophthalmol* **103**: 366–74.

Narda R, Magnavita N, Sacco A, *et al.* (1990) Chronic conjunctivitis in arc welders. *Med La* **81**: 399–406.

National Society to Prevent Blindness. *Fact Sheet (1980)*. New York: National Society to Prevent Blindness, 1980.

Norn M, Franch C. (1991) Long term changes in the outer part of the eye in welders. Prevalence of spheroid degeneration, pingueculae, pterygium and corneal cicatrices. *Acta Ophthalmol* **69**: 382–86.

Percival SPB. (1972) A decade of intraocular foreign bodies. *Br J Ophthalmol* **56**: 454–61.

Pruett RC, Weiter JJ, Goldstein RB. (1987) Myopic cracks, angioid streaks, and traumatic tears in bruch's membrane. *Am J Ophthalmol* **103**: 537–43.

Purtscher O. (1910) Noch unbekannte Befunde nach Schadel-trauma. *Ber Versamml Dtsch Ophthalmol* **13**: 1295–99.

Reynard M, Minkler DS (1983) Cataract extraction in the sympathetic eye. *Arch Ophthalmol* **101**: 1701–703.

Rodman HI (1963) Chronic open angle glaucoma associated with traumatic dislocation of the lens. *Arch Ophthalmol* **69**: 445–54.

Roper-Hall MJ. (1954) Review of 555 cases of intraocular foreign body with special reference to prognosis. *Br J Ophthalmol* **38**: 65–99.

Roper-Hall MJ. (1965) Thermal and chemical burns. *Trans Ophthalmol Soc UK* **85**: 631–53.

Rosenbaum JJ, Tammaro J, Robertson JE. (1991) Uveitis precipitated by non-penetrating ocular trauma. *Am J Ophthalmol* **112**: 392–95.

Ross WH. (1981) Traumatic retinal dialysis. *Arch Ophthalmol* **99**: 1371–74.

Ross WH. (1991) Retinal dialysis: lack of evidence for a genetic cause. *Can J Ophthalmol* **26**: 309–12.

Rousell DF. (1979) *Eye protection*. Birmingham: Royal Society for Prevention of Accidents.

Sabates R. (1988) Choroiditis compatible with the histopathological diagnosis of sympathetic ophthalmia following cyclocryotherapy of neovascular glaucoma. *Ophthal Surg* **19**: 176–82.

Scott JA. (1988) The computation of temperature rises in the human eye induced by infrared radiation. *Phys Med Biol* **33**: 243–57.

Shein OD, Hibberd PL, Shingleton BJ, *et al.* (1988) The spectrum and burden of ocular injury. *Ophthamology* **95**: 300–305.

Shock JP, Adams D. (1985) Longterm visual acuity results after penetrating and perforating ocular injuries. *Am J Ophthalmol* **100**: 714–18.

Slingsby JG, Forstot SL. (1981) Effect of blunt trauma on the corneal endothelium. *Arch Ophthalmol* **99**: 1041–43.

Smiddy WE, Hamburg TR, Kracher GP, Gottsch JD, Stark WJ. (1989) Contact lenses for visual rehabiliation after corneal laceration repair. *Ophthalmology* **96**: 293–98.

Smith RE, Kelly JS, Harbin TS. (1974) Late macular complications of choroidal ruptures. *Am J Ophthalmol* **77**: 650–58.

Sneed SR, Weingeist TA. (1990) Managements of siderosis bulbi due to a retained iron-containing foreign body. *Ophthalmology* **97**: 375–79.

Spaeth GL. (1967) Traumatic hyphaema, angle recession, dexamethasone hypertension and glaucoma. *Arch Ophthalmol* **78**: 714–21.

Sternberg PL, De Juan E, Michaels RG, Auer C. (1984) Multivariate analysis of prognostic factors in penetrating ocular injuries. *Am J Ophthalmol* **98**: 467–72.

Tawara A. (1986) Transformation and cytotoxicity of iron in siderosis bulbi. *Invest Ophthalmol Vis Sci* **27**: 226–36.

Taylor HR, West SK, Rosenthal FS, Munoz B, Newland HS, Emmett EA. (1989) Corneal changes associated with chronic UV irradiation. *Arch Ophthalmol* **107**: 1481–84.

Tesluck GC, Spaeth GL. (1985) The occurrence of primary open angle glaucoma in the fellow eye of patients with unilateral angle cleavage glaucoma. *Ophthalmology* **92**: 904–11.

Thomas JET, Ayyar DR. (1972) Systemic fat embolism. A diagnostic profile in 24 patients. *Arch Neurol* **26**: 517–23.

Thomas MA, Parrish RK, Feuer WJ. (1986) Rebleeding after traumatic hyphaema. *Arch Ophthalmol* **104**: 206–10.

Tönjun AM. (1966) Gonioscopy in traumatic hyphaema. *Acta Ophthalmol* **44**: 650.

Tönjun AM. (1968) Intraocular pressure and facility of outflow late after ocular contusion. *Acta Ophthalmol* **46**: 886–908.

Van Johnson E, Kline LB, Skalka HW. (1987) Electrical cataracts: a case report and review of the literature. *Ophthal Surg* **18**: 283–85.

Vernon SA, Yorston DB. (1984) Incidence of ocular injuries from road traffic accidents after introduction of seatbelt legislation. *J R Soc Med* **77**: 198–200.

Wainwright PR, Whillock MJ. (1990) Measurement and mathematical models in the assessment of optical radiation hazards to the eye. *J Radiol Prot* **10**: 263–69.

Watts MT. (1988) A study into the effectiveness of varying forms of eye protection. *J Soc Occup Med* **38**: 98–100.

Weene LE. (1985) Recurrent corneal erosion after trauma: a statistical study. *Ann Ophthalmol* **17**: 521–24.

Williams DF, Mieler WF, Abrams GW, Lewis H. (1988) Results and prognostic factors in penetrating ocular injuries with retained intraocular foreign bodies. *Ophthalmology* **95**: 911–16.

Winter FC. (1955) Sympathetic uveitis: a clinical and pathological study of the visual result. *Am J Ophthalmol* **39**: 340–47.

Wolf SM, Zimmerman LE. (1962) Chronic secondary glaucoma associated with retrodisplacement of iris root and deepening of the anterior chamber angle secondary to contusion. *Am J Ophthalmol* **54**: 547–63.

Wood CM, Richardson J. (1990) Indirect choroidal ruptures: aetiological factors, patterns of ocular damage and final visual outcome. *Br J Ophthalmol* **74**: 208–11.

Zyon VM, Burton TC. (1980) Retinal dialysis. *Arch Ophthalmol* **98**: 1971–74.

21

Injury to the lids and orbital contents: post-traumatic enophthalmos and diplopia

Geoffrey E Rose, John P Lee

Introduction

The eyelids and orbit can be affected by head and facial trauma in several ways: the tissues may be damaged by laceration (either directly or through disruption of the orbital bones), by contusional injury, or by the spread of soft tissue infections. The effect of injury on the physiological function of the eyelids and orbital structures (and, indirectly, on visual function) is largely dependent upon the degree of damage to mobile structures within the eyelids and orbit, whereas cosmesis is dependent also upon the extent of damage to static structures, such as the orbital rim and walls.

Injury to the eyelids

Injury to the lids is generally by direct sharp laceration or by tearing as a result of shearing forces; such tears typically occur at the medial end of the lid (the weakest point) and are often associated with canalicular laceration.

Clinical assessment of eyelid injury

Early assessment

After ocular adnexal injury, it is most important first to determine the potential vision and whether the globe is intact. With extensive lid injury and swelling the lids may be unopenable, and it may be possible only to ascertain whether perception of light is present. Repair of a ruptured globe takes priority, because the manipulation for repair of the eyelids or lacrimal drainage system may further injure a hypotonic globe.

A plain radiograph at soft tissue density may be valuable when an intraorbital foreign body is suspected. This can be supplemented by thin-section CT scan if necessary. Magnetic resonance imaging is indicated later if intraorbital wood is suspected, but the presence of ferromagnetic materials must be excluded. An early CT scan, without preceding plain films, is advisable where orbital fracture or significant head injury has occurred.

At both the initial and late assessment of periocular injury, the position and extent of lacerations should be recorded, with particular reference to involvement of the lid margins or the lacrimal drainage canaliculae. Tissues are often displaced immediately after adnexal injury and may give the appearance of tissue loss. It is important that no tissue should be sacrificed at the time of repair, as it is most unusual for significant necrosis to occur in these structures.

Late assessment

The amount of lid movement, closure and degree of corneal protection should be recorded immediately after injury, after repair, and in the late assessment of such injuries. The corneal protection afforded by the lids is also influenced by the contour and application of the eyelid margin on the globe, the state of the strength of Bell's phenomenon (an involuntary deviation of the eyes, generally upwards, with lid closure) and by the range of ocular movements. These should be gauged at later examination, together with any lack of eyelid closure (lagophthalmos), both on gentle and on forced closure.

If lagophthalmos is present, or if symptoms (such as grittiness or intermittent sharp pain) are suggestive of corneal exposure, then the cornea should be examined in detail for evidence of epithelial exposure, vascularization or inflammation.

Lacrimal drainage is best assessed by the rate of clearance of a marker from the tear line, and by its recovery from the nose. A tiny portion of a drop of 2% fluorescein solution should be applied by capillary action to the posterior margin of the lower eyelid and clearance of this nonirritant solution noted after five minutes. A difference between the two sides or marked persistence of dye at this time, especially if there is an increased tear line on the affected side, is good evidence of delayed tear clearance. Dye recovery from the nose may be accomplished by asking the patient to blow the nose into a clean tissue or by placing a moist cotton bud at the nasolacrimal duct opening under the inferior turbinate. The results for nasal dye recovery are poorly reproducible and, whereas the test is helpful when recovery is positive, it is not conclusive if recovery fails.

Management of eyelid injury

Early management

The management of ocular adnexal injuries takes second place to that of major head or systemic injury and generally does not warrant emergency surgery. Early treatment with antibiotics and tetanus prophylaxis should be considered and the ocular safety maintained with topical lubricants and moisture chambers. Pressure dressings or eye pads should be avoided.

The acute treatment of eyelid injuries (after repair of any rupture of the globe) is aimed at protecting the eye, but is often limited by extensive swelling and bruising. Such repair involves approximation of torn conjunctiva, reconnection of a disinserted levator muscle (if recognizable), alignment and suturing of the lid margin or canthi, and, finally, closure of skin lacerations.

If both eyelids are missing, the primary repair should be aimed at closing conjunctival remnants over the cornea and placement of a split thickness skin graft on to this surface. A later cautious opening of this ocular cover may be attempted.

Repair of the lid margin, if medial to the lacrimal puncta, may require canalicular repair.

Many methods have been described, some of which present a significant hazard to intact parts of the lacrimal drainage system. It is extremely important, therefore, that canalicular repair does not jeopardize undamaged lacrimal tissues, especially the partner canaliculus or the common canaliculus. A single intact canaliculus is sufficient to provide baseline tear drainage and will often cope with reflex tearing. Repaired canaliculi tend to be of limited function and better lacrimal drainage may be achieved if the distal canalicular remnant is united with the conjunctival sac, rather than attempting an unreliable and time consuming canalicular anastomosis.

Late management

Late reconstructive surgery is frequently required, as complete primary repair may be impossible if tissue displacement, bruising or swelling prevents the accurate identification or apposition of tissues. Late deformities which often necessitate repair include notches of the lid margin (Figure 21.1), residual ptosis (Figure 21.2) and lacrimal obstruction with medial canthal injuries (Figures 21.1 and 21.3).

Misalignment or notches of the eyelid margin may be repaired by opening or excision of the defect and accurate repair. Transposition flaps or free grafts may be required where there has been a significant loss of tissue.

Aberrant or misdirected lashes cause irritation through abrasion of the cornea and present a significant risk of infection. Where the misdirected lashes are few, they can be treated conveniently by electrolysis or cryotherapy. If related to a notch,

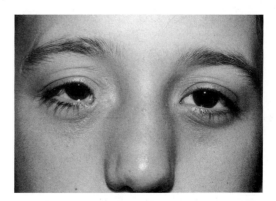

Figure 21.1. Medial canthal dystopia, inner canthal rounding, lower lid notch and lacrimal drainage obstruction occurring after a childhood dog bite.

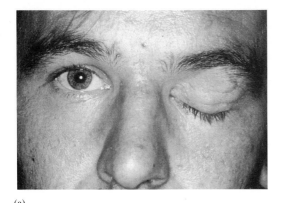

(a)

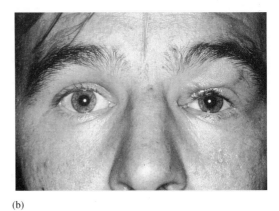

(b)

Figure 21.2. (**a**) Complete ptosis due to disinsertion of the levator muscle during avulsion of the upper eyelid. (2) (**b**) The lid position and cosmesis are improved after repair of the disinsertion, but eyelid movement is still impaired.

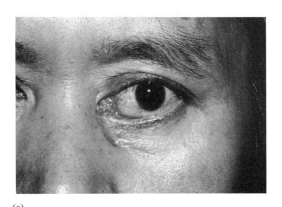

(a)

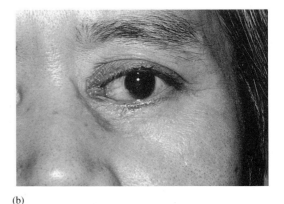

(b)

Figure 21.3. (**a**) Cicatricial ectropion after medial canthal injury. (**b**) The lid position has been improved somewhat by posterosuperior fixation of the lower tarsus and skin grafting performed during lacrimal drainage surgery.

they may be excised during the secondary repair of the notch. More extensive misdirection of the lashes is best treated as for the surgical correction of entropion.

Canthal malposition, or dystopia, may occur with midfacial fractures and may necessitate late correction (Figures 21.3 and 21.4a). Lacrimal drainage surgery provides an opportune time to repair medial canthal dystopia, although the results may be limited by fibrosis, especially in the concavity of the inner canthus (Figure 21.3b).

Epiphora (watering) after adnexal injury may result from many causes, which commonly include lid malposition (with spillover of tears), lagophthalmos (with corneal exposure and reflex lacrimation), canalicular stenosis after laceration, and nasolacrimal duct occlusion after midfacial fractures. Epiphora can almost always be cured or improved by lacrimal or oculoplastic surgery. Some such patients require placement of a canalicular bypass tube (Figure 21.4b).

Outcome after eyelid injury

The eyelids protect the globe and, together with lacrimal drainage, help to maintain the smooth corneal surface required for good visual function. They also have a prominent role in cosmesis and the psychology of interpersonal relations.

Functional effects of eyelid injury

Injury or loss of the lid margin is liable to distortion of lid contour and misdirection of the lashes, with accompanying chronic ocular

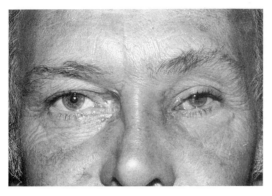

(a)

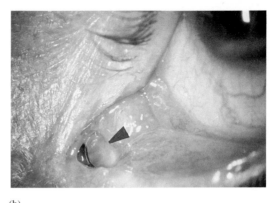

(b)

Figure 21.4. (**a**) Persistent medial canthal dystopia after major injury. (**b**) A glass Lester Jones canalicular bypass tube (arrow) is present at the inner canthus.

discomfort. Reduced lid closure, movement or blinking causes accumulation of tear film debris and corneal epithelial irregularity. Both of these impair vision. Likewise, abnormal lacrimal drainage affects vision, particularly in bright light or with night-time driving, and predisposes to secondary ocular infection.

The visual field may be significantly restricted where the palpebral aperture is reduced by ptosis or canthal rounding. This often causes functional difficulty at the extremes of gaze, as when driving a vehicle in reverse or when crossing a road.

All changes affecting the ocular surface or tear film carry a particular hazard in the presence of reduced ocular motility or an anaesthetic (neurotrophic) cornea. In such circumstances there is a great risk of infective keratitis and endophthalmitis, with possible blindness or loss of the eye.

Cosmetic deformity after eyelid injury

With no loss of periocular tissues and an accurate repair, there may be almost no visible scarring; the only noticeable cosmetic deficit may be an alteration of ocular closure or blink frequency. Full thickness periocular injuries, especially those parallel to the lid margin, may cause gross tissue oedema that can persist for a particularly long time.

A persistent cosmetic deformity is inevitable where loss of lid margin has occurred. The deformity typically constitutes a smaller palpebral aperture, rounded canthi, inadequate lashes and reduced movement of the eyelid.

Where primary or secondary eyelid repair has necessitated the replacement or transposition of skin, there generally follows a cosmetically noticeable blemish due to a contracture of transplanted tissues or a slight mismatch of the thickness and colour of the skin flaps. The reduced compliance of lids repaired with such grafts or flaps inevitably produces a cosmetically noticeable reduction in both voluntary movements and reflex blinking. This blemish is often highlighted by changes secondary to chronic exposure of the ocular surface: a chronically red eye, corneal opacities, or a marked accumulation of tear film debris.

Loss of the eyelashes or eyebrow hairs produces a cosmetic deformity that is poorly concealed by transplantation of hair-bearing tissues. Attempts to recreate lashes often result in misdirection of the false lashes, secondary corneal abrasions and chronic discomfort.

In addition to impairment of vision, reduced lacrimal drainage causes social embarrassment and

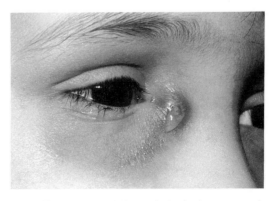

Figure 21.5. Cutaneous drainage of a lacrimal sac mucocoele arising after midfacial fracture.

occupational difficulties not only due to an overfull tear film, spillover onto the cheek with skin excoriation, and wetting of glasses, but also as a result of the discharge of infected material from a lacrimal sac mucocoele. A post-traumatic communication between the drainage system (typically the lacrimal sac) and the skin is generally associated with intermittent discharge of mucus or tears from an inflamed fistula (Figure 21.5).

Effect of eyelid injury on activities of daily living

Adnexal injury in which there is a residual functional deficit or cosmetic blemish inevitably has a significant effect upon the life of an individual. Treatment is generally protracted and may require multiple operations, with disruption of the patient's personal life and employment. Their personal and social interactions are affected permanently, and the ability to continue employment or the prospect for re-employment is generally reduced. The necessity for chronic ocular medication or long-term medical care may be inconvenient, expensive or embarrassing.

Injury to the orbit and post-traumatic enophthalmos

Injury to the orbital tissues presents a particular risk to optic nerve function, most commonly due to compression by inflammatory oedema or haematoma, but occasionally due to direct avulsion or severance of the nerve. Damage to the extraocular muscles or their innervation may cause a transient or permanent restriction of ocular ductions and, in binocular patients, diplopia. Likewise, damage to levator palpebrae or its nerve is associated with ptosis (Figure 21.2a).

Expansion of the orbital volume after a blow-out fracture of the orbital floor or medial wall is a common cause of post-traumatic enophthalmos, although it remains uncertain whether atrophy of fat and other soft tissues (Rootman and Neigel, 1988; Soll, 1982) contributes to this problem (Kronish *et al.*, 1990). The extent of post-traumatic enophthalmos may not become apparent for many months, until after the acute oedema has resolved.

Assessment of orbital soft-tissue injury

Early assessment

As with eyelid injury, assessment of the globe and potential visual function is of paramount importance after orbital injury. A compromise of optic nerve function may be present where visual acuity is reduced without adequate cause from other ocular injuries, such as corneal abrasions or retinal oedema. A relative afferent pupillary defect would be expected in unilateral cases. Marked restriction of eye movements and increased resistance of the intact globe to ballottement are generally seen with orbital oedema or haematoma sufficient to impair optic nerve function.

Late assessment

Enophthalmos is a posterior positioning of the globe relative to the other eye, although a difference of less than 2 mm may result from errors in the method of measurement (Jones *et al.*, 1986). Comparison with the normal eye allows for the natural variation

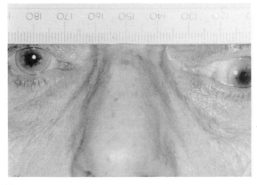
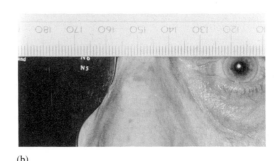

(a)   (b)

Figure 21.6. (**a**) Apparent inferolateral displacement of the left globe due to hypo-exotropia. (**b**) Cover testing, during fixation of the left eye, reveals the true position.

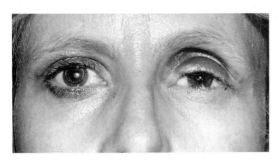

Figure 21.7. Patient with left postenucleation socket syndrome showing volume deficiency, ptosis and discharge from the socket.

in the prominence of the globes relative to periocular bony landmarks. The most commonly used of these is the lateral orbital rim. Lateral canthal displacement due to injury may complicate such measurements. Displacement of the globe, both vertically and horizontally, should be recorded and a cover test used during measurement if a manifest squint is present (Figure 21.6).

Orbital wall injury may be present if there is periorbital sensory loss, particularly in the territories of the infraorbital and zygomatic nerves. Abnormal ocular movement or a latent or manifest squint may follow orbital injury (see later section on motility disturbance).

Where there has been a great loss of orbital tissues, due to enucleation, evisceration or partial exenteration, the socket may display features of the 'postenucleation socket syndrome' (PESS). A grossly phthisical eye may also simulate this syndrome. The features of PESS due to volume deficiency are a sunken ('enophthalmic') look, a deep upper eyelid sulcus, ptosis, and backward tilting of any ocular prosthesis due to gravitation of

orbital tissues (Figure 21.7). An oversized prosthesis, often fitted to compensate for volume deficiency in the PESS, contributes to other characteristics. These are displacement and poor motility of the prosthesis; inadequate lid closure, causing chronic discomfort; entropion and adherence of the lashes to the prosthesis; giant papillary conjunctivitis with mucoid discharge; and lower eyelid laxity associated with instability of the artificial eye.

Ptosis after orbital soft tissue injury may result from volume deficiency (Figure 21.7), severance of the levator muscle (Figure 21.2a), or haematoma and secondary fibrosis within the muscle or its aponeurosis.

Management of orbital injury

Early management

The early treatment of orbital injury is similar to that for eyelid injury. In particular, systemic antibiotic therapy should be considered with all open injuries, including those with communication solely to the sinuses.

Where optic nerve compromise appears due to intraorbital haematoma, orbital imaging should be arranged prior to early exploration of the orbit. Very high dose systemic steroids, generally given with appropriate prophylaxis against gastric ulceration, may be of benefit when optic nerve impairment is due to diffuse orbital oedema or in cases of direct optic neuropathy. The value of optic canal decompression remains controversial (Goldberg, 1991; Warren and Kuppersmith, 1992).

The treatment of injuries to the orbital rim, walls and midface are discussed in other chapters. Displacement of the canthi is largely corrected during such corrective midfacial surgery.

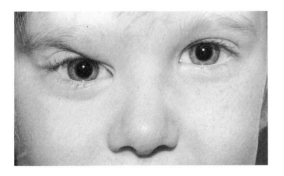

(a)

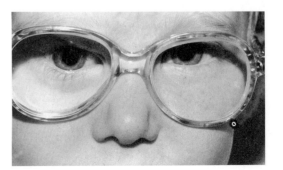

(b)

Figure 21.8. (**a**) A downward displacement of the right globe and orbit is camouflaged (**b**) by the use of a base-down prism in the right spectacle lens and a base-up prism in the left lens. (Photographs used with parental consent.)

Late management

Late rehabilitation after orbital injury is largely directed at improvement in canthal position, lacrimal reconstruction and the reduction of enophthalmos or other features of PESS.

In many patients, canthal position can be improved during lacrimal reconstruction (Figure 21.3) or with lateral canthal surgery. Where gross displacement of the canthi or palpebral aperture cannot be corrected, optical devices may be used to camouflage the problem (Figure 21.8).

Mild enophthalmos, often associated with a slight ptosis, may be camouflaged with appropriate spectacle correction (Figure 21.9) or by the use of a thin scleral shell. The shell may be clear if a

sighted eye is present, or painted if the underlying eye is disfigured.

For more marked enophthalmos, especially with a blow-out fracture and restriction of inferior rectus action, consideration should be given to exploration of the orbital floor and implantation of an appropriate material (Figure 21.10). The principal surgical risks (Hawes and Dortzbach, 1994), of worse motility and diplopia, visual loss, sensory loss to the cheek, and lower eyelid retraction, although small, should be explained to such patients. Where prior enucleation or evisceration has been performed, a secondary intraconal implant provides very effective enhancement of orbital 'tissue' volume. Extraconal dermis fat grafting may be considered if a deep upper lid

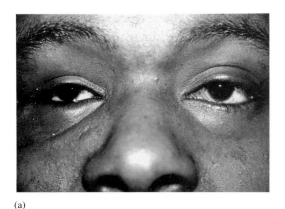

(a)

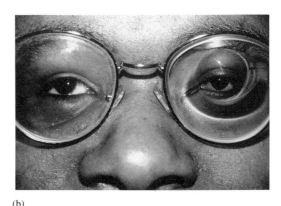

(b)

Figure 21.9. (**a**) The signs of right volume deficiency are lessened (**b**) by reducing, on the enucleated side, the 'balance' spherical correction required by this high myope.

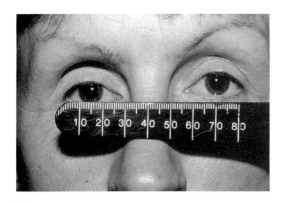

(a)

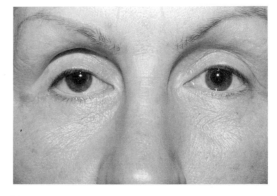

(b)

Figure 21.10. Right hypoglobus and upper eyelid sulcus deformity after orbital floor blow-out fracture, (**a**) before and (**b**) 12 days after repair through a subciliary incision.

sulcus persists after both intraconal ball implantation and orbital floor implantation.

After surgery for enhancement of orbital tissue volume, lateral canthal suspension may be used for correction of lower eyelid sagging, and a new prosthesis fitted (with accurate positioning of the iris and pupil). Finally, the upper lid position can be adjusted with anterior approach resection of the levator muscle/aponeurosis.

To camouflage differences between the two sides after performing all possible surgery on the injured side, consideration may be given to operating upon the uninjured side. Reduction upper lid blepharoplasty or retractor recession are particularly useful for hiding residual signs of volume deficiency or ptosis. The risks of such surgery on the uninjured side, although small, should be clearly explained to the patient.

Outcome after orbital injury

Injury to the orbital soft tissues is often associated with abnormalities of ocular balance or eye movements, with both functional and cosmetic consequences. More extensive damage, to orbital bones or with loss of the eye, produces a marked cosmetic blemish requiring a long-term psychological adaptation.

Functional effects of orbital injury

Ocular motility and binocular functions may be disturbed with orbital injury. Ptosis, due to reduced levator muscle action, is often observed. If binocular function is affected, this will significantly impair the patient in employment, home life and leisure activities (see following section on motility disturbance).

Changes in the position of the canthi tend to inhibit eyelid closure and tear flow across the ocular surface, leading to exposure keratopathy, reduced vision or epiphora.

Wearing a cosmetic shell or an artificial eye is frequently associated with an abnormal blink pattern, with incomplete lid closure or with chronic discharge from the socket, in some cases with discomfort. Wherever an ocular device is worn there is a greater risk of ocular surface infection and the inconvenience of its treatment. This risk extends to endophthalmitis and possible visual loss if a cosmetic shell is worn over a sighted eye.

Blow-out fractures and other injuries to the sinuses may affect air flow through the nose and predispose to recurrent sinusitis or orbital cellulitis. Materials implanted for the repair of such injuries may increase the long-term risk of infective complications (Mauriello *et al.*, 1994). Likewise, foreign materials implanted for the volume enhancement have a continued risk of exposure or extrusion, although this risk is extremely low with meticulous surgical technique (Woog *et al.*, 1994).

Cosmetic effects of orbital injury

Cosmetic deformity is always present after orbital injury. With relatively mild injury there may be visible changes in ocular balance and motility, or in the position and movement of the upper and lower eyelids.

Injuries to the orbital rim may be treated effectively with open reduction, internal fixation and osteoplastic techniques. However, treatment of displaced canthi is not so successful. Scar tissue formation, particularly at the concavity of the inner canthus, tends to draw the structure away from its ideal location, leaving a cosmetic blemish (Figures 21.3 and 21.4).

With adequate enhancement of orbital volume and lining, most of the static features of PESS can be largely hidden. However, volume enhancement may be associated with inadequate lid closure, inflammation of the socket mucosa and continued chronic discharge from the socket.

The extremes of movement of an ocular prosthesis are limited by the conjunctival fornices of a socket, the fornices being smallest where an eye has been removed. There is, therefore, always a marked limitation of 'eye' movements with either an artificial eye or a shell. This important cosmetic defect, and its psychological consequences, cannot be avoided.

Effect of orbital injury on activities of daily living

In the same way as eyelid injury, orbital injuries have a profound effect upon the daily lives of affected individuals. The presence of an ocular prosthesis adds further to the burden of facial injury. Any such device requires daily care and regular professional maintenance or replacement. This can be time consuming and expensive. Most patients are very aware of the abnormal appearance and movements of an artificial eye or shell, in particular, of limitations in the treatment of the static and dynamic aspects of the postenucleation socket syndrome.

Motility disturbance and diplopia after injury

The most common cause of diplopia following blunt head injury is cranial nerve palsy. Local trauma to the orbit may, however, cause motility disturbance in several ways. Individual extraocular muscles may be disinserted or ruptured; there may be intramuscular or intraorbital haemorrhage and oedema; the trochlear apparatus may be compromised; or the muscles or their fascial attachments may be trapped in orbital fracture sites.

Types, assessment and treatment of injuries affecting ocular motility

Disinsertion or rupture of an extraocular muscle

Such cases are rare and are due typically to a penetrating injury of the orbit with, for example, a broken drill bit, hook or other sharp-pointed instrument.

The initial assessment will demonstrate severe limitation of ocular rotation in one direction and may also show a stump of muscle still attached to the globe. Most avulsions occur in the belly of the muscle and not at the insertion on to the globe. The muscular injury can generally be shown on a CT scan or on MRI. This may be supplemented by MRI in different positions of gaze to further elucidate the site of the damage.

Such cases should be explored as soon as local swelling and oedema clear. The fascial attachments are often readily identifiable and provide a guide to localizing the proximal portion of the muscle towards the orbital apex. Reattachment, either of the two avulsed ends or of the sheath to the globe, is often successful in restoring reasonable anatomical function, but many such patients require later planned strabismus surgery to get the best ocular rotations.

Intramuscular or intraorbital haemorrhage and oedema

Direct or indirect orbital injury can be associated with extensive bruising and haemorrhage within the extraocular muscles. Bruising near the supraorbital fissure (Rootman and Neigel, 1988) has been demonstrated in many cases of fatal road traffic accidents and, under these circumstances, it is not surprising that there is often a disturbance of ocular motility. This generally resolves over a few weeks. The inferior rectus, because of its inferior and somewhat exposed position, is probably the most commonly affected muscle. A downgaze deficit following local orbital trauma, particularly that associated with fracture of the inferior rim or zygoma, is not unusual.

The best management of such patients is to await spontaneous improvement. During this phase, it may be of considerable value to ask patients to perform duction exercises: the patient is asked to keep the head still and to follow the tip of a pencil or a finger into the extremes of gaze, with instructions to move the eyes towards the position in which they may be showing a deficit of movement. There is a strong clinical impression that such activities are of value and they certainly represent something for the patient to do whilst awaiting spontaneous recovery. Some authorities have suggested the use of systemic steroids, but no controlled trial has been undertaken.

Damage to the trochlear apparatus

The trochlea is a complex structure in the superonasal angle of the orbit, through which the superior oblique tendon passes before bending posteriorly and temporally to insert into the superotemporal quadrant of the posterior part of the globe. Helveston (1982) has shown that the trochlea is a complex sliding joint with a number of tubular structures that move within one another (Figure 21.11). If damage occurs to the trochlea, there is no longer free movement of the tendon and the patient exhibits a post-traumatic acquired Brown's syndrome. Relaxation of the superior oblique tendon is impossible, and the eye is unable to move superonasally in normal ocular rotation. In severe cases, the patient must adopt a head posture of chin elevation and head tilt for ocular fixation.

Such cases were very common when seat belt wearing was not compulsory and the majority of car windscreens consisted of toughened glass. In a typical road traffic accident of that period, patients would be thrust forcefully on to the broken spikes of glass protruding from the bottom of the windscreen and present with multiple horizontal cuts around the face, particularly in the region of the eyes and in the brow area. In most cases of post-traumatic Brown's syndrome, pieces of windscreen glass would be found in the region of the trochlea. Although these may be readily removed, it is extraordinarily difficult to improve ocular

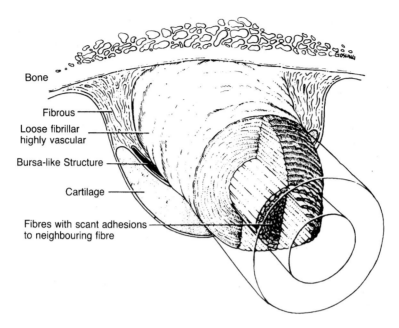

Bone

Fibrous

Loose fibrillar
highly vascular

Bursa-like Structure

Cartilage

Fibres with scant adhesions
to neighbouring fibre

Figure 21.11. Structure of the trochlea. (Reproduced from Helveston (1982).)

motility after this particular injury. It has been shown that there is only limited improvement in the field of single vision and most of these patients are left with a significant deficit of ocular movement (Aylward *et al.*, 1992). With the advent of laminated windscreens and compulsory seat belt wearing, such cases have become less common in recent years.

Muscle or fascial entrapment at the site of orbital fracture

With a blow-out fracture of either the floor or medial orbital wall, neighbouring orbital connective tissues may become prolapsed through and incarcerated into the fracture site. Initially, it may be hard to distinguish the motility disturbance after a blow-out fracture from that due to local oedema. The signs characteristic of blow-out fractures become apparent after a time. There is a limitation of movement, typically of elevation in floor fractures and abduction in those of the medial wall. This is associated with retraction of the globe on attempted movement in these directions, and sometimes with elevation of intraocular pressure. Overaction of the synergistic muscles of the other eye may be seen.

Management of orbital blow-out fractures

The management of these fractures remains controversial (Manson and Iliff, 1991; Putterman, 1991). Some advocate surgical intervention within 14 days of injury, with exposure of the fracture site, release of the prolapsed orbital tissues and repair of the fracture using a variety of materials. Silicone rubber, bone grafts, lyophilized cartilage and other materials have been used for this purpose. The orbital floor may be explored through a lid incision, where the fracture is approached from above and tissue freed. Alternatively, using a Caldwell–Luc approach through the maxillary antrum, the fracture is opened, tissues reduced from below and the orbital floor elevated and temporarily maintained in its correct position by means of maxillary packing with gauze or a balloon. There is no evidence that either of these surgical approaches has a particular advantage. Both may cause further damage to the infraorbital nerve, whose function is often compromised in such patients (Norman *et al.*, 1982).

Others recommend that, in the majority of patients, blow-out fractures should be reviewed until the clinical signs stabilize. The appropriate extraocular muscle surgery may then be undertaken to minimize the defect and give the patient the best possible field of single vision. Proponents of this approach recognize that the motility in most blow-out fractures improves spontaneously and that, in many patients, early surgery is not capable of giving normal ocular motility. In many such patients, the fibrosis consequent upon orbital and intramuscular haemorrhage will continue to limit ocular motility, despite early repair (Helveston, 1977; Metz, 1983).

At present, neither of these views has the greater credence and a controlled investigation of the results after early surgery, compared with late (or no) surgery, is required. Many patients with blow-out fracture are managed without the involvement of ophthalmologists and adequate documentation of the pre- and postoperative morbidity is often lacking.

Quantification of subjective deficit in post-traumatic diplopia

The characteristics of strabismus are conventionally described in terms of the angle of deviation in various positions of gaze. This may be given in degrees or prism dioptres (one degree equals approximately two prism dioptres). In acquired strabisums with marked incomitance (different in the various positions of gaze), the deviation may be measured in all positions of gaze. The various angles of squint are, however, generally inadequate to describe the patient's problems and various other techniques have been devised to describe the disability.

The Hess Chart

The Hess chart is based on the principle of ocular projection. If the eyes are pointing in the same direction and are shown dissimilar images (such as red and green lights), each retina will project the light to the same point in space and the patient will superimpose the red and green targets. If, however, the gaze is towards a position in which one eye has deficient movement, then, if the eye with the deficient movement is the reference, there will be a subjective tendency to place the target seen by the other, unaffected eye at an excessively peripheral point. This occurs because the effort involved in moving the deficient eye will lead to an increased effort (and therefore increased movement) of the normal eye. When the reference is the normal eye, however, there will be an underplacement of the projected image seen by the abnormal eye and this will be recorded as an underaction. A blow-out fracture of the orbital floor leads to a characteristic Hess chart (Figure 21.12), in which the good eye appears to have

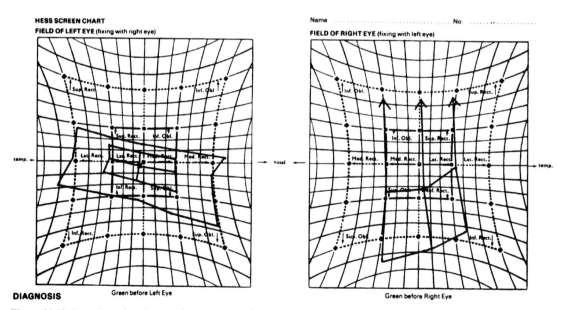

Figure 21.12. Hess chart after blow-out fracture of the left orbital floor. The vertical movements of the left globe are restricted, whereas those of the right eye are exaggerated relative to the left.

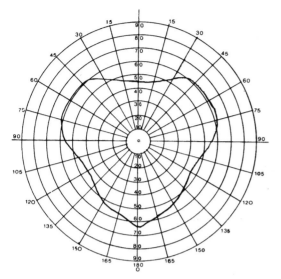

Figure 21.13. Limits for the normal field of binocular single vision.

trolled conditions of testing facilitate repetition by investigators in other institutions and sequential comparisons of motility.

The field of binocular single vision

If the main symptom is diplopia, it may be possible to chart the field of binocular single vision by immobilizing the patient's head in a perimeter and establishing the area over which the eyes are incapable of fusing the target image (that is, the field of diplopia). The type of perimeter is unimportant, but on all types it is imperative to establish a normal range for the field of binocular single vision (Figure 21.13).

Clearly, some positions of gaze are of greater importance and, for most persons, the straight ahead and downgaze positions are particularly valuable in everyday life. Reading, eating and walking up or down stairs are, for instance, all done with the eyes in the midgaze or downgaze positions. Various 'weighted' fields of single vision have been described in an attempt to quantitate the patient's disability when the field of binocular single vision is reduced. Such methods have found favour in the documentation of such cases. The binocular field is measured, an appropriate transparent grid (Figure 21.14a) is placed upon the field and the percentage deficit is calculated by the number of weighted areas within which the patient can see a single image (Figure 21.14b). Again, this allows for a

overactions, because its movement is being compared with the deficient movement of the affected eye, and the affected eye appears to show marked underactions because its movement is being compared with that of the normal eye.

The Hess chart is performed at a standard distance of one metre and is, therefore, an accurate record of a patient's ocular movements and secondary changes in ocular motility. The con-

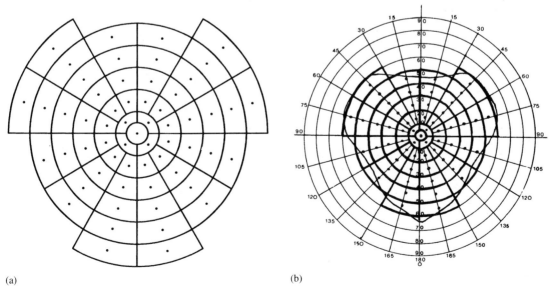

(a) (b)

Figure 21.14. A transparent grid (**a**) may be used for scoring the field of binocular single vision as a percentage of the normal area (**b**).

reproducible check on whether the situation is improving or deteriorating and also allows for quantification of the defect for the purposes of legal and other settlements.

Long-term disability following orbital trauma

It has been reported in a long-term study of orbital trauma that patients often suffer significant social disability (Kousoulides *et al.*, 1993). Twenty-four patients were reviewed between five and eight years after blow-out fractures. Most patients who had undergone spontaneous improvement had no significant alteration in their working or leisure activities, but, in the more serious cases requiring orbital or strabismus surgery, it was found that there was substantial disability. On average it took such patients 15 months to return to full working activities and, even then, 35% of patients complained of significant short-term psychological disturbances, including marital difficulties and problems with confidence. In the long term, 18% of patients needed to change their occupations to less responsible, and frequently less well paid, posts; 12% of patients were unable to return to driving, and five patients (29%) had to give up or change sporting activities, including membership of the Territorial Army.

Thus, major injury to the eyelids, lacrimal drainage apparatus and the bony orbit or orbital soft tissues may cause not only a persistent cosmetic disability but also long-term social and functional disabilities.

References

Aylward GW, Lawson J, McCarry B, Lee JP, Fells P. (1992) The surgical treatment of traumatic Brown's syndrome. *J Pediatr Ophthalmol Strabismus* **29**: 276–83.

Goldberg RA. (1991) Diagnosis and surgical management of fractures of the orbit and optic canal. *Curr Opin Ophthalmol* **2**: 633–38.

Hawes MJ, Dortzbach RK. (1994) Blow-out fractures of the orbital floor. In: Dortzbach RK, editor. *Ophthalmic plastic surgery. Prevention and management of complications.* New York: Raven Press, 195–210.

Helveston EM. (1982) Structure of the trochlea. *Ophthalmology* **89**: 124–33.

Helveston EM. (1977) The relationship of extraocular muscle problems to orbital floor fractures: early and late management. *Trans Am Acad Ophthalmol Otolaryngol* **83**: 660–62.

Jones IS, Jakobiec FA, Nolan BT. (1986) Patient examination and introduction to orbital disease. In: Duane TD, editor. *Clinical ophthalmology.* Philadelphia: Harper and Row, **2**: 15.

Kousoulides L, Fells P, Lee JP, Hague S, Aylward GW. (1993) Blow-out fractures: a study of the long term morbidity of patients with and without surgical treatment. In: Kaufmann, editor. Trans 21st Meeting ESA.

Kaufmann H. (1993) Transactions 21st Meeting of European Strabismological Association. Salzburg, 217–22.

Kronish JW, Gonnering RS, Dortzbach RK, *et al.* (1990) The pathophysiology of the anophthalmic socket: Part two. Analysis of orbital fat. *Ophthal Plast Reconstr Surg* **6**: 88–95.

Manson PN, Iliff N. (1991) Management of blow-out fractures of the orbital floor: II. Early repair for selected injuries. *Surv Ophthalmol* **35**: 280–92.

Mauriello JA, Hargrave S, Yee S, Mostafavi R, Kapila R. (1994) Infection after insertion of alloplastic orbital floor implants. *Am J Ophthalmol* **117**: 246–52.

Metz HS. (1983) Restrictive factors in strabismus. *Surv Ophthalmol* **28**: 71–83.

Norman JE, Dan NG, Rogers PA. (1982) Post-traumatic infraorbital neuropathy. *Orbit* **1**: 259–64.

Putterman AM. (1991) Management of blow-out fractures of the orbital floor: III. The conservative approach. *Surv Ophthalmol* **35**: 292–98.

Rootman J, Neigel J. (1988) Trauma. In: Rootman J, editor. *Diseases of the orbit. A multidisciplinary approach.* Philadelphia: Lippincott, 504–23.

Soll DB. (1982) The anophthalmic socket. *Ophthalmology* **89**: 407–23.

Warren FA, Kupersmith MJ. (1992) Controversies in management of traumatic and ischemic injury to the anterior visual pathways. *Curr Opin Ophthalmol* **3**: 571–74.

Woog JJ, Angrist RC, White WL, Dortzbach RK. (1994) Enucleation, evisceration and exenteration. In: Dortzbach RK, editor. *Ophthalmic plastic surgery. Prevention and management of complications.* New York: Raven Press, 251–68.

Section III

Ear, nose and throat

22

Temporal bone trauma: auditory, vestibular and facial nerve disorders after head injury

D A Moffat, R H Ballagh

Introduction

In the late twentieth century, trauma remains a significant cause of morbidity and mortality. Road traffic accidents, interpersonal violence, and industrial, domestic and athletic injuries all ensure that the sequelae of trauma commonly present to the medical practitioner and surgeon. Head injury is one of the most frequently suffered traumatic events; over 500 000 head injuries occur annually in the UK. Seventy-five thousand new patients with persisting postconcussive symptoms present each year in Canada (Barber, 1969).

Symptoms of an injury to the temporal bone and its contents occur in 25–30% of head injuries (Gurdjian, 1969). The male to female ratio is 3 : 1 because the male group is more prone overall to traumatic injuries (Wright *et al.*, 1969). The most common cause of temporal bone injury is motor vehicle accidents.

Up to 7% of head-injured children suffer temporal bone fractures (Mitchell and Stone, 1973), the majority occurring in children younger than five years old (McGraw and Cole, 1990). The most common aetiology for paediatric temporal bone fractures is falling (43%), followed by road traffic accidents (31%) (McGuirt and Stool, 1992).

Traumatic injuries to the temporal bone are therefore common and mostly occur in children and young people. A classification of temporal bone trauma is included in Table 22.1.

Blunt trauma

Fracture injuries

A fracture of the skull base is the result of sudden intense contact between a solid object and the head. The middle cranial fossa is involved in 60–80% of basal skull fractures. The temporal bone forms two-thirds of the floor of the middle cranial fossa; it is therefore not surprising that it is the most commonly injured bone in the base of the skull (Hagan and Cole, 1964). The temporal bone is made up largely of dense bone, and intense

Table 22.1. Classification of temporal bone trauma

Blunt trauma
   Fracture injuries
   Nonfracture injuries
     Blast injuries
     Injuries caused by water under pressure
Penetrating trauma
   Foreign bodies
   Surgical trauma
   Stab and gunshot wounds
Whiplash trauma
Barotrauma
   Injuries caused by water pressure
   Injuries caused by air pressure
Thermal trauma
Radiation injury
Acoustic trauma

mechanical forces must be present to distort it. The presence of numerous foramina, an irregular surface, and numerous thin osseous panels explains the frequency with which this otherwise solid bone is prone to fracture. The air-containing spaces of the temporal bone are surrounded and strengthened by bony buttresses, the anatomy of which are relatively constant. Consequently, there are predictable patterns of temporal bone fracture.

Types of temporal bone fracture

The classification of temporal bone fractures into longitudinal and transverse is attributed to Ulrich (1926). McHugh (1959) formalized the classification and added a third group: 'mixed' temporal bone fractures. Recently, a fourth pattern of 'oblique' temporal bone fractures has been added (Ghorayeb and Yeakley, 1992).

Longitudinal temporal bone fracture

The 'longitudinal' temporal bone fracture is one whose lines run parallel to the petrous ridge (i.e. the longitudinal axis of the bone) (Figure 22.1). According to most standard textbooks, the longitudinal type constitutes approximately 85% of temporal bone fractures (Cannon and Jahrsdoerfer, 1983; Harwood-Nash, 1970). In the paediatric age group, this proportion is even higher, with one series demonstrating that longitudinal fractures made up 95% of temporal bone fractures suffered by those under the age of 18 years (McGuirt and Stool, 1992). Twenty-three per cent are bilateral (Grove, 1947).

The blow that results in a longitudinal temporal bone fracture usually originates lateral to the skull, with the impact directly on to the temporal or parietal region. To understand the injury, consider the fracture to begin in the squamous temporal bone and continue towards the petrous apex, coursing around the dense bone of the otic capsule. The 'classical' longitudinal fracture is described as beginning in the superior temporal squamosa, passing anteroinferiorly to reach the postero-superior roof of the external auditory canal (EAC), then spreading medially across the roof of the middle ear, disrupting the tegmen tympani and possibly dislocating the incudomalleolar joint. The fracture then disrupts the medial wall of the middle ear in the region of the geniculate ganglion. It bypasses the otic capsule and runs anterior to the carotid canal. The fracture plane then courses

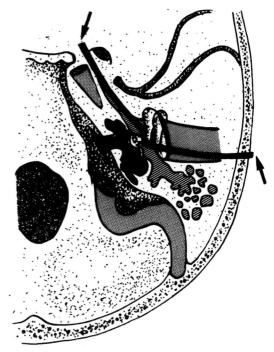

Figure 22.1. Diagrammatical representation of a longitudinal fracture of the temporal bone. The fracture line is along the longitudinal axis of the petrous bone (heavy line indicated by black arrows).

anteromedially, toward the clivus, between the carotid artery and the foramen spinosum (i.e. between the petrous and the sphenoid bones).

A posterior variant is described by Harwood-Nash (1970), originating in the posterior parietal region in the area of the transverse dural venous sinus and sigmoid sinus and extending medially from the tegmen to involve the otic capsule or the jugular foramen.

The structures that are most commonly disrupted in these fractures are the tympanic membrane, the roof of the middle ear, and the contents of the petrous apex. Hearing loss is common following this injury; it is usually a conductive or mixed hearing loss. Sensorineural hearing loss is relatively uncommon, but if it does occur it is usually a mild high frequency loss, maximal at 3000–4000 Hz. This hearing loss is thought to arise from the effect of labyrinthine concussion and not from the disruption of the inner ear by the fracture (Schuknecht, 1974).

The conductive hearing loss experienced in this fracture is often temporary, arising from blood in the external and middle ear, and from soft tissue swelling. Persistent conductive hearing loss is usually the result of ossicular disruption. The most common type is an isolated incus or incudostapedial dislocation. Ossicular dislocation may also resolve spontaneously, due to minimal displacement of the incus.

These fractures invariably result in laceration of the roof of the external auditory canal and, often, the tympanic membrane. Blood from the middle ear will present in the EAC, leading to the dictum that bloody otorrhoea following head injury represents a longitudinal temporal bone fracture until proven otherwise. If the dura is disrupted, cerebrospinal fluid (CSF) leak may occur through a disrupted tegmen tympani, resulting in CSF otorrhoea or otorhinorrhoea.

Vestibular disorders are unusual following longitudinal fracture; when present, they are usually mild and temporary. Spontaneous nystagmus is rare.

The facial nerve is usually spared in fractures of this type, with a 20% incidence of facial paralysis. Most fractures extend along the fallopian canal rather than across it. When the nerve is injured, the fracture line usually involves the fallopian canal in its tympanic portion, in the region of the geniculate ganglion, or, less commonly, in the mastoid portion (Fisch, 1974; Gobman *et al.*, 1989; Lambert and Brackmann, 1984). Facial weakness following these fractures is usually incomplete and is most often delayed, secondary to oedema rather than to disruption of the nerve.

Transverse temporal bone fracture

The 'transverse' temporal bone fracture is one that runs at right angles to the longitudinal axis of the petrous bone (Figure 22.2). This pattern represents 15–30% of temporal bone fractures (Cannon and Jahrsdoerfer, 1983; Harwood-Nash, 1970; Proctor *et al.*, 1956). Such fractures are caused by a blow to the occiput, or, less commonly, by a direct frontal blow. Those transverse fractures caused by a frontal blow will most often be accompanied by a fracture of the floor of the anterior cranial fossa. Transverse fractures have a higher immediate mortality than longitudinal fractures, and a require a greater force to generate them.

The 'classical' transverse temporal bone fracture begins in the posterior cranial fossa, usually in the region of the foramen magnum. It then extends through the jugular foramen and courses across the petrous pyramid and the floor of the the middle cranial fossa to the region of the foramen lacerum or foramen spinosum. This fracture traverses the otic capsule or the internal auditory canal (IAC).

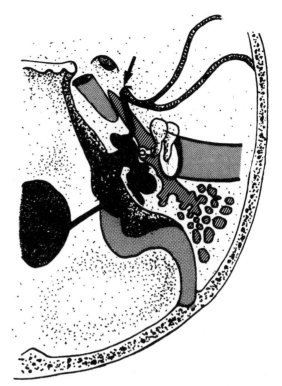

Figure 22.2. Diagrammatical representation of a transverse fracture of the temporal bone. The fracture line is perpendicular to the longitudinal axis of the petrous bone (heavy line indicated by black arrows).

The hearing loss associated with transverse fractures is usually sensorineural, due to disruption of the integrity of the labyrinth or the neurovascular bundle in the IAC. The fracture may disrupt the lateral wall of the otic capsule and extend to the medial wall of the middle ear, occasionally through the oval or round windows, resulting in middle ear haemorrhage and the clinical finding of haemotympanum.

Vertigo with spontaneous nystagmus and post-traumatic dysequilibrium is common following transverse temporal bone fracture. Facial nerve paralysis is also common (50%), and is more often immediate and more severe than that seen in longitudinal fracture. This is due to the fact that the orientation of the fracture line is perpendicular to the course of the facial nerve and the nerve is therefore more vulnerable to complete transection.

Mixed

Severe crushing injuries to the skull base can result in multiple fractures, involving a combination of several of the routes described for classical longitudinal and transverse injuries.

Oblique temporal bone fracture

Recently, the advent of high resolution CT scanning of the skull base has resulted in a reinvestigation of the patterns of temporal bone fractures. Aguilar *et al.*, (1987) analysed a large series of temporal bone fractures and found that a high percentage (68%) did not fall into the classically defined longitudinal and transverse categories. Instead, these fractures were orientated obliquely across the petrous pyramid. Ghorayeb and Yeakley (1992) reported a study of 150 temporal bone fractures and found that the oblique fracture was actually the most common pattern, occurring in 75%. The classically described longitudinal fracture pattern was seen in only 3%. The oblique fracture runs in the same direction as the longitudinal fracture when viewed from above, but has a different pattern of fracture lines on the external aspect of the skull if viewed laterally. The fracture line extends from the temporal squama posteriorly, and then downward across the mastoid cortex to the region of Henle's spine. The EAC is split longitudinally by the fracture into an upper and a lower half. Anteriorly, the fracture crosses the petrotympanic fissure and extends into the mandibular (glenoid) fossa. The fracture line in the middle fossa and petrous apex is indistinguishable from a longitudinal fracture.

Other fractures of the temporal bone

Fractures of the anterior wall of the EAC can occur in conjunction with injuries to the mandible. Unrecognized injuries in this area can result in the late complication of EAC stenosis, while early recognition often results in an easily accomplished reduction of the fracture. Late recognition of this lesion presents the otologist with a difficult reconstruction, often requiring the use of local skin flaps or split thickness skin grafts.

An unusal type of temporal bone fracture involves the mastoid process alone. Such a fracture may open into the EAC and middle ear and may involve the mastoid segment of the facial nerve (McHugh, 1959).

Clinical assessment of temporal bone fractures

As with any traumatic injury, the initial management of the patient presenting with a possible temporal bone fracture involves the assessment and maintenance of the airway, the stabilization of possible cervical spine injury, the control of haemorrhage, and a comprehensive evaluation of potential life-threatening injuries. Wherever possible, given the patient's other injuries and neurological status, a full clinical evaluation of the injury should be undertaken as soon as possible. Concomitant neurological injury is a bad prognostic factor and should be excluded as quickly as possible. This is particularly true in the paediatric population. In one reported series, up to one-third of children with intracranial injuries associated with temporal bone fractures died (McGuirt and Stool, 1992).

Hearing loss is a common complaint following blunt temporal bone trauma. An accurate history may reveal potential risk factors for significant injury to the hearing apparatus. These risk factors include: (1) unconciousness, and (2) bleeding from the ear, which, when occurring with (3) subjective hearing loss, has been been called the 'traumatic conductive triad' (Hough and Stuart, 1968).

Unconsciousness occurs in the vast majority of patients who suffer temporal bone fractures (Grove, 1947; Hough and Stuart, 1968). Bleeding from the ear is the hallmark of a longitudinal fracture; in this injury, such bleeding is usually brief in duration and mild in severity. Persistent bloody otorrhoea should alert the physician to the possibility of a vascular injury or CSF leak. Bleeding from the ear is unusual in transverse fractures, as the tympanic membrane is commonly left intact. Severe bleeding occurs in only 15% of temporal bone fractures, and, by draining down the eustachian tube, can compromise the airway (Hough and Stuart, 1968). Death caused by temporal bone fracture is unusual, but, when it occurs, it is most frequently the result of exsanguination (Pollanen *et al.*, 1992). Laceration of the internal carotid artery with bleeding through the fracture to the middle ear is the pathological mechanism of these catastrophic events.

Vertigo and dysequilibrium occur as sequelae of head injury, with or without a fracture of the temporal bone. Seventeen per cent of children suffering a temporal bone fracture will have vestibular symptoms (McGuirt and Stool, 1992). The head-injured patient should have a thorough evaluation of the history and a full neurotological examination when the neurological status allows. This should include an examination for spontaneous and positional nystagmus, including the Dix–Hallpike manoeuvre. This examination is considerably enhanced by the use of Frenzel's lenses (20 dioptre lenses which abolish the patient's visual fixation while magnifying the eye movements as seen by the observer).

Every patient with a head injury should have an otoscopic examination as soon as possible after the injury. The status of the external canal wall and tympanic membrane should be determined, and otomicroscopic removal of debris should be undertaken. This debris may be an external source of bacterial contamination and acts as a culture medium for bacterial multiplication. Irrigation of the EAC is absolutely contraindicated, as this greatly increases the likelihood of ascending infection and contamination of the central nervous system. Any fluid emanating from the EAC should be considered as possible CSF, and an attempt should be made to collect some for analysis. This is often difficult because of the small quantities available for sampling, but even a drop of bloody otorrhoea on a tissue may demonstrate a 'halo' sign, or a central red blood patch surrounded by a clear ring of watery fluid, heralding the presence of CSF in the otorrhoea. Ecchymosis over the mastoid region, or 'Battle's sign', is often indicative of blood in the air-filled spaces of the temporal bone. Tuning fork testing should be performed in all patients; this may give important clues as to the nature of any hearing loss.

A full examination of the cranial nerves should be conducted as soon as the patient's condition permits. The most critical of these is the evaluation and documentation of the function of the seventh nerve.

Radiological assessment

When the patient is stable enough for the test, a high resolution computed tomographic (CT) scan of the head should be undertaken. Fracture lines may be seen and the nature of the fracture identified (Figure 22.3). Unless there is suspected intracranial or vascular involvement, there is no need for the use of contrast. Temporal bone fractures can be difficult to detect and describe, even in the presence of good CT equipment and competent appraisal. One clue to such cryptic injuries may be the presence of air in the temporomandibular joint. This finding is seen in 20% of temporal bone fractures and should be evaluated in every case of a suspected fracture and equivocal CT scan examination (Betz and Weiner, 1991). The finding of free air in the labyrinth, or a 'pneumolabyrinth', has been described in a patient with a transverse temporal bone fracture (Weissman and Curtain, 1992). Recently, it has been suggested that conventional tomography may be a useful adjunct in the radiological assessment of

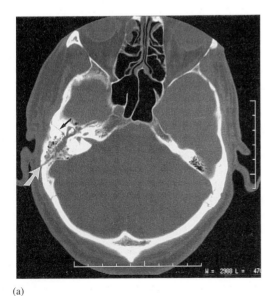

(a)

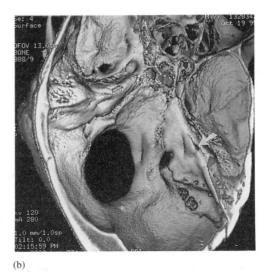

(b)

Figure 22.3. (**a**) Transaxial CT scan demonstrating a longitudinal fracture (white arrow) and a transverse fracture (black arrow) of the right temporal bone. (**b**) Three dimensional CT reconstruction of the same patient demonstrating the longitudinal fracture (white arrow).

those patients in whom the surgeon's index of clinical suspicion for a temporal bone fracture is high and the CT results are negative (Goligher and Lloyd, 1990).

In severe blunt and penetrating trauma, an assessment of the vascular structures of the temporal bone may be necessary. The most common vascular lesion of the skull base following trauma is occlusion of the jugular bulb and transverse sinus, which may be identified by lack of contrast enhancement on CT scan, or by an absence of 'flow-void' on MRI. Impingement on or injury to the carotid artery can be identified using carotid arteriography or digital subtraction angiography. Traumatic carotid aneurysms and arteriovenous malformations are identified in this way. An unusual complication of skull base trauma is a caroticocavernous fistula, which requires carotid angiography for diagnosis and can be treated with balloon occlusion.

Hearing loss

Audiometry

All patients suspected of having sustained significant trauma to the temporal region should have thorough audiometrical testing, including an assessment of pure-tone thresholds, speech discrimination, and impedance for both ears. This is particularly relevant for patients with immediate, total facial nerve weakness in whom facial nerve decompression surgery is being considered, as hearing loss is a common complication of this procedure (May and Klein, 1983). Preoperative assessment of hearing is therefore imperative. Other more advanced audiological tests such as auditory brain stem response testing and electronystagmography (ENG) may also be indicated.

In one study, 60% of patients with temporal bone fractures had a post-traumatic hearing loss. Of these, 43% were conductive, 52% were sensorineural, and 5% were mixed (McGuirt and Stool, 1992).

Injuries to the conductive hearing apparatus

External auditory canal and tympanic membrane injuries

In these patients, careful otomicroscopic debridement is carried out and an inspection of the EAC and tympanic membrane is undertaken. The ear canal may be narrowed by fracture of the anterior canal wall associated with trauma to the mandible. Fracture lines, lacerations, protruding bone or displaced ossicles may be seen in the EAC. Abnormalities of the EAC are almost always associated with further, deeper temporal bone injuries. The most frequent finding in a longitudinal fracture is a laceration of the meatal skin and bony disruption of the posterosuperior EAC, in the region of the notch of Rivinus. Since many of these patients are referred to the otolaryngologist late (months or even years after the injury), careful examination may reveal healed fracture lines, which are often visible as step deformities in the region of the notch of Rivinus. The tympanic membrane is frequently torn in the posterosuperior quadrant, and a paper patch may be placed over this to aid healing, even at the time of the original examination under the microscope (Guerrier *et al.*, 1965). Tos (1973) observed that most perforations were spontaneously healed by three weeks and that all were healed by three months. Spontaneous healing of tympanic membrane perforations in children is just as likely to occur as in adults, with 78% healed at three weeks postinjury and 96% at six months reported in one large series (McGuirt and Stool, 1992).

The presence of a haemotympanum without rupture of the tympanic membrane or laceration of the EAC is suggestive of a transverse temporal bone fracture.

Middle ear injuries

Over half of traumatic injuries to the ossicular chain are due to blunt temporal bone trauma sustained in automobile accidents (Hough, 1970). This is seen predominantly in younger patients, with 50% of ossicular chain injuries occurring in children younger than 13 years of age, and 70% in persons aged 21 and younger.

In those patients with a conductive hearing loss following trauma to the temporal bone, the most common injury is incudostapedial joint separation, which occurred in 82% of patients in one study (Hough and Stuart, 1968). The incus may be massively dislocated (57%), and the stapedial arch may be fractured (30%) in these cases. Fractures of the malleus are uncommon. Multiple sites of ossicular disruption are observed in one-third of these patients. Late post-traumatic ankylosis and tympanosclerosis are common, occurring in up to 25% of these injuries. Cholesteatoma is another late complication in 9%, presumably through the entrapment of squamous epithelium through a tympanic membrane perforation, behind a healed tympanic membrane perforation, or within a fracture line itself.

The incudostapedial joint

This is the area of the ossicular chain most vulnerable to damage by traumatic forces, regardless of the direction or origin of that force. This area is commonly disrupted as a result of foreign body insertion into the ear canal and by forces transmitted during skull fractures. The possible forces that can be exerted in this region include severe transmitted vibratory energy from the impact itself, tortional forces resulting in twisting of the incudostapedial joint by momentary movement of the attached regional bone masses, the inertial forces inherent in the ossicular chain, and the action of the tympanic muscles when sudden tetanic contraction occurs during trauma (Hough, 1959).

Massive dislocation of the incus

The incus has the weakest ligamentous and soft tissue attachments of the three ossicles. It is therefore not surprising, given all the potential forces exerted on it during skull base trauma, that it may become completely detached. The dislocated incus has been observed in remote parts of the middle ear and mastoid or trapped within a fracture line; it may even be extruded through a fracture line to be discovered in the EAC (Hough and Stuart, 1968). McHugh (1963) discovered an incus in the middle cranial fossa and a malleus jammed into the eustachian tube orifice. For this to occur, there must be a brief moment during the traumatic incident during which the fracture is at least as wide as the body of the incus, demonstrating the massive forces that must have been necessary for such a derangement to occur. This is confirmed by the experimental work of Gurdjian and Webster (1958), who performed high speed cinefilms of blows to the skull and demonstrated that a fracture line opens widely at the moment of injury at a site distant from the impact.

Other ossicular abnormalities

The same forces involved at the level of the incudostapedial joint may be transmitted to the arch of the stapes and result in fractures in this area. This is particularly true of mixed longitudinal/transverse fractures, where forces are maximal in the region of the medial wall of the middle ear (Hough and McGee, 1991). Injuries to the stapes were four times less common than injuries to the incus in the series of Tos (1973). Malleus abnormalities are rare, given the well secured location of this ossicle as part of the tympanic membrane and its firm ligamentous attachments to the anterior and superior walls of the epitympanum. Injuries to the malleus are usually associated with massive trauma, and other ossicular abnormalities are almost always present (Wright *et al.*, 1969).

Treatment

The treatment for ossicular disruption is exploratory tympanotomy and repair of the ossicular defect. It is often possible to replace the displaced incus in its original position, and stabilize it with gelfoam and fibrin glue. This is the most satisfying result surgically and usually renders the best hearing result, but, unfortunately, late adhesion formation may draw the replaced incus away from its anatomical position months after the repositioning procedure and this may account for the redevelopment of late conductive hearing losses.

If the incus or the head of the stapes is damaged by the fracture, it may be necessary to perform an ossiculoplasty. The body of the incus is often the best raw material for such a reconstruction, as it can be sculpted to an appropriate size microscopically and replaced into the patient, in the fashion of a Wullstein Type IIb tympanoplasty over the stapedial head, or a Wullstein Type IIc technique in the case of the stapedial arch fracture. In one clinical series of patients presenting with conductive hearing loss following temporal bone fracture, closure of the air–bone gap to 10 dB or less was achieved in 78% (Hough and Stuart, 1968); it was equal to or better than the pretrauma hearing in 45%.

Ossicular fixation is relatively common as a late sequel of skull base trauma, and is due to the extensive scarring and new regional bone formation involved in healing temporal bone fractures. Hyperostosis may result in the fusion of the head of the malleus and incus, and fixation of these to the tegmen tympani. Tympanosclerosis may cause a similar fixation of the ossicular chain, particularly in the region of the attic. These lesions are treated by mobilization or ossicular replacement. Occasionally, stapedectomy is necessary for lesions that cause significant footplate immobilization.

Prognosis of traumatic conductive hearing loss

In one series, 75% of patients suffering a mild conductive hearing impairment following temporal bone fracture regained normal hearing (McGuirt and Stool, 1992). Of those with a moderate conductive loss, 43% resolved completely with no intervention. A conductive hearing loss persisting for longer than six weeks after trauma and exceeding 30 dB is an indication for surgical exploration (Wennmo and Spandow, 1993).

Injuries to the sensorineural hearing apparatus

Inner ear injuries

The pathological basis for inner ear injuries when temporal bone fracture is absent is thought to be due to 'labyrinthine concussion' (neuroepithelial damage in the inner ear caused by the force of a head injury). Auditory impairment may result from hair cell damage in the organ of Corti due to the transmission of high energy vibration (Schuknecht, 1969). The spectrum of sensorineural hearing loss following such concussive injuries is similar to that seen in noise exposure, and is centred around 4000 Hz. The severity of the hearing loss is related to the severity of the traumatic injury and the concussive forces at work during the event (Schuknecht, 1950).

Treatment

Aural rehabilitation in the form of fitting of a hearing aid may be appropriate for those patients suffering a permanent incomplete loss of sensorineural hearing. The indications for this are the same as for stable sensorineural hearing loss of any aetiology.

The advent of cochlear implantation has provided an additional means of possible rehabilitation for those rare patients who suffer bilateral complete audiovestibular injuries in skull base fractures and has been successfully employed in several of these individuals (Jenkins *et al.*, 1989). Successful aural rehabilitation is not always achieved, however, leading several authors to advocate strict patient selection criteria for cochlear implantation following skull base fracture (Morgan *et al.*, 1994). The majority of patients suffering from this problem have had bilateral transverse temporal bone fractures, an injury that can damage the inner ear and eighth nerve. An electrodiagnostic assessment of the integrity of the spiral ganglion and the eighth nerve is essential in all of these patients. Electrode insertion can be complicated by bony derangement and by labyrinthitis

ossificans as a result of the trauma itself or of post-traumatic infection. A preoperative high resolution CT scan of the temporal bones is needed to anticipate and plan for these difficulties.

Prognosis of traumatic sensorineural hearing loss

In one large series, all patients who suffered a transverse temporal bone fracture had complete and permanent sensorineural hearing loss in the affected ear (Tos, 1971).

In the same series, 59% of patients suffering a longitudinal temporal bone fracture had a conductive hearing loss, 4% had a pure sensorineural hearing loss and 4% had a mixed loss. The hearing returned to normal in the majority of these, with 63% doing so in the first six weeks. Over the long term, 80% of patients had a complete return to normal hearing and, of the remainder, 13% had ossicular disruptions amenable to surgical repair, 4% had a mixed loss, and 4% had a persisting sensorineural hearing loss. Other series indicate that the incidence of sensorineural hearing loss following longitudinal temporal bone fracture may be higher initially, with figures ranging from 10% to 24% (Barber, 1969; Podoshin and Fradis, 1975), but the same trend towards spontaneous resolution is seen. This trend was also seen in a large series of paediatric temporal bone fractures, with 50% resolving in less than three months and 50% exhibiting a persistent stable loss at six months following the trauma.

Dural defects

Concomitant fracture of the floor of the middle cranial fossa and its associated dura can result in a CSF leak into the middle ear. The incidence of CSF otorrhoea in one large series of 1800 patients was 1.4% (Canniff, 1971), although it has been reported to be as high as 11.5% (Brawley and Kelly, 1967). The resulting leak usually ceases spontaneously, and conservative care is indicated in the majority of patients. Most authors agree, however, that leaks lasting longer than two weeks require surgical exploration and repair (Hough and McGee, 1991). Purulent inflammation of the middle ear is a common sequel of temporal bone trauma (Hough and Stuart, 1968). It is important to be vigilant for the early signs of ascending central nervous system infection. The incidence of meningitis in patients with CSF otorrhoea is relatively high: 20% in the series of Canniff (1971) representing all ages, and

24% in a similar series of children (MacGee *et al.*, 1970).

The use of prophylactic antibiotics has been the subject of conflicting studies and reports. Brawley and Kelly (1967) reported that none of the 35 patients they treated with antibiotic prophylaxis developed meningitis. Tos (1973) reported that meningitis developed in 8% of 113 patients treated with antibiotic prophylaxis and 5% of 80 patients who were not so treated. Most authors now agree, therefore, that the use of antibiotics prophylactically is not helpful in these injuries. Moreover, the theoretical disadvantage of the possible emergence of resistant bacterial strains by antibiotic prophylaxis provides another reason to hold these medications in reserve for actual clinical evidence of evolving meningitis. As a result of the breakdown of the normal protective anatomical barriers in temporal bone fractures, such intracranial infections can be rapidly progressive and difficult to control even when the bacterial spectrum has not been affected by previous antiobiotic use (Perlman, 1939).

The diagnosis of a CSF leak can be difficult to confirm. Intrathecal injection of fluorescein or a radioactive carrier substance may be useful when spinal fluid is suspected to be leaking from the external auditory canal. Fluorescein is visible under an ultravioet light, or, in the case of a radioactive carrier, packing can be placed in the ear canal to be analysed under a gamma camera for radioactivity. If CSF otorhinorrhoea is suspected, these same procedures can be performed using intranasal inspection for fluorescein or pledget placement for analysis in a department of nuclear medicine to confirm the diagnosis.

Most CSF leaks close spontaneously within 7–10 days postinjury. If CSF drainage persists beyond this point, active intervention is usually required. A lumbar drain is the first step in management in the otherwise healthy patient. If the leak is profuse, or if it fails to close with these conservative measures, surgical exploration should be undertaken. The floor of the middle fossa is the most likely site of leakage in temporal bone fractures. The choice of a transmastoid or an intracranial middle fossa repair depends upon the personal preference of the surgical team. If an intrancranial exploration is planned, the repair may be intradural or extradural. The preference of the authors is the intracranial-extradural repair for the majority of these surgical lesions.

Many temporal bone fractures heal with a fibrous union only; this may break down and lead

to the late complication of intracranial infection (Ward, 1969).

Large dural defects in association with a loss of the osseous integrity of the temporal bone may result in encephalocoele or meningoencephalocoele formation. These are usually the late sequelae of temporal bone fractures or subsequent infection with loss of bone. A soft tissue mass may be seen in the superior EAC, the middle ear, or in the surgical defect of a canal wall down mastoidectomy. The management of these lesions includes early recognition, radiological confirmation, and surgical reconstruction. The goal of surgery is to reconstitute the barrier between the central nervous system and the respiratory mucosa of the middle ear and the mastoid, or of the skin of the mastoid bowl. A combined approach through the mastoid and through the middle cranial fossa is usually necessary. Obliteration of the mastoid is one option in the surgical treatment of these lesions (Moffat *et al.*, 1994).

Vertigo and dysequilibrium

Injuries to the temporal bone may be associated with mechanical disruption of any or all parts of the vestibular system, from the labyrinth to the vestibular nuclei of the brain stem. These disruptions may be partial or total, immediate or delayed, short lived or permanent. This provides for a spectrum of symptoms that can be a challenge to diagnosis and treatment. Moreover, these injuries are often compounded by concomitant injuries to those elements of the central nervous system involved in balance and eye movement co-ordination, such as the cerebellum and higher cortical centres

Benign paroxysmal positional vertigo is a relatively common complaint following severe head trauma, and may be the most common post-traumatic syndrome of labyrinthine injury (Barber, 1965). Schuknecht (1969) believes that free floating particles become dislodged within the endolymph of the vestibule during the violent events of labyrinthine concussion. These free floating particles, which have mass and move under the influence of gravity, will therefore stimulate the affected inner ear in response to positional changes. This theory is strongly supported by the findings of Parnes and Price-Jones (1993). They have suggested that the aetiology of the majority of cases of benign paroxysmal positional vertigo may be free floating particles in the posterior semicircular canal, and that the repositioning of these particles into the utricle results in resolution of the vertigo in 68% of patients. This represents an improvement over the natural history of this disorder as described by Berman and Fredrickson (1978). Thirty-four per cent of workmen with minor head injuries (no fracture, less than three hours post-traumatic amnesia) complained of vertigo, although only 40% had objective findings to support the diagnosis of a labyrinthine injury. Of those with hard physical findings, 60% had symptoms lasting longer than five years after the traumatic injury. Fifty per cent of patients with major head injuries (skull base fractures, post-traumatic amnesia greater than three hours) complained of vertigo. Objective evidence of an inner ear disorder was present in 65% of these and 75% still had symptoms more than five years after the original incident.

Spontaneous nystagmus following head injury is always significant and is almost always the result of an acute injury to the labyrinth. ENG recording with the eyes closed or with the use of Frenzel's lenses greatly enhances the ability of the clinician to detect a spontaneous nystagmus (Barber, 1969). Nystagmus is usually paralytic soon after the injury, beating away from the affected side, but may beat toward the affected side weeks to months after the injury, as recovery of peripheral vestibular function occurs following central compensation (Lange and Kornhuber, 1962).

Thirteen per cent of people remember vertigo after a longitudinal fracture of the temporal bone (Hough and Stuart, 1968), but few suffer long-term vertiginous symptoms. A transverse fracture of the temporal bone may result in disruption of the integrity of the labyrinth itself; it is usually associated with a sudden and complete loss of vestibular function on the involved side. The patient experiences a period of severe vertigo until central compensation occurs. Bilateral vestibular injury is an unusual outcome in temporal bone trauma. It is almost always the result of bilateral transverse fractures and results in permanent oscillopsia and long-term disability in the majority of subjects (Hough, 1970).

Central vestibular compensation may be delayed by the patient's other bodily or central nervous system injuries. Visual disturbance or proprioceptive impairments will further impede the process of central compensation. The new physiotherapeutic modality of vestibular rehabilitation has been shown to enhance central compensation and reduce the incidence of chronic balance disorders resulting from head injury. Attention tends to be focused on auditory rehabilitation, but few centres concentrate on the vestibular rehabilitation of patients with inner ear disorders. Vestibular rehabilitation programmes have recently been developed that integrate the clinical and audiological investigation with a comprehensive assessment of the balance system and the patient's general state of fitness (Shepard *et al.*, 1990). A programme of specific exercises is then designed for the patient by the medical and physiotherapy teams, the goal of which is improved central compensation for vestibular asymmetry and improved attention to nonvestibular balance clues. Whilst vestibular rehabilitation is not tremendously helpful for patients with rapidly changing vestibular outputs, such as a patient suffering frequent vertiginous episodes, it is helpful for patients with relatively static vestibular function. It is very helpful for patients with poorly compensated unilateral vestibular hypofunction and for patients with bilateral vestibular hypofunction (Telian *et al.*, 1990).

Fluctuating vestibular symptoms are most commonly the result of a perilymphatic fistula (an abnormal leakage of perilymph from the inner ear into the middle ear). While some authors dispute this entity as a cause of spontaneous hearing loss and vertigo, most would argue that mechanical trauma and barotrauma are recognized causes of this lesion. The diagnosis is a clinical one, made on the basis of a history of fluctuating vertigo, fluctuating hearing loss, and possibly tinnitus. The 'fistula test' is a physical sign in which positive pressure is introduced into the external auditory canal, in the form of simple tragal pressure or by using a Siegles pneumatic speculum or an audiometric impedance probe. A positive 'subjective' response of vertigo or dysequilibrium may be experienced by the patient. Close observation of the eye movements may yield a positive 'objective' response, which classically includes a conjugate deviation of the eyes away from the affected side, followed by a horizontal nystagmus beating toward the affected side (irritative nystagmus). The treatment for this is exploratory tympanotomy and soft tissue plugging of the round and oval windows, and any other areas suspicious of possible perilymphatic leakage.

Endolymphatic hydrops is an unusual outcome of temporal bone trauma, which may also result in fluctuating vestibular sympoms. When the vestibular acqueduct is involved in the traumatic injury, secondary endolymphatic hydrops may occur. An association has been noted between Menière's disease and trauma, either physical or acoustic (Paparella and Mancini, 1983). The chronological sequence of events in certain patients suggests that trauma may have had a role to play in the genesis of Menière's-related symptoms. Trauma may produce biochemical dysfunction in the cells of the membranous labyrinth, or it may simply cause the release of debris into the endolymph, which could then obstruct the endolymphatic duct and sac (Paparella and Mancini, 1983).

'Acute' endolympathic hydrops has been seen in the cochlea of a patient who died shortly after a blunt traumatic temporal bone injury that did not result in fracture (Murakami *et al.*, 1990). Delayed endolymphatic hydrops occurs when Menière-like symptoms develop in an ear that has been previously deafened. This distinctive entity typically affects young adults; in one study, the mean age at clinical presentation was 32 years (LeLiever and Barber, 1980). The latency between the onset of deafness and the onset of vertigo is from one to 68 years, with an average of 23–28 years (LeLiever and Barber, 1980). The aetiology of the original hearing loss does not appear to have an effect on the development of delayed endolymphatic hydrops. This disorder has been described in ears deafened by temporal bone fracture (Rizvi and Gibbin, 1979). One interesting report implicates heavy noise exposure and acoustic trauma in the development of delayed endolymphatic hydrops in a group of professional soldiers (Ylikoski, 1988).

Facial nerve paralysis

The facial nerve, with its important somatic motor function, and its lesser functions of taste, secretomotor and somatic sensation, is at great risk during head injury. Of the cranial nerves, the facial nerve travels the greatest distance through a confined bony canal. It is therefore particularly vulnerable to injury during skull fracture. It is the second most commonly injured cranial nerve in trauma.

Complete paralysis of the facial nerve following head injury is pathognomonic of a temporal bone fracture (Hough and Stuart, 1968). Facial nerve injuries are seen in 15% of adults (Tos, 1973) and in 6–21% of children with temporal bone fractures (McGuirt and Stool, 1992; Mitchell and Stone, 1973). While unilateral facial nerve weakness is of major concern, 0.8–1% of these patients will present with bilateral weakness (Wormald *et al.*, 1991), which is a devastating problem that presents particular difficulties in prognostic electrodiagnostic testing and management.

According to one series, longitudinal temporal bone fracture was associated with complete facial paralysis in 19.3% of patients (Hough and Stuart, 1968). One-third of these recovered spontaneously without surgical intervention. The remaining two-thirds experienced incomplete return of facial function, with most suffering noticeable facial weakness during movement, synkinesis, facial tics or mass movement. A longitudinal fracture rarely causes total lysis of the facial nerve, because the fracture is orientated parallel to the path of the nerve, resulting in a sudden stretching force being applied to it.

Transverse temporal bone fractures are associated with a far greater incidence of facial nerve injury (approximately 50%). This is due to the fact that the fracture is perpendicular to the path of the seventh nerve, resulting in shearing of its connective tissue elements. There is a greater likelihood of the nerve being completely transected in transverse fractures.

Decisions about the management and prognosis of facial nerve injuries in temporal bone fractures are influenced by several factors. The most important of these is the nature and timing of the onset of facial paralysis. In those head-injured patients who develop facial palsy, approximately one-half will have immediate onset paralysis. In those patients in whom it is difficult to determine when the onset of facial paralysis occurred, it is best to treat them as though they had immediate onset paralysis (McHugh, 1963). Immediate-onset facial paralysis has a greater chance of resulting in long-term disruption of facial nerve function and permanent weakness than paralysis that is delayed in onset.

Those injuries that are delayed in onset are usually the result of local post-traumatic phenomena in the region of the fracture, such as oedema, haemorrhage and ischaemia. Most injuries will become manifest within five days of the head trauma, and up to 94% will recover full function within six to eight weeks of the injury (Griffin *et al.*, 1979). If recovery does not become apparent after three weeks, the chance of complete recovery diminishes.

Site of injury

In a skull base fracture, the assumption that a single fracture site identified in one part of the temporal bone is the sole site of the facial nerve injury may be incorrect. Fisch (1974) found that when the facial nerve did not recover after a considerable period of time, the lesion was most often located in the geniculate ganglion area.

Lambert and Brackmann (1984) reported 21 patients with longitudinal temporal bone fractures, all of whom had injuries in the perigeniculate region. Four of the same patients, however, had associated fractures involving the facial nerve in either the tympanic or mastoid segments. Based on a report of a patient with a longitudinal temporal bone fracture, it has been suggested that Wallerian degeneration appears to originate in the labyrinthine segment of the seventh nerve, at the meatal foramen (Grobman *et al.*, 1989). A CT scan can be helpful in determining the orientation of a temporal bone fracture, but most authors caution against relying solely on this in diagnosing the site of facial nerve injury or in planning surgical decompression of the nerve. Gadolinium DTPA-enhanced MRI is often useful in demonstrating enhancement of the injured segment of the the facial nerve.

Topognostic testing

Topognostic testing is sometimes helpful in determining the site of a facial nerve injury. The Schirmer test and stapedial reflex test are recommended by some authors as a means of preoperative localization of the site of a seventh nerve injury, but electrogustometry and submaxillary gland flow testing are of less diagnostic value (Hough and McGee, 1991).

Schirmer test
In this technique, two strips of paper are folded and placed in the lower conjunctival fornix for five minutes. Lambert and Brackmann (1984) describe an abnormal Schirmer's test as being a decrease of lacrimation of 75% or more on the affected side as measured by the amount of paper soaked by tears on each side, or a bilateral decrease in lacrimation (less than 10 mm for both sides at five minutes). The latter may be due to the fact that unilateral injury to the geniculate ganglion can paradoxically cause a bilateral reduction in tearing.

Stapedial reflex testing
This is accomplished at the time of impedance testing, and should be part of the comprehensive audiometrical evaluation indicated for all patients with facial nerve weakness following head trauma. If the stapedial reflex is absent in the face of normal hearing, then the site of the lesion is likely to be between the geniculate ganglion and the stapedius muscle. If the reflex is present, then the site of the lesion is distal to the stapedius muscle.

Electrical testing

The question that is of paramount importance to the otolaryngologist is which facial nerve palsies will recover and which will not. In the past two decades, this question has led to the development of electrical tests to determine the status of the facial nerve and predict its potential for recovery. The electrical tests which offer the most useful information are the maximal stimulation test (MST) and electroneuronography (ENoG).

The minimal excitability test determines the minimal current necessary to stimulate muscle movement when applied to a branch of the facial nerve. The Hilger nerve stimulator was designed for use in this test. A comparison was made between the normal and abnormal sides, and a difference of 3.5 mA or greater between the two sides was thought to be significant and an indication for surgical decompression of the facial nerve (Alford *et al.*, 1970). The MST was first described by May *et al.* in 1971 and represents an evolution of the minimal excitability test. The MST also utilizes the Hilger nerve stimulator at the highest setting tolerated by the patient, usually 5 mA or greater. The response of the involved side is compared with the normal side and evaluated as an equal, reduced or absent response. May *et al.* (1971) found this test to be more accurate in predicting facial nerve outcome following injury. They reported that 88% of patients with a normal MST response had complete recovery of facial nerve function, while those with a reduced response had a 73% chance of full recovery. Of those with no MST response, only 27% returned to completely normal function (May *et al.*, 1976). It is interesting to note that the MST is of no value up to 72 hours postinjury. Normal values are obtained prior to this time, even in facial nerves that have been completely transected.

ENoG was described by Esslen (1977) and popularized by Fisch (1981). ENoG records the actual compound action potential of the facial nerve following stimulation. May *et al.* (1981) have used the term 'evoked electromyography' (or EEMG), which is probably more accurate, because it is the compound action potentials of muscle fibres that are measured. The stimulating electrode is placed on the skin over the stylomastoid foramen and a supramaximal stimulation is applied, to ensure that all functioning nerve fibres are stimulated. The recording electrode is placed in the region of the nasolabial fold, which has been shown to be the optimal site for this electrode

(Gutnick *et al.*, 1990). The stimulus is gradually increased in magnitude until there is no further increase in the amplitude of the response. Again, the normal side is compared with the abnormal side. The amplitude loss on the involved side is directly proportional to the degree of degeneration taking place in the nerve. Therefore, if the amplitude of the affected side is 25% of the normal side, a 75% degeneration has occurred in the abnormal facial nerve. May (1980) recommended surgery when the amplitude of the affected side was 25% of that of the normal side. Esslen (1977) has shown, however, that the majority of patients with less than 90% degeneration will have complete recovery of facial nerve function, prompting the majority of authors to advocate the figure of 10% or less amplitude of the affected side compared with the normal as a more appropriate indicator for surgical decompression. Fisch (1974, 1980) has recommended surgical intervention within three weeks in patients in whom a traumatic injury has resulted in 90% amplitude reduction by ENoG testing within six days of the injury. These guidelines have been modified by the recent work of Lieberherr *et al.* (1990), in which the injuries of 82 patients with temporal bone fractures and facial palsies were retrospectively reviewed. Current recommendations are for operative exploration as soon as the patient's condition permits in cases of immediate paralysis with greater than 90% degeneration.

Like the MST, ENoG is not useful for at least 72 hours postinjury, and most authors advocate that testing should begin on the third or fourth day following the trauma.

Magnetic stimulation of the intracranial portion of the facial nerve has recently been described, and has the advantage of providing a stimulus originating proximal to the temporal bone (Cramer and Kartush, 1991). Magnetic stimulation of the motor cortex is even possible; varying magnetic fields induce in-depth electrical currents that initiate neural depolarization (Barker *et al.*, 1985). The potentials generated have a similar character to those of ENoG, leading some to call it 'magnetic evoked neuromyography' or MNoG. The latencies are longer, given the greater distance across which the impulse is transmitted; an analysis of these latencies supports the idea that the root entry zone is the site of stimulation of MNoG (Seki *et al.*, 1990). The principal disadvantage of this modality, however, is the lack of clinical studies demonstrating its repeatability and its value in providing an accurate indication

of the prognosis of a facial nerve injury (Cramer and Kartush, 1991).

Electromyography is not helpful in the evaluation of facial paralysis of recent onset. It does not demonstrate denervation potentials until 8–10 days after denervation has occurred (Esslen, 1976). All electrical testing is therefore limited by the fact that it cannot provide an indication of the status of the facial nerve in the immediate postinjury state.

Surgery for traumatic facial nerve paralysis

The facial nerve may be compressed by impinging bone fragments or by local haematoma. It may be partially or totally disrupted by a fracture. The surgeon should be prepared for any of these possibilities when exploring such a patient, and should be skilled in the microsurgical techniques of nerve decompression, nerve grafting, and nerve rerouting and transposition.

The facial nerve should be explored through both the middle ear and the mastoid. A cortical mastoidectomy is performed in the usual way, with care being taken to note any fracture lines or areas of bone compression. Great care should be taken to preserve the EAC wall, as taking it down can significantly impair the management of any posttraumatic or postsurgical CSF leaks. The aditus and antrum are exposed and the second genu of the facial nerve is skeletonized. The posterior incudal ligament is divided and the body of the incus is gently reflected laterally. Through this approach, the tympanic portion of the facial nerve can be visualized and gently exposed, as far as the geniculate ganglion. The otologist should be prepared to explore and expose the nerve from the geniculate ganglion to the stylomastoid foramen and also to explore the nerve from the geniculate ganglion to the porus acousticus of the IAC via the middle cranial fossa approach if any possibility exists that the site of injury is in this region. This is especially true if no lesion is discovered in the tympanic or mastoid portions of the nerve. It must be remembered that the transmastoid decompression is carried out first, followed by the middle fossa approach, since the latter carries a higher morbidity.

Immediate onset facial paralysis following traumatic injury is an indication for surgical exploration and surgical decompression as soon as the patient's condition permits (Kettle, 1950), especially if ENoG evidence indicates greater than 90%

neuronal degeneration (Lieberherr *et al.*, 1990). Early surgical intervention will improve the final facial nerve outcome in immediate onset facial palsy from temporal bone trauma. Many physicians outside the field of otolaryngology are unaware of the importance of early facial nerve decompression surgery. Immediate onset facial nerve palsy associated with total sensorineural hearing impairment, usually the result of a transverse temporal bone fracture, is best explored through a transmastoid/translabyrinthine exposure of the seventh nerve from the porus acousticus to the stylomastoid foramen (Hough and McGee, 1991). This provides the best visualization of the nerve and optimizes exposure for nerve grafting or transposition. Immediate post-traumatic facial nerve palsy associated with intact hearing is best explored progressively, starting with an assessment of the tympanic and mastoid segments, followed by an exploration of the IAC if indicated.

Delayed onset facial paralysis following traumatic injury should be followed clinically and electrodiagnostically at regular intervals. If neuronal degeneration occurs, facial nerve decompression may be indicated. In a patient with greater than 90% degeneration with total sensorineural hearing impairment, transmastoid/translabyrinthine exploration of the entire length of the facial nerve in the temporal bone is indicated (Hough and McGee, 1991). In a patient with electrodiagnostic criteria for a facial nerve decompression and intact hearing, progressive exploration and decompression of the nerve through the middle ear and mastoid is indicated, followed by IAC exploration, although this is rarely necessary in these patients. The finding of Wallerian degeneration in the labyrinthine segment of the facial nerve in a longitudinal temporal bone fracture (Grobman *et al.*, 1989) indicates that middle fossa decompression may be necessary for optimal outcome, and should be considered in surgical planning (Felix *et al.*, 1991).

Another form of facial nerve injury due to temporal bone trauma is observed in the neonatal period. Harris *et al.* (1983) divided neonatal facial palsy into two types: conditions acquired during or soon after birth, and conditions that result from developmental disorders. The majority are due to blunt trauma to the nerve during delivery. This injury is thought to be due either to the shearing effect of forceps on the nerve as it exits the stylomastoid foramen (which is quite laterally placed and vulnerable in the skull base of a neonate), or through compressive injury by forceps

on the bone surrounding the vertical/mastoid portion of the fallopian canal. The prognosis of these injuries is very good, with approximately 90% of all acquired paralyses resolving spontaneously given time (Falco and Ericksson, 1990). Given that some of the remaining children will actually have a congenital deformity, such as an agenesis of the seventh nerve (Saito *et al.*, 1994), the consensus of opinion is that surgery is not indicated for the vast majority of infants with facial paralysis (Stenner, 1984).

Nonfracture blunt injuries

Blast injuries

The sudden massive pressure changes that result from explosions may have devastating effects on the ear. In an explosion, there is a short positive pressure phase, lasting milliseconds, followed by a longer-lived negative phase. The energy of each phase of the blast wave is equal, but the force vector is opposite for each phase (Kerr and Smyth, 1987).

Tympanic membrane injury in the pars tensa is common in blast injury, but chronic suppuration following this is less common than with perforations caused by pressurized water or welding trauma (Hough and McGee, 1991). The majority heal spontaneously. Kerr and Byrne (1975) reported that 83% of 66 perforated tympanic membranes caused by one explosion healed spontaneously. The implantation of squamous epithelium deep to the tympanic membrane results in the late complication of cholesteatoma formation in up to 12% (Seaman and Newell, 1971).

Ossicular chain injuries are unusual following an explosion. Inner ear injuries, however, are common, and sensorineural hearing loss and vertigo are frequent complaints. Most patients sustaining a significant blast injury will have a temporary hearing loss, known as a 'temporary threshold shift'. This phenomenon may result in quite severe hearing loss and is most marked immediately after the explosion, but usually resolves spontaneously within 24 hours (Kerr and Byrne, 1975). Hearing loss lasting longer than 24 hours is likely to be permanent. Tinnitus is also a sequel of blast injury and mirrors the severity and duration of the sensorineural hearing loss. Vertigo is usually temporary and resolves spontaneously in the majority of cases; those that do not improve should be suspected of having a perilymph fistula.

Injuries caused by water under pressure

The effects of water entering the ear under pressure can be devastating. Diving is the commonest cause of these injuries (48%), followed closely by water-skiing (30%) (Hough and McGee, 1991). Damage to the ear can also be iatrogenic. Syringing of the ear may cause tympanic membrane perforation, especially when the full force of the jet of water is directly on to the tympanic membrane. Caloric testing in patients with atrophic tympanic membranes can result in the same lesion. This trauma can easily be prevented by directing the water jet against the posterior EAC during irrigation.

Acute injuries from a sudden rush of pressurized water into the ear include tympanic membrane perforation (pars tensa), which is the commonest such injury, ossicular disruption, and rupture of the oval window annular ligament or round window membrane. The late complications of this include otitis media and cholesteatoma. Otitis media may be acute, subacute or chronic. Chronic otorrhoea develops in as many as 50% of these patients, and results in incudostapedial joint necrosis in a large number. Cholesteatoma occurs in 5% of this patient population (Hough and McGee, 1991).

Prevention is easily accomplished with occlusive ear plugs. Treatment of the actual injury is conservative. Even large perforations may heal if given time, appropriate otomicroscopical toilet and medical treatment. Surgical repair is indicated in those perforations that fail to close spontaneously in three to six months.

Penetrating temporal bone trauma

Foreign bodies

The EAC has several features that are protective against accidental foreign body insertion. These include its location deep in the conchal bowl, its protective coarse hairs and cerumen at its meatus, its narrow width and tortuosity, and its sensitive sensory innervation. Despite this, foreign body trauma via the ear canal remains one of the commonest presenting complaints in this specialty.

This is a largely paediatric problem; 73% of patients with foreign body trauma are children (Hough and McGee, 1991). Tympanic membrane perforations are very common, usually occurring posteriorly and often involving a large portion of the surface area of the drum. Ossicular injuries are also common, with more than 50% of ear explorations demonstrating significant ossicular disruption. The spectrum of these injuries is similar to that of temporal bone fractures. Occasionally, a foreign body can cause inner ear damage, either through subluxation of the stapes and disruption of oval window integrity or by trauma to the round window region.

Surgical trauma

The chorda tympani nerve is frequently disrupted during middle ear surgery, sometimes resulting in a disorder of taste and salivary secretion on the affected side, although such complaints are uncommon even after significant trauma to the nerve (Kerr and Smyth, 1987).

The jugular bulb is occasionally injured during transcanal tympanotomy procedures, as its bony covering in the floor of the middle ear may be deficient. Packing the area is frequently all that is required to alleviate the situation. Less frequently, a dehiscent carotid artery may be injured during middle ear surgery, an injury that may, on occasions, lead to a stroke, or death.

The facial nerve is at risk during surgery almost anywhere in the temporal bone and parotid regions. A thorough knowledge of the anatomy of the temporal bone and the facial nerve and its variations is essential before the junior surgeon is allowed to undertake even the most simple of middle ear procedures.

Stab and gunshot wounds

Other penetrating injuries in the temporal bone region include stabbing injuries and gunshot wounds. A stab wound is the result of a low energy mechanical blow and is unlikely to result in appreciable damage to the osseous integrity of the temporal bone. Sharp edged weapons will often glance off the temporal bone and damage the surrounding soft tissues. This is particularly important in the region of the skull base and zone III of the neck, as many critical vascular and neurological structures exist in this area and may be disrupted.

Gunshot wounds are the commonest cause of penetrating injury to the temporal bone. These wounds are the result of high energy mechanical blows and cause significant bone and soft tissue destruction and the deposition of foreign material in the wound. The effect depends upon the mass and velocity of the bullet. The kinetic energy (KE) imparted to the head can be expressed as $KE = 1/2\ MV^2$, in which M equals the mass of the bullet and V is its velocity. The effect also depends on the direction in which the missile comes in contact with the skull, and the course the projectile takes after it enters the temporal bone or the soft tissue of the skull base region. Harder missiles, such as copper-jacketed bullets, tend to penetrate deeply into the skull and remain intact, while softer missiles like lead bullets break up the soft tissue on entry and penetrate less deeply. The ipsilateral infraorbital region is the most common entrance site for gunshot wounds involving the temporal bone (Adkins and Osguthorpe, 1991).

As many as one-third of gunshot wounds to the temporal bone will result in significant, life-threatening injuries to the vascular structures contained within, and to the underlying central nervous system (Adkins and Osgunthorpe, 1991). Arteriography and CT scanning or MRI are mandatory investigations once the patient has been stabilized. Wounds should then undergo surgical exploration by the otoneurosurgical team, with debridement and, exploration of the facial nerve and middle ear. Soft tissue and bone reconstruction should be undertaken as for gunshot wounds elsewhere in the head. When the facial nerve is injured, it is usually in the tympanic or mastoid segments; these patients will have a concomitant conductive hearing loss.

Gunshot will remain in the temporal bone for some time after the original injury. One report by Kerr (1967) described a patient whose injury involved loss of the tympanic membrane and who had retained gunshot in the middle ear. This patient suffered the complication of erosion of the tegmen tympani and a subsequent herniation of a meningoencephalocoele into the middle ear. The presence or discovery of retained foreign material in the middle ear at any time following the injury is an indication for exploration and debridement (Kerr and Smyth, 1987).

Whiplash

The term whiplash injury refers to a sudden extension and/or flexion of the neck resulting from rapid acceleration and/or deceleration. These injuries are most commonly the result of sudden acceleration from a stopped position when a standing vehicle is struck by a moving one, usually when the standing vehicle is struck from the rear and the sudden acceleration causes neck extension. They are relatively rare in side collisions, where lateral flexion is the predominant movement (McNab, 1971). The complaints generated by such injuries are numerous, and litigation may result. Many people continue to complain of chronic symptoms generated by the whiplash, even years after the acute injury and the litigation surrounding it are over (Gotten, 1956). Aural symptoms following whiplash include deafness and tinnitus, and, more commonly vertigo and dysequilibrium, which are usually associated with neck pain. The symptoms may be elicited by certain head positions or neck movements, leading to the term 'cervical vertigo'.

The aetiology of 'cervical vertigo' is likely to be the disruption by the neck lesion of spinovestibular input and cervical proprioception. Other potential causes include irritation of the vertebral sympathetic plexus, disruption of the regional blood supply, direct irritation by the neck lesion of the periarterial plexus of the vertebral and basilar arteries, and compression of the subclavian artery and its tributary, the vertebral artery, by neck muscles in spasm (i.e. scalenus anterior) (Lee, 1987).

Symptoms often begin weeks or even months after the injury. They include headache, rotary vertigo, syncope, tinnitus and hearing loss (usually the low frequencies), nausea and vomiting, and visual symptoms such as flashing lights. One-third of patients will manifest a supraclavicular bruit on physical examination (Lee, 1987). It can be difficult to exclude functional causes of these symptoms, especially when matters of legal compensation arise.

Treatment is conservative, including bed rest, anti-inflammatory drugs and splinting for early injuries. Patients with chronic symptoms should receive instruction in proper posture and neck exercises, and should be given physiotherapy, cervical traction, neck immobilization with a collar, and local heat and massage.

Barotrauma

Barotrauma is defined as the pathophysiological effect of changes in ambient pressure affecting the air containing spaces of the temporal bone.

Injuries caused by water pressure

The majority of barotrauma injuries are related to scuba diving.

Ear canal

If air is trapped in the ear canal, and the ambient pressure is changed, EAC barotrauma can occur. This is most commonly the result of occlusive ear plug use, but may also occur with cerumen or foreign body impaction. Conditions that narrow the ear canal, such as the EAC exostoses that occur commonly in divers, will predispose the patient to this problem.

If air is trapped in the ear canal and the ambient pressure is increased, the relative pressure of the trapped air drops. This results in a 'reverse ear squeeze', which causes intense otalgia, haemorrhage into the skin of the ear canal, which can coalesce and expand into subepithelial blebs, and tympanic membrane rupture.

Middle ear

Barotrauma of the middle ear, called a 'middle ear squeeze', is experienced on descent whilst diving, and occurs because of failure to equalize the middle ear pressure with the increasing ambient pressure. This is the most common diving-related aural barotrauma, and is also the most common diving-related injury (Dickey, 1984). It occurs in up to 30% of novice divers and 10% of experienced divers. As the diver descends, aural pressure is the first symptom, during which time the tympanic membrane is retracted into the middle ear. Middle ear mucosal haemorrhage and bleb formation is common, and tympanic membrane rupture may occur. A pressure differential of 90 mmHg or more between the ambient pressure and the middle ear can result in locking of the eustachian tube, in which case it cannot be opened by the Valsalva manoeuvre (Taylor, 1959). Farmer and Thomas (1976) reported that a pressure differential of 500 mmHg will result in tympanic membrane rupture, which is experienced at a depth of 17.4 feet in salt water, and that ruptures can occur in depths as little as 4.3 feet of water. If the tympanic membrane ruptures, a caloric response stimulating the labyrinth can result in vertigo. This can be a distressing and life-threatening event, but usually abates after several minutes and does not recur on ascent.

An unusual occurrence following middle ear barotrauma is facial nerve paralysis, known as 'alternobaric facial nerve paralysis'. This rare entity occurs on ascent and is thought to be due to ischaemic changes in a dehiscent segment of the facial nerve in the middle ear. It is temporary and reverses spontaneously in the majority of subjects.

Inner ear

Vertigo has been experienced by as many as 50% of divers at some point in their lives (Lundgren *et al.*, 1974). In 'alternobaric vertigo', hearing loss and tinnitus do not occur, but the patient is suddenly seized by vertigo that lasts minutes to hours. This phenomenon results from relative overpressure of the middle ear (Inglestedt *et al.*, 1974) and the diver's inability to equalize the pressure in the middle ear. This causes a change in the pressure of the inner ear fluids.

Perilymph fistula is a recognized entity that causes fluctuating dizziness and deafness following otic barotrauma. The initial treatment of a patient with a perilymph fistula is bed rest (Singleton *et al.*, 1978). The fistula should be explored and repaired as soon as possible to preserve sensorineural hearing and stabilize vestibular function (Becker and Parell, 1979).

Air pressure injuries

Most aural barotrauma resulting from air travel occurs during descent, since the pressure of the air in a pressurized aeroplane is less than atmospheric at ground level. Alternobaric vertigo may occur on ascent. The vertical distance travelled in air must be greater to experience the same pressure changes as in water. For example, an 18 000 feet vertical change in altitude accomplishes the same change in pressure as a vertical move of only 16.5 feet in salt water.

Thermal trauma

Welding injuries

The EAC is a protective structure that prevents the migration of hot slag to the tympanic membrane and middle ear in the majority of affected subjects. The most common injury is therefore an EAC burn and otitis externa. Usually, no permanent damage is caused.

Tympanic membrane perforation is an uncommon but recognized complication of welding activity. This is less likely to regenerate spontaneously than other traumatic tympanic membrane perforations, due to ingrowth of avascular scar tissue. In the middle ear, ossicular chain damage is rare. Complications of aural slag injury include chronic otitis media, which occurs in up to 85% of affected ears (Hough and McGee, 1991).

Radiation injury

The ear is at risk during radiation exposure to the head and neck region. This is particularly true of therapeutic radiation for nasopharyngeal carcinoma and other skull base tumours. The most common clinical presentation is eustachain tube dysfunction, resulting in a middle ear effusion and a conductive hearing loss. Placement of a ventilating tube in the affected ear is often required.

Osteoradionecrosis of the temporal bone is claimed to be an unusual result of radiotherapy (Guida *et al.*, 1990), but otologists believe it to be more common than was once thought. Symptoms of this disorder include hearing loss (conductive, sensorineural, or mixed), otalgia, otorrhoea and sequestration of bone. The complications of temporal bone osteoradionecrosis include cranial neuropathy and intracranial infection. Treatment includes systemic antibiotics, local wound care, and debridement of devitalized tissue, including bony sequestra. Reconstruction of extensive debridement defects in the form of the importation of vascularized tissue or mastoid obliteration are occasionally required. Hyperbaric oxygen has provided some limited benefit in the treatment of this entity (Guida *et al.*, 1990).

Sensorineural hearing loss and vestibular injury are reported, although some authors feel that the association between inner ear dysfunction and radiotherapy is speculative (Kerr and Smyth, 1987).

Acoustic trauma

Injury to the inner ear by loud noise is a well recognized form of aural trauma. Acute acoustic trauma injuries follow the same course as the blast injuries and labyrinthine concussive injuries described above. Chronic exposure to high noise levels causes sensorineural hearing loss, and the characteristic audiogram of an individual affected by this condition demonstrates bilateral sensorineural hearing loss, which is usually symmetrical and maximal at 4000 Hz. Tinnitus is a common complaint. The diagnostic testing and aural rehabilitation is as for sensorineural hearing loss of any aetiology.

Conclusions

Trauma to the head is common, sudden and often devastating for the patient. It often has profound and lasting physical and psychological sequelae. The resulting deterioration in quality of life for the individual and the family can wreak havoc at home and in the work place, and has far reaching implications for society as a whole.

It is important to realize that more people are killed and injured in road traffic accidents than by any other cause. The major risk to health between the ages of one and 34 is now automobile accidents. Almost 75% of these involve the head. When the head is severely injured, the ear is the most frequently damaged sensory organ. Direct trauma to the ear in closed head injuries therefore constitutes an area of correctable aural pathology, in which the injuries are numerous and complex and vary enormously depending on the type and degree of the physical forces involved.

The importance of these injuries is therefore undeniable. The hitherto prevalent misconception that any permanent hearing loss secondary to skull trauma must be due to sensorineural damage and therefore irreparable must be banished for ever. In the past, otologists were seldom consulted about head injuries that involved hearing loss; even if they were, it was usually at a later stage when life-threatening injuries had been treated. Otologists must be an integral part of the head injuries team. The benefit of their expertise should be sought at the outset if the morbidity from head injury is to be reduced and the concomitant improvement in quality of life realized.

References

Adkins WY, Osguthorpe JD. (1991) Management of trauma of the facial nerve. *Otolaryngol Clin North Am* **24**: 587–611.

Aguilar EA, Yeakley JW, Ghorayeb BY, *et al.* (1987) High resolution CT scans of temporal bone fractures: association of facial paralysis with temporal bone fractures. *Head Neck Surg* **9**: 162–66.

Alford BR, Jerger JF, Coats AC, *et al.* (1970) Neurodiagnostic studies in facial paralysis *Ann Oto Rhinol Laryngol* **79**: 227–33.

Barber HO. (1965) Dizziness and head injury. *Can Med Assoc J* **92**: 974–78.

Barber HO. (1969) Head injury: audiological and vestibular findings. *Ann Otol Rhinol Laryngol* **78**: 239–52.

Barker A, Jalinous R, Freeton I. (1985) Noninvasive magnetic stimulation of the human motor cortex. *Lancet* **i**: 1106–107.

Becker GD, Parell GH. (1979) Otolaryngologic aspects of scuba-diving. *Otolaryngol Head Neck Surg* **87**: 569–72.

Bergman JM, Fredrickson JM. (1978) Vertigo after head injury: five year follow-up *J Otolaryngol* **7**: 237.

Betz BW, Weiner MD. (1991) Air in the temporomandibular joint fossa: CT sign of temporal bone fracture. *Radiology* **180**: 463–66.

Brawley BW, Kelly WA. (1967) Treatment of basal skull fractures with and without cerebrospinal fistulae. *J Neurosurg* **26**: 56–61.

Canniff JP. (1971) Otorrhoea in head injuries. *Br J Oral Surg* **8**: 203–10.

Cannon CR, Jahrsdoerfer RA. (1983) Temporal bone fractures: review of 90 cases. *Arch Otolaryngol* **109**: 285–88.

Cramer HB, Kartush JM. (1991) Testing facial nerve function. *Otolaryngol Clin North Am* **24**: 555–70.

Dickey LS. (1984) Diving injuries. *J Emerg Med* **1**: 249–62.

Esslen E. (1977) *Facial nerve surgery*. Birmingham: Aesculapius, 93–100.

Falco NA, Eriksson E. (1990) Facial nerve palsy in the newborn: incidence and outcome. *Plast Reconstr Surg* **85**: 1–4.

Farmer JC, Thomas WG. (1976) Ear and sinus problems in diving. In: Strauss RM, editor. *Diving medicine*. New York: Grune and Stratton, 109–33.

Felix H, Eby TL, Fisch U. (1991) New aspects of facial nerve pathology in temporal bone fractures. *Acta Otolaryngol* **111**: 332–36.

Fisch U. (1974) Facial paralysis in fractures of the petrous bone. *Laryngoscope* **84**: 2141–54.

Fisch U. (1980) Management of intratemporal facial nerve injuries. *J Laryngol Otol* **94**: 129–34.

Fisch U. (1981) Surgery for Bell's palsy. *Arch Otolaryngol* **107**: 1–11.

Ghorayeb BY, Yeakley JW. (1992) Temporal bone fractures: longitudinal or oblique? The case for oblique temporal bone fractures. *Laryngoscope* **102**: 129–34.

Gobman LR, Pollack A, Fisch U. (1989) Entrapment injury of the facial nerve resulting from longitudinal fracture of the temporal bone. *Otolaryngol Head Neck Surg* **101**: 404–409.

Goligher JE, Lloyd GAS. (1990) Fracture of the petrous temporal bone. *J Laryngol Otol* **104**: 438–39.

Gotten N. (1956) Survery of 100 cases of whiplash injury after settlement of litigation. *JAMA* **162**: 865–67.

Griffin JE, Altenau MM, Schaefer SD. (1979) Bilateral longitudinal temporal bone fractures: a retrospective review of seventeen cases. *Laryngoscope* **89**: 1432–35.

Grobman LR, Pollak A, Fisch U. (1989) Entrapment injury of the facial nerve resulting from longitudinal fracture of the temporal bone. *Otolaryngol Head Neck Surg* **101**: 404–408.

Grove WE. (1947) Hearing impairment due to craniocervical trauma. *Ann Otol* **56**: 264–70.

Guerrier Y, DeJean Y, Serrou B. (1965) Les surdites de transmission dans les traumatismes fermes du crane. *Otorhinolaryngologie* **1**: 11–65.

Guida RA, Finn DG, Buchalter IH, *et al.* (1990) Radiation injury to the temporal bone. *Am J Otol* **11**: 6–11.

Gurdjian ES. (1969) Head injury exhibit at World Congress of Neurological Sciences. *Med Post* **5**: 2–4.

Gurdjian ES, Webster JE. (1958) *Head injuries*. Boston: Little.

Gutnick HN, Kelleher MJ, Prass RL. (1990) A model of waveform reliability in facial nerve electroneurography. *Otolaryngol Head Neck Surg* **103**: 344–50.

Hagan PJ, Cole J. (1964) Medical management of injuries to the temporal bone and its contents. *Med Clin North Am* **48**: 1605–17.

Harris JP, Davidson TM, May M, *et al.* (1983) Evaluation and treatment of congenital facial paralysis. *Arch Otolaryngol* **109**: 145–51.

Harwood-Nash DC. (1970) Fractures of the petrous and tympanic parts of the temporal bone in children: a tomographic study of 35 cases. *Am J Roentgenol Radiother Nucl Med* **110**: 598–607.

Hough JVD. (1959) Incudostapedial joint separation. *Laryngoscope* **69**: 644–64.

Hough JVD. (1970) Surgical aspects of temporal bone fractures. *Proc R Soc Med* **63**: 245–52.

Hough JVD, McGee M. (1991) Otologic trauma. In: Parapella MM, *et al.* editors. *Otolaryngology*. London; Saunders, 1137–60.

Hough JVD, Stuart WD. (1968) Middle ear injuries in skull trauma. *Laryngoscope* **78**: 899–937.

Inglestedt S, Ivarsson A, Tjernstrom O. (1974) Vertigo due to relative overpressure in the middle ear. *Acta Otolaryngol* **78**: 1–14.

Jenkins H, Chmeil R, Jerger J. (1989) Speech tracking in the evaluation of a multichannel cochlear prosthesis. *Laryngoscope* **99**: 177–86.

Kerr AG. (1967) Gunshot injury of the temporal bone – a histological report. *J Ir Med Assoc* **162**: 446–48.

Kerr AG, Byrne JET. (1975) Concussive effects of a bomb blast on the ear. *J Laryngol Otol* **89**: 131–43.

Kerr AG, Smyth GDL. (1987) Ear trauma. In: *Scott-Brown's otolaryngology*, 5th edition. Somerset: Butterworths,

Kettle K. (1950) Peripheral facial palsy in fractures of the temporal bone. *Arch Otolaryngol* **51**: 25–41.

Lambert PR, Brackmann DE. (1984) Facial paralysis in longitudinal temporal bone fractures: a review of 26 cases. *Laryngoscope* **94**: 1022–26.

Lange G, Kornhuber HH. (1962) Zur bedeutung peripherund zentralvestibularer Storungren nach Kopftraumen. *Arch Ohr Nas Kehlkopfheilk* **179**: 366.

Lee KJ. (1987) The vestibular system and its disorders: Part II. In: Lee KJ, editor. *Essential otolaryngology, head and neck surgery*. New York: Medical Examination Publishing, 113–28.

LeLiever WC, Barber HO. (1980) Delayed endolymphatic hydrops. *J Otolaryngol* **9**: 375–80.

Lieberherr U, Schwarzenbach D, Fisch U. (1990) Management of severe facial nerve paralysis in temporal bone fracture – a review of 82 cases. In: Castro D, editor. *Facial Nerve.* Amsterdam: Kugler & Ghedini, 285–89.

Lundgren CE, Tjernstrom O, Ornhagen H. (1974) Alternobaric vertigo – a diving hazard: an epidemiological study. *Undersea Biomed Res* **1**: 251–58.

MacGee EE, Cauthen JC, Brackett CE. (1970) Meningitis following acute traumatic cerebrospinal fluid fistula. *J Neurosurg* **33**: 312–17.

May M. (1980) Facial nerve paralysis. In: Paparella MM, Shumrick DA, editors. *Otolaryngology*, 2nd edition. London: Saunders, 1680–704.

May M, Klein SR. (1983) Facial nerve decompression complications. *Laryngoscope* **93**: 299–305.

May M, Harvey JE, Marovitz WF, *et al.* (1971) The prognostic accuracy of the maximal stimulation test compared with that of the nerve excitability test in Bell's palsy. *Laryngoscope* **81**: 931–38.

May M, Hardin WB, Sullivan J, *et al.* (1976) Natural history of Bell's palsy: the salivary flow test and other prognostic indicators. *Laryngoscope* **86**: 704–12.

May M, Blumenthal F, Taylor FH. (1981) Bell's palsy: surgery based upon prognostic indicators and results. *Laryngoscope* **91**: 2092–103.

McGraw BL, Cole RR. (1990) Paediatric maxillofacial trauma. Age-related variations in injury. *Arch Otolaryngol Head Neck Surg* **116**: 41–45.

McGuirt, WF, Stool SE. (1992) Temporal bone fractures in children: a review with emphasis on long-term sequelae. *Clin Paediatr* **31**: 12–18.

McHugh HE. (1959) The surgical treatment of facial paralysis and traumatic conductive deafness in fractures of the temporal bone. *Ann Otol* **68**: 855–89.

McHugh HE. (1963) Facial paralysis in birth injury and skull fractures. *Arch Otolaryngol* **78**: 443.

McNab I. (1971) The 'whiplash syndrome.' *Orthop Clin North Am* **2**: 389–403.

Mitchell DP, Stone P. (1973) Temporal bone fractures in children. *Can J Otolaryngol* **2**: 156–62.

Morgan WE, Coker NJ, Jenkins HA. (1994) Histopathology of temporal bone fractures: implications for cochlear implantation. *Laryngoscope* **104**: 426–32.

Murakami M, Ohtani I, Aikawa T, *et al.* (1990) Temporal bone findings in two cases of head injury. *J Laryngol Otol* **104**: 986–89.

Paparella MM, Mancini F. (1983) Trauma and Menière's syndrome. *Laryngoscope* **93**: 1004–1012.

Parnes LS, Price-Jones RG. (1993) Particle repositioning maneuver for benign positional vertigo. *Ann Otol Rhinol Laryngol* **102**: 325–31.

Perlman HB. (1939) Process of healing in injuries to the capsule of the labyrinth. *Arch Otolaryngol* **29**: 287–305.

Podoshin L, Fradis M. (1975) Hearing loss after head injury. *Arch Otolaryngol* **101**: 15–18.

Pollanen MS, Deck JHN, Blenkinsop B, *et al.* (1992) Fracture of the temporal bone with exsanguination: pathology and mechanism. *Can J Neurol Sci* **19**: 196–200.

Proctor B, Gurdjian ES, Webster JE. (1956) The ear in head trauma. *Laryngoscope* **66**: 16–59.

Rizvi SS, Gibbin KP. (1979) Effect of transverse temporal bone fracture on the fluid compartment of the inner ear. *Ann Otol Rhinol Laryngol* **87**: 797–803.

Saito H, Takeda T, Kishimoto S. (1994) Neonatal facial nerve defect. *Acta Otolaryngol (Suppl)* **510**: 77–81.

Schuknecht HF. (1950) A clinical study of auditory damage following blows to the head. *Ann Otol* **59**: 331–36.

Schuknecht HF. (1969) Mechanism of inner ear injury from blows to the head. *Ann Otol* **78**: 253–62.

Schuknecht HF, editor. (1974) *Pathology of the ear.* Boston: Harvard University.

Seaman RW, Newell RC. (1971) Another etiology of cholesteatoma. *Arch Otolaryngol* **94**: 440–42.

Seki Y, Krain L, Yamada T, *et al.* (1990) Transcranial magnetic stimulation of the facial nerve: recording technique and estimation of the stimulated site. *Neurosurgery* **26**: 286–90.

Shepard NT, Telian SA, Smith-Wheelock M. (1990) Habituation and balance retraining therapy: a retrospective review. *Neurol Clin North Am* **8**: 459–75.

Singleton G, Karlan M, Post K, Bock D. (1978) Perilymph fistulas: diagnostic criteria and therapy. *Ann Otol Rhinol Laryngol* **87**: 797–803.

Stenner E. (1984) Indications for facial nerve surgery. *Adv Otorhinolaryngol* **34**: 214–26.

Taylor GD. (1959) The otolaryngologic aspects of skin and scuba diving. *Laryngoscope* **69**: 809–59.

Telian SA, Shepard NT, Smith-Wheelock M, *et al.* (1990) Habituation therapy for chronic vestibular dysfunction: preliminary results. *Otolaryngol Head Neck Surg* **103**: 89–95.

Tos M. (1971) Prognosis of hearing in temporal bone fractures. *J Laryngol Otol* **85**: 1147–55.

Tos M. (1973) Course and sequelae of 248 petrosal fractures. *Acta Otolaryngol* **75**: 353–54.

Ulrich K. (1926) Verletzungen des gehororgans bei Schadelbasisfrakturen. (Eine histologische und klinissche Studie). *Acta Otolaryngol (Suppl)* **6**: 1–150.

Ward PH. (1969) The histopathology of audiological and vestibular disorders in head trauma. *Ann Otol* **78**: 227–38.

Weissman JL, Curtain HD. (1992) Pneumolabyrinth: a computed tomographic sign of temporal bone fracture. *Am J Otolaryngol* **13**: 113–14.

Wennmo C, Spandow O. (1993) Fractures of the temporal bone – chain incongruities. *Am J Otolaryngol* **14**: 38–42.

Wormald PJ, Sellars SL, DeVilliers JC. (1991) Bilateral facial nerve palsies: Groote Schuur Hospital experience. *J Laryngol Otol* **105**: 625–27.

Wright JW, Taylor CE, Bizal JA. (1969) Tomography and the vulnerable incus. *Ann Otol* **78**: 263–79.

Ylikoski J. (1988) Delayed endolymphatic hydrops syndrome after heavy exposure to impulse noise. *Am J Otol* **9**: 282–85.

23

Trauma to the external and middle ear

Marcus D Atlas, John E Fenton

Introduction

Twenty years ago, the majority of trauma cases affecting the head and neck were due to road traffic accidents, sports and occupational injuries, but in recent years the relative incidence has fallen. This is due to the increase in drug and gang-related violence, as well as child and spouse abuse (Holt, 1992). There has been a 66% increase in cases of child abuse during a recent eight-year period (1980–1988) in the USA (Willner *et al.*, 1992).

This chapter deals specifically with trauma and the consequences of trauma to the external and middle ear.

Pinna

The pinna is an exposed part of the human anatomy and is therefore susceptible to injury. Trauma to the pinna is common and may be classified as blunt, sharp or thermal. These injuries can be further subdivided by the severity of the injury (Table 23.1).

The lateral surface of the auricle is covered by tightly adherent layers of skin and perichondrium. Haematoma auris or othaematoma occur most frequently after repeated injuries to the ear, such as in wrestling or boxing. The mechanism of injury is a shearing force that separates the cartilage from the overlying perichondrium (Templer and Renner, 1990). A haematoma collects between the perichondrium and the cartilage if the injury is sufficient to cause tearing of the perichondrial blood vessels. The resultant haematoma usually

presents as a firm painful swelling on the lateral surface of the pinna, obscuring the normal contours, but a medial haematoma is almost always associated with complete fracture of the cartilage (Kirsch and Amedee, 1991). The blood supply of the cartilage is via the perichondrium; therefore a seroma or haematoma may compromise the blood supply. A small collection of blood usually forms granulation tissue and then dense fibrous tissue, which results in a mild, painless deformity. A larger collection may organize and result in a more

Table 23.1. Classification of auricular injury

Blunt
  Ecchymosis
  Seroma
  Haematoma

Sharp
  Abrasion
  Simple laceration (greater or less than 2 cm)
  Complex laceration
  Lobule
  Near-total avulsion
  Amputation

Thermal burns (chemical/electrical)
  First degree: erythema and oedema of skin, involving only the epidermis
  Second degree: blister formation and weeping, destroys epidermis, portion of dermis
  Third degree: full thickness of the skin
  Fourth degree: irreversible loss of skin and cartilage

Cold
  Frostbite
  Gangrene

noticeable deformity but the presence of avascular necrosis of the cartilage causes marked deformity of the ear. This is often termed 'cauliflower or wrestler's ear'.

Bilateral auricular haematomata in children are considered a manifestation of child abuse (Willner *et al.*, 1992). Another manifestation of child abuse is the 'tin ear syndrome', which is a triad of auricular bruising, haemorrhagic retinopathy and ipsilateral subdural haematoma with severe cerebral oedema, caused by a blow to the side of the head and ear (Leavitt *et al.*, 1992).

Sharp injuries of the auricle vary from insignificant abrasions to total amputation. Large partial avulsions may survive on the most tenuous of skin pedicles.

Burns of the head and neck involve the pinna in more than 50% of patients (Kirsch and Amedee, 1991). The burns are classified using the recognized criteria, with the addition of a fourth degree indicating cartilage involvement (Table 23.1). It may be difficult to differentiate between second and third degree burns and a number of features detailing the type of incident have to be recorded. Electrical and chemical burns result in the most tissue damage, followed in decreasing order of severity by flames, liquids, immersion in water, scalds and flash burns. The features that help to categorize burns are the appearance of the lesion, the presence or absence of sensation, the course of the healing process and other tests using various substances such as dyes.

The damage should be recorded on a diagram with reference to the extent (in percentage terms) relative to the whole pinna in blunt or thermal trauma, and to the size of the wound in cases of sharp trauma.

Management

It is almost impossible to restore the normal appearance of the pinna following significant trauma. The best management is the avoidance of injury. Wrestlers, boxers and rugby forwards should be required to wear protective headgear. The treatment of choice for all but very small auricular haematomas is a cosmetically appropriate incision in a hidden area, carried out under aseptic conditions, and the evacuation of the blood clot with reapposition of the perichondrium. The prevention of recurrence and of infection is vital, and is achieved using bolster splints with through and through sutures.

Abrasions should be cleansed frequently and antibiotic ointment applied to prevent infection. The area should be covered with a skin graft if a significant amount of skin is avulsed from the lateral surface with exposure of perichondrium. Skin grafts will not survive over bare cartilage and pedicled flaps may have to be used. Small (less than 2 cm) lacerations of the pinna can be repaired primarily without any difficulty. Lacerations of the auricle that extend through the skin, cartilage and perichondrium should be resutured in layers. Primary reattachment should be attempted following near-total avulsion of the pinna as a small pedicle may provide an adequate blood supply (Clemons and Severeid, 1993).

An amputated pinna should be cleansed and stored in a solution of iced saline and an antibiotic. The patient should be placed on intravenous antibiotics and many authors advocate low dose or full heparinization. The subcutaneous placement of de-epithelized cartilage and conversion of the avulsed segment into a retroauricular composite graft, is probably the optimal treatment in cases of amputation treated more than four hours following an injury (Kirsch and Amedee, 1991). Reconstruction of the pinna using various prostheses can also be performed.

The treatment aims following burns to the pinna are to preserve skin and to prevent infection. The burned pinna is very susceptible to the development of chondritis if debridement is too aggressive and it is advisable to remove loose necrotic tissue only.

Complications

The principal complications of auricular trauma (Table 23.2) are deformity and disfigurement due to loss of cartilage and a combination of fibrosis or cartilage necrosis (Clemons and Severeid, 1993).

Infections of the pinna are divided into stage 1 (perichondritis) and stage 2 (chondritis) (Clemons and Severeid, 1993). Perichondritis is a soft tissue

Table 23.2. Complications of auricular trauma

Infection
    Stage 1:   perichondritis
    Stage 2:   chondritis

Keloid

'Cauliflower ear'

infection that has not yet violated the perichondrium and occurs prior to abscess formation. Chondritis refers to cartilage infections with abscess formation and cartilage necrosis. Perichondritis manifests as a painful erythematous pinna with oedema and sparing of the lobule. The quinalone antibiotics (ciprofloxacin) are the treatment of choice for this condition, as the antibacterial activity includes the usual organisms causing pinna infections (*Pseudomonas* and *Staphyloccus*).

Chondritis can result from all forms of auricular injury; the risk of infection is increased considerably when the overlying skin of the pinna is penetrated or lacerated. Auricular perichondritis and perichondrial abscesses are recognized complications of the fashionable 'high' ear piercing (Widick and Coleman, 1993). Ear piercing of auricular cartilage carries the risk of implanting micro-organisms and the reduced vascular supply in this area adds to the risk of infection.

Chondritis has been reported in up to 20% of all ear burns (Skedros *et al.*, 1992). The onset of infection is usually insidious and can often take three to five weeks to develop. It is characterized by dull pain followed by erythema, oedema, increasing temperature and tenderness. This can lead to suppuration with destruction of the cartilaginous structure. *Pseudomonas* is the most common organism, and has been isolated in 80–95% of cultures (Skedros *et al.*, 1992). The prevention of chondritis involves the avoidance of pressure, the removal of all hair in the vicinity, and cleansing with antibacterial soap followed by the application of topical antibiotics. Systemic antibiotics have little effect on chondritis once it has developed. Some authors recommend local instillation or irrigation with antibiotics (Afelberg *et al.*, 1974; Stevenson, 1964) or iontophoresis (Templer and Renner, 1990). The debridement of infected cartilage should be conservative with respect to the extent of tissue removal.

Keloid formation is a complication of ear lobe injury that may be a result of lacerations, burns or ear piercing. Various forms of treatment have been suggested, including repeated triamcinalone injections and laser excision.

Measurement of outcome

The pinna performs only marginal functions of augmenting sound delivery and sound localization (Templer and Renner, 1990). Individuals losing the auricle are more concerned with the cosmetic defect and with support for eyewear or a hearing aid.

External auditory canal

The examination of the external auditory meatus for evidence of trauma should document the presence of bleeding or cerebrospinal fluid leakage. The size and site of a laceration or haematoma should be recorded diagrammatically. The circumference of the bony canal should be assessed carefully for a step deformity, which indicates a fracture. The tympanic membrane should also be examined.

The incidence of casualty attendance due to foreign bodies in the external canal ranges from 1 in 219 to 1 in 1792 of all patients registering at accident and emergency departments (Bressler and Shelton, 1993). The type of foreign body may include anything that fits into the ear canal including insects, beads, crayons and cotton wool (Figure 23.1).

The epithelium of the osseous portion of the external canal is delicate and sometimes even minimal trauma, such as the use of cotton buds, can result in a haematoma. The lining of the cartilaginous canal is tougher and haematoma is less common. Extensive lacerations due to knife injuries, bites or road traffic accidents may sever the external canal and result in stenosis.

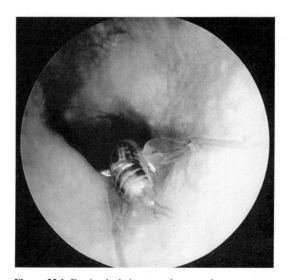

Figure 23.1. Foreign body in external ear canal.

Fractures involving the bony canal can occur following trauma. These are often in association with more obvious and life-threatening injuries, and as a consequence, may be overlooked or ignored. The force of trauma that is sufficient to fracture the temporal bone occurs when the head collides with an immovable object such as in a road traffic accident. Similar forces occur when a missile is directed against the head, such as a bullet from a gun (Kinney, 1992).

Fractures involving the temporal bone are divided into longitudinal, transverse and mixed. The line of a longitudinal fracture of the temporal bone is in the long axis of the petrous bone and involves the roof of the bony external canal, the tympanic cavity and parts of the inner ear (Figure 23.2). These fractures usually result from trauma to the lateral aspect of the head. Posterior fractures extend through the mastoid air cells, external ear canal and tegmen tympani, posterior to the cochlea and labyrinth (Roche, 1975). A bony deformity of the external meatus may be obvious and bleeding may be a presenting sign if the canal skin is lacerated. Any bleeding or leakage of clear fluid from the external canal following head injury indicates the presence of a fracture of the temporal bone until proven otherwise. Ecchymosis of the postauricular area (Battle's sign) is indicative of a temporal bone fracture and usually develops within 24 hours of the injury. Anterior canal wall fractures

occur following posterior dislocations of the mandible and may result in bony occlusion of the canal.

High resolution CT scanning with bone algorithms has become the standard investigation for localization of trauma within the temporal bone. Any significant fracture should be detected with axial and coronal imaging.

Management

A fracture of the bony meatus may need reduction or excision of the displaced fragment, but involvement of the middle ear, facial nerve or the inner ear usually dictates the type of treatment. Early treatment is required because displaced fragments may cause stenosis of the canal. Management of a posterior dislocation of the mandible involves relocating the displaced bone anteriorly and stenting of the external canal.

Foreign bodies in the external canal may produce lacerations of the meatal skin, ossicular dislocation, perforation of the tympanic membrane, otitis externa, haematoma and facial palsy (Bressler and Shelton, 1993).

Complications (Table 23.3)

External auditory canal stenosis

Localized proliferation of fibrous tissue, forming webs in the external auditory canal, may follow injuries by corrosives or foreign bodies. Treatment using local methods such as cautery and topical antibiotics are notoriously unsuccessful and most, ultimately, require a canal-widening procedure. A soft tissue stenosis may result from local lacerations, especially complete transection of the external canal. The stenosis can range from mild narrowing to complete occlusion. The formation of a 'false fundus' or complete stenosis occurs when there is a circumferential loss of epithelium and

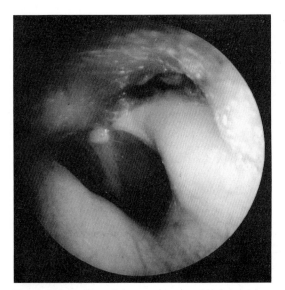

Figure 23.2. Fracture of the petrous temporal bone involving superior external canal and middle ear, causing haemotympanum.

Table 23.3. Complications of external auditory canal trauma

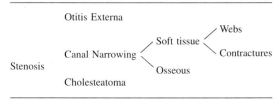

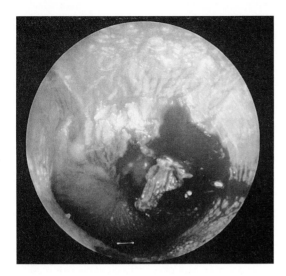

Figure 23.3. Traumatic tympanic membrane perforation.

fibrosis of the ear canal. Exact figures on the incidence of post-traumatic external auditory canal stenosis are not available in the literature. The surgical treatment requires excision of the soft tissue stenosis, bony canal enlargement and a split-skin graft. Obliteration of the mastoid and middle ear cavities may have to be performed for severe disruption of the canal wall (Kveton, 1987). Surgical correction of acquired external auditory canal stenosis is often difficult to achieve but success rates of up to 82% (McDonald *et al.*, 1986) have been reported.

External auditory canal cholesteatoma

A variety of injuries of the temporal bone can lead to the development of cholesteatoma, but there is no typical temporal bone injury that predisposes to cholesteatoma formation (Strohm, 1986). Post-traumatic cholesteatoma is a rare late complication of a fractured temporal bone (Bottrill, 1991) and probably occurs more often than has been described in the literature. The incidence has been estimated as 5.7% of all longitudinal temporal bone fractures and 6.1% of all injuries to the bony canal wall (Strohm, 1986). Cholesteatoma can occur long after the injury, and cases have been reported occurring up to 12 years following trauma (Freeman, 1983). Cholesteatoma can also occur in the absence of a fracture, due to the epithelium between the site of a stenosis and the tympanic membrane continuing to desquamate, leading to entrapped keratin debris. This creates an ear canal

cholesteatoma that gradually enlarges and progressively erodes surrounding bone and soft tissue (McKennan and Chole, 1992). A causal relationship between trauma and cholesteatoma is difficult to prove, especially when there is a lengthy time gap between the events. The clinical features that support a traumatic aetiology of a cholesteatoma in a patient with a history of head injury are: an aerated mastoid; an unusual site; formation adjacent to the fracture line; or formation deep to post-traumatic external canal stenosis. A cholesteatoma may be presumed to be present before the injury in the absence of a wide fracture line and in the presence of a sclerotic mastoid (Kerr and Smyth, 1987).

Measurement of outcome

The objective in management of trauma to the external canal is to attain normal hearing and a self-cleansing ear that is free of infection.

Haemotympanum

Haemotympanum is defined as a middle ear cavity containing blood in the presence of an intact ear drum (Figure 23.4). This is as a result of bleeding into the middle ear cavity due to a temporal bone fracture or to ossicular trauma. Haemotympanum

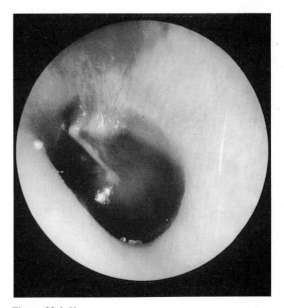

Figure 23.4. Haemotympanum.

may be evident when the stapes is the only ossicle involved in the injury (Bellucci, 1983). Clinically the tympanic membrane (TM) appears blue-red and there is a moderate conductive hearing loss of approximately 40 dB. The haemotympanum usually resolves spontaneously in between six weeks and three months.

Tympanic membrane perforation

Traumatic perforation of the TM (Figure 23.4) has been estimated to occur in 1.4–8.6 per 100 000 population (Kristensen, 1992).

TM perforations almost invariably involve the pars tensa and the majority are reported to occur in either the anteroinferior (Lindemann *et al.*, 1987; Strohm, 1986) or posteroinferior quadrants (Ludman, 1988). The posterosuperior quadrant of the pars tensa contains a higher proportion of elastic fibres than the other parts and is therefore less likely to perforate (Jensen and Bonding, 1993). The TM is more susceptible to traumatic rupture if the structure has been scarred or is atrophic. TM perforations are more common in older patients.

The classification of traumatic TM perforations is based on the causative mechanism (Table 23.4). The most frequent causes are self-induced injury during attempts to clean the external canal, or a slap against the ear (Lindemann, 1987). Traumatic TM perforations during childhood, especially repeated events, are considered a manifestation of child abuse and have been described in association with Meadow's syndrome or 'Munchausen's by proxy' (Leavitt *et al.*, 1992). A traumatic ear drum perforation can occur due to compression of fluid in the external auditory canal following water-sports such as waterpolo or water-skiing. Scaldings by hot water, and oil, plastic and particles from grindstone or welding tasks are typical examples of thermal causes of TM ruptures (Strohm, 1986). Longitudinal fractures of the temporal bone may cause a tear of the ear drum when they involve the tympanic ring. TM perforation is the most common otological finding following lightning injuries (Jones *et al.*, 1991).

The clinical features of TM perforation include otalgia, blood-stained or mucopurulent otorrhoea, hearing loss, tinnitus, or a history of trauma. All patients should be attended to, in the acute phase, by an otolaryngologist. The perforation should be recorded diagrammatically, noting the quadrant(s) and the percentage of the TM involved. Air compressive ruptures are single and are either radially directed slits or triangular in shape. Fluid compression produces rounded edges that are often not blood-encrusted when examined (Strohm, 1986). The characteristic feature of lightning injuries is a complete disintegration of the TM (Redleaf and McCabe, 1993). The additional factors that must be assessed in the management of traumatic perforations are the mechanism of injury, the hearing status, the presence or absence of infection, and the presence of skin flaps.

The initial management is nonsurgical and most clinicians advocate observation and possibly prophylactic oral antibiotics. Antibiotic eardrops should be added to the treatment regimen if infection is present. Spontaneous healing should take place within four to six weeks (Glasscock and Cueva, 1991) but has been reported at up to 10 months (Kronenberg *et al.*, 1988). Large epithelial flaps folded into the middle ear should be approximated under general anaesthesia. Myringoplasty should be considered if the perforation has failed to heal after about two or three months. Any associated ossicular discontinuity should also be repaired at that time.

Complications

Chronic otitis media is more common following thermal, blast and water pressure-induced perforations. Ear discharge has been reported in 50% of patients who received water-sport injuries (Hough, 1980). Otitis media can also be induced by penetrative injuries, when retained foreign material, such as bullet fragments, also predispose to infection. Oral antibiotics and ear drops should be used following thermal perforation, especially those due to welding sparks and hot liquids. Patients with retained foreign material in the ear should undergo an exploratory tympanotomy and tympanoplasty once the otorrhoea has settled (Glasscock and Cueva, 1991).

Table 23.4. Classification of tympanic membrane trauma

Penetrating
Air pressure
  Nonblast
  Blast
Fluid pressure
Thermal
Fractures of the temporal bone
Lightning

The rim of a traumatic perforation tends to fold medially and may adhere to the promontory or incudostapedial joint (Strohm, 1986).

Faulty healing of the TM can result in the formation of a thin atrophic membrane covering the perforation. This is called a 'replacement membrane'. Post-traumatic cholesteatoma can result from a perforated TM. The two theories of development are: ingrowth of epithelium in posterosuperior perforations; and spalling, which is middle ear implantation of myringeal epithelial cells. This is especially likely to occur secondary to blasts, which are associated with large central perforations (Kristensen, 1992). Epithelial cysts have been found in the middle ear following the spontaneous healing of an ear drum after blast-induced injuries (Kerr and Byrne, 1975). Cholesteatoma has been described following post-traumatic eustachian tube obstruction resulting from a longitudinal temporal bone fracture (Strohm, 1986). The implication of trauma in the development of a cholesteatoma is difficult to prove and the features of post-traumatic external canal cholesteatoma discussed in the previous section apply here also.

The extent of the conductive hearing loss in an ear with a ruptured TM and a normal ossicular chain is directly related to the size, not the site, of the perforation. The average hearing loss ranges from 12–28 dB (Browning, 1986). The mean conductive hearing loss in a study of nonexplosive blast injury of the TM was 11.2 dB (Berger *et al.*, 1994).

Prognosis

About 80% of all traumatic ruptures diagnosed within two weeks of the injury, will heal spontaneously (Kristensen, 1992). The likelihood of complete healing is increased by the presence of a highly pneumatized mastoid air cell system but does not appear to be affected by increasing age or by the site of the perforation (Kristensen, 1992). Primary spontaneous healing can take up to 10 months to occur (Kronenberg *et al.*, 1988), but there is no way, at present, of predicting accurately the amount of time required for perforations to heal. Ultimately, 94.8% of nonblast injuries heal spontaneously, compared with 80–83% of blast injuries (Berger *et al.*, 1994). Lightning injuries demonstrate a remarkable ability to heal spontaneously despite the extreme damage to the TM (Redleaf and McCabe, 1993).

The procedure of myringoplasty is successful in 85.3% of cases following TM rupture (Strohm, 1986).

The ossicular chain

Trauma to the ossicular chain occurs in 23% of all temporal bone fractures and in approximately 2% of all cases of blunt skull trauma (Strohm, 1986).

The classification of ossicular damage is dependent on the site and type of injury (Table 23.5). The injury may be a dislocation, fracture or fixation (fibrous or osseous) of the ossicle. The damage may be further subclassified by the site.

The most commonly affected ossicle is the incus and the most frequently found defect is a dislocation of the incudostapedial joint. The incus is the most vulnerable ossicle for displacement, and 80% of persistent post-traumatic conductive hearing loss is due to subluxation of this ossicle (Ludman, 1988). A fracture dislocation of the stapes is the most frequently encountered abnormality in ossicular trauma associated with a penetrating injury (Kinney, 1992). Post-traumatic fixations are rare and usually involve the mallear head (Strohm, 1986).

Blunt skull trauma is the most frequent cause of ossicular chain injuries, but the precise mechanisms are not certain. Hough and Stuart (1968) have proposed that they may be due to: tetanic contractions of the middle ear muscles; vibrations from strong impulses; inertia secondary to acceleration/deceleration of the head; or when the middle ear walls are split by a temporal bone fracture and the fragments move apart. The

Table 23.5. Classification of ossicular chain trauma

Dislocation	Incudostapedial joint	
	Malleoincudal joint	
	Incus/stapes/malleus	
Fracture	Stapes	Crura
		Neck
	Incus	Long process
	Malleus	Handle
Fixation	Fibrous/adhesions	Malleus
		Incus
		Stapes
	Osseous	Incus
		Annular ligament
		Mallear head ligaments
		Incudal fossa ligaments
Combined injuries		

formation of new bone between the ossicle and the middle ear wall around a fracture line causes osseous ossicular fixation. Fixations develop gradually and surgical management has been required for hearing loss acquired many years after the injury. The average time lapse is 16 years (Strohm, 1986).

Ossicular damage can occur in the absence of a temporal bone fracture or a perforated TM. Otoscopic examination fails to provide a diagnosis of ossicular trauma in more than 50% of all skull injuries (Strohm, 1986). The major clinical feature is of a conductive hearing loss but the degree of impairment varies greatly; it may be less severe if fibrous adhesions have formed between the fragments. An injury to the ossicular chain must be suspected if a traumatic perforation involves the posterosuperior quadrant of the ear drum. Tinnitus may occasionally be associated with a pure middle ear lesion (Strohm, 1986).

Pure-tone audiometry provides documentation of the type and degree of hearing loss. Impedance testing and tympanometry are helpful, but not diagnostic of a particular type of ossicular chain discontinuity (Strohm, 1986). High resolution CT scans of the middle ear are able to detect abnormalities of the mallear head and the body and long process of the incus, but can only reveal 60% of stapes superstructure abnormalities and 33% of the disorders affecting the malleal manubrium (Fuse *et al.*, 1992). A definitive diagnosis can be made only at exploratory tympanotomy.

Management

A conductive hearing loss persisting for three months after trauma, and with no evidence of middle ear fluid, requires surgical exploration. The treatment is ossiculoplasty and the type of reconstruction is dependent on the injury. Homograft or allografts are utilized to reconstruct the ossicular chain, but discussion of the reparative techniques employed is not within the scope of this chapter. Some patients elect to have no treatment for a mild hearing loss and others successfully use a hearing aid.

Complications

Conductive hearing loss is the principal middle ear complication of ossicular trauma and is best treated with an ossiculoplasty. Ossicular trauma may compromise the minimal blood supply to the long process of the incus and result in delayed necrosis and conductive hearing loss (Kerr and Smyth, 1987). Incudostapedial joint separation as a result of delayed necrosis of the incus was discovered in over 50% of patients in a study of trauma to the middle ear. The majority of these findings were in association with chronic otitis media (Hough, 1980). Another study by Berger *et al.* (1994) did not find any cases of chronic otorrhoea or necrosis of the long process, which suggests that delayed necrosis of the long process of the incus is an uncommon complication in the absence of an associated chronic inflammation. A fracture or subluxation of the stapes may cause a perilymph fistula. Tinnitus may develop following ossicular damage and can be a permanent finding, depending on the degree of concussive injury to the inner ear (Bellucci, 1983). The consequences of inner ear trauma will be discussed in another chapter. There are no available figures in the literature that allow estimation of the incidence of tinnitus following middle ear injury.

Measurement of outcome/prognosis

The operative hearing results are excellent and usually better than ossiculoplasty in chronic otitis media. The probability is good of a conductive hearing loss of less than 20 dB following surgical repair. Ossicular reconstruction that requires repositioning of a luxated stapes is expected to result in a conductive hearing loss greater than 20 dB (Strohm, 1986). The results of tympanoplasty types II and III have been reported by Strohm (1986) resulting in a persistent air–bone gap of 0–35 dB (mean 13 dB).

Barotrauma

Barotrauma (Figure 23.5) occurs when the middle ear pressure fails to equalize with the external air pressure as a result of failure of the eustachian tube to function properly. The failure of the eustachian tube to relieve negative middle ear pressure is called 'locking'. This occurs when there is a pressure difference of 80 mmHg or more. This pressure is too great for the normal opening of the eustachian tube by muscular action and the persistence of reduced middle ear pressure causes damage. The most frequent causes of barotrauma

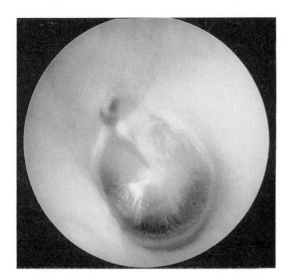

Figure 23.5. Barotrauma causing redness along manubrium of malleus.

are changes of altitude during flying or changes in depth during diving.

The classification of barotrauma is based on the severity of otoscopic findings on examination (Table 23.6). Ossicular dislocation or discontinuity can also result from severe pressure (Bellucci, 1983).

Clinical symptoms are usually absent or minimal in the first two grades but can be severe following grade 3 or 4 trauma. The clinical features include otalgia, hearing loss, tinnitus and vertigo.

Table 23.6. Classification of barotrauma (Igarashi *et al.*, 1993)

Grade 0	Normal
Grade 1	Retraction with redness in pars tensa and along the manubrium
Grade 2	Retraction with redness of the entire tympanic membrane
Grade 3	Same as grade 2 plus evidence of a middle ear effusion or haemotympanum
Grade 4	Tympanic membrane perforation

Barotrauma is prevented by the avoidance of flying with an upper respiratory tract infection, the avoidance of sleeping during descent, the use of topical nasal vasoconstrictors before descent, and autoinflation. The treatment of middle ear barotrauma includes simple observation, eustachian tube catheterization and myringotomy.

Acknowledgement

The authors thank Dr B Black for the kind permission to publish his still photography of the ear.

References

Afelberg DB, Waisbren BA, Masters FW, *et al.* (1974) Treatment of chondritis in the burned ear by the local instillation of antibiotics. *Plast Reconstr Surg* **53**: 179–83.

Belluci RJ. (1983) Traumatic injuries of the middle ear. *Otolaryngol Clin North Am* **16**: 633–50.

Berger G, Finkelstein Y, Harell M. (1994) Non-explosive blast injury of the ear. *J Laryngol Otol* **108**: 395–98.

Bottrill ID. (1991) Post-traumatic cholesteatoma. *J Laryngol Otol* **105**: 367–69.

Bressler K, Shelton C. (1993) Ear foreign-body removal: a review of 98 consecutive cases. *Laryngoscope* **103**: 367–70.

Browning GG. (1986) *Clinical otology and audiology.* London: Butterworths, 7–22.

Clemons JE, Severeid LR. (1993) Trauma. In: Cummings CJ, Fredrickson JM, Harker LA, Krause CJ, Schuller DE, editors. *Otolaryngology – head and Neck Surgery*, 2nd edition; vol. 4. St Louis: Mosby Year Book, 2865–71.

Freeman J. (1983) Temporal bone fractures and cholesteatoma. *Ann Otol Rhinol Laryngol* **92**: 558–60.

Fuse T, Aoyagi M, Koike Y, Sugai Y. (1992) Diagnosis of the ossicular chain in the middle ear by high-resolution CT. *Journal of Oto-Rhino-Laryngology and its Related Specialties* **54**: 251–54.

Glasscock ME, Cueva RA. (1991) Traumatic tympanic membrane perforation. In: Hill Britton B, editor. *Common problems in otology.* St Louis: Mosby Year Book, 200–203.

Holt GH. (1992) A commentary on violence. *Arch Otolaryngol Head Neck Surg* **118**: 580.

Hough JVD. (1980) Otologic trauma. In: Paperella MM, Shumrick DA, editors. *Otolaryngology*, 2nd edition; vol. 2. Philadelphia: Saunders, 1656–79.

Hough JVD, Stuart WD. (1968) Middle ear injuries in skull trauma. *Laryngoscope* **78**: 899–937.

Igarashi Y, Watanabe Y, Mizukoshi K. (1993) Middle ear barotrauma associated with hyperbaric oxygenation treatment. *Acta Otolaryngol (Stockh)* **504**: 143–45.

Jensen JH, Bonding P. (1993) Experimental pressure induced rupture of the tympanic membrane in man. *Acta Otolaryngol (Stockh)* **113**: 62–67.

Jones DT, Ogren FP, Roh LH, Moore GF. (1991) Lightning and its effects on the auditory system. *Laryngoscope* **101**: 830–34.

Kerr AG, Byrne JET. (1975) Concussive effects of bomb blast on the ear. *J Laryngol Otol* **89**: 131–43.

Kerr AG, Smyth GDL. (1987) Ear trauma. In: Booth JB, editor. *Scott-Brown's Otolaryngology*, vol. 3. Otology. London: Butterworths, 172–84.

Kinney SE. (1992) Violence and the ear and temporal bone. *Arch Otolaryngol Head Neck Surg* **118**: 581–83.

Kirsch JP, Amedee RG (1991) *Management of external ear trauma. J LA State Med Soc* **143**: 13–16.

Kristensen S. (1992) Spontaneous healing of traumatic tympanic membrane perforations in man: a century of experience. *J Laryngol Otol* **106**: 1037–50.

Kronenberg J, Shoshan J, Modan M, Leventon G. (1988) Blast injury and cholesteatoma. *Am J Otol* **9**: 127–30.

Kveton JF. (1987) Obliteration of mastoid and middle ear for severe trauma to the temporal bone. *Laryngscope* **97**: 1385–87.

Leavitt EB, Pincus RL, Bukachevsky R. (1992) Otolaryngologic manifestations of child abuse. *Arch Otolaryngol Head Neck Surg* **118**: 629–31.

Lindemann P, Edstrom S, Granstrom G, *et al.* (1987) Acute traumatic tympanic membrane perforations. *Arch Otolaryngol Head Neck Surg* **113**: 1285–87.

Ludman H. (1988) Diseases due to trauma or physical agents. In: Ludman H, editor. *Mawson's diseases of the ear*, 5th edition. London: Hodder and Stoughton, 305–21.

McDonald TJ, Facer GW, Clark JL. (1986) Surgical treatment of stenosis of the external auditory canal. *Laryngoscope* **96**: 830–33.

McKennan KX, Chole RA. (1992) Traumatic external auditory canal atresia. *Am J Otol* **13**: 80–81.

Redleaf MI, McCabe BF. (1993) Lightning injury of the tympanic membrane. *Ann Otol Rhinol Laryngol* **102**: 867–69.

Roche J. (1975) Fractures of the temporal bone involving the ear. *Australas Radiol* **19**: 317–25.

Skedros DG, Goldfarb IW, Slater H, Rocco J. (1992) Chondritis of the burned ear: a review. *Ear Nose Throat J* **71**: 359–62.

Stevenson EW. (1964) *Bacillus pyocyaneus* perichondritis of the ear. *Laryngoscope* **74**: 255–59.

Strohm M. (1986) Trauma of the middle ear. *Adv Otorhinolaryngol* **35**: 1–248.

Templer J, Renner MD. (1990) Injuries of the external ear. *Otolaryngol Clin North Am* **23**: 1003–18.

Widick MH, Coleman J. (1992) Perichondrial abscess resulting from a high ear-piercing – case report. *Otolaryngol Head Neck Surg* **107**: 803–804.

Willner A, Ledereich PS, de Vries EJ. (1992) Auricular injury as a presentation of child abuse. *Arch Otolaryngol Head Neck Surg* **118**: 634–37.

24

Nasal fractures

Ian S Mackay and P M J Scott

Introduction

The nose has a position of prominence in the centre of the face. This makes it vulnerable to trauma. Any resultant cosmetic deformity is likely to be conspicuous. To optimize outcome following nasal injury and to avoid complications requires early assessment, followed by reduction of the fracture as necessary. The main measure of outcome is the cosmetic appearance of the nose. This is a very subjective measure and makes generalizations about prognosis difficult.

Epidemiology

The nose is one of the most commonly fractured bones in the body (Facer, 1975). Nasal bone fractures represent 39% of all facial fractures (Lundin *et al.*, 1973). In 63% of cases the nasal fracture is isolated (Mayell, 1973). In Denmark, the incidence of nasal fractures is estimated at 53.2 per 100 000 population per year (Illum *et al.*, 1986). In Cardiff, the incidence of all nasal injuries is 500 per 100 000 population (Clayton and Lesser, 1986). Of all the nasal injuries assessed in an ENT department, 40–50% are fractures that require further treatment (Illum, 1986; Murray and Maran, 1980). Males are up to four times more likely to have a nasal fracture than females, and the peak incidence is in the age group 20–30 years (Illum *et al.*, 1983; Mayell, 1973; Murray and Maran, 1980; Murray *et al.*, 1984). This high incidence in young males is largely the result of sports-related trauma, road accidents, and assaults (Illum *et al.*, 1983; Lundin *et al.*, 1973; Mayell, 1973; Murray and Maran, 1980).

Clinical assessment

Initial assessment

The ideal time to assess a nose is immediately following the injury. More often, the examination is performed some time later, by which time there is soft tissue swelling and bruising preventing accurate assessment of nasal contours. The main aim of this assessment is to exclude or treat any acute complication of the injury. It is important to take a history and examine the patient to exclude any significant head injury or other bony or soft tissue injury. The nose is then inspected and palpated in a good light. The inside of the nose should also be examined.

Specific injuries to be diagnosed and treated at this stage are epistaxis, soft tissue injury, and septal haematoma.

Epistaxis

Minor epistaxis is commonplace and implies mucosal injury and that the fracture is compound. As osteomyelitis is very rare, antibiotic treatment is not required routinely. Although minor epistaxis will settle, more major, and occasionally life-threatening, epistaxis can occur. This may require resuscitation, nasal packing and urgent referral to an otolaryngologist.

Soft tissue injury

Cuts in the skin over the nasal bones are common. Again they imply a compound fracture but can be successfully managed by wound toilet and primary suture.

Septal haematoma

Septal haematoma is an uncommon but important complication of nasal fracture. The incidence is 2–6% (Becker, 1948; Illum *et al.*, 1983). Fracture of the nasal septum leads to a subperichondrial haematoma, which strips the perichondrium from the cartilage and deprives the septum of nutrition. If not drained, although the haematoma will gradually resolve, the cartilage necroses and nasal support is lost. This leads to sagging of the nasal dorsum, and a saddle deformity. It can also result in a septal perforation, which can crust and bleed, causing distress to the patient. If an undrained haematoma becomes infected, the process of cartilage destruction is accelerated. Early drainage of the haematoma can often avoid these complications (Facer, 1975). As it is a painful procedure, it is best performed under general anaesthesia. Clinically, a haematoma is likely if the patient complains of total nasal obstruction, either unilaterally or bilaterally. On examination, a soft bulging nasal septal swelling blocking the airway is usually seen if the nasal tip is elevated with the examiner's thumb.

Radiology

Although a radiograph is often taken as part of the assessment of nasal injury, as long ago as 1948 Becker questioned the value of radiology. By taking radiographs of skulls, De Lacey *et al.* (1977) have shown how difficult it is to discriminate between the normal bony markings and nasal fractures. Thus, management of nasal injury is based on clinical grounds, and radiology of nasal fractures adds little or nothing to the assessment (Clayton and Lesser, 1986; de Lacey *et al.* 1977; Illum *et al.*, 1983; Mayell, 1973). However, if

other fractures of the facial skeleton are suspected, the appropriate radiograph examination should then be requested.

Second assessment

When the swelling has subsided, the patient should be reviewed. This second assessment is usually performed 7–10 days after the injury. A check for any other injuries should be made and a septal haematoma excluded. The nasal shape is then assessed to plan further management. If, when the swelling has settled, there is an obvious change in nasal shape, a displaced nasal fracture can be diagnosed. The patient is then offered reduction of the fracture to minimize the cosmetic deformity.

Fracture classification

Becker (1948) has described a classification of nasal fractures. Both Illum *et al.* (1983) and Murray and Maran (1980) have found that this was of no value in deciding treatment or assessing outcome.

Structural pathology

Postmortem studies have been made of the pathology of nasal fractures by striking cadavers and then dissecting the face (Harrison, 1979; Murray *et al.*, 1986). These have shown that nasal bone fractures are often associated with a fracture of the nasal septum. This occurs where the bony and cartilaginous parts of the septum join (Figure 24.1)

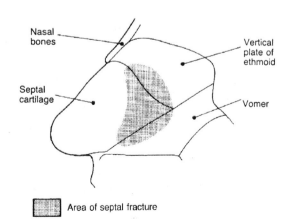

Figure 24.1. The nasal septum.

and is more likely if the nasal bones are displaced by greater than half the width of the nasal bridge (Murray *et al.*, 1986).

Management

Closed reduction

Closed (simple) reduction of the nasal bones involves digital manipulation and instrumentation to disimpact and realign the septum and nasal bones (Becker, 1948; Renner, 1991). This can be performed under local or general anaesthetic with equal success (Cook *et al.*, 1989; Waldron *et al.*, 1989; Watson *et al.*, 1988).

Open reduction

It is possible to treat a septal injury at the same time as nasal manipulation. If septoplasty or submucous resection of the septum is performed concurrently with manipulation, this is referred to as 'open reduction'. It has been suggested that overlapping septal fractures impart deforming stresses on the nasal bones, leading to persisting deformity despite manipulation (Murray *et al.*, 1986).

Outcome

Appearance

Due to the prominence of the nose, the cosmetic appearance is the most important measure of outcome. Illum (1986) has studied simple closed reduction and followed 106 patients over a three-year period. Of 53 treated by simple nasal reduction and assessed at three years, 77% were happy with the appearance of their noses and 87% were satisfied with the overall result. This compares well with two other series. Mayell (1973) asked 44 patients their assessment of the nasal shape following manipulation and noted that none was concerned by the appearance. Dickson and Sharpe (1988) assessed 60 patients and noted that 41 (83%) were satisfied with the outcome. However, when results were based on the surgeon's assessment of the cosmetic appearance, simple reduction gave much poorer results, with 50–90% of the surgeons being unhappy with the appearance (Dickson and Sharpe, 1986; Mayell, 1973; Murray and Maran, 1980). This disparity can be partly

explained. Illum (1986) noted that 29% of a group of uninjured patients had nasal deformities and Mayell (1973) obtained a history of prior deformity in 30% of those with a nasal fracture. Thus, when shape is assessed by a surgeon after manipulation, it would appear that a false assumption is made that the nose was straight prior to injury.

It has been suggested that open reduction gives better results than closed reduction. From a total of 1325 patients, Murray *et al.* (1984) selected 84 for open reduction and found a significantly better appearance at three months postoperatively than in a similar number who underwent closed reduction. Harrison (1979), likewise, showed a superior result after open reduction than after closed reduction in a small group of patients. These very selective studies, however, have not persuaded the majority of surgeons that open reduction is the standard treatment for a fractured nose, although there are patients in whom it should be considered.

Nasal deformity occurs in 58% of patients who have not suffered nasal trauma. Of these, 9% complain of nasal obstruction (Illum, 1986). Following nasal fractures, septal deformities are present in 40–60% of patients, and 25–40% complain of nasal obstruction (Illum, 1986; Mayell, 1973).

Nasal fracture in children

Up to 50% of all nasal injuries occur in children (Barrs and Kern, 1980; Goode and Spooner, 1972). The initial assessment of the injury is the same as for adults, but a general anaesthetic may be required for a thorough assessment, particularly if there is any suspicion of a septal haematoma (Moran, 1977).

Unlike in adults, many injuries are minimally displaced 'greenstick' fractures and do not require reduction (Goode and Spooner, 1972). As growth of the nose and midface is determined by the nasal septum (Pirsig, 1977), any damage to it, either by injury or by overzealous reduction, can lead to subsequent nasal deformity (Moran, 1977). Accordingly, any surgery undertaken for nasal fractures in children should be as conservative as possible.

Further surgery

The final result of a nasal fracture is judged by the nasal shape and the degree of nasal obstruction. If a patient is unhappy with the shape of the nose it is possible to alter it by rhinoplasty, provided that a reasonable time from injury has elapsed to allow the scarring and fibrous tissue to mature. If nasal obstruction is a significant problem, septal surgery can be offered to improve the airway. Again, a reasonable time should have elapsed after the injury.

References

Barrs DM, Kern EB. (1980) Acute nasal trauma; emergency room care of 250 patients. *J Fam Pract* **10**: 225–28.

Becker OJ. (1948) Nasal fractures. An analysis of one hundred cases. *Arch Otolaryngol* **48**; 344–61.

Clayton MI, Lesser THJ. (1986) The role of radiography in the management of nasal fractures. *J Laryngol Otol* **100**: 797–801.

Cook JA, McRae DR, Irving RM, Dowie LN. (1990) A randomized comparison of manipulation of the fractured nose under local and general anaesthesia. *Clin Otolaryngol* **15**: 343–49.

Dickson MG, Sharpe DT. (1986) A prospective study of nasal fractures. *J Laryngol Otol* **100**: 543–51.

Facer GW. (1975) Management of nasal injury. *Postgrad Med* **57**: 123–26.

Goode RL, Spooner TR. (1972) Management of nasal fractures in children. A review of current practices. *Clin Paediatr* **11**: 526–29.

Harrison DH. (1979) Nasal injuries: their pathogenesis and treatment. *Br J Plast Surg* **32**: 57–64.

Illum P, Kristensen S, Jorgensen K, Brahe Pedersen C. (1983) The role of fixation in the treatment of nasal fractures. *Clin Otolaryngol* **8**: 191–95.

Illum P. (1986) Long-term results after treatment of nasal fractures. *J Laryngol Otol* **100**; 273–77.

de Lacey GJ, Wignall BK, Hussain S, Reidy JR. (1977) The radiology of nasal injuries: problems of interpretation and clinical relevance. *Br J Radiol* **50**: 412–14.

Lundin K, Ridell A, Sandberg N, Ohman A. (1973) One thousand maxillo-facial fractures and related fractures at the ENT clinic in Gothenburg. *Acta Otolaryngol* **75**: 359–61.

Mayell MJ. (1973) Nasal fractures. Their occurrence, management and some late results. *J R Coll Surg Edinb* **18**: 31–36.

Moran WB. (1977) Nasal trauma in children. *Otolaryngol Clin North Am* **10**: 95–101.

Murray JAM, Maran AGD. (1980) The treatment of nasal injuries by manipulation. *J Laryngol Otolaryngol* **94**: 1405–10.

Murray JAM, Maran AGD, Mackenzie IJ, Raab G. (1984) Open v closed reduction of the fractured nose. *Arch Otolaryngol* **110**: 797–802.

Murray JAM, Maran AGD, Busuttil A, Vaughn G. (1986) A pathological classification of nasal fractures. *Injury* **17**: 338–44.

Pirsig W. (1977) Septal plasty in children: influence on nasal growth. *Rhinology* **15**: 193–95.

Renner GJ. (1991) Management of nasal fractures. *Otolaryngol Clin North Am* **24**: 195–213.

Watson DJ, Parker AJ, Slack RWT, Griffiths MV. (1988) Local versus general anaesthetic in the management of the fractured nose. *Clin Otolaryngol* **13**: 491–94.

Waldron J, Mitchell DB, Ford G. (1989) Reduction of fractured nasal bones; local versus general anaesthesia. *Clin Otolaryngol* **14**: 357–59.

25

Laryngeal and tracheal injury

Nicholas Stafford, R M Rudd

Laryngeal Trauma

The introduction of seat belt legislation for motorists has led to a significant reduction in the incidence of laryngeal trauma. The majority of cases now seen are the result of deliberate trauma (e.g. strangulation, stabbing, bullet trauma), accidental inhalation of smoke or chemical fumes, or iatrogenic damage to the larynx. Intubation of the larynx can result in dislocation of one of the arytenoid cartilages, whilst thyroidectomy, other neck surgery or certain cardiopulmonary procedures can result in damage to one, or both, recurrent laryngeal nerves.

Direct physical trauma to the larynx can result in long-term morbidity, especially laryngeal stenosis, in three ways. First, a displaced fracture of one or more laryngeal cartilages will often result in serious disruption of the airway and phonatory mechanism. Secondly, even if there is no alteration to the cartilaginous framework, the larynx has several spaces, or potential spaces, into which submucosal haemorrhage can occur. Whilst a bleed into Reinke's space will usually reabsorb spontaneously, haemorrhage into one of the paraglottic spaces or into the pre-epiglottic space is likely to result in chronic laryngeal stenosis unless recognized and dealt with during the acute period after injury. Lastly, mucosal adhesions will often occur between raw mucosal surfaces. Not only may this occur after microlaryngoscopic surgery for laryngeal papillomatosis but it is also an almost inevitable development in the badly traumatized larynx if the mucosal tears are not closed surgically.

The larynx has three basic functions, all of which must be appraised when examining a patient following laryngeal trauma. These functions are:

1. Provision of an adequate airway;
2. Protection of the airway;
3. Phonation: production of a voice.

Each function should be assessed separately when preparing a medical report on a patient who has suffered from trauma to the upper airway.

Provision of an adequate airway

A history of stridor and/or dyspnoea on slight or moderate exertion indicates significant narrowing of the airway. If there is any doubt or suspicion that the patient may be overplaying the symptoms, then an exercise tolerance test should be undertaken. In severe cases, the symptoms will be evident at rest or on slight exertion. In these patients, a tracheostomy may be required.

If the appearance of the larynx cannot be assessed easily by indirect laryngoscopy, the patient should undergo fibreoptic laryngoscopy. However, clinical examination may give a misleading impression regarding the extent of the damage sustained. Conventional coronal plane tomography, CT scanning and MRI all provide useful additional information, particularly in those patients in whom more than one level of the larynx is affected. Xeroradiography is a valuable technique for assessing the grossly disrupted or stenosed larynx but is not available in many centres.

Direct endoscopic examination of the upper airway should be avoided if at all possible; the problem of the shared airway and the possibility of postendoscopy oedema create the risk of serious airways obstruction, necessitating tracheostomy.

Occasionally, a patient will have an obstructive problem at more than one level in the airway. Indeed, there may be coincidental chronic obstructive airways disease. In such situations it may be difficult to know to what extent the patient's symptoms are related to post-traumatic changes in the upper airway as opposed to pre-existing chronic pulmonary disease. The flow volume loop provides a graphic record of airflow rate during maximal respiration and expiration at different lung volumes, and can differentiate between extrathoracic and intrathoracic airways obstruction (Brookes and Fairfax, 1982). In the presence of obstruction of both portions of the upper airway, the loop will indicate the contribution made by the obstruction at each site.

Protection of the airway

An incompetent larynx is almost always the result of damage to one or both recurrent laryngeal nerves. In terms of treatment, it is a far more difficult problem to deal with than obstruction of the larynx. The voice is characteristically weak and 'breathy' and the cough may be bovine. Coughing attacks during meals or, in more extreme cases, recurrent chest infections should alert the physician to the probability of aspiration.

Indirect or fibreoptic laryngoscopy will provide information about cord mobility and glottic closure. If both cords are fully mobile then significant aspiration will not occur. Occasionally, damage to the external branch of the superior laryngeal nerve, usually a result of thyroid surgery, may cause slight aspiration by disrupting the afferent arm of the cough reflex.

Radiological assessment of the swallow may be necessary, in which case the radiologist must be forwarned about the problem. Videofluoroscopy will provide more information about the mechanism of aspiration than will a conventional barium swallow.

Phonation

For most patients, disorders of phonation are the most troublesome symptom. It takes very little structural change to upset the finely balanced function of the vocal cords; even a poorly performed excision biopsy of a cord nodule can result in permanent hoarseness.

Subjective assessments of the voice employ a scale or grading system by which the patient's voice can be scored (Greene and Mathieson, 1989). The 'GRBAS' scale evaluates hoarseness on five scales: grade (i.e. degree of voice abnormality) and if rough, breathy, asthenic or strained. Evaluation is subjective and requires training, as do other voice profiles such as Vocal Profile Analysis (VPA). VPA establishes a phonetic description of voice quality; phonation types are classified as harshness, whispery, breathiness, creaky, falsetto and modal. For medicolegal purposes, neither these nor other perceptual assessments of voice are adequate alone. One or both should be combined with objective assessment of vocal function. Such techniques include videostroboscopy and electrolaryngography (electrogluttography).

Videostroboscopy

Only gross disorders of vocal cord movement are discernable by indirect or fibreoptic laryngoscopy because the cords vibrate too rapidly for the eye to detect the individual vibratory cycle. The problem can be overcome by using a stroboscope synchronized to the vibratory cycle (Konrad *et al.*, 1981). The flash sequence can be adjusted so that the vocal cord appears to stand still. A rigid or fibreoptic laryngoscope can be used to deliver the stroboscopic illumination. The technique enables minor degrees of cord malfunction to be diagnosed (e.g. mild cord oedema or cord weakness secondary to nerve damage). As with other objective techniques, videostroboscopy provides both physician and patient with a permanent record of laryngeal function at any one time.

Electrolaryngography (electrogluttography)

This technique allows noninvasive monitoring of vocal cord activity during speech (Hanson *et al.*, 1983). It can assess cord vibration and voice pitch and intensity but only provides information concerning the two cords together; it does not provide specific information about functional impairment of one particular cord. This is of little importance with regard to voice assessment but it means that the technique may not be helpful in providing an accurate diagnosis.

Acoustic output

Acoustic signal analysis provides an indirect measure of the vibratory patterns of the vocal cords as well as of the shape of the vocal tract and changes in that shape over time. Specific features of the voice can be characterized: shimmer (cycle to cycle variation in amplitude); jitter (cycle to cycle variation in time); and signal-to-noise ratio. Along with electrolaryngography, signal analysis provides a reproducible record of vocal tract function.

Electromyography

Laryngeal electromyography (EMG) provides information about the nerve supply to, and activity in, the intrinsic muscles of the larynx (Schaefer, 1991a). Its chief role is in the detection of viable recurrent laryngeal nerve innervation of the thyro-arytenoid muscle after iatrogenic vocal cord paralysis. From a clinical viewpoint, it is often difficult to differentiate between vocal cord paralysis and cricoarytenoid joint fixation or dislocation. Dislocation of the joint is an occasional sequel to intubation or endoscopy. EMG will allow the distinction to be made without resort to direct endoscopy.

The functions of the larynx and pharynx are inextricably related. Not only are they anatomically contiguous but they also share the same nerve supply and are lined by a continous epithelium. Disruption of normal pharyngeal function should therefore be considered in a patient who has pathology relating to the voice or airway. Videofluoroscopy is the investigation of choice in any patient in whom dysfunction of the swallow is a possibility. In patients in whom stricture formation has occurred in the hypopharynx, indirect or fibreoptic pharyngoscopy will often fail to demonstrate the abnormality. In such situations, direct pharyngo-oesophagoscopy under general anaesthesia will be necessary.

Outcome

Maran *et al.* (1981) reported the results of acute laryngeal trauma sustained by 44 patients. Surgical intervention was required in only 50% of these patients, none of whom underwent long-term treatment for a chronically stenosed airway. The early recognition and treatment of severe injury to the larynx improved subsequent morbidity and decreased by a factor of three the chance of the patient having to have a permanent tracheostomy.

Schaefer (1991b) discussed the 'state of the art' treatment of acute external laryngeal injuries. He recommends fibreoptic assessment of the larynx, with or without CT scanning, unless there is impending airways obstruction, in which case an emergency tracheostomy, under local anaesthesia, is mandatory. Clinical or CT evidence of disruption of the laryngeal mucosa or cartilaginous framework were also indications for tracheostomy, followed by direct endoscopic assessment and open exploration of the larynx. Unstable fractures or disruption of the anterior commissure mucosa are both considered as indications for stenting the larynx (using a McNaught Keel or silicone tube).

Tracheal trauma

Tracheal injury may occur in a number of ways: as a result of penetrating or blunt trauma; as a result of the inhalation of hot or caustic gases or liquids; or as a result of therapeutic endotracheal intubation. The symptoms and disability arising from tracheal injury are generally similar whatever the cause, but the management and outcome differ to some extent according to the mode of injury and the age of the patient.

Symptoms following tracheal injury

If a tracheal injury heals satisfactorily, then no long-term symptoms or disability are likely to ensue. Problems arise when there is narrowing of the tracheal lumen, either as a result of damage to the cartilaginous rings, which normally support the trachea, or as a result of stricture formation due to fibrous scar tissue at the site of the injury. Damage to the cartilaginous rings can lead to inward collapse of the tracheal wall, resulting in narrowing of the lumen, which will vary with the phase of respiration. A fibrous stricture tends to lead to fixed narrowing of the trachea. Mild narrowing of the trachea results in breathlessness, which is only evident on strenuous exertion. Severe narrowing of the tracheal lumen will not only produce much worse exertional dyspnoea but may also lead to severe respiratory distress at rest, with difficulty in clearing secretions from the airway. This in turn may result in an increased risk of lower respiratory tract infection.

Mild degrees of tracheal narrowing do not generally merit treatment, but moderate and severe stenoses usually require treatment to re-establish a wider tracheal lumen. In some cases, removal of the stenosis or reconstruction of the trachea may not be possible and the patient may require a permanent tracheostomy. Whilst this does not usually cause significant impairment of respiratory function it may lead to permanent problems with voice production.

Assessment of tracheal injury

The functional severity of tracheal narrowing may be assessed by simple lung function tests, including spirometry and flow volume loop studies. A CT scan may help to demonstrate the severity and extent of tracheal narrowing. Views in expiration as well as in inspiration should be obtained in patients with tracheal narrowing due to inward collapse following damage to cartilaginous rings. Bronchoscopic assessment will usually be necessary if any treatment is under consideration. Bronchoscopy under local anaesthesia is preferable in order to allow observation of variations in the shape and size of the tracheal lumen during spontaneous respiration.

Mechanisms of injury

The trachea is most commonly involved in penetrating wounds of the neck, resulting from knife or gunshot assaults. Conservative management is successful in the majority of patients and surgery for late complications is only occasionally necessary (Ngakane *et al.*, 1990). Blunt injury is rather more likely to cause long-term problems. If the injury is not too extensive, surgical repair may be carried out. With more severe injuries the trachea is intubated and the trachea allowed to heal. Following extubation it will soon become evident whether a stenosis requiring subsequent surgical repair has occurred.

Post intubation injuries

Intubation of the trachea with an endotracheal tube is required not only for most surgical procedures performed under general anaesthesia but also in the management of patients with respiratory failure who require assisted ventilation. Until relatively recently, prolonged endotracheal intubation was not uncommonly followed by permanent damage to the trachea resulting from pressure necrosis of the tracheal wall mucosa. Modern techniques and equipment – in particular the advent of the lower pressure cuffed tube – have substantially reduced the incidence of such injuries, although they still occur occasionally. Patients requiring long-term assisted ventilation are generally provided with a tracheostomy, which has certain mechanical and physiological advantages over an oral or nasal tube. Whilst the incidence of long-term tracheal damage is also reduced it may still occur.

Damage to the trachea may take the form of a stenosis with or without damage to the cartilaginous rings. Granuloma formation at the site of the tracheostomy is a common problem. These rarely present a serious management problem; they can be removed by a variety of bronchoscopic techniques including laser therapy. Damage to the cartilaginous rings and the formation of benign fibrous strictures can produce a more serious problem, which may require surgical reconstruction of the trachea. Conservative methods of management include repeated dilatation and stenting of the tracheal lumen; they are not generally successful for anything other than mild stenoses. Moderate and severe degrees of stenosis are best managed by surgical reconstruction. This usually involves resection of the affected segment of the trachea, followed by reanastomosis of the cut ends. Such a technique is best handled by an expert. In a series of 203 patients treated by reconstructive surgery, the long-term result was classified as good in 83% and satisfactory in 10% (Grillo, 1979). In occasional cases that are not amenable to reconstructive surgery, a permanent stent may be inserted. A stent is commonly made of steel wire, its inner surface becoming epithelialized with time. The long-term durability of such stents is uncertain; most are used in the management of malignant strictures. However, their use should be considered where other techniques are inappropriate or have proven unsuccessful.

Following reconstructive surgery, there is some risk of re-stenosis. This will usually occur at a relatively early stage; if it does not become evident within a year of surgery, the risk of subsequent development is very small. If the residual tracheal lumen is smaller than normal the patient will be left with some impairment of respiratory function. This is unlikely to worsen with the passage of time. Substantial narrowing of the trachea may also lead to some impairment of the clearance of secretions from the bronchial tree and hence some increase in the risk of respiratory infection.

The management of tracheal stenosis in childhood is more difficult because of the smaller tracheal diameter. As the trachea is still growing, reconstructive surgery is commonly delayed, being employed only when conservative measures have failed. In a proportion of patients, long-term tracheostomy may be necessary. In one series of 55 surviving patients, 80% were eventually able to manage without a tracheostomy (Wever *et al.*, 1991).

Tracheal burns

Similar injuries may result from the inhalation of hot gases in burns victims and from the inhalation of toxic chemicals, such as acids and alkalis. Such tracheal injuries are commonly associated with similar injuries to the larynx. The incidence of stricture formation in survivors is high.

These injuries are often very difficult to deal with, as they involve a considerable length of the trachea, rendering resection of the area impossible. Approaches to management include tracheal stenting and/or permanent tracheostomy. Gaissert *et al.* (1993) reported a series of 18 cases of tracheal stenosis following inhalation injury. In the long term, half the patients were able to manage without any device in their tracheas.

References

Brookes GB, Fairfax AJ. (1982) Chronic upper airway obstruction: value of the flow volume loop examination in assessment and management. *J R Soc Med* **75**: 425–34.

Gaissert HA, Lofgren RH, Grillo HC. (1993) Upper Airway Compromise after inhalation injury. Complex structures of the larynx and trachea and their management. *Ann Surg* **218**: 672–78.

Grillo HC. (1979) Surgical treatment of post intubation tracheal injuries. *J Thorac Cardiovasc Surg* **78**: 860–75.

Greene MCL, Mathieson L, editors. (1989) Dysphonia: Classification and perceptual assessment. In: *The Voice and its Disorders*. London: Whurr Publications, 86–90.

Hanson DG, Gerratt BR, Ward PH (1983) Glottographic measurement of vocal dysfunction: a preliminary report. *Ann Otol Rhinol Laryngol* **98**: 541–49.

Konrad HR, Hople DM, Bussen J. (1981) Use of strobofibrescopic video recording of vocal fold vibration. *Ann Otol Rhinol Laryngol* **90**: 398–400.

Maran AGD, Murray JA, Stell PM, Tucker A (1981) Early management of laryngeal injuries. *J R Soc Med* **74**: 656–60.

Ngakane H, Muckart DJ, Luvuno FM. (1990) Penetrating visceral injuries of the neck: results of a conservative management policy. *Br J Surg* **77**: 908–10.

Schaefer SD. (1991a) Laryngeal electromyography. *Otolaryngol Clin North Am* **24**(5): 1053–57.

Schaefer SD. (1991b) The treatment of acute external laryngeal injuries. *Arch Otolaryngol Head Neck Surg* **117**: 35–39.

Wever TR, Connors RH, Tracy TF. (1991) Acquired tracheal stenosis in infants and children. *J Thorac Cardiovasc Surg* **102**: 29–34.

Section IV

Maxillofacial trauma

26

Fractures in the maxillofacial region: a general introduction

Hugh Cannell

Introduction

Injuries to the facial region can occur through all forms of trauma. This generally means blunt trauma but it can also include crush and perforating injuries.

Injuries to the facial bones or to the jaws involve the part of the body by which other people recognize us and by which we recognize ourselves. In particular, injuries to the so-called 'high points' of the face will necessarily involve considerable distortion of appearance. The high points are: the forehead; the area around the eyes; the prominences of the cheek bones; the nose; and the prominence of the front of the chin. Very accurate reduction of fractures in these regions is always necessary to restore normal appearance. After they have been reduced, it then becomes possible to achieve some reduction of other smaller and thinner pieces of bone and thereby achieve pre-accident harmony of the face.

Studies in various countries have confirmed that, whilst blunt trauma to drivers of cars through road traffic accidents has declined, there are still large numbers of injuries associated with pedal cyclists, motor-cyclists and pedestrians. Unbelted car occupants may also sustain injuries to the facial bones. The ratio of men to women injured is 2.8:1. Most injuries occur to those in the second decade of life. Perkins and Leyton (1988) reported a 75% drop in maxillofacial trauma cases in front seat occupants after seat belt legislation was introduced in the UK.

Vetter *et al.* (1991) reported that, in their region of the USA, road traffic accidents remained the principal cause of facial injuries (40%), whilst personal violence contributed 37% and sports-associated causes about 9% of the total. They noted that, of 274 injuries to the middle one-third of the face, 33% were zygomaticomaxillary complex fractures, while the orbital area constituted 26%, maxillary fractures 23%, nasal fractures 8%, and isolated zygomatic arch fractures only 4%.

An increase in personal violence leading to facial injuries has been reported in many countries (Karyouti, 1987; Khan, 1988; Kooray *et al.*, 1992; Sanhey and Ahuja, 1988; Timoney *et al.*, 1990). In Greece, Stylogian *et al.* (1991) reported that road traffic accident was the predominant cause of fractures in children. Although middle third fractures accounted for only 4% of their 147 cases it was noted that in the majority of these, seat belts were not used.

Many injuries to the facial region are associated with alcohol abuse, especially those to the mandible and cheek bones. Sports-associated injuries may vary from region to region and between countries, according to the season of the year, but may account for 15–50% of all facial injuries.

Mechanisms of injury

The facial bones and jaws have a tolerance to blunt trauma. Some of the original work concerning the resistance of the facial skeleton to various forms of trauma was carried out by the American Civil Aviation Authority (Swearingen, 1965). There have been many studies since, including those carried out by the automobile industry. The facial bones with the least tolerance to blunt trauma are the bridge of the nose and the rib-like zygomatic arches. These are closely followed by the bones in and around the orbit. By contrast, the thick frontal bone can withstand a very large and prolonged force if this is distributed across the whole bone. Figure 26.1 demonstrates some comparisons between tolerances of the various facial bones. The forces shown are comparative, as the amount of energy necessary to fracture an individual bone will depend upon the area of impact, the mass of the impacting object and the duration of the loading force. Thus, the force of a blow necessary to produce an injury is reduced when the speed of the blow, for the same mass, impacts over a longer time. The avoidance response to a perceived blow (e.g. a punch) takes about 70 ms to become operational. Most facial bone fractures occur after the force (acceleration) is applied to about 2.54 cm^2 for 3–4 ms.

The thicker facial bones act as struts to the main bulk of the face. The mandible, with its curved shape and double joint to the base of the skull, transmits any forces from the point of the chin to the area of the temporomandibular joint, but is protected by the thin condylar neck from transmitting those forces directly to the brain. The firm and relatively unyielding tooth tissues act as wedges when compressive forces are applied to the jaws. This often results in fractures next to the roots of the longest or the deepest buried teeth. Since the thin bones of the air sinuses form a large part of the middle third of the face, they break into many fragments and cannot necessarily be reduced with accuracy. It is even more important, therefore, that the firmer buttress bones of the face are reduced with precision.

Gunshot wounds are capable of causing extensive facial injuries. The degree of injury sustained is dependent upon the momentum of the missile and its flight characteristics, as well as any associated shock waves through blast from high explosives. Facial injuries from so-called baton rounds or rubber bullets, as used for riot control, cause similar injuries to any other form of blunt trauma (Marshall, 1986). The pattern and stream of pellets from cartridges fired from shotguns cause maximum damage at short ranges (e.g. in suicides or assaults). The muzzle velocity of the pellets may be up to 259 m/s. At ranges of less than 6 m, the shot stream will be very dense and avulsion of tissues is inevitable. Marshall (1986) stated that a velocity of only 103 m/s was all that was necessary for a pellet to be able to penetrate the globe.

Missiles from weapons with a low muzzle velocity may have poor flight characteristics, and yawing and tumbling actions may produce large entry wounds but no exit wounds. Damage to bone is less likely and secondary missile effects uncommon except after strikes at very short ranges. The momentum of missiles from weapons with high muzzle velocities is sufficient to shatter facial bones and create secondary missile effects but, according to Marshall (1986), massive soft tissue loss at gaping exit wounds is not a feature of injuries to the region. Presumably, the large forces generated at

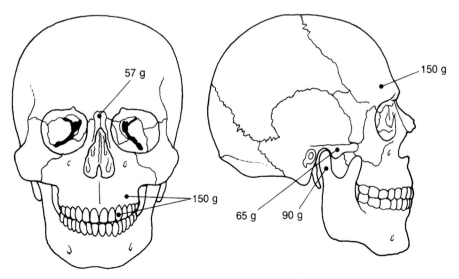

Figure 26.1. Tolerances of some facial bones to impacting forces over a few milliseconds (Swearingen, 1965).

impact are partly dispersed by the volumes of the oral cavity and the air sinuses. Blast injuries associated with rocket or shell fragments of high momentum may create severe shredding of the facial tissues and multiple fragments in bone (Al-Shawi, 1986). Excellent descriptions of these types of injuries as encountered in the maxillofacial region have been given by Shuker (1988, 1990).

Relevance of any pre-existing conditions

The shape of the face and its prominences often dictate the pattern of fracture, for example, after a frontal impact. Prominent upper front teeth may first take the force of a blow to the area of the mouth and become fractured or otherwise damaged. The facial sinuses expand throughout a person's life. In children, they are very small. For example the maxillary sinus arises as a pea-shaped evagination on the lateral side of the nose. As the upper teeth erupt, particularly the premolars and molars, the size of the maxillary sinus increases by lateral pneumatization. The frontal sinuses also tend to expand gradually with age. Thus the size and shape of the sinus determines the patterns of facial fractures and the response of the facial skeleton to trauma. In general, it is unusual for children, with their small air sinuses, to have fractures in the middle third of the face. Older patients may show considerable damage and displacement of fractures for the same amount of trauma, as the bones covering their facial sinuses are large in area and very thin.

Occasionally, the thickness of the bone may determine the severity and pattern of the fracture. It is unusual, but by no means rare, to find extreme variations in the thickness of bone. Those with thin bones are more likely to have severely displaced fracture patterns after trauma. There are also some systemic conditions in which the trabecular pattern of the bone and its texture are altered. It is not within the remit of this text to consider each of these, but sufficient to note that systemic disease may affect fracture patterns.

First aid and its effect on outcome

All primary care as first aid or as other emergency interventions to an injury sustained to the face and the jaws must first be concerned with the restoration of the airway. Any forces that have distracted facial bones may also have reduced the size and patency of the nasal or oral airways. Sometimes both airways are affected. Emergency first aid should therefore be directed to providing an airway. A displaced maxilla will usually be found to have been deviated downwards and backwards. This is because, when fractured from its neighbouring bones, the middle one-third of the face slides backwards down the inclined plane of the skull base. The displacement is particularly marked if the entire face has been detached from the base of the skull. The manoeuvre of choice for first aid is to insert two fingers behind the hard palate, or such of it as remains. The maxillary fractures are then reduced by gentle traction downwards and forwards and finally upwards.

Badly displaced or comminuted mandibles can be reduced manually at the same time and nearby intact teeth can be used to help to hold severely comminuted fragments approximately in line by means of thread or wire wound around them.

After the airway, breathing, and circulation of the patient have been restored and stabilized, any displaced facial bones can be held in place by temporary means until definitive or temporary operative procedures can be undertaken. A description of first aid to the posteriorly displaced maxilla in the multiply-injured patient, as used by the Royal London Hospital team, was reported by Cannell et al. (1993). In their patients, a previously displaced maxilla was temporarily maintained in the reduced position by the insertion of McKesson-type wedge-shaped hard rubber props, placed firmly into the most posterior part of the gap between the jaws or teeth. This produced an upwards pressure on the facial bones in relation to the base of the skull and acted as a counterforce to the downwards pressure exerted due to the weight of the bones. Nasal Epistats (Xomet-Treace, Bristol-Myers Squibb Co., Jacksonville, FL 32216) could then safely be inserted, inflated with saline and nasomaxillary, nasoethmoidal or nasal haemorrhage controlled. Nasal Epistats, it was advised, should not be used without first wedging a fractured maxilla with intra oral props, as their inflation was found to distract maxillary fractures and cause bleeding rather than control it.

Failure to disimpact a posteriorly placed maxilla, central middle third of the face or frontal naso-ethmoidal region as soon as possible, may result in the need for delayed treatment by facial bone osteotomies. Delays in the reduction and stabilization of maxillofacial injuries are, in the author's view, less acceptable now that both temporary stabilization and minimally invasive internal fixation techniques are readily available.

First aid to displaced orbital bones and to the zygomaticomaxillary complex are considered in the appropriate chapter. In brief, any injury that involves actual or potential damage to the globe of the eye must be assessed by a senior clinician, preferably an ophthalmic surgeon. Failure to seek an expert opinion may result in unnecessary loss of vision.

The outcome of treatment of complex craniofacial trauma in the multiply-injured patient may be dependent upon the severity of other life-threatening injuries. For example, subdural haematoma, diffuse brain injury, increases in intracranial pressure, haemopneumothoraces, fractures of the spine, and bleeding from abdominal organs or single or multiple organ failure may each require treatment so urgently that definitive management, or even temporary stabilization, of facial fractures should be postponed. Under these conditions, it has been suggested that maxillofacial treatment may best be limited to simple soft tissue wound closure (Marcione and Gonty, 1993).

Marcione and Gonty (1993) have described three levels of care. Level one is definitive surgical management of combined intra- and extracranial injuries. Level two is when the patient's condition does not allow definitive treatment and intervention is directed towards prevention of infection. In level three, there is no facial trauma management as the patient's condition is critical and death a possibility. The protocols used at the Royal London Hospital do not necessarily agree with these principles and, in our view, even in the multiply-injured patient with a very poor prognosis, some attempt ought to be made to reduce facial fractures early.

A firm case for early maxillofacial surgical intervention in patients with fewer injuries has been made by Hayter and Cawood (1993). They reported that miniplate osteosynthesis of the facial skeleton had important advantages in that inter-maxillary fixation was then not required and the patient's safety was thereby improved due to the reduced risk to the airway.

More recently, Cannell *et al.* (1996) have produced evidence that, even with badly displaced fractures of the maxillofacial region leading to recurrent oral or upper airway bleeding in the multiply injured, these should be reduced and fixed by means of internal fixation techniques such as miniplates or stainless steel plates. At the same time, the oral cavity and throat should be explored so that any lacerations under the tongue or in the back of the mouth can be diagnosed and treated. This form of early operation can also assist in determining the cause of bleeding when haemoptysis or haematemesis is a feature. Operations that commence within the so called 'golden hour' may involve many different disciplines. The priorities between the disciplines may change during the operation, so that the role of the maxillofacial surgeon, instead of being limited to minimal soft tissue closure, may become expanded so that grossly mobile and severely displaced fragments of facial bone are reduced and stabilized at the time of maximum opportunity (i.e. at the first emergency operative stage).

Soft tissue management

Treatment of lacerations is an important part of the preliminary work of a maxillofacial surgeon, as the outcome of failure to treat at this early stage may be severe scarring. Most facial lacerations should be regarded as contaminated. If less than four hours old they should be closed by primary suture after careful cleaning, but slight wound edge freshening may be necessary. If over 24 hours old, some wound edge excision will certainly be necessary. Every laceration should be explored to its depth and any bone beneath it probed to make sure that there are no underlying fractures. Any tattered skin edges should be preserved if possible and only very limited excision should be performed even on facial wounds more than 24 hours old. Cleansing of contaminated wounds can be done with hydrogen peroxide, Milton's solution diluted with 40 parts of water, antiseptic solutions, or plain soap and water. Wounds contaminated with road dirt should be treated by scrubbing with a soft nylon brush and copious irrigation. Interrupted, deep, catgut sutures should be used to approximate muscles and subcutaneous tissues. The skin should then be brought together to evert the edges, using 4/0 or 5/0 material. The vertical mattress suture causes slight eversion of the skin edges and therefore produces the best results.

Emergency treatment of high velocity gunshot wounds

High velocity (momentum) wounds to the maxillofacial region usually result in gross tissue destruction, with shredding of soft tissues and comminution of bone. The patency of the airway is highly likely to have been compromised after blast injuries (Shuker, 1988) and laryngeal obstruction may have occurred, especially in closed wounds (Al-Shawi, 1986). Apart from endotracheal intubation or tracheostomy, the nasal airway remnant can be encouraged to reform, as well as be kept patent, by suitably placed plastic tubes (Shuker, 1988). The mucosa should be sutured to skin edges, dead muscle conservatively excised and local skin flaps advanced to cover defects.

Even the smallest of comminuted bone fragments, if attached to some periosteum, should be preserved and Kirschner-type wire used to stabilize them. At the same time, soft tissue remnants can be expanded by the use of stretching devices and every effort made to achieve closure of defects and reformation of the oral cavity (Shuker, 1990).

Soft tissues: surgical incisions and scars

Incision lines for surgery of the face are designed to be along Langer's lines. This means that, on movement of the face, the scar tends to be in the natural creases of the skin and should therefore be minimally visible. Scars from lacerations to the face may cut across natural lines and remain conspicuous. To allow for maximum improvement, they should be left for at least one year subsequent to the injury. Occasionally, some small amount of tissue loss or deep scarring causes very conspicuous secondary deformity. The most common example is ectropion of the lower eyelid. Depressed scars may indicate deep tissue loss or irregular suturing of deeper layers. A reddened, angry-looking scar may indicate the presence of a foreign body or stitch abscess. A broad scar may indicate that the laceration has cut across the natural lines of the skin and muscle and is being pulled and exaggerated. After 12 months, each facial scar should be reassessed, and excised and revised as necessary.

Small losses of the facial skin can normally be concealed by undermining to obtain an approximation of the residual skin edges. Larger areas of tissue loss, such as occur after blast injuries or gunshot wounds, may require early management by replacement of the skin and deep tissue. This can be achieved by means of split skin (Wolff grafts) for small areas and for larger areas by means of local advancement flaps using adjacent facial muscles. Still larger areas of skin or muscle loss can be minimized by the use of axial flaps from the chest, such as the pectoralis major or deltopectoral flap. Flaps raised from the chest may be of insufficient length to reach up onto the face. In general, axial flaps from the chest are unlikely to be useful if the tissue defect for restoration is superior to the occlusal line of the upper teeth.

Free flaps using microsuturing of feeder vessels can now be used for the replacement of major tissue loss. A useful donor site for the facial region is the radial forearm flap.

Chronic complications in soft tissue

Degloving-type mucosal tears, typically of the lower anterior region of the mouth, produce a loss of sulcus depth. Vestibuloplasty-type epithelial inlays may be necessary later. Facial and lip scars, oro-antral fistulae or nasal fistulae, salivary fistulae, cellulitis, tetanus, chronic wound infection, foreign bodies (e.g. teeth), nonunion, actinomycosis and myositis ossificans may each occur as late complications.

Reasonable expectations of outcome

The majority of facial injuries caused by blunt trauma have a good prognosis. The exceptions to this occur where there is soft tissue or bony loss as a consequence of the trauma or where there has been very extensive destruction, such as after a gunshot wound or after sharp trauma to the globe of the eye. Facial scars may be a problem and, as has been explained, later revision may be necessary. Provided that treatment of all maxillofacial injuries is undertaken at the earliest opportunity compatible with other injuries, the eventual outcome should be good. Occasionally, more complicated injuries may result in permanent disability.

Treatment options affecting outcome

Modern methods of management of facial bone and jaw fractures now include direct reduction of facial buttress bones at open operation. The fractures are then fixed in the ideal position by means of malleable titanium or steel miniplates. Extra-oral methods of fixation are less common but are occasionally still used. Whether the treatment is by internal or external skeletal fixation, its success rests entirely upon the accurate and stable approximation of the buttress facial bones.

References

Al-Shawi A. (1986) Experience in the treatment of missile injuries of the maxillofacial region in Iraq. *Br J Oral Maxillofac Surg* **24**: 244–50.

Cannell H, Silvester KC, O'Regan MB. (1993) Early management of multiply injured patients with maxillofacial injuries transferred to hospital by helicopter. *Br J Oral Maxillofac Surg* **31**: 207–12.

Cannell H, Paterson A, Loukota R. (1996) Maxillofacial injuries in multiply injured patients. *Br J Oral Maxillofac* **34**: 303–308.

Hayter JP, Cawood JI. (1993) Functional case of mini plates in maxillofacial surgery. *J Oral Maxillofac Surg* **22**: 91–96.

Karyouti SM. (1987) Maxillofacial injuries at Jordan University Hospital. *Int J Oral Maxillofac Surg* **16**: 262–65.

Khan A. (1988) A retrospective study of maxillofacial injuries to the facial skeleton in Harare, Zimbabwe. *Br J Oral Maxillofac Surg* **26**: 435–39.

Marcione RD, Gonty GR. (1993) Principles of management of complex craniofacial trauma. *J Oral Maxillofac Surg* **51**: 535–42.

Marshall WG. (1986) An analysis of firearm injuries to the head and face in Belfast 1969–1977. *Br J Oral Maxillofac Surg* **24**: 233–43.

Perkins CS, Layton SA. (1988) The aetiology of maxillofacial injuries and the seat belt law. *Br J Oral Maxillofac Surg* **26**: 353–63.

Sawhney CP, Ahuja RB. (1988) Facio maxillary fractures in Northern India. A statistical analysis and review of management. *Br J Oral Maxillofac Surg* **26**: 430–34.

Shuker ST. (1988) Intra-nasal stabilisation for severe nasal war injuries. *J Cranio Maxillo fac Surg* **16**: 120–25.

Shuker ST. (1990) Severe lower lip disfigurement resulting from war injuries. *J Cranio Maxillofac Surg* **18**: 304–309.

Stylogianni L, Arsenopouls A, Patrikiou A. (1991) Fractures of the facial skeleton in children. *Br J Oral Maxillofac Surg*, **29**: 9–11.

Swearingen JJ. (1965) Tolerance of the human face to crash impacts. (USA Report AM 65–20.) Oklahoma City, OH: Federal Aviation Agency, Civil Aeromedical Research Institute, 1–24.

Timoney N, Saiveau M, Pinsolle EJ, Shepherd J. (1990) Comparative study of facial trauma in Bristol and Bordeaux. *J Cranio Maxillofac Surg* **18**: 154–57.

Vetter JD, Topazian RG, Goldberg MH, Smith DG. (1991) Facial fractures occurring in a medium sized metropolitan area; recent trends. *Int J Oral Maxillofac Surg* **20**: 214–16.

27

Frontonasal and ethmoidal fractures

John L B Carter

Introduction

The terminology used to describe injuries to this area of the face is complex and may be confusing. In the management of frontonasal and ethmoidal trauma, several specialties may overlap with the result that the relative importance of various aspects of injury may become exaggerated to the detriment of the patient as a whole.

Fractures affecting the area at the junction of the face and forehead, where the root of the nose separates the orbits, are complicated to manage. The sturdy external appearance of the nasal and frontal bones in this region belies the hollow cavities of the paranasal sinuses within the bones on either side of the nose. Growth of the face is accompanied by progressive pneumatization within the bones (Figure 27.1). This results in an increasing volume of the paranasal sinuses throughout life.

Although fractures in this region are particularly likely to affect the frontal and ethmoidal sinuses

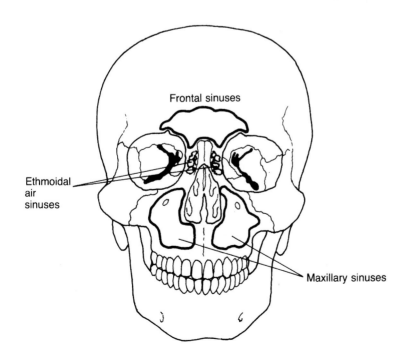

Figure 27.1. Frontonasal region.

they may also be associated with disruption of the sphenoidal and maxillary sinuses. The frontal, ethmoidal and maxillary sinuses all communicate with the nasal cavity. The bridge of the nose supports the medial canthal ligaments, which maintain the soft tissue structures so important for the normal appearance of this area of the face.

Between the upper and lower attachments of the pulleys supporting the eyes to the nose (medial canthal ligaments) lies the lacrimal sac. This facilitates the normal drainage of tears, necessary for the natural lubrication of the conjunctiva. Between the frontal lobes of the brain and the roof of the nose lies the cribriform plate. Through its multiple perforations pass the fine branches of the olfactory nerve, transmitting the sensation of smell which is so important, in addition, in fulfilling taste perception.

Mechanisms of injury

Extreme direct force, such as the kick of a horse, produces impaction of the nasal bridge with collapse of the less robust ethmoidal bone beneath. Similarly, a direct blow to the forehead may fracture the inner plate of bone lining the frontal sinus, raising the possibility of meningitis or of brain abscess.

Severe indirect injury to the middle face including the bridge of the nose (Le Fort II and III level) may also include elements extending into the frontal or ethmoidal regions.

Severity of injury

Collapse of the nasal root can be likened to failure of the poles supporting a ridge tent, with resulting spread of the walls. Spreading of the skin between the eyes results in loss of tension in the medial canthal ligament, and, as a consequence, the unsightly appearance of telecanthus or hypertelorism.

The indices of severity of frontonasal and ethmoidal fractures include the degree of comminution and the degree of displacement. Injuries to structures other than the bone (e.g. olfactory nerve, canthal ligaments and lacrimal drainage), penetration and contamination will also affect the severity of injury and the ability to recover. Associated injuries to the eyes or to the brain will determine the relative importance of these fractures as a contribution to the overall severity of the injury.

High velocity injuries predictably inflict greater damage to bone and soft tissues with massive disruption of supporting structures. Haemorrhage due to rupture of the anterior or posterior branches of the ethmoid arteries can be severe.

Signs and symptoms

Serious fractures of the frontonasal and ethmoidal region may be difficult to isolate from coexisting fractures of the skull vault or the middle face. In the latter injuries, it is true to say that all Le Fort II and III fractures and some nasal fractures share characteristic signs and symptoms. In some cases it is a matter only of terminology about how a fracture in the region around the root of the nose is classified.

Al-Qurainy *et al.* (1991) studied ocular injuries associated with midfacial fractures and found surface damage to the eyelids and conjunctiva to be the most common ophthalmological injuries associated with naso-orbito-ethmoidal fractures, although displacement of the eye and damage to the nasolacrimal apparatus were also noted. They suggested that all patients sustaining a midfacial fracture associated with a significant decrease in visual acuity, either pre- or postoperatively, should have an early review by an ophthalmologist.

Hypertelorism may be disguised by the gross swelling so typical of midfacial bruising. An objective measure of the intercanthal distance (normally some 33–36 mm) may give a guide to disruption of the canthi, as may clinical or radiological observation of upturning of the tip of the nose, or increased nasolabial angulation.

Any damage to the globes must be carefully assessed, as must any complaint of reduced visual acuity or smell.

Relevance of pre-existing conditions to outcome

The size of the frontal sinuses is subject to natural variation. Bilateral asymmetry or midline confluence are well described and may influence both injury and recovery.

Any pre-existing disability of sight or smell will influence and exaggerate the effect of injuries in the frontonasal region. Problems with vision and lacrimal drainage occur more frequently with advancing years, but, in the younger patients, these are mainly secondary to laceration of the nasolacrimal duct as a consequence of fractures of the facial skeleton (Zapala *et al.*, 1992). Management is surgical, by recanalization. This requires a precise technique and is often delayed for months or years following the trauma.

Any slight variation in normal appearance between the eyes can become grossly exaggerated by bone disruption or by scarring in this region, and any predilection to allergic irritation of sinus or lacrimal flow may be worsened.

Investigations

The routine radiological assessment of craniofacial trauma is by a 'skull series'. In this, three plain radiographs are intended primarily to identify fractures to the skull vault. Just as these views usually exclude much of the lower jaw, so they may also fail adequately to illustrate the fronto-nasal region. The use of an occipito frontal 25% projection (Trapnell, 1985) may overcome this deficit and should be considered if this injury is suspected.

Unrecognized nasal and fronto-ethmoidal complex fractures are a major source of cosmetic and functional deficit. Failure properly to define and treat these fractures may result in hypertelorism, epiphora and dacrocystitis.

Nowadays, high definition CT scanners are widely available in the United Kingdom. It is now becoming routine for an emergency CT scan to be performed whenever clinical circumstances permit (Kassell *et al.*, 1983). This is undoubtedly the investigation of choice to obtain the maximum information on frontonasal and ethmoidal fractures, as it includes, as plain radiographs can not, detail of soft tissue, especially in the orbital region. In severe midfacial and naso-ethmoidal injuries, comminution is common (Figure 27.2) and unrecognized injury is difficult to correct at a later date (Russell *et al.*, 1990). When these fractures are suspected they are best investigated by CT.

Treatment options

The timing of surgery in the repair of frontonasal fractures is a major determinant of successful outcome. Although, historically, there was resistance by neurosurgeons to early maxillofacial intervention, it is now increasingly recognized that with modern antibiotics, aseptic techniques and modern anaesthesia, these objections have been largely overcome. Danford *et al.* (1993) advocate early combined surgery 'to achieve improved functional and aesthetic results and to reduce the length of hospital stay'. Such patients have often had a primary brain injury. The traditional approach has been to wait 7–14 days after the trauma to allow resolution of facial swelling before undertaking the definitive repair. In the selection of patients suitable for early surgery, it is critical to avoid exacerbating any brain injury, or operating on patients who may ultimately succumb or remain severely disabled.

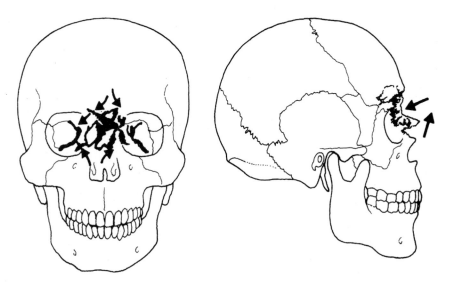

Figure 27.2. Frontonasal fractures.

Persistent leakage of cerebrospinal fluid (CSF) was previously cited as a reason to delay fronto-nasal and maxillofacial skeletal reconstruction, whereas it now appears more likely that early repair of the bony injury will shorten the period of CSF leakage. The development of intracranial infection is particularly likely in fractures that involve the posterior wall of the frontal sinus.

Ionnades *et al.* (1993) studied 71 patients and found fractures involving both the posterior wall and the anterior wall of the frontal sinus in 26. All received primary treatment within 6–12 hours of injury. Of 10 patients with a posterior wall fracture but without displacement, two developed meningitis and a further one patient, 18 months later, an infected cyst (mucopyelocoele) causing osteomyelitis of the frontal bone. In fractures of the posterior wall, they recommended cranialization and blocking the frontonasal duct to obliterate the cavity.

The choice of approach incisions, especially bicoronal flaps, may have a significant effect on a patient's appreciation of the postoperative appearance, particularly in males, where failure to account for future baldness may leave permanent and unsightly scars. The complications of access flaps are well recorded by Mitchell *et al.* (1993), and include frontalis paresis, numbness and wound infection. Other surgical approaches have been described (Bowerman, 1985). The choice must depend on particular circumstances such as the suitability of existing lacerations and the length of delay before surgery.

However, effective treatment of the fractured bones, together with reattachment of the medial canthi, makes an open surgical approach mandatory if accurate repositioning of tissues is to be achieved. The use of stainless steel wires has now largely been superseded by small plate osteosynthesis. In these techniques, the prescription of appropriate antibiotics is particularly important.

Prediction of outcome

Assessment of the quality of recovery after frontonasal fractures should include a comparison of the cosmetic appearance following surgery with photographs taken prior to injury. Olfactory and visual function and assessment of lacrimal drainage are also important determinants of outcome. Late infection of sinus origin is a well recognized complication although the place of the sinus obliteration in its elimination is still debated.

Degree of disability

Sensory disability is particularly severe if the sense of smell is lost as a consequence of frontonasal fractures. For many people the enjoyment of life is highly dependent upon a normal sense of smell and taste (Huizing, 1988). Up to 80% of frontonasal fractures result in a disturbance of the sense of smell (Philip *et al.* 1992). Extensive injuries are frequently associated with unconsciousness. Consequently, although impairment of the sense of smell can often be attributed to the fracture itself causing disruption of the olfactory nerve fibres as they pass through the cribriform plate, associated cerebral lesions may also be implicated, affecting different levels of the pathway of olfactory perception (Zusho, 1982). In more than half of the patients with a disturbance of smell, a simultaneous impairment of taste was reported. Although very little is known about the cerebral processing of gustatory information, it is recognized that taste is initiated by olfaction (Snow, 1983).

Cosmetic deformity is very obvious in this region of the face, especially where scarring of the facial skin or altered underlying bone symmetry is present or when muscle tone and activity is reduced and unbalanced.

Contour abnormalities produce related disturbances of facial landmarks, such as the eyebrows and forehead, especially where fractured bone fragments have not been replaced or accurately repositioned after craniotomy.

Risk of future complications

The consequences of nonunion of a fracture after initial healing include persistent CSF leak, infection and the complications of any subsequent treatment required.

A deterioration in the quality of sight or smell may not be detected for many months, especially when serious concussion has delayed recovery. Difficulty or discomfort with wearing spectacles is a commonly overlooked complication of these injuries.

Prognosis

Prognosis is determined by the degree of disability persisting after optimal recovery has been achieved. The local consequences of a frontonasal fracture may be complicated by neurological and psychological morbidity. The potential for post-traumatic epilepsy from an associated head injury must also be considered.

If untreated or inadequately treated, fronto-nasal-ethmoidal injuries may result in residual deformity of the nasal crest, the orbitonasal angle, dystopy of the medial canthus, alteration of the continuity of the lacrimal passages, or a reduction in the patency of the nasal airway. Any of these problems is likely to require secondary surgical correction.

References

Al Qurainy IA, Stassen LFA, Dutton GN, *et al.* (1991) Midfacial fractures and the eye. *British Journal of Oral Maxillo Facial Surgery* **29**: 291–301.

Bowerman JE. (1985) Fractures of the middle third of the facial skeleton. In: Rowe NL, Williams J, editors. *Maxillofacial injuries*, vol. 1. Edinburgh: Churchill Livingstone, 387.

Danford M, Palmer JD, Lang D, Neil-Dwyer G. (1993) Selection of patients for early combined repair of craniofacial trauma [abstract]. *Br J Oral Maxillofac Surg* **31**: 56.

Huizing EH. (1988) Nose and society. *Rhinol Suppl*, **7**: 9.

Ionnades T, Freihofer HP, Frienz J. (1993) Fractures of the frontal sinus; a rationale of treatment. *Br J Plast Surg* **46**: 208–14.

Kassell EE, Noyek AM, Cooper PW. (1983) CT in facial trauma. *J Otolaryngol* **12**: 2–15.

Mitchell DA, Barnard NA, Bainton RJ, (1993) An audit of 50 bitemporal flaps in primary facial trauma. *J Craniomaxillofac Surg* **21**: 279–83.

Philip A van Damme, Freihofer HPM. (1992) Disturbances of smell and taste after high central midface fractures. *J Craniomaxillofac Surg* **20**: 248–50.

Russell JL, Davidson MJC, Daly BD, Corrigan AM. (1990) Computed tomography in the diagnosis of maxillofacial trauma. *Br J Oral Maxillofac Surg* **28**: 287–91.

Snow JB. (1983) Clinical problems in chemosensory disturbances. *Am J Otolaryngol* **4**: 224.

Trapnell DH. (1985) Diagnostic radiography. In: Rowe NL, Williams J, editors. *Maxillofacial injuries*, vol. 1. Edinburgh: Churchill Livingstone, 135.

Zapala J, Bartkowski AM, Bartkowski SB. (1992) Lacrimal drainage system obstruction: management and results obtained. *J Craniomaxillofac Surg* **20**: 178–83.

Zusho H. (1982) Post traumatic anosmia. *Arch Otolaryngol* **108**: 90.

28

Zygomaticomaxillary complex and orbital fractures

Hugh Cannell

Mechanisms of injury

The region of the zygoma, with its complex pattern of suture lines to neighbouring bones, is easily damaged by blunt or penetrating trauma. The high points of the face that protect the globe of the eye are the supraorbital ridges, the nose, the orbital rims inferiorly, and, laterally, the buttresses of the zygomatic bones. Displacement of any or all of these structures by a fracture therefore exposes the globe to the risk of injury. This risk remains until the fractures of zygomaticomaxillary complex (ZMC) and orbit are reduced (Figure 28.1).

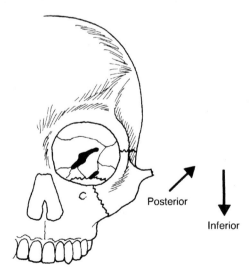

Figure 28.1. ZMC fracture sites and the most common directions of displacement.

The concept of hemispheric dominance is an important one in any consideration of fractures in and around the orbit. Hitchin and Shuker (1973) confirmed their clinical impression that the majority of zygomatic injuries, if caused through interpersonal violence, were to the left side of the injured patient. They postulated that predominance of left-sided injury was because most assailants were right handed. When an assailant confronts an intended victim there is a tendency to aim a blow to the recipient's left side. As soon as an intended recipient, who is also likely to be right handed, realizes that acceptance of a blow is inevitable, there is a tendency to turn away to protect the 'master' side (i.e. the right) and hence accept the blow on the left or nondominant side.

Injuries to the thin bones around the orbital cavity easily occur after direct or indirect violence. Displacement and comminution into very small fragments is often found. Where the bones are thicker, laterally at the zygomaticofrontal suture and superiorly at the supraorbital ridge, and in the male where there are more marked and rougher prominences of the bones, there is a greater resistance to injury.

Despite some thickening of the lateral bony border of the orbit, the globe of the eye is less well protected from injury on the lateral side than from any other direction. This is due to the slightly more posterior position of the processes of the zygomatic and the frontal bones, than the remaining planes of the bones of the orbit (Sischer, 1960). The supraorbital ridges, especially in the male, afford the best protection superiorly, whilst the good lateral vision of the human eye is provided at the expense of indifferent lateral protection against globe injury.

So-called 'trapdoor' or 'blow-out' fractures occur in the very thin bones separating the medial side of the orbit from the ethmoid air sinus and the floor from the maxillary air sinus (antrum of Highmore). The mechanism of a pure 'blow-out fracture' is that of compression of the globe of the eye by an object smaller than the bones guarding the circumference of the orbit. Since the globe can be considered as a fluid-filled capsule, any compressive forces will be transmitted via the periorbital fat to the containing bony walls. The walls may then fracture in their weakest areas, for example where expansion of the maxillary air sinus has hollowed out to a depth of 0.5 mm the minor thickenings of bone around the course of the infraorbital nerve within its canal. Fists or rounded blunt instruments, or the balls used in sports, have all been implicated in blow-out fractures of the orbit (Figure 28.2).

Injury may likewise produce alterations in the volume of the bony orbit. Compression, for example after a crushing injury, will result in exophthalmos. More commonly, the displaced bones increase the available space for the contents of the orbit and the classic 'sunken eye' or enophthalmic appearance is produced. Avulsion of the medial palpebral ligament, or bilateral displacement of the bone to which it is attached, results in an increase in the intercanthal distance (normally 33 mm in the adult) and the appearance of traumatic telecanthus (Rowe, 1981). Since it is also inevitable that comminution of the medial walls of the orbits has occurred, then the orbital telecanthus may be complicated by increased orbital volume producing an enophthalmos, or by a crushed orbit producing exophthalmos.

Single or multiple defects of the orbital walls, with comminution, may also occur within the main fracture patterns associated with multiple facial bone injuries. In general, the higher the degree of force causing the injury, the more likely it is that bony defects of the orbital walls will occur.

Other types of orbital injury may be due to damage to the canthal ligaments. In particular, injuries to the lateral side of the bony orbit may result in a torn lateral canthal ligament or its detachment, together with a significant displaced fragment of bone. Similarly, injuries to the central nasal ethmoidal region, and therefore the medial side of the bony orbit, may involve the medial canthal ligament. Such medial injuries may require a canthopexy and, laterally, an adjustment of the lateral canthal ligament for height by stabilization of the bony fragment after open operation.

Other injuries may involve the nasolacrimal apparatus. The lacrimal gland itself may have been injured by lacerations and should be repaired. The drainage is on the medial side of the eye through the nasolacrimal ducts, which drain into the lateral wall of the nose. Scarring or blockage of the ducts may result in epiphora. These injuries are best treated early, before scarring has interfered with the line of the drainage duct. A dacrorhinocystotomy or similar operation should be undertaken.

Nerve damage is frequent, especially to the infraorbital nerve. This nerve is easily damaged either in the floor of the orbit or near its exit on the anterior wall of the maxilla at the infraorbital foramen. Similarly, the supratrochlear and/or supraorbital nerve may be damaged in orbital roof injuries, which are often associated with frontal bone fractures.

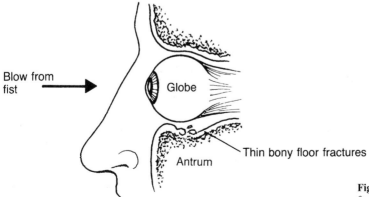

Figure 28.2. Trapdoor or so-called 'blowout' fracture of orbit.

Relevance of pre-existing conditions

Untreated, displaced, malunited fractures of the bones in and around the cheek and orbit will greatly increase the risk of further injury. In particular, if the globe of the eye is left unprotected by displacement of the guarding high points, then permanent loss of vision becomes a probability in the event of further injury.

In the older age groups, the diminished masticatory forces following the loss of teeth will lead to expansions of the air sinuses and even to hollowing out of the zygomatic buttress, the pterygoid region and the floor of the orbit. Decreases in the substance of the bones of the calvarium takes place by resorption of the outer surfaces, whilst facial bones resorb from the inner surface in relation to air sinuses (Sischer, 1960).

The frontal sinus also enlarges with age and in response to reductions in masticatory function. Fractures of the ZMC and orbital region in the elderly may therefore be more comminuted and displaced than those occurring in younger patients.

Clinical and radiological assessment

An injury to the ZMC or orbit places the patient at risk from diminished visual acuity or blindness. A careful examination of the eye should be followed by a test of visual acuity. Thereafter, sequential tests of acuity, ocular mobility, and pupil size and reaction should be recorded, as should the patient's neurological status.

Radiographs are less useful if marked periorbital swelling is present. In particular, fractures of the thin bones of the orbital walls may be masked by oedema, although fractures of the thicker bones of the ZMC will normally be visible. Russell *et al.* (1990) recommend high resolution CT scanning for the demonstration of orbital injuries and for injuries to the frontal and nasoethmoidal regions. In their study, they revealed a large number of soft tissue injuries of the orbit, which required immediate treatment. They noted that splaying of the lateral walls of the nasoethmoidal region into the medial part of the orbital cavity after injury was responsible, or could become responsible, for such conditions as ocular hypertelorism, dacrocystitis and epiphora, as well as direct damage to the globe.

Apart from a high resolution CT scan, if necessary taken in several planes, it is useful to have plain radiographs as supplementary views of injuries to the lateral middle third of the face. The occipitomental projection demonstrates the middle one-third of the face particularly well and the angle of projection can be altered to demonstrate preferentially the upper one-third of the face. Rotational tomograms, including hypercycloidal tomograms of the ZMC region and orbits are often used. If the patient is unconscious or has to lie flat due to multiple injuries, then specialized apparatus such as the 'Zonarc' tomograph machine or the newer CT scanners can be used to image the region.

Management of injuries

The early management of a single facial injury confined to the ZMC is expectant until any gross periorbital and facial oedema has settled. Apart from the usual period of observation for head injury, the reasons for delaying surgical treatment for definitive fracture reduction of the ZMC regions are the presence of significant orbital oedema and the presence of other injuries with greater treatment priorities. Occasionally, early referral of an injured patient may allow the reduction of a displaced ZMC fracture before much periorbital swelling has taken place. It is more often the case that both the ZMC and the orbital bones have been injured and, as a consequence, orbital oedema has occurred.

Thus, the early management of injuries to the bones within and around the orbit is that of careful sequential observations, and of surgical intervention at the right moment. Commonly, considerable swelling occurs within a few hours of injury. This may result in proptosis of the globe. Occasionally there may also be an associated retrobulbar haemorrhage. Over 90% of injured patients will show some impairment of visual acuity or of eye mobility. The key to successful management is therefore to await resolution of the swelling and yet to intervene early enough to minimize any damage to orbital contents that may have become trapped by sharp bony fragments in the walls or the floor of the orbit (Figure 28.1).

Reasonable expectations of outcome

The success of any treatment following ZMC or orbital fracture and any associated globe injury, depends entirely upon the speed of diagnosis and therefore upon co-operation between maxillofacial and ophthalmic surgeons. This teamwork concept is particularly important if moderate to severe injuries to the globe have occurred or are likely to occur, especially as a result of developing haemorrhage.

Al-Quirainy *et al.* (1991a–d) considered that both early surgical reconstruction of the bones around the orbit, and conservative management for disorders of motility, contribute to a satisfactory outcome. One of the outcomes they measured was diplopia (Al-Quirainy, 1991c), which recovered within a matter of a few hours to one week in 25% of the 363 patients in their series. In a further 29.2% it recovered in one to four weeks and 25% suffered from diplopia for between one and six months; 11.1% of their patients recovered within 7–12 months and only 6.9% complained of diplopia for more than 12 months. Blow-out fractures of the orbit were particularly likely to be associated with sustained diplopia; their study showed that blow-out fractures contributed to diplopia in 58.3% of patients. In addition, 2.8% of their 363 patients developed palsy of a cranial nerve. There were two patients with sixth cranial nerve palsy and one with third nerve palsy. Spontaneous recovery of each of these took place within seven months. No case of fourth nerve palsy was found but the remaining patients had the seventh cranial nerve affected, possibly due to penetrating injury.

The disabilities that may occur after failure to repair accurately the ZMC and/or bones of the orbit are severe. These can be divided into those affecting the globe, those affecting surrounding anatomical structures, and those affecting the bones. Some of those affecting the globe have already been discussed and it should be noted that a few patients will have permanent impairment of visual acuity or blindness, permanent diplopia, the 'orbital apex' syndrome affecting the second, third, fourth, fifth and sixth cranial nerves, or the 'superior orbital fissure' syndrome affecting the third, fourth, fifth and sixth cranial nerves.

A poor outcome may also be due to the cosmetic effects of damage to the globe itself or to the soft or hard tissues around it. Injuries such as blow-out fractures and comminution of the walls or floor of the orbit. This may result in an enophthalmic appearance. The upper eyelid looks drooped and the patient is often described as having a ptosis. This is due to the deepening of the fornix of the eye and of the supratarsal fold, which is associated with enophthalmos, due to the changed position of insertion of the levator palpebrae superioris muscle

into an inwards and inferiorly displaced globe (Rowe, 1981). It used to be thought that periorbital fat, which normally acts as a cushion around the globe may become affected by necrosis due to delayed loss of blood supply. If this occurred, the fat underwent liquefaction and, with subsequent scarring and fibrosis, became greatly decreased in volume. A delayed enophthalmos may occur, usually within three months or so of any original injury which increases available space for the globe of the eye.

The level of the pupil may also drop compared with the other side. A rough test for this is to attempt to line up the pupil levels with the line of the occlusion of the teeth. These two planes should be approximately parallel. A drop in level is most likely to happen in association with a displaced fracture of the lateral wall of the orbit, which results in a lowering of ocular level on that side, due to displacement of the insertions of the suspensory (Lockwood's) ligament of the globe.

Temporary concussional effects, alterations in the volume of the orbit, disturbance or trapping of the intraocular muscles (particularly those of elevation), a lowered ocular level, and central neurological damage, can each cause diplopia. An acceptable but approximate measure of diplopia is the Hess chart, as recorded by an orthoptist. However, it is the author's experience that more minor degrees of diplopia, especially diplopia due to head injury, may not be measurable by Hess charting but patients may still complain of this symptom.

Al-Quarainy *et al.* (1991a–d) found that 90% of their patients who had sustained trauma to the midfacial region had ocular injuries of varying severity. Fortunately, 63% sustained only minor or transient injuries, 16% had moderately severe injuries to the globe, and 12% had severe injuries. Of 27 patients with comminuted malar fractures, nine had severe injuries to the globe. Blow-out fractures of the orbital walls occurred in 16.7% of these patients. They found that comminuted malar fractures (ZMC) were associated with the most severe ocular and motility defects. It was stressed that all injuries to the area carried a high risk of damage to the globe. Minimal degrees of injury, which were not referred for ophthalmic assessment, were those involving eyelid swelling or bruising, conjunctival chemosis, post-traumatic neuralgia or anaesthesia, subconjunctival haemorrhage, small corneal abrasions, mild reduction of visual acuity with recovery, mild failure of accommodation, mild comotio retini, and orbital emphysema. The more serious injuries to the globe, which required referral for ophthalmic opinion, were enophthalmos, lacerations of the conjunctiva, traumatic changes to the papilla or iris, damage to the lens, cataract, severe failure of accommodation, moderate reduction of acuity, and moderate or severe comotio retini, as well as choroidal tears, vitreous floaters, traumatic pigmentary retinopathy and nasolacrimal damage. Very urgent referrals were required for proptosis, retrobulbar haemorrhage, corneal damage with puncture wounds, scleral injury, hyphaema, angle recession, lens dislocation, subluxation or rupture of the capsule, severe reduction in acuity, loss of vision, or visual field loss. Choroidal tears involving the macula, vitreous haemorrhage, retinal detachment or tears with optic nerve injuries were found to be of great significance. If any of these signs were present after injury then the outcome for the patients with ZMC or orbital injuries was very much worse. In particular, retrobulbar haemorrhage is a very serious complication, which may rapidly produce blindness. According to Wood (1989), it rarely occurs at the time of the injury, but can do so soon after or even be delayed in development. Bailey *et al.* (1993) found that monocular blindness following midfacial surgery for any reason was extremely rare. They found an incidence of 0.03–0.04% after reviewing 1405 cases of surgical procedures involving the facial skeleton. The pathophysiological cause of the haemorrhage was reported to be obscure, but the bleeding into the closed intraconal space produced an increase in intraocular pressure and a progressive loss of visual acuity, probably from retinal vessel impairment and decreased perfusion pressure. Uncorrected, the increased intraocular pressure ultimately leads to ischaemia with retinal or optic nerve infarction. Surgical management is by decompression of the cone of the ocular muscles via the infraorbital, or occasionally by the supraorbital, approach (Rowe, 1981). Medical management, if carried out early enough, may avoid the risks of surgery. According to Wood (1989), the onset of acute pain in the globe ipsilateral to any ZMC or orbital injury, or headache, nausea and progressive loss of visual acuity, are signs of probable retrobulbar haemorrhage. In their series, a reduction in intraocular pressure was achieved by aggressive treatment with mannitol, acetazolamide and hydrocortisone. Improvement of visual acuity followed and, finally, full recovery of vision.

Impairment of visual acuity was found to be the single most sensitive predictor for any form of ophthalmic injury by Al-Qurainy *et al.* (1991a,b,d). Their visual acuity code was based on five categories ranging from 0 (6/6 or better) to 4 (no perception of light). They noted that comminuted malar fractures were likely to be associated with the most severe ocular and motility defects. Their prospective survey studied 100 patients with midface fractures and had a sensitivity value of 93.4% and specificity value of 89%. Only one patient who warranted referral to an ophthalmologist was missed by their system and protocol, whereas nine others (false positives) were incorrectly classified as warranting referral.

Lee (1983) has found that cranial nerve palsies, including those cranial nerves subserving ocular motility functions, occur in from 3% to 71% of closed head injuries following road traffic accidents. Further evidence that central connection damage may occur after injury to the head and face has been reported by Larkin *et al.* (1993). Delayed conduction along one optic nerve resulted in four of their patients incorrectly appreciating moving objects. This phenomenon was considered to be due to a temporal mismatch of interpretation between the two optic pathways. This defect is termed the Pulfrich phenomenon. It was identified after the patients became inexplicably frightened by car travel. They were found to perceive oncoming traffic as moving in a shallow curve towards them. Correction of the disability was achieved by provision of a tinted lens for the normal eye.

Outcome following injury

Nerve damage

The infraorbital nerve is the most frequently damaged as a result of injuries to the ZMC and orbital regions. Some clinicians believe that any neurological defect should be reassessed one year after injury and state that post-traumatic neuralgia, dysesthaesia, or even complete anaesthesia, is relatively common. Whilst agreeing that damage was often present soon after injury, Taicher *et al.* (1993) studied recovery of sensation of the infraorbital nerve after various treatments, including a comparison of open versus closed fracture reduction. They found an open reduction and direct fixation of displaced fractures with wire or miniplate osteosynthesis had the best prognosis, with 70% improvement after 12 months. The difference between the groups was identified by testing only pain sensation. Two-point discrimination, light touch and temperature difference were not assessed.

Damage that affects the pupillary light reflex may be temporary, with good recovery, or may be permanent. The latter is likely if the oculomotor nerve has been stretched beyond repair by herniation of the uncus through the tentorium cerebelli, or if the optic nerve has been divided (Rowe, 1981). An oculomotor nerve palsy is usually permanent. Post-traumatic iridoplegia rarely persists, but some degree of irregular dilatation may be present for many months following injury to the ZMC or orbit.

Rowe (1981) was optimistic about the prognosis of patients with the superior orbital fissure syndrome. Despite the ptosis, dilated pupil and immobility of the globe, he favoured a conservative approach and predicted partial or even complete recovery after one year. However, if the optic nerve was damaged then blindness was likely to be permanent.

Diplopia

Ilzuka *et al.* (1991) noted in their study that persistent diplopia following zygomatic fractures correlated significantly with orbital floor defects of greater than 10 mm in diameter and with the presence of comminuted fractures. They noted that overcorrection in terms of height seemed to be necessary. They used polydiaxone (PDS) material to overlay floor defects. This was eventually replaced by bone, and gave a satisfactory outcome. Delayed management of orbital injuries, especially of diplopia, may also involve bone grafting. This is particularly necessary in delayed management or revision procedures when osteotomy has to be undertaken. Grafts of cartilage, lyophilized bone, autologous bone and alloplastic materials such as PDS have been used. In the author's experience the Tessier marginotomy procedure is particularly suitable for delayed management of severe orbital floor injuries involving correction of diplopia.

Reconstruction of orbital walls and floor

Outcome may be poor following severely comminuted injuries of the bony orbit. The best results are achieved by early reconstruction. As has already been mentioned, many different materials have been used for reconstructive purposes. Titanium mesh sheets are suggested for orbital floor defects of up to 2.5 cm in size (Sugar *et al.*, 1992). Children with blow-out fractures of the orbit of the 'trapdoor' variety should undergo definitive exploration and treatment as soon as possible after injury (Derton *et al.*, 1992). Enophthalmos inevitably results from increases in orbital volume which cannot be corrected.

Lacrimal drainage defects: outcome

Outcome following obstruction of the lacrimal drainage system is good, with 83% of post-traumatic patients having complete recovery. Zirpallah *et al.* (1992) recorded post-traumatic obstruction of the drainage system in 45 of 70 patients with naso-orbital maxillary or ZMC fractures. The typical problems they encountered were epiphora, discomfort in wearing spectacles or contact lenses, and recurrent infections of the eyelid, conjunctiva, lacrimal sac or nasolacrimal duct. Dacrocystorhinostomy by canalicular intubation was used in 31 of their 45 patients. Zirpallah *et al.* (1992) also found that coexisting injuries of the visual system were common, including laceration of the eyelids, damage to the medial palpebral ligament, ptosis, diplopia and orbital fractures. Where possible, primary operation by canalicular anastomoses after intubation of the nasolacrimal duct and primary closure was undertaken at the time of treatment of the fracture. Drainage tubes were left *in situ* for three months.

The delayed management of deformity

Flattening of the malar prominence is a cosmetic defect that is easily noticed. Similarly, retropositions of the lateral portion of the orbit or defects of the zygomatic arch are noticeable. Very accurate reduction and reconstruction of the bones around the orbit is necessary for protection of the globe. Diplopia and enophthalmos will occur unless they are placed accurately in position. If malunion has occurred, full zygomatic osteotomies may be necessary. Autologous bone should be placed behind all osteotomy cuts. In the author's experience, on-lay grafts tend to resorb over time and are unsatisfactory.

Other problems that may occur in reconstructing the areas around the orbit and zygoma are due to the thin surface skin and the thin depth of tissue over the osteosyntheses. Many miniplates, or even wire osteosyntheses, have subsequently had to be removed if they became uncomfortable. Too rapid drilling without sufficient cooling or sufficient smoothing of the holes may lead to ring sequestra at the common operative sites on the lateral side of the orbit or the orbital rim. These can be a cause of much late pain and discomfort. Persistent oro-antral or oronasal fistulae, with maxillary sinusitis or even pansinusitis, may occur after fractures of the zygomatic bones. An untreated fracture of the zygomatic arch may lead to ankylosis of the arch to the coronoid process of the mandible, with con-sequent limitation of jaw movement.

Risk of long-term complications

Long-term complications are most likely to occur when the cranial nerves of the orbital complex have been affected. Some may never recover. In addition, impairment of the drainage of the lacri-mal apparatus, or such severe damage to the orbit that restitution and reconstruction is impossible, may result in permanent cosmetic deformity and disability, including loss of sight. As a con-sequence, the long-term prognosis of these injuries may be poor. Although some further surgery can usually be undertaken, this may involve further surgical scars. Occasionally, alloplastic materials, such as silastic and Teflon, are extruded from the floor of the orbit. This complication has been reported by Brown and Banks (1993). These authors also noted that any alloplastic material is a potential source of irritation and subsequent infec-tion, even if chemically inert. Maxillary sinusitis may very well be the precipitating cause of such an event. If this is considered likely, autogenous cartilage can be used for the augmentation of defects of the zygomatic area. Pffeifer and Gun-dlach (1989) recorded a series of 52 patients who had received transplantation of cartilage to the face; 25 had a good result, 25 an acceptable result and a further 2 a poor result.

References

Al-Qurainy IA, Titterington DM, Dutton GN, Stasson LFA, Moos KF, El-Attar A. (1991a) Mid-facial fractures of the eye; the development of a system detecting patients at risk of eye injury. *Br J Oral Maxillofac Surg* **29**: 363–67.

Al-Qurainy IA, Titterington DM, Dutton GN, *et al.* (1991b) Mid-facial fractures of the eye; the development of a system detecting patients at risk of eye injury: a prospective evaluation. *Br J Oral Maxillofac Surg* **29**: 683–89.

Al-Qurainy IA, Dutton GN, Stasson LFA, Moos KF, El-Attar A. (1991c) Diplopia following mid-facial fractures. *Br J Oral Maxillofac Surg* **29**: 302–307.

Al-Qurainy IA, Dutton GN, Stasson LFA, Moos KF, El-Attar A. (1991d) The characteristics of mid-facial fractures associated with ocular injury: a prospective study. *Br J Oral Maxillofac Surg* **29**: 291–301.

Bailey WK, Kud PC, Evans LS. (1993) Diagnosis and treatment of retrobulbar haemorrhage. *J Oral Maxillofac Surg* **51**: 700–82.

Brown EA, Banks P. (1993) Late extrusion of alloplastic orbital floor implants. *Br J Oral Maxillofac Surg* **31**: 154–57.

Derton K. Wijngaarde R, Hesse J, de Jong PT. (1992) Influence of age on the management of blow-out fractures of the orbital flows. *Int J Oral Maxillofac Surg* **20**: 330–36.

Hitchin AD, Shuker ST (1973) Sork observations on zygomatic fractures in the Eastern region of Scotland. *Br J Oral Maxillofac Surg* **11**: 114–17.

Ilzuka P, Nikkonem P, Parku P, Lindquist D. (1991) Reconstruc-tion of orbital floor by use of polydiaxonone (PDS plate). *Int J Oral Maxillofac Surg* **20**: 83–87.

Larkin EB, Dutton BNP, Herron G. (1993) Impaired perception of moving objects following mid-facial trauma [abstract]. *Br J Oral Maxillofac Surg* **30**: 341.

Lee J. (1983) Ocular mobility consequences of trauma and their management. *Br Orthop J* **14**: 26.

Pfeifer P, Gundlach KKH. (1987) Residual deformities: frac-tures of the zygomatic complex. In: Rowe NL, Williams JL, editors. *Maxillofacial injuries*, vol. 2. London: Churchill Livingstone, 821.

Rowe NL. (1981) Surgical anatomy of the orbit. Anatomy of the orbit, salivary glands and neck. In: Cannell H, editor. Proceedings of the British Association of Oral Surgeons Consultants' Study Day, 1980. London: British Association of Oral Surgeons, 12–36.

Russell JL, Davidson MJC, Daily BD Corrigan AM (1990) Computed tomography and diagnosis of maxillofacial trauma. *Br J Oral Maxillofac Surg* **28**: 281–91.

Sischer H. (1960) *Oral anatomy.* St Louis: Mosby.

Sugar AW, Kuraikose M, Wallshaw ND. (1992) Titanium mesh in orbital wall reconstruction. *Int J Oral Maxillofac Surg* **21**: 140–44.

Taicher S, Ardecian L, Sammett N, Yoshani Y, Caffe I. (1993) *Int J Oral Maxillofac Surg* **22**: 339–41.

Wood CM. (1989) The medical management of retrobulbar haemorrhage complicating facial fractures – a case report. *Br J Oral Maxillofac Surg* **27**: 291–95.

Zirpallah J, Bartkowska A, Bartkowski JB. (1992) Lacrimal drainage system obstruction; management and results of change in 70 patients. *J Cranio Maxillofac Surg* **20**: 178–83.

29

Maxillary fractures

Hugh Cannell

Introduction

It is unusual for a maxillary fracture to be found in isolation after an injury. When it does occur, it is usually the result of a direct blow to the maxilla, often, in the author's experience, as a result of interpersonal violence. More commonly, fractures of the upper jaw are associated with fractures of the nose, nasoethmoid and frontal regions, zygomaticomaxillary complex (ZMC) and orbit. In addition, in patients with severe trauma after impacts of high momentum to the facial region, there may be mandibular fractures and thus disturbances of the occlusion of both jaws.

A simple classification of fractures of the middle one-third of the face was proposed by Rene Le Fort in 1901. He noted that the fracture patterns were broadly related to the weak areas of bone supporting the buttresses (bony pillars) and, in the case of fractures next to the base of the skull, were through the weakest areas of the buttresses. Le Fort's classification suggested three main levels of fracture pattern. The lowest level was Le Fort I. This approximately corresponds to the dento-alveolar and basal bone of the maxilla becoming separated from the remainder of the upper jaw across the floor of the nose (Figure 29.1). The two higher levels, Le Fort II and III, very approximately describe the separation of a larger piece of the middle third of the face from the cranial base at levels just below (Le Fort II) and just above (Le Fort III) the zygomatic bone. Even a cursory examination of the typical radiographic views for demonstration of facial fractures will disclose many more than the main Le Fort classification

fracture lines. Surgical exploration of a person with fractured facial bones will disclose that the fracture patterns that affect the buttress bones are connected by a crazy paving of multiple cracks in the comminuted, smaller and thinner facial bones bordering the air sinuses. The Le Fort levels are

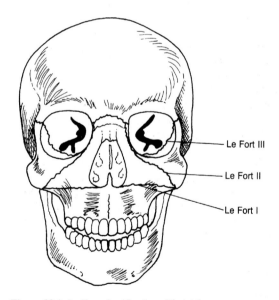

Figure 29.1. Le Fort classification of facial fractures.

I   Horizontal fracture of lower part of maxilla, generally at the floor of the maxillary sinus;
II Pyramidal fracture involving the maxillary, nasal, lacrimal, ethmoid and sphenoid bones; the vomer and nasal septum may also be involved;
III Transverse fracture involving the nasal bones, orbit and malar bone.

therefore useful as a broad description, although not an accurate account of what has actually been fractured and displaced.

Relative frequency of maxillary fractures

The relative frequency of occurrence (i.e. presentation at a maxillofacial unit) of patients with injuries to the middle one-third of the face was reported by Schuchardt *et al.* (1966), Rowe and Killey (1968), Vincent-Townend and Langdon (1985) and Timony *et al.* (1990). The results are shown in Table 29.1.

Timony *et al.* (1990) showed that rates per annum of a fracture at any site in the maxillofacial region ranged from 18/100 000 population in Bordeaux to 33/100 000 population in Bristol. The absolute incidence cannot be assessed with any accuracy because of variations in the referral bases and less accurately predictable populations. The high frequencies of severe maxillary fractures reported by Cannell *et al.* (1993) were in a small number of patients ($n = 34$) during one year of operation of a specialized helicopter medical evacuation service.

Mechanism of injury

The mechanism of injury is usually blunt trauma. Occasionally, cases of blast injury from industrial explosions are seen. Gunshot wounds may also contribute to the incidence.

Comminuted fractures with impaction of fragments are found most commonly after high speed road traffic accidents, especially if the car occupants are unrestrained by seat belts, or after falls or jumps of greater than 20–30 ft (approximately 6–9 m). For a complete understanding of such fractures, the accompanying injuries should also be described. These may include severe comminution about the orbits and separate levels of fracture from one side of the face to another. Thus, a combination of a Le Fort I and a Le Fort II-type injury is quite common. Other associated injuries are likely to be severe. The more extensive the facial fracture, the more likely it is that there will be a concomitant head injury.

The severity of injury increases with the speed of a road traffic accident or with the degree of personal violence encountered. For example, a kick from a leg weighing 30–40 lb (13.6–18.1 kg) can create extensive damage to facial bones, particularly if the foot that does the striking is covered with boots with metal caps or with pointed ends to the sole. The severity of the injury is increased still further if one considers that there is a degree of whip and elasticity not only in rotation about the assailant's hip but also about the knee and ankle. Kicks to the face and head can and do result in death.

Relevance of pre-existing conditions

The relevance of any pre-existing conditions is typically that of the associated multiple injuries. Most usually, associated neurosurgical injuries are responsible for delays in treatment of maxillofacial injuries. Sailer (1985) quotes a residual deformity rate in maxillary injuries of about 70% at the Zurich Clinic. This high figure is likely to have included patients with severe brain damage, who were consequently not available for early management by the maxillofacial surgeon. In the UK, residual maxillary deformity after injury is uncommon, reflecting the availability in most areas of specialized maxillofacial surgeons. When cases of residual deformity do occur, they nearly always arise in patients in whom there has been a delay before definitive treatment can be undertaken. It is still possible, although fortunately unusual, for

Table 29.1. Frequency of maxillary fractures[a]

Authors and year	% Le Fort I	% Le Fort II	% Le Fort III
Schuchardt *et al.*, 1966	18.5	23.4	1.2
Rowe and Killey, 1968	4.3	8.4	3.6
Vincent-Townend and Langdon, 1985	6	7	3
Timoney *et al.*, 1990	8.2	8.2	8.2
Cannell *et al.*, 1993	3	21	21

[a]Some patients in each group may have had maxillary fractures at more than one level.

patients with severe combined intracranial and maxillofacial injuries to languish in neurosurgical units for many months before they are considered well enough to have their facial fractures treated. If the most severely displaced facial fractures are reduced at early operation, much residual deformity can be avoided.

Outcome

Except in the multiply injured and the brain damaged, in whom intervention to reduce maxillary facial fractures was considered to be impractical, the expected outcome should be excellent.

Treatment options affecting outcome

Maxillary fractures may be treated by extraskeletal or internal skeletal fixation. External fixation is now becoming less common due to the wide availability of miniplates for direct internal fixation of any fractured upper or midfacial bones. Occasionally, a degree of rotation of the maxilla can be missed even at a careful primary surgical intervention. This is particularly likely to occur if the patient had a malocclusion before the accident or has missing teeth, so that the occlusal guide to reduction is unhelpful. More usually, impacted buttress bones, typically the ZMC, may have to be reduced at open operation when a degree of impaction leading to a reduction of midfacial height can be seen. A comminuted fractured mandible may also complicate the reduction of a fractured maxilla; in turn this may lead to occasional misjudgements resulting in rotations and incorrect vertical height.

Sailer (1985) commented that restoration of the normal occlusion did not automatically guarantee the restoration of the original relationship between the various thirds of the face. Because the middle one-third of the face may have become comminuted with impaction and with overriding of fragments, then vertical height may be easily lost, but must be restored for a favourable outcome. This problem of impaction has led to the modern treatment of complex cases of the fractured middle one-third by open reduction and the fixation of the reduced fragments by miniplate osteosynthesis.

In hospitals that treat multiply-injured patients, it is common to find an oral endotracheal tube in place for the first few days after the injury. If so, examination of the mouth and oral cavity may not be very easy and, if the area is very swollen, it is sometimes impossible. In these circumstances, and where there are associated head or chest injuries, it is recommended that tracheostomy should be considered. This will allow proper inspection of the oral cavity and any necessary reduction of maxillary bones by direct intervention followed by intermaxillary fixation.

External skeletal fixation

External skeletal fixation can be by means of plaster head caps (although these are now rarely used), by halo frames, such as the Berkshire or Crewe halo frame, or by pins and rods. Many forms of external skeletal fixation have attachment rods screwed to a plate on a splint cemented to the teeth. A problem that may occur with external fixation and which affects outcome is loosening of the pins or screws of the halo frame. This may be due to insufficient tightening, to poor positioning, to a lack of electrical insulation leading to galvanic action, or to poor resistance to infection in the patient (e.g. in diabetics). Loose pins or screws can then lead to scars and deformity at the anterior hairline. Supraorbital pins, if loose, will cause scars at the lateral sides of the eyebrows.

Internal skeletal fixation

Because internal skeletal fixation is now the treatment of choice in facial injuries, accurate reduction and fixation of the fractures is now possible. The judicious use of dental casts, or of photographs of the patient prior to the injury, followed by achievement of symmetry of the buttress bones, will normally result in accurate reduction.

The older techniques of reduction of residual maxillary deformity depended upon slow movement of the maxilla into the correct position. This was often carried out by elastic traction or even by means of extraoral fixation, for example to a Balkan beam. Such techniques are now rarely used, because most interventions can take place in the first two to five weeks after injury. In the early stages after trauma it may be possible to break open a forming malunion or nonunion and reposition the maxilla into its proper height and place. Occasionally, a patient can be so critically ill that treatment has to be deferred and, after about three weeks to one month, it is certain that a malunion will take place.

Degree of disability

The degree of disability following malunion can be of the function of the jaws or of appearance and may be severe. As personal appearance is of great importance to the patient and to the relatives, it is the duty of the maxillofacial surgeon to consider maxillary osteotomies for correction of any residual deformity. In their simplest forms, these can be segmental osteotomies of parts of the occlusal plane in the upper jaw. Occasionally, a posterior part of the upper jaw can be impacted upwards after injury and may then be associated with an oro-antral fistula. This displacement can easily be reduced by segmental surgery and the oro-antral fistula closed at the same time. Zaccariades *et al.* (1993) postulate a 14-day window for the treatment of fractures of the upper and middle facial third. They suggest that definitive surgery should be undertaken within this time in order to avoid the necessity for secondary operations and the significant risk of leaks of cerebrospinal fluid or chronic disease of the air sinuses, with a consequent high risk of infection of the sinuses and brain.

Treatment of residual maxillary deformity

Any osteotomy for residual maxillary deformity will require suitable bone grafts and plating in order to hold the repositioned maxilla in place. The best graft is autologous bone. This can be harvested from the iliac crest or ribs. Of particular importance is the stabilization of a maxilla that has to be repositioned in a forward direction. Autologous bone can be placed as grafts at the pterygoid region. Any alteration in height of the maxilla requiring bone grafts, should be treated with plates, with the plate also being screwed into the graft. At this stage, it is also possible to introduce endosseous implants to the grafted area and leave them buried for later use.

Russell *et al.* (1990) have commented that in the treatment of this complication, sound preoperative planning is necessary. Nowadays this can be achieved by means of a computer-assisted reconstruction of a three-dimensional model of the face or facial skeleton.

Apart from segmental osteotomies for dento-alveolar structures, various classical osteotomies are available for the correction of mid-face residual deformities. These are the Le Fort I, Le Fort II, and, finally, the bicoronal scalp flap approach to the Le Fort III osteotomy. Where ocular hypertelorism has occurred as a result of the injury, then a combined craniofacial approach is necessary.

Such osteotomies may have to be combined with other surgery, for example to repair calvarial defects. Titanium cranioplasties have been used, and have proved an ideal material for the restoration of such defects (Joffe *et al.*, 1993).

References

Cannell H, Silverster KC, O'Regan MB. (1993) Early management of multiply injured patients with maxillofacial injuries transferred to hospital by helicopter. *Br J Oral Maxillofac Surg* **31**: 207–12.

Joffe JM, Aghabeigi D, Harris M. (1993) Retrospective study of 66 titanium cranioplasties. *Br J Oral Maxillofac Surg* **31**: 140–48.

Le Fort R. (1901) Étude expérimentals sur les fractures de la mochoire supériere. *Rev Cheo* **23**: 208.

Rowe NL, Killey HC. (1968) Fractures of the facial skeleton, 2nd edition. Edinburgh: Churchill Livingstone.

Russell JL, Davidson MJC, Daily BD, Corrigan AM. (1990) Computed tomography and diagnosis of maxillofacial trauma. *Br J Oral Maxillofac Surg* **28**: 287–91.

Sailer HF. (1985) Residual maxillary deformities. In: Rowe NL, Williams JLL, editors. *Maxillofacial injuries*. Edinburgh: Churchill Livingstone, 831–42.

Schuchardt K, Schwenzer N, Rotthe B, Lendtradt J. (1966) Urascheei Kaufrgkeit und lokalisation der fractures ges ge sichtesschadels. *Fortschr Kiefer Gesichtchir* **11**: 1.

Timoney N, Saiveau M, Pinsolle J, Shepherd J. (1990) A comparative study of maxillofacial trauma in Bristol and Bordeaux. *J Cranio Maxillofac Surg* **18**: 154–57.

Vincent-Townend JL, Langdon JD. (1985) Appendix. In: Rowe NL, Williams JLL, editors. *Maxillofacial injuries*, vol. 2. Edinburgh: Churchill Livingstone, 999–1014.

Zaccariades N, Bazattis M, McAliss A. (1993) Post-traumatic osteotomies of the jaw. *Int J Oral Maxillofac Surg* **22**: 328–31.

30

Injury to the temporomandibular joint

Paul F Bradley

Introduction

Applied anatomy

The anatomy of the joint can be divided into the following components.

Bony articulating surfaces

The moving part of the mandible, the condyle, articulates with a hollow on the base of the skull termed the glenoid fossa. In front of the fossa is a bony prominence called the eminence. The articulating surfaces are lined with 'wear and tear' fibrocartilage. The basic movements of the joint are:

1. Hinge movements: these allow the jaw to swing open and closed;
2. Gliding or translatory movements: these allow the condyle to move downwards and forwards along the eminence.

A combination of hinging open and gliding forward is necessary to incise food between the front teeth, as the lower incisors lie behind the upper incisors so that there would not be contact in a simple hinge movement alone.

The insubstantial anatomical dimensions of the condyle make it vulnerable in trauma to the mandible, so that fracture in this region represents around 25–35% of all mandibular fractures (Rowe and Killey, 1968). The most common site of fracture is in the subcondylar region between the neck (the position of attachment of the capsule) and the mandible proper level with the most inferior point of the sigmoid notch anteriorly. The condylar head is another site of fracture involving that part that lies within the capsule (intracapsular fracture). This site is very important because it poses a real risk of ankylosis of the joint i.e. union between the condylar head and the glenoid fossa, which prevents movement. The condylar neck itself is a third site. An important clinical classification of condylar fractures is that of MacLennan (1952), who looked at the relationship of the fractured fragment to the remainder of the mandible and gave four main categories:

1. *No displacement*;
2. *Fracture deviation* Here there is simple angulation of the condylar process to the major fragment. An example of this is the 'greenstick' fracture of childhood.
3. *Fracture displacement* Here there is some degree of overlap of the condylar process and the major mandibular fragment.
4. *Fracture dislocation* This is where the head of the condylar process has been completely disrupted from the glenoid fossa. This has considerable clinical importance because the condylar head is pulled forwards and medially by the lateral pterygoid muscle, thereby allowing foreshortening or telescoping of the vertical ramus of the mandible due to the pull of the elevator muscles of the pterygomasseteric sling. This causes premature contact of the back molar teeth on the affected side, with inability of the rest of the teeth to meet fully (dental malocclusion). Lindahl (1977) proposed a more comprehensive classification suitable for research purposes.

Interarticular disc (meniscus) and capsule

A fibrocartilaginous disc lies between the articulating surfaces and is attached peripherally to the fibrous tissue of the joint capsule, which links the two surfaces. The disc has two thickenings running transversely across it, namely an anterior band and a thicker posterior band (approximately 3 mm thick); in normal function, the latter should lie between the transverse ridge of the condyle and the highest concavity of the fossa (Juniper, 1990). A very important component of the disc is its posterior part, termed the bilaminar zone. This is made up of a lower dense layer and an upper elastic layer. It is the latter that is responsible for the passive return of the disc after protrusive movements. The bilaminar zone is an area prone to injury, whereby the disc may not move smoothly with the condyle, producing clicking noises (reciprocal clicking), or, alternatively, it may stay in a forward position where it can cause locking of the joint i.e. a blockage to full forward movement and opening (acute closed lock).

Related muscles

The position of the lower jaw is determined by the reciprocal movement of the elevator or closing muscles (masseters, medial pterygoids and temporalis) and the depressor or opening muscles (the suprahyoid muscles, particularly digastrics and mylohyoid). Two muscles assist opening by causing protrusion or forward movement of the condyle over the eminentia, namely the lateral pterygoid muscle and the anterior fibres of the temporalis. The lateral pterygoid is particularly important in this respect in that it is attached to the anterior aspect of the neck of the condyle and also has a small slip, which is inserted into the anterior aspect of the disc; it is therefore capable of causing a co-ordinated protrusive movement of both the condyle and the disc together. It should be noted that, although there is a muscular mechanism for bringing the disc forward, recoil of the disc relies entirely on the elastic components of the bilaminar zone.

Related nerves

The auriculotemporal nerve, a branch of the second division of the trigeminal nerve, winds its way round the back of the neck of the condyle to provide sensation over the area of the temple. This nerve gives off the main nerve supply to the joint over its back surface, namely a rich leash of fibres termed the posterior articular nerves. They provide a plexus of nerve endings in relationship to the bilaminar zone. The auriculotemporal nerve may occasionally be injured in trauma to the region, producing numbness over the temple and sometimes aberrant or gustatory sweating at meal times (Frey's syndrome). The temporal and zygomatic branches of the facial nerve are related to the anterior aspect of the joint and are at risk during surgical exposure of the joint via the preauricular route (Al-Kayat and Bramley, 1979). The temporal branch is particularly prone to damage as it runs forward and upwards to cross the midpoint of the zygomatic arch to reach the frontalis muscles (which are responsible for wrinkling the forehead and elevating the eyebrows when looking upwards).

Mechanism of injury

The following are common patterns of injury or disturbance to the temporomandibular joint, which produce either bony injury and/or internal derangement of the disc.

Direct blow

A direct blow to the preauricular region may produce a fracture of the condyle, usually in the subcondylar or neck regions. This is particularly likely to occur with a relatively localized impact, as from a metal rod or bottle end; a more diffuse impact, as from a fist or boot, is more likely to fracture the vertical ramus itself. The degree of displacement of the condyle depends on the force of the blow so that there may be no displacement, a fracture deviation, a fracture displacement or a fracture dislocation, with the latter being related to the most severe impact.

Indirect blow

A diffuse blow to the opposite body of the mandible, as by a fist or boot, may cause a direct fracture of the mandible. It is also likely to transmit its force to the opposite side, causing a fracture of the condyle (the so-called indirect or contrecoup injury).

Fall causing impact to region of the chin

Experiments with cadaveric material (Fonseca, 1974) have shown that it is easier to produce condylar fractures after axial blows to the mandible while the mouth is open than with it closed. Fonseca pointed out a relatively high incidence of condylar fractures in road traffic accidents, speculating that at the moment of impact, the mouth is likely to be open, either to scream or in fright. This can be contrasted with the low incidence of condylar fractures in boxing, where the boxer uses a mouth protector and has a tendency to keep the teeth clenched into the soft material. Falls are an important example of such impacts and it is possible to divide these into two categories:

1. *Parade ground-type fall.* This is exemplified when a soldier on parade has a syncope and falls on to the chin. This kind of impact can also occur with a fall from any kind of medical collapse e.g. diabetic hypoglycaemic attack, myocardial infarction or cerebrovascular accident. In all of these it is likely that the mouth is flaccid and open at the time of the attack. A typical pattern is one of a direct fracture of the mandibular parasymphyseal area combined with bilateral fractures (often fracture dislocations) of both condyles.
2. *Fall with mouth closed.* This may occur in falls from a significant height (e.g. from the upper storey of a building) or in epileptic attacks in which the jaw is closed in the tonic phase. Here, the teeth are frequently fractured (longitudinal-type fractures involving the roots). Lindahl (1977) has pointed out that, in this instance, the condylar fractures are usually of the intracapsular type.

Stretching and tearing of internal structures of the joint

A connection is now recognized between whiplash injury (cervical extension–flexion) and internal derangement of the temporomandibular joint (Roydhouse, 1973). The mechanism is postulated to be a stretching and tearing of the posterior and polar attachments of the disc in the cervical hyperextension phase (as in a rear end collision) when the unsupported head accelerates less quickly than the body and there is a downward and forward displacement of the disc–condyle complex. This is under the influence of the supra- and infrahyoid muscles, which are unable to lengthen quickly enough. This tearing action on the bilaminar zone of the disc is followed by a crushing impact on the already traumatized posterior attachment structures by their impingement between the condyle and the glenoid fossa in the cervical hyperflexion stage. This is caused by the ultimate deceleration as the car involved strikes the vehicle or object in front or the brakes are applied. Internal derangement of the joint has been demonstrated by arthrography in 22 of 25 subjects with temporomandibular joint symptoms after whiplash injury (Weinberg and Lapointe, 1987). Mannheimer *et al.* (1989) stressed the importance of the recognition of this possibility in whiplash injuries, to allow early therapeutic intervention. Therapies that could be envisaged would be a short period of intermaxillary fixation to allow repair, or possibly physical therapy in the form of ultrasound (Bradley, 1987). There is, however, as yet no evidence that such treatment can prevent the ultimate sequelae of internal derangement of the joint in such patients.

Other ways in which the vulnerable bilaminar zone may be damaged are by means of a wide, prolonged opening, such as in a yawn or the type of movement that sometimes occurs in sporting endeavours (e.g. reaching for a high shuttle in badminton). In these instances, the subject may suddenly feel a sharp pain in the joint, indicating tearing of the internal structures. Wide prolonged opening of the jaw, as during dental treatment or during intubation for a general anaesthetic, also appears to be capable of causing similar, if less severe, effects. The usual result here is a painful joint for some weeks afterwards, although occasionally internal derangement can occur. Damage to the posterior attachments of the disc can also occur due to overloading of the joint as in parafunction e.g. grinding the teeth at night (Bruxism) or in lack of posterior occlusal support in which the patient has lost the back molar teeth and does not have any form of denture replacement, thereby throwing stress on to the disc itself. A combination of both factors would be particularly damaging.

Dislocating forces

A strong tractional force on the mandible may pull the condylar heads out of the fossae in such a way that they lodge in that position. The commonest dislocation is in an anterior position (Heslop, 1956), where the condyles come over the eminentiae with the mouth wide open, the chin protruded and no teeth occluding. This can occur with a wide yawn, during prolonged dental treatment, or in forced opening during a general anaesthetic. It is most likely to happen in patients who have naturally lax ligaments. Such patients will often have noticed episodes of subluxation whereby the condyles come out but they are able to reposition them by themselves; dislocation is where the patient is unable to rectify the situation. Such patients will usually be able to achieve an opening gap between their incisor teeth above the usual upper limit of 40 mm and will often have other joints that demonstrate hypermobility (e.g. clicking finger joints, shoulders or knee caps).

If such an anterior dislocation is not recognized, muscle spasm of the elevator groups can occur quite rapidly making reduction by the usual Hippocratic method of downward and backward pressure on the jaw impossible without a general anaesthetic, an aid to relaxation in the form of intravenous sedation, or a local anaesthetic to the motor branches of the affected muscles. Such dislocation may only come to light months after the event, particularly in edentulous patients. Fordyce (1965) reviewed the literature and pointed out that manual reduction using appliances such as mouth gags; although generally difficult after a month from the time of the dislocation, can be successfully accomplished after as long a period as six months, although sometimes operation is necessary.

Rarer variants of dislocation are anterolateral (Morris and Hutton, 1957), posterior (Helmy, 1957), lateral (Allen and Young, 1969) and lastly superior (Zecha, 1977). Superior dislocation, although very rare, is of considerable clinical importance in that it involves a fracture of the glenoid fossa, allowing the condyle to be pushed upwards into the cranial cavity. This appears to be associated with a particularly small rounded type of condyle, which fails to impinge on the margins of the glenoid fossa. It is significant that seven of ten reported patients were female.

Degree of disability

The possibility of an injury to the temporomandibular joint should be borne in mind in anyone who has had a direct impact over the preauricular region or has suffered a hard blow over the opposite side of the mandible that was capable of producing an indirect injury (Figure 30.1). Patients who have experienced a whiplash injury should be kept under review as far as their joints are concerned so that appropriate therapy may be given should it appear that they have suffered an internal derangement. In acute traumatic cases, bleeding from the ear may arouse the suspicion that there has been a posterior dislocation of the condyle into the external auditory meatus, while the observation of Battle's sign (bruising over the mastoid process area) will arouse the suspicion of a concomitant fracture of the temporal bone. The usual patterns of disability observed in the acute injury are:

1. *Signs of joint hypofunction* (Figure 30.1a) If there has been damage either to the bony or to internal structures of the joint there is likely to be a triad of features:
   a. Pain in the joint area on opening;
   b. Limitation of opening of the jaw, secondary to the pain; normal jaw opening involves a gap (interincisal clearance) of 30–40 mm between the anterior incisor teeth and this will be reduced;
   c. Deviation to the affected side on opening; a disturbance to the joint is likely to affect the function of the lateral pterygoid muscle on that side so that when the patient opens the jaw it deviates towards the side of injury.
   The presence of one or more features of this triad will throw suspicion on a possible injury to the joint.
2. *Premature contact on the molar teeth on one side* (Figure 30.1b) This form of malocclusion of the teeth (posterior gagging) is commonly associated with a unilateral fracture dislocation of the condyle. The condyle is pulled medially and forwards by the lateral pterygoid muscle so that the vertical ramus of the jaw is telescoped under the action of spasm of the elevator muscles, producing an effective shortening and making the teeth meet prematurely at the back on that side.
3. *Premature contact on molar teeth on both sides (anterior open bite)* (Figure 30.1c) This sign is seen in bilateral fracture dislocation of the condyles where telescoping of both vertical rami occurs.
4. *Failure of any teeth to occlude* (Figure 30.1d) This occurs in bilateral dislocation where the heads of the condyles have been brought forward of the eminentia. The lower jaw will appear prominent (pseudo class III appearance). This appearance is easy to recognize in patients with teeth but may be difficult in those who are edentulous, although it will be revealed if the dentures are put in place, when they will fail to occlude.

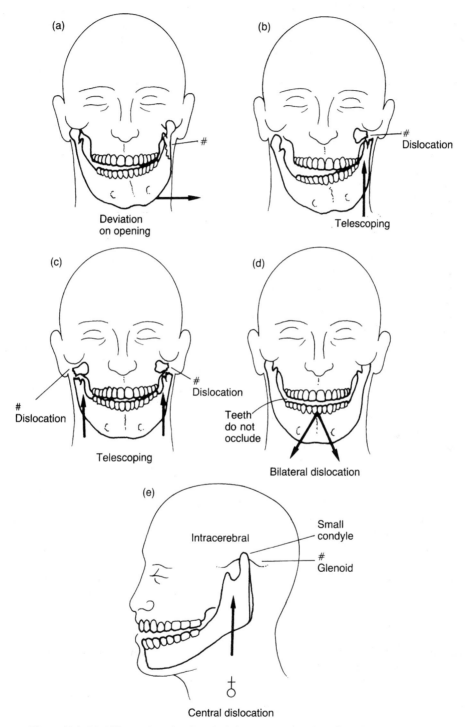

Figure 30.1. Disability: (**a**) hypofunction (deviation on opening); (**b**) unilateral molar contact; (**c**) bilateral molar contact; (**d**) failure to occlude (anterior dislocation); (**e**) absolute immobility (central dislocation, i.e. superior).

5. *Absolute immobility of lower jaw* (Figure 30.1e) This sign may be observed in the rare central dislocation of the condyle where this structure has perforated the glenoid fossa to enter the cranial cavity. In this instance, the lower jaw cannot be moved and this should arouse suspicion of this serious situation.

The presence of any of these patterns of signs would indicate the need for radiological investigation of the joints.

Investigation: imaging examinations

1. *Conventional radiographs* In general two radiographs films at right angles to each other should be undertaken, such as an orthopantomogram, or a lateral oblique to give a lateral view and a PA of the mandible, or a reverse Towne's view in that plane. Transcranial views of the temporomandibular joints may also be helpful.
2. *Tomography* Where conventional radiographs have not been definitive or are not possible due to the difficulty of turning a patient face downwards, conventional tomography, either in the coronal or sagittal planes, may provide useful information (Ekerdal, 1973).
3. *CT Scanning* If scanning is being undertaken for other head and neck injuries then it may be relevant to include the region of the joint. Raustia *et al.* (1990) have demonstrated that a CT scan gives a good definition of the relationship of the condyle to the mandibular fossa. For this reason, it is particularly indicated for suspected central dislocations of the condyle, where it will also demonstrate the presence of any related intra- or extradural haematoma.
4. *Magnetic resonance imaging (MRI)* Surface-coil MRI has permitted a significant advance in the diagnosis of internal derangement of the temporomandibular joint (Harms *et al.*, 1985; Schellhas and Wilkes, 1989). It is possible to visualize the meniscus clearly and also the associated muscles of mastication. It is likely that in the future this investigation will be indicated more frequently as for example in patients of whiplash injury in whom internal derangement is suspected.
5. *Arthrography* By introducing a contrast medium into the upper and lower joint spaces, it is possible to visualize the position of the meniscus in internal derangement (Wilkes, 1978). However, this method is not suitable for use in the acutely-injured patient. It is likely to be used less frequently in the future (as it is somewhat trying for the patient) now that MRI is available, although the two methods can be combined (Schellhas *et al.*, 1988).

Risk of future complications

The principal long-term complications of importance are:

Ankylosis of the joint

This is the development of significant or complete limitation of movement of the joint by bone or fibrous tissue. This is obviously a serious complication but fortunately only a small proportion of patients are at risk. The factors involved have been summarized by Laskin (1978):

1. *Site and type of fracture* As might be expected, bony ankylosis is most commonly associated with intracapsular fracture (Figure 30.2a,b), so that it is very important to recognize this variant. The risk is not present with the majority of fractures that involve the subcondylar or neck regions, except in the rare circumstance of when there is such gross telescoping of the vertical ramus (due to the lack of posterior teeth) that the condylar stump comes into contact with the glenoid fossa. Extra-articular ankylosis (i.e. away from the joint) can occur when there is a combined fracture of the zygomatic arch and the coronoid process of the mandible, which lies anterior to the joint. In this instance, it is very important to reduce the fractured zygoma so that it is out of contact with the coronoid (Figure 30.2c).
2. *Age of the Patient* The majority of patients who develop ankylosis sustain their injuries before the age of 10 years (Topazian, 1964). In children the condyle is very bulbous and liable to intracapsular fracture.
3. *Duration of immobilization of the lower jaw* In the presence of an intracapsular fracture, it is generally taught that the lower jaw should not be immobilized for more than about 10 days, as movement is felt to discourage bone growth. Experimental work in primates has, however, failed to produce ankylosis by this means after artificially produced condylar fractures (Mackey *et al.*, 1980). Immobilisation is therefore felt to be a contributory factor rather than the primary cause.

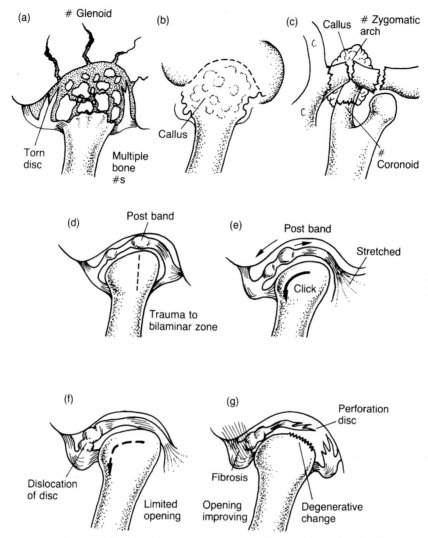

Figure 30.2. Future complications: (**a**) intracapsular fracture; (**b**) intra-articular ankylosis; (**c**) extra-articular ankylosis; (**d**) normal joint; (**e**) reciprocal clicking; (**f**) acute closed lock; (**g**) chronic closed lock.

4. *Damage to the intra-articular disc* The disc normally acts as a barrier to bony union after condylar fracture. Animal experiments have shown that this structure needs to be removed to allow ankylosis in experimental animals (Wheat *et al.*, 1977). It has been difficult to obtain data on the meniscus in acute injuries in humans, but MRI scanning offers the opportunity of obtaining such information, as yet however, present scanning regimens are rather prolonged for use in the acutely-injured patient.

Defective development of the mandible

In the group of patients at risk from intracapsular fracture and ankylosis (i.e. children under the age of 10 years), there is a potential risk to the development of the mandible on the affected side. At one time it was felt that the condylar cartilage acted as a growth centre in the same way as an epiphyseal plate in a long bone, but it is now realized that this is not the site of primary growth of the mandible, but it merely allows the condylar head to stay in the glenoid fossa as the mandible develops downwards and forwards with the demands of the functional matrix (Moss, 1968). Excision of the condyle in developing Rhesus monkeys does, however, result in less growth of the height of the ramus and preangular notching, although anteroposterior development still takes place (Choukas *et al.*, 1966). However, in the human situation, if ankylosis takes place, the immobile condyle may tether the mandible, preventing it participating in the functional matrix and thereby creating some disturbance to anteroposterior growth. It is therefore important to operate early to relieve the ankylosis in such situations, in order to allow mandibular development.

Persistent internal derangement

If the bilaminar zone of the meniscus (Figure 30.2d) has been torn and does not unite, then a sequence of changes may be set in train:

1. *Reciprocal clicking* (Figure 30.2e) After opening and protrusion, the meniscus may fail to return completely to its normal position so that during the next excursion it is positioned anteriorly to its normal place, causing a click as the condyle moves past the prominent posterior band.
2. *Acute closed lock* (Figure 30.2f) The tendency of the meniscus to be displaced forward as seen in reciprocal clicking may be accentuated to transform into the condition of acute closed lock, in which the meniscus stays in a forward, and often medial, position. In this instance, the click disappears and the patient is unable to open more than about 20 mm interincisal clearance. The mandible deviates to the affected side markedly on opening.
3. *Chronic closed lock* (Figure 30.2g) If acute closed lock is not remedied, as by surgery or, occasionally, by forced lavage of the joint to break down any adhesions, the patient may proceed to chronic closed lock. The anteriorly displaced meniscus becomes fibrosed in the anterior position and contracts so that opening improves a little, but not to normal. The bilaminar zone is stretched over the condyle; with time this disc tends to wear through to produce a perforation. Once the protective role of the disc is lost between the joint surfaces, wear of the fibrocartilage will occur and eventually result in the exposure of bone. This results in a characteristic sound or crepitus heard by the patient during mandibular excur-

sions (often described 'like the noise of sandpaper') and by the clinician particularly if a stethoscope is used. The condyle will eventually show degenerative signs, which may comprise lysis of the head, osteophyte formation, reactive sclerosis and, occasionally, pseudocyst formation i.e. osteoarthritis.

Other untoward features

1. *Persistent pain* Persistent pain may occasionally follow any condylar injury, despite extensive treatment. It can sometimes be difficult to determine whether this is organic in nature or whether it is associated with the acute 'stress' of an injury and may need psychiatric help and psychotropic medication.
2. *Persistent deviation on opening* This may be observed in any patient who has had an injury to the temporomandibular joint. The incidence varies in different reported series, but Konstantinovic and Dimitrijevic (1992) found an incidence of around 7% in two groups of patients with condylar fractures, one of whom had been treated conservatively and the other surgically. These are particularly good results and the author feels that the results of McLennan (1952) of 16% after conservative treatment are more representative, although slight deviation has been reported in one series in as many as 23% of patients (Lachner *et al.*, 1991). Such persistent deviation is more likely to occur after fracture dislocation. It is probably of little significance in most patients except for those professionals who require very precise mandibular function e.g. singers, musicians and actors (Bradley, 1994).

Treatment options affecting outcome

For a condylar fracture there are three main treatment options:

Functional

This comprises advocating a soft diet, analgesics as required and a gentle regimen of exercises focused on centring the mandible on opening to remedy deviation once pain is lessening. This kind of regimen may reasonably be used for a patient with a unilateral fracture dislocation who can attain a normal dental occlusion (it is usual to wait for about 48 hours to allow muscle spasm to settle before assessment) and who is not experiencing excessive pain.

Conservative regimen

This comprises securing the two jaws together by intermaxillary fixation for a period to allow muscle spasm to settle down. The means of intermaxillary fixation may be arch bars, eyelet wires (Ivy loops), or Gunning-type denture splints in edentulous patients. Ten days is usually an adequate period for unilateral fractures but four to six weeks may be necessary in patients with bilateral fracture dislocation and an anterior open bite. Indications for conservative treatment in the form of intermaxillary fixation may be summarized as:

1. Patients who have persistent malocclusion at 48 hours after injury;
2. Patients who have excessive pain at 48 hours after injury;
3. If there is a fracture without any displacement, it may be argued that it would be best to put the patient into fixation for about 10 days to ensure that it does not convert to a fracture dislocation, when morbidity would be more likely. This is particularly so in patients who are likely to experience another episode of trauma to the joint.

Surgical reduction of fracture and immobilization

The absolute indications for surgery have been well summarised by Zide and Kent (1983):

1. Fracture dislocation of the condyle into the middle cranial fossa;
2. The impossibility of obtaining adequate occlusion by closed reduction due to locking by the condylar fragment;
3. Lateral fracture dislocation of the condyle;
4. Invasion by a foreign body (e.g. gunshot wound). This category would include most compound fractures of the condyle where some degree of debridement and surgical toilet is indicated.

They also suggest relative indications for open reduction. These may be summarized as those patients in whom there is an association with comminuted midface fractures necessitating reconstruction of a mandibular platform, medical conditions in which intermaxillary fixation is contraindicated (such as severe respiratory disease) or cases with a very unstable occlusion.

In those patients in whom surgery has been used to reduce a fractured condyle, a variety of methods of fixation can be used, but the use of miniplates appears to be the method of choice. They may be inserted through an extraoral route (e.g. Stewart and Bowerman, 1991) or via an intraoral incision (e.g. Lachner *et al.*, 1991).

In patients in whom internal derangement is diagnosed early, as with MRI scanning, there is as yet no clear cut consensus on the best management. Where such internal derangement occurs in combination with condylar fractures Chuong and Piper (1988) have described the immediate repair of a discal injury. Under the microscope, the anteriorly displaced disc is released, often simply by the process of a transecting joint space adhesions, although additional release of the epimysium of the lateral pterygoid muscle may be necessary or removal of a wedge of posterior disc attachment with repair.

Reasonable expectations of outcome

The following general statements may be made with regard to injuries of the temporomandibular joint:

1. The major complication of condylar fracture is ankylosis. This principally occurs in a small and predictable group of patients, namely those with intracapsular fractures and under 10 years of age. In this group, it is important to institute functional treatment i.e. movement after not more than 10 days to discourage intra-articular bone formation. If this is done, the outcome appears to be good. If limitation of movement does occur despite functional treatment, then it is relevant to carry out condylectomy and replacement with a costochondral junction graft (rib with a cartilage cap), which is capable of undergoing adaptive remodelling with the growth of the patient (James, 1994).
2. Patients in this risk group should be kept under regular review at six monthly intervals for about two years and then yearly until mandibular development is complete at the age of about 16 in the female and 18 in the male.
3. Conservative treatment of condylar fractures has been shown in large series to produce relatively satisfactory results, although approx-

imately 20% of patients will have some sort of residual disability in the form of deviation on opening to the affected side or clicking (MacLennan, 1952).

4. The indications for surgical repositioning of the condyle have now been established in an absolute sense. It has still not been established however by properly designed trials whether surgical reduction gives better results than conservative treatment in the case of a unilateral fracture dislocation.

5. The remarkable remodelling process after fracture dislocation in children emphasizes that surgical reduction is not indicated in this age group (Lindahl and Hollender, 1977). This faculty persists, but with a lesser degree of certainty, into the teenage years.

6. Patients with a history of any injury to the temporomandibular joint area must be kept under review to detect an internal derangement. MRI scanning may be indicated to confirm a malpositioning of the meniscus. The best form of early treatment is not yet fully established. Consideration should be given to arthroscopy, which allows visualization of the problem area, the breakdown of adhesions and some limited opportunities for intra-articular repair procedures or open surgery, which permits disc repositioning.

References

Al-kayat A, Bramley PA. (1979) A modified pre-auricular approach to the temporomandibular joint and malar arch. *Br J Oral Surg* **17**: 91–103.

Allen FJ, Young AH. (1969) Lateral displacement of the intact mandibular condyle. A report of five cases. *Br J Oral Surg* **7**: 24–30.

Bradley PF. (1987) Conservative treatment for temporomandibular joint pain dysfunction. *Br J Oral Maxillofac Surg* **25**: 125–37.

Bradley PF. (1994) Injuries of the condylar and coronoid process In: Rowe NL, Williams JLL, editors. *Maxillofacial injuries*, vol. 1. Edinburgh: Churchill Livingstone, 405–39.

Choukas NC, Tota PD, Guccione JM. (1966) Mandibular condylectomy in the rhesus monkey. *J Oral Surg* **24**: 422–32.

Chuong R, Piper MA. (1988) Open reduction of condylar fractures of the mandible in conjunction with repair of discal injury: a preliminary report. *J Oral Maxillofac Surg* **26**: 257–63.

Ekerdal O. (1973) Tomography of the temporomandibular joint: correlation between tomographic image and histological sections in a three dimensional system. *Acta Radiol* **329**: 1–107.

Fonseca GD. (1974) Experimental study on fractures of the mandibular condylar process. *Int J Oral Surg* **3**: 89–101.

Fordyce GL (1965) Long standing bilateral dislocation of the jaw. *Br J Oral Surg* **2**: 222–5.

Harms JE, Wilk RN, Wolford LM, Chiles DG, Milam S. (1985) The temporomandibular joint: magnetic resonance imaging using surface coils. *Radiology* **157**: 133–6.

Helmy M. (1957) Rare type of dislocation of the temporomandibular joint. *Egypt Dent J* **3**: 27–9.

Heslop IH. (1956) Fracture of the midline of the mandible associated with complete unilateral dislocation of the jaw. *Br J Plast Surg* **9**: 129–31.

James D. (1994) Injuries of the temporomandibular joint in children. In: Rowe NL, Williams JLL, editors. *Maxillofacial injuries*, vol. 1. Edinburgh Churchill Livingstone, 439–55.

Juniper R. (1990) Surgery for internal derangement. In: Norman JE de B, Bramley P, editors. *A textbook and colour atlas of the temporomandibular joint*. London: Wolfe, 176–86.

Konstantinovic VW, Dimitrijevic V. (1992) Surgical versus conservative treatment of unilateral condylar process fractures: clinical and radiological evaluation of 80 patients. *J Oral Maxillofac Surg* **50**: 349–52.

Lachner J, Clanton JT, Waite PD. (1991) Open reduction and internal rigid fixation of subcondylar fractures via an intraoral approach. *Oral Surg Oral Med Oral Pathol* **71**: 257–62.

Laskin DM. (1978) Role of the meniscus in the aetiology of post-traumatic temporomandibular joint ankylosis. *Int J Oral Surg* **7**: 340–5.

Lindahl L. (1977) Condylar fractures of the mandible: I. Classification and relation to age, occlusion and concomitant injuries of teeth and tooth supporting structures and fractures of the mandibular body. *Int J Oral Surg* **6**: 12–21.

Lindahl L, Hollender L. (1977) Condylar fractures of the mandible: II. A radiographic study of remodelling processes in the temporomandibular joint. *Int J Oral Surg* **6**: 153–65.

MacLennan WD. (1952) Consideration of 180 cases of typical fractures of the mandibular condular process. *Br J Plast Surg* **5**: 122–8.

Mannheimer J, Attanasio R, Cinotti WR, Pertes R. (1989) Cervical strain and mandibular whiplash effects upon the craniomandibular apparatus. *Clin Prev Dent* **11**: 29.

Markey AJ, Potter BE, Moffett BC. (1980) Condylar trauma and facial symmetry: an experimental study. *J Maxillofac Surg* **8**: 38–51.

Morris EE, Hutton CE. (1957) Unusual luxation of mandibular condyle. Report of a case. *J Oral Surg* **15**: 332–3.

Moss ML. (1968) The primacy of functional matrices in orofacial growth. *Dent Pract* **19**: 65–73.

Raustia AM, Pyhtianene J, Okiarinan KS, Attonen M. (1990) Conventional radiographic and computed tomographic findings in cases of fracture of the mandibular condylar process. *J Oral Maxillofac Surg* **48**: 1258–62.

Rowe NL, Killey HC. (1968) *Fractures of the facial skeleton*. Edinburgh: Livingstone, 179–80.

Roydhouse RH. (1973) Whiplash and temporomandibular dysfunction. *Lancet* **i**, 1394–5.

Schellhas KP, Wilkes CH. (1989) Temporomandibular joint inflammation: comparison of MR fast scanning with T_1 and T_2 weighted imaging techniques. *Am J Neuroradiol* **10**: 589–94.

Schellhas KP, Wilkes CH, Omlie MR. (1988) The diagnosis of temporomandibular joint disease: two compartment arthrography and MR. *Am J Neuroradiol* **9**: 579–88.

Stewart A, and Bowerman JE. (1991) A technique for control of the condylar head during open reduction of the fractured mandibular condyle. *Br J Oral Maxillofac Surg* **29**: 312–5.

Topazian RG. (1964) Aetiology of ankylosis of temporomandibular joint. Analysis of 44 cases. *J Oral Surg* **22**: 227–33.

Weinberg S, Lapointe H. (1987) Cervical extension–flexion injury (whiplash) and internal derangement of the temporomandibular joint. *J Oral Maxillofac Surg* **45**: 653–6.

Wheat PM, Evaskus DS, Laskin DM. (1977) Effects of temporomandibular joint meniscectomy in adult and juvenile primates. *J Dent Res* **58** (special issue): B139–45.

Wilkes CH. (1978) Arthrography of the temporomandibular joint in patients with the TM pain dysfunction syndrome. *Minn Med* **61**: 645–52.

Zecha J. (1977) Mandibular condyle dislocation into the middle cranial fossa. *Int J Oral Surg* **6**: 141–6.

Zide MF, Kent JN. (1983) Indications for open reduction of mandibular condyle fractures. *J Oral Maxillofac Surg* **41**: 89–98.

31

Fractures of the mandible

John L B Carter

Introduction

The mandible articulates with the base of skull via the temporomandibular joints. Injuries to the joints and teeth carry specific associations of sufficient importance to be the subject of separate chapters.

After any significant injury, fractures of the mandible may occur at any site, on either side. They frequently affect one site on the side of direct injury (ipsilateral) and another site on the opposite (contralateral) side. Dental injuries may occur in isolation but often accompany fractures of both the mandible and the maxilla.

The bone of the mandible represents the scaffolding infrastructure of the lower one-third of the face. The size and symmetry of this area relative to the face as a whole has significant social, cosmetic and sexual connotations. These must balance harmoniously to maintain an aesthetic 'norm'.

The types of fractures suffered by children, their special management and possible future implications during growth merit specific and separate consideration from adults. According to a study by Thoren *et al.* (1992), the decisive age limit seems to be 10 years. After this age, the aetiologies and fracture types become similar to those occurring in young adults. According to Stylogianni *et al.* (1991) fractures of the mandible represent more than 80% of all fractures of the facial skeleton in children.

The current classic English language text is *Maxillofacial injuries*, edited by Rowe and Williams (1985), which developed in part from *Fractures of the facial skeleton*, edited by Rowe and Killey and first published in 1968. The dramatic changes in the management of such injuries during the intervening two decades have been more than matched since 1985 by clinical developments and improvements in imaging techniques.

Basic anatomy

Skeleton

The common sites of mandibular fracture are the subject of regional variation, but Hopkins (1985) has reported the following:

- The condyles (31%): at or below the joint articulation;
- The angle (20%): from the lower border towards the third molar tooth area where the body and ramus merge;
- The body (20%): which bears the premolar and molar teeth;
- The symphysis (11%): is rarely fractured in the midline but more commonly just laterally in the parasymphyseal region;
- The parasymphyseal region (13%): bearing the lateral incisors and canine teeth.
- The ramus (1%): between the condyle and the angle, also includes the coronoid process;
- The alveolus (4%): this portion of the bone is not a separate anatomically identifiable structure but rather that portion of the mandibular bone which supports the teeth and their adnexae during dental development and the roots of the teeth so long as they persist. Alveolar bone resorbs most quickly in disease affecting the teeth and following tooth loss (Figure 31.1).

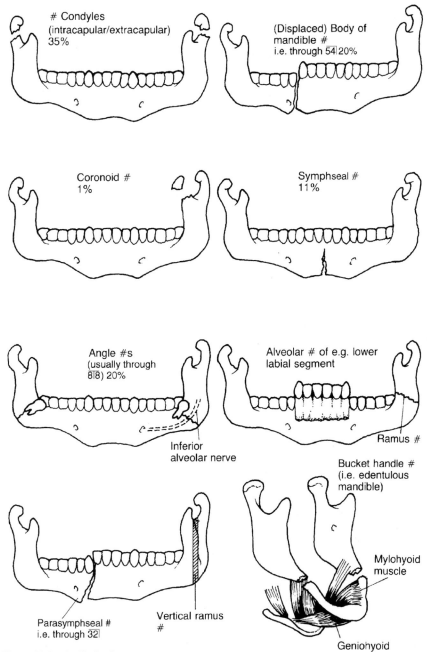

Figure 31.1. Mandibular fractures.

Nerves

The mandible conducts a canal from the ramus to the mental foramen, which contains the inferior dental nerve and its associated artery and vein. A distracted fracture across this canal usually results in altered sensation of the lower front teeth (and their associated mucosal cover), and of the lower lip and chin skin on the same side as the displaced fracture. In one study of such fractures, mental nerve sensation was reduced in 15% of patients with one fracture site, in 28% of those with two fractures and in over 30% of those with three or more (Adi *et al.*, 1990). The degree of initial injury and subsequent treatment will influence whether there is a temporary or permanent loss of sensation.

The term neuropraxia implies diminished sensation of an intact nerve resulting from bruising, which should recover. Although no identical study has been carried out on fracture patients, Takeuchi *et al.* (1994) considered transient mental nerve paraesthesia after mandibular sagittal split osteotomy and found a mean delay to recovery time of 179 ± 75 days.

Neurotmesis implies absolute sensory loss, usually resulting from division of the nerve bundle. This may be permanent or take up to 18 months to recover. If it is temporary, maximal recovery should not be assessed until at least one year after injury.

The lingual nerve and, rarely, the facial nerve may also be involved.

Blood vessels

Haemorrhage from the vessels within the inferior dental canal can be severe and may be difficult to arrest. Bleeding may also occur from the lingual and facial arteries or veins. If contained in the surrounding tissues it causes swelling and discoloration. If bleeding occurs from torn mucosa and/or skin, large amounts of blood or clots can lead to airway obstruction and breathing difficulties, especially where conscious responses are reduced from concurrent injury, illness, drugs or alcohol.

Soft tissues

Nearby structures that are less commonly involved with mandibular fractures include the salivary gland ducts and the enveloping soft tissues (Brookes, 1988).

Mechanism of injury

Fractures of the mandible arise from assaults (around 50% of victims know their assailant; Bailey *et al.*, 1988), sport (Hill *et al.*, 1985), falls and road traffic accidents (Rogers *et al.*, 1992). Social patterns and legislative changes, such as the 'drink driving' and 'seat belt' laws, affect injury

statistics. Telfer *et al.* (1991) commented in particular on the overall reduction in maxillofacial injuries, particularly fractures of the mandible, between 1977 and 1987.

On some occasions, predictable patterns of fractures occur with particular forces and directions of impact. Imaging and other investigations and knowledge of the mode of injury may enable the practitioner to recognize a particular type of fracture, for example the classical 'guardsman's' fracture resulting from a fall onto the chin, with consequent fractures at the parasymphyseal region and both condylar necks.

Fractures may result from direct or indirect injury and different patterns result from blunt or penetrating wounds (Figure 31.2).

The incidence of fracture of the mandible in children differs from that in adults and, although in children they represent less than 10% of all mandibular fractures in most reported series (Thoren *et al.*, 1992), the implications for growth may be particularly important.

Injury severity and outcome

Injuries without skin laceration or obvious bleeding can appear trivial and, if the diagnosis is missed, this can have deleterious consequences. The degree of initial disruption of tissues will determine the extent of consequential damage, but subsequent timing and treatment will determine whether or not maximal recovery is achieved. Fortunately, most patients with a fractured mandible benefit from early referral to oral and maxillofacial specialists who have undergone dental, as well as surgical, training. Inexperienced assessment may lead to a fracture being overlooked in the presence of more obvious injury. This can result in a delay in diagnosis, with an increased risk of avoidable complications.

The severity of such fractures of the mandible are assessed by the degree of comminution at the fracture margins, the site of fracture, injuries to structures other than the bone (e.g. nerves, teeth), penetration and contamination.

Associated injuries will determine the relative importance of mandibular fractures as a contribution to the overall severity of the injury.

High velocity injuries inflict predictably greater damage to bone and soft tissues, with massive disruption of supporting structures (Al Shawi, 1986; Marshall, 1986).

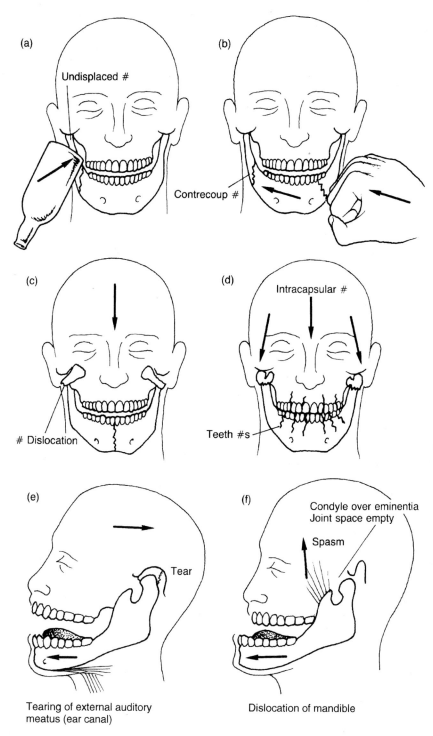

Figure 31.2. Mechanism of injury: **(a)** direct blow; **(b)** indirect blow; **(c)** 'parade ground' fall; **(d)** fall from height, teeth closed; **(e)** whiplash (bilaminar zone tear); **(f)** dislocation.

Significant signs and symptoms in mandibular fracture

The cardinal signs of any fracture (i.e. pain, swelling and loss of function) are usually present in mandibular fractures. Specific signs that may also occur include malocclusion, palpable step deformity of both margins, sensory changes in the lower lip, and missing or damaged teeth.

Any looseness of teeth may suggest a fracture confined to the tooth-bearing alveolar part of the bone or a fracture of dental roots, below the gingival margin. However, it must be pointed out that pre-existing periodontal disease affects most adults to some degree and may be a significant cause of loose teeth.

A discontinuity of the dental arches is often accompanied by bleeding under the nearby mucosa in the mouth and may be a useful indicator to the need for more detailed investigation including radiograph examination.

The symptoms specific to a fracture of the mandible will usually include pain at the fracture site, awareness of a changed pattern of biting, difficulty with chewing, and altered sensation around the lower lip, lower incisor and canine teeth, and gum on the side ipsilateral to the injury.

Relevance of pre-existing conditions to outcome

The loosening of teeth so often associated with a fracture of the tooth-bearing part of the bone must be properly assessed before consideration is given to pretraumatic disease, the progress of which may simply have been accelerated by injury.

The failure of matched tooth approximation between the dental arches of the upper and lower jaws is termed malocclusion. Many patients who suffer a fracture of the mandible may have a pre-existing abnormal occlusion, which may even predispose them to this injury. Some people are unaware of a malocclusion until an injury focuses their attention upon it (Winstanley, 1984).

The loss of teeth without proper restoration of the occlusion is common, as is the failure of certain teeth to develop or erupt into good alignment in the mouth. The specialty of orthodontics exists specifically to correct such malalignments. A complaint of malocclusion after mandibular fracture should be investigated carefully to ascertain any previous dental condition. On rare occasions, such questioning may elicit the existence of previous dental casts, which may shed light on previous occlusal status.

Mandibular fracture occurs more commonly at sites where bone strength is least able to withstand an impact. This occurs naturally, but may be compounded by pre-existing weakness due to bone disease or atrophy.

The term pathological fracture implies a pre-existing disease affecting the bone at a fracture site. In the mandible, it may be specifically related to the presence or absence of teeth or cysts, or, more rarely, tumours or other bone-weakening diseases such as osteogenesis imperfecta.

The ability of bone to repair can be influenced by systemic disease (e.g. predisposition to infection), nutritional deficiency, chronic debility and discontinuity of the fracture margins. Excessive movement across the fracture during the repair may result in delayed union or nonunion.

Investigations

A clinical diagnosis of a fracture of the mandible should be confirmed by radiography as soon after injury as circumstances allow. Classically, radiographs are taken across the fracture site in at least two planes at right angles to each other and should always include the joints at each end of the bone concerned.

In practice, delaying treatment of a fractured mandible to await better quality imaging may be in the patient's best interest, provided a reassessment occurs when the patient's clinical condition has stabilized. The most commonly used radiographic technique is a panoral view (orthopantomogram). This gives a single plate image of a topographic slice of the whole of the lower jaw and much of the upper jaw. The imaging equipment necessary for this is not universally available; in such cases the so-called lateral oblique (properly 'oblique lateral') views of the mandible provide acceptable alternatives. In either event, further views in the anteroposterior and/or lateral planes should also be taken. When standard 'head injury' radiographs are requested in the casualty situation, they are intended to allow the examination of the skull vault and will not necessarily include the mandible.

Special radiographic investigations for fracture-related problems in the lower jaw, particularly for teeth close to the fracture site, include intra-oral periapical and occlusal views. Special views of the teeth and joints will not be considered further in this chapter but are covered in detail elsewhere. Helpful information may also be gained from CT scans (Davidson *et al.*, 1991), MRI and various dye enhancement techniques, but these are also beyond the scope of this chapter.

Radiography of the chest may be helpful if teeth or prostheses have been lost at the time of the accident, are unaccounted for and may have been inhaled (Ong *et al.*, 1988).

Treatment options affecting outcome

Conservative management

The decision not to operate or intervene in the management of a fracture does not imply lack of treatment. In many instances, the natural repair processes of the body are quite capable of responding to injury more appropriately than any other treatment option. In surgical intervention, the primary aim is to help healing and speed recovery. All interventions carry risks and the duty of the surgeon is to ensure that, in assisting healing, fewer complications are likely than by not intervening. Provided a fracture is minimally displaced, comfortable and unlikely to become infected, then no further treatment may be necessary.

Conservative treatment of a mandibular fracture may include the prescription of analgesic drugs and antibiotics and perhaps splint support of the arch (Niimi *et al.*, 1989). In Britain, the term would not usually include intermaxillary fixation.

Surgical management

Operations to treat fractures of the mandible do not necessarily require general anaesthesia. Concurrent medical problems may contraindicate this.

Minimally displaced fractures are often treated by simple stabilization. Sometimes this may only require the 'lassoing' together of healthy teeth on either side of the fracture.

More frequently the upper jaw will be splinted to the lower jaw by intermaxillary fixation (IMF) (Figure 31.3). The methods of achieving the attachment of devices to the teeth and between the jaws are legion but share the common requirement of achieving optimal interdigitation of natural or artificial teeth between the upper and lower jaws so that the ends of the mandibular fracture are held

closely together. This technique applies indirect fixation to the fracture and has been used to good effect for decades. Intermaxillary fixation may be achieved by attaching eyelet wires, buttons, arch bars or cap splints to the teeth of the upper and lower jaws, then linking these together by vertical loops. A specific constraint on the use of IMF for prolonged periods exists if there is an associated condylar fracture (this topic is explored more fully elsewhere).

When performed well, IMF should ensure the minimum chance of postoperative malocclusion but does inconvenience patients, who often complain bitterly during the three to six weeks that the jaws are held together. Oikarinen *et al.* (1993) point out that, although prolonged sick leave may result from this treatment, its costs compare favourably with those of direct surgical fixation.

In the edentulous mandible, the patient's own dentures may be adapted, and wired directly to the upper and lower jaws to permit intermaxillary fixation by then wiring the dentures, or 'Gunning' splints, together.

The choice between splinting fractures and open direct surgical repair is often most difficult with the edentulous mandible. The thin shaft of bone may require supplementary grafting and, particularly with bilateral fractures of the body of the edentulous mandible (which can produce 'bucket handle' deformity), direct fixation with screwed plates is increasingly practised.

Significant displacement, comminution or contamination of the mandibular fracture routinely requires open reduction and direct fixation. Where segments of the mandibular bone have been lost together with teeth, making IMF impractible, there are still indications for the use of external pin fixator devices.

Modern biocompatible materials and effective antibiotics have made early operative intervention the favoured choice of treatment in most developed countries. Brown *et al.* (1991) have audited the use of IMF compared with miniplate osteosynthesis and found little difference between overall costs or clinical variables.

Direct bone healing (osteosynthesis) can occur when close approximation of fracture ends is achieved under direct vision. This was initially performed by transosseous wires, usually requiring extraoral skin incisions, later to be followed by metallic mesh trays into which bone graft fragments could be inserted.

The requirement for external skin incisions for the treatment of large numbers of mandibular

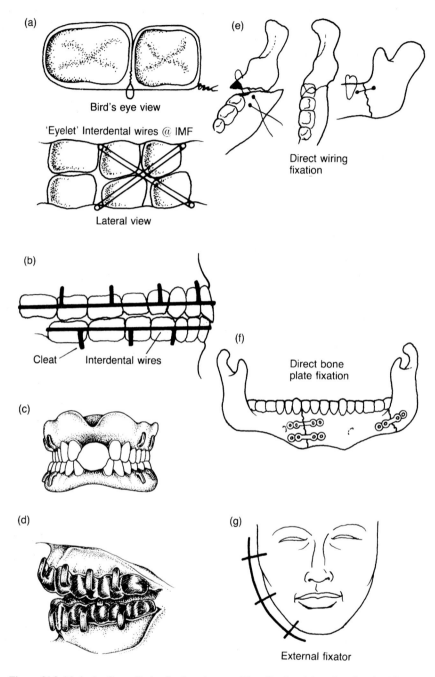

Figure 31.3. Methods of mandibular fixation. *Intermaxillary fixation*: **(a)** eyelet wires (requires a good number of teeth and good occlusion); **(b)** arch bars (preformed, custom made, i.e. Jelenko, Erich); **(c)** Gunnings splints, i.e. dentures without teeth wired around jaws; **(d)** silver cap splints – cemented on plus circummandibular wires (sometimes) i.e. 'James Bond jaws'. *Direct fixation* (transosseous techniques, usually in addition to intermaxillary fixation): **(e)** upper border wire (intraoral approach); **(f)** plating, i.e. 'Champy'/'Halls', may not need intermaxillary fixation; **(g)** external pin fixation.

fractures has largely béen superseded by the technique of mandibular osteosynthesis by miniature screwed plates via a buccal approach (Champy *et al.*, 1978). In this paper, the authors developed a scientific argument to show that the stresses across fracture lines at different sites in the mandible where miniplates were used would not exceed the mechanical qualities of such small plates during the healing phase, as long as certain biomechanical principles were observed. In summary, provided two plates are used at the front of the jaw where torsional forces are greatest and single plates elsewhere, satisfactory healing can occur in the majority of mandibular fractures without the need for IMF or external skin incisions (Cawood, 1985).

In 1986, Champy *et al.* made a series of recommendations to reduce postoperative complications. Although most of his recommendations are now current practice, his suggestion that osteosynthesis should be carried out within 12 hours of injury has been strongly contested (Smith, 1991) and is in practice often unrealistic.

Uglesic *et al.* (1993) state that the optimum time for treating mandibular fractures is within 72 hours, but, in fractures older than seven days, they still recommend miniplate fixation.

In recent years the main impetus of research in the treatment of mandibular fractures has been concerned with modifications of the design of the bone plates and with quality standards (Carter, 1992), especially with regard to miniaturization (Schmelzeisen *et al.*, 1992), and with the arguments for and against stainless steel or titanium from which the plates and screws are constructed (Millar *et al.*, 1990). Controversy continues throughout Europe about whether or not either or both materials need to be removed after healing of the fracture (this is not current practice in UK; Brown *et al.*, 1989) and whether or not more significant occlusal problems occur as the result of not using IMF.

Biodegradable materials for future plate and screw construction are now under development (Obwegeser, 1994) as is consideration of the use of bone morphogenetic protein as a biological glue to enhance the rate of bone repair (Sailer and Kolb, 1994).

Outcome indicators

Assessment of the quality of recovery after fractures of the mandible requires consideration of the occlusion, the facial and dental appearance, masticatory function, and complications of the treatment method, as well as the complications that might reasonably be associated with the original injury.

The frequency and severity of dental injuries in association with mandibular fractures has been studied (Oikarinen *et al.*, 1993), which reveals that the treatment of tooth loss or crown fracture can be time-consuming and expensive. Dental trauma and occlusal disturbances are complications that may require more attention after the accident than the mandibular fracture itself.

Degree of disability

Disability in fractures of the mandible implies reduction or loss of the normal functions related to the bone and its associated tissues.

Numbness in the lower lip is particularly disabling, with dribbling or speech impediments as not uncommon consequences. Alteration in appearance is particularly prominent in injuries affecting the lower face, especially where scarring of the facial skin or altered underlying bone symmetry is present or when muscle tone and activity is reduced and unbalanced. Contour abnormalities of a fractured bone may produce related disturbances of dental occlusion and/or of the range of joint movements. These are considered in more detail in the appropriate chapters.

Risk of future complications

The delayed consequences of mandibular fractures after the initial healing has occurred include malocclusion, masticatory inefficiency, speech impediment and complications of the treatment method. The long-term viability of injured teeth can be extremely difficult to predict with any degree of accuracy and the variety of possible treatment options, especially the increasing availability of osseo-integrated implant systems, make the likely financial consequences of such injuries extremely significant.

Prognosis

Prognosis is determined by the degree of disability persisting after optimal recovery has been achieved. The purely physical consequences of such an injury will be complicated by the patient's increased awareness of the area of injury, and the social and psychological consequences of the injury. These factors need also to be considered when assessing the prognosis.

Fortunately, the vast majority of mandibular fractures cause little disturbance to external appearance. Occasionally, severe occlusal malalignment does occur, such as massive anterior open bite, but this is usually amenable to secondary surgical correction.

The current popularity of plate fixation undoubtedly raises the possibility of increasing the demand for the removal of the plates after fracture healing. The current practice in the UK is only to remove plates that become infected, provoke wound dehiscence, or cause palpable deformity.

Rarely, injury to a sensory nerve leads to intractable causalgic pain. This may respond to drugs such as carbamazepine or merit direct ablation with cryotherapy, chemical injection of alcohol, or nerve section. Despite these various attempts at treatment, there are unfortunately still many patients in whom the pain persists.

References

Adi M, Ogden GR, Chisholm DM. (1990) Analysis of mandibular fractures in Dundee, Scotland (1977–1985). *Br J Oral Maxillofac Surg* **28**: 194–200.

Al-Shawi A. (1986) Experience in the treatment of missile injuries of the maxillofacial region in Iraq. *Br J Oral Maxillofac Surg* **24**: 244–51.

Bailey BMW, Carr RJ, Bermingham DF, Shepherd RG. (1988) A comparative study of psychosocial data on patients with maxillofacial injuries in an urban population – a preliminary study. *Br J Oral Maxillofac Surg* **26**: 199–205.

Brookes CN. (1988) Facial nerve paralysis complicating bilateral fractures of the mandible: a case report and review of the literature. *Br J Oral Maxillofac Surg* **26**: 149–55.

Brown JS, Trotter M, Cliffe J, Ward-Booth RP, Williams ED. (1989) The fate of miniplates in facial trauma and orthognathic surgery: a retrospective study. *Br J Oral Maxillofac Surg* **27**: 306–16.

Brown JS, Grew N, Taylor C, Millar BG. (1991) Intermaxillary fixation compared to miniplate osteosynthesis in the management of the fractured mandible: an audit, *Br J Oral Maxillofac Surg* **29**: 308–12.

Champy M, Lodde JP, Schmitt R, Jaegar JH and Muster D (1978) Mandibular osteosynthesis by miniatute screwed plate via a buccal approach. *J Maxilloface Surg* **6**: 14.

Champy M, Pape HD, Gerlach KL and Lodde JF (1986) The Stasbowz miniplate osteosynthesis. *Oral and Maxillo-Facial Surg* **2**: 19–43.

Carter JLB. (1992) The use of bone plates in Maxillofacial surgery. In: *Debrett's book of surgery*. London: Sterling Publications Ltd, 47–50.

Cawood JI. (1985) Small plate osteosynthesis of mandibular fractures. *Br J Oral Maxillofac Surg* **23**: 77–92.

Davidson MJC, Daly BED, Russell JL. (1991) The use of computed tomography in the management of facial trauma by British oral and maxillofacial surgeons. *Br J Oral Maxillofac Surg* **29**: 80–82.

Hill CM, Crosher RF, Mason DA. (1985) Dental and facial injuries following sports accidents of 130 patients. *Br J Oral Maxillofac Surg* **23**: 268–75.

Hopkins R. (1985) In: Rowe NL, Williams JLL, editors. *Maxillofacial injuries*. Edinburgh: Churchill Livingstone, 232–92.

Marshall WG. (1986) An analysis of firearm injuries to the head and face in Belfast 1969–1977. *Br J Oral Maxillofac Surg* **24**: 233–44.

Millar BG, Frame JW, Browne RM. (1990) A historical study of stainless steel and titanium screws in bone. *Br J Oral Maxillofac Surg* **28**: 92–95.

Niimi M, Mizuna A, Nakuna Y, Motegi K. (1989) Reduction and fixation of jaw fractures using acrylic splints. *Br J Oral Maxillofac Surg* **27**: 321–29.

Obwegeser JA. (1994) Bioconvertable screws made of allogenic cortical bone for osteosynthesis following sagittal split ramus osteotomy without postoperative immobilisation. *J Craniomaxillofac Surg* **22**: 63–75.

Oikarinen K, Ignatius E, Silvennoinen U. (1993) Treatment of mandibular fractures in the 1980s. *J Craniomaxillofac Surg* **21**: 245–50.

Oikarinen K, Ignatius E, Kaupi I, Silvennoinen U. (1993) Mandibular fractures in Northern Finland in the 1980s – A ten year study. *Br J Oral Maxillofac Surg* **31** (1): 23–28.

Ong TK, Lancer JM, Brook IM. (1988) Inhalation of a denture fragment complicating facial trauma. *Br J Oral Maxillofac Surg* **26**: 511–14.

Rogers S, Hill JR, Mackay GM. (1992) Maxillofacial injuries following steering wheel contact by drivers using seatbelts. *Br J Oral Maxillofac Surg* **30**: 24–13.

Rowe NL, Killey HC. (1968) *Fractures of the facial skeleton*. Edinburgh: Churchill Livingstone.

Rowe NL, Williams JLL, editors. (1985) *Maxillofacial injury*. Edinburgh: Churchill Livingstone.

Sailer HF, Kolb E. (1994) Application of purified bone morphogenetic protein (BMP). *J Craniomaxillofac Surg* **22**: 2–11.

Schmelzeisen R, McIff T, Rahn B. (1992) Further development of titanium miniplate fixation for mandibular fractures. *J Craniomaxillofac Surg* **20**: 251–56.

Smith WP. (1991) Delayed miniplate osteosynthesis for mandibular fractures. *J Craniomaxillofac Surg* **29**: 73–77.

Stylogianni L, Arsenopoulos A, Patrikiou A. (1991) Fractures of the facial skeleton in children. *Br J Oral Maxillofac Surg* **29**: 9–12.

Takeuchi T, Furusawa K, Hirose I. (1994) Mechanism of transient mental nerve paraesthesia in sagittal split mandibular ramus osteotomy. *Br J Oral Maxillofac Surg* **32**: 105–109.

Telfer MR, Jones GM, Shepherd JP. (1991) Trends in the aetiology of maxillofacial fractures in the United Kingdom (1977–1987). *Br J Oral Maxillofac Surg* **29**: 250–56.

Thoren H, Iizuka T, Hallikainen D, Lindquist C. (1992) Different patterns of mandibular fractures in children. *J Craniomaxillofac Surg* **20**: 292–96.

Uglesic V, Virag M, Alginovic N, Macan D. (1993) Evaluation of mandibular fracture treatment. *J Craniomaxillofac Surg* **21**: 251–57.

Winstanley RP. (1984) The management of fractures of the mandible. *Br J Oral Maxillofac Surg* **22**: 170–78.

32

Injuries to the teeth

Hugh Cannell

Mechanism of injury

Most injuries to the teeth occur as a result of direct violence. Blows from fists, blunt instruments, elbows and feet can each produce shattered and painful teeth. More complex injuries, possibly involving the dento-alveolar structures and the facial bones, may be found after deliberate violence, road traffic accidents, or falls.

A frequent cause of injuries to the teeth is through participation in sports, particularly contact and team sports. The frequency of this injury as a contribution to maxillofacial injury from all causes may be up to 16% (Lees and Gaskell, 1976). Bollam and Wanneumacher (1974) reported a sports-related incidence in Germany of up to 40% and Cathcart (1968) in the USA has noted that up to 50% of participants in sport have tooth injuries. Horse riding, in all its forms, places participants at particular risk from injuries affecting the teeth (Lie and Lucht, 1977). Falls, blows from the horse's head and from accidents with the riding crop, can each cause tooth fracture or loss.

Severity of injury

The severity of injury is increased if there is a rapid deceleration. This is likely to occur after falls of over 20 ft (approx. 6 m). The face may hit the knees after a jump, or the face and teeth may hit a hard, unyielding surface. If the lower jaw is violently closed against the upper jaw, many, or even all, of the teeth may be shattered and split longitudinally. This form of dental injury is almost impossible to restore and may necessitate a complete dental clearance.

Almost any severity of injury to the mouth may result in cracks in or chipping of the brittle enamel surfaces of the teeth. In addition pre-existing dental restorations may be damaged. Injuries may be confined to the enamel of the teeth or may involve both the enamel and the sensitive underlying dentine, with immediate pain as a result. More severe pain may occur where the enamel, dentine and the pulp of the tooth are broken off to gum level. More difficult to diagnose may be vertical or horizontal cracks without displacement of the fractured segments of the root of the tooth. In addition, teeth may be avulsed, intruded, extruded or dislocated within their sockets. Any of these injuries may eventually result in a loss of vitality of the teeth, as may injuries to the enamel, dentine or pulp.

Injuries to the deciduous teeth of children have a better prognosis as they are shed naturally when the permanent dentition erupts. Unfortunately, severe injuries to a child's mouth may cause permanent effects, such as a dilaceration upon the soft, partly calcified, partly formed permanent successors. Damage to underlying permanent teeth is particularly likely to occur if a deciduous tooth is intruded or loses its vitality and becomes infected.

An excellent treatise on injuries to the teeth of both children and adults has been published

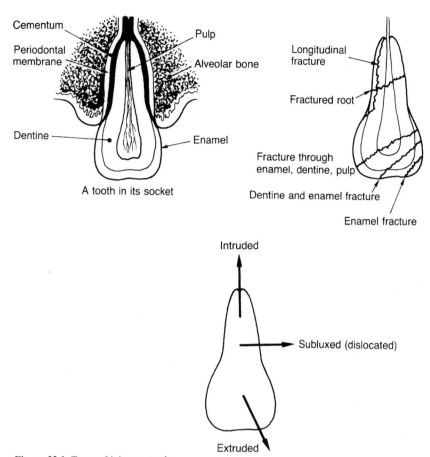

Figure 32.1. Types of injury to teeth.

(Andreasen, 1979). It is highly recommended for further reading and for probability tables of outcome after injury.

The severity of damage in sports-associated injury can be reduced by as much as 43% by wearing some form of carefully constructed mouth guard (Nicholas, 1976). American football players are required to wear face and mouth guards and consequently have fewer dental injuries than players in many other team sports, for example basketball or hockey. They even have fewer dental injuries than boxers (Jones, 1979). Figure 32.1 illustrates the various types of dental injury.

Relevance of pre-existing conditions

Those with prominent teeth are more likely to injure them. Figure 32.2 shows some types of occlusion in which the teeth are prominent. In the

USA, some sportsmen with prognathic mandibles, and therefore with especially prominent lower teeth, are prevented from playing contact sports.

Impacted and unerupted teeth form a line of weakness in the jaws. Forces that strike the jaws may be dispersed and absorbed in the bone until they come up against a hard, unyielding tooth. Under these conditions, the tooth may act as a wedge, resulting in fractures in the line of the tooth, especially those lying deep in the bone. The area of the lower wisdom tooth and lower canine (cuspid) are sites where mandibular fractures are often found (Figure 32.3).

Teeth and implants

Pre-existing restorative work of the teeth may be of the utmost importance in determining outcome after injury. A patient with extensive bridgework

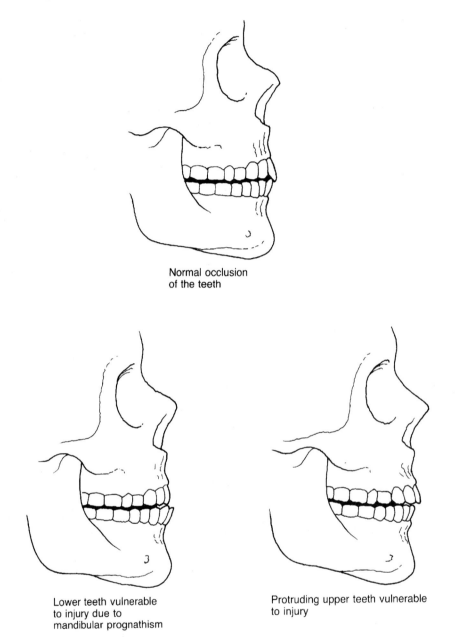

Normal occlusion
of the teeth

Lower teeth vulnerable
to injury due to
mandibular prognathism

Protruding upper teeth vulnerable
to injury

Figure 32.2. Vulnerability of teeth not in natural occlusion: **(a)** normal occlusion; **(b)** lower teeth vulnerable to injury due to mandibular prognathism; **(c)** upper teeth vulnerable to injury.

may have paid as much as £1000 ($2400) per tooth for each restoration. The crown is often only the cosmetic coat of the restored tooth. Beneath it may be other types of restorative work, such as a root filling. Similarly, on top of a previously prepared stump there may be a gold core with only the porcelain outer cosmetic crown making the whole

look like a natural tooth. Several teeth may be linked together as a dental bridge in order to span a gap where a tooth has previously been lost. There may also be complicated attachments into gold or other metal inlays, which, in turn, hold partial dentures in place. Nowadays, more and more patients may have endosseous implants *in situ* as

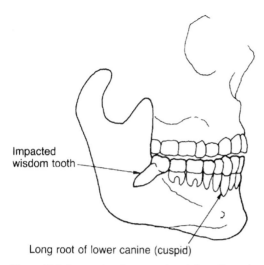

Impacted
wisdom tooth—

Long root of lower canine (cuspid)

Figure 32.3. Impacted or long rooted teeth form lines of weakness compared with remainder of body of mandible.

replacements for missing teeth. In these, the implant is a titanium- or ceramic-based screw fitting, which becomes integrated with the bone of the jaws. Fractures of tooth restorations based upon implants must necessarily have a poor outcome; it is likely that an implant will be lost if it is involved in a fracture line. In particular, the implant, although osseo-integrated, would be likely to act as a wedge in the same way as a buried tooth, and thus create a higher chance of a fracture at that site.

A previous fracture of the jaws with an osteosynthesis still in place may also constitute a line of future weakness. In particular, there seems to be a loss of elasticity in the jaw if bone miniplates are left *in situ*. The elasticity of any metal is unlike that of bone and is unable to cope with sudden distortions. Wire osteosyntheses are less likely to suffer from this trouble, but, from time to time, they apparently 'come to the surface' and the adjacent area may have to be disturbed in order to remove the wire.

If a tooth has been affected by a nearby fracture of the jaw, then not only may the tooth be lost at the time but, if it is retained, it may be responsible for later complications, including local infection, nonunion of the fracture and osteomyelitis. Improvements in oral hygiene and the availability of antibiotics have made this less likely but it is still possible.

Berger *et al.* (1992) have conducted a 15-year retrospective survey. They advise that, in general, teeth involved in a fracture line of the mandible should be retained. They excluded from their survey teeth that were obviously very damaged by decay or by the original trauma, those with marked periodontal bone loss and those in which apical changes were present. In contrast, impacted teeth, including wisdom teeth, were utilized. They reported that sometimes the wisdom teeth had to be removed later. The authors also noted that whilst many teeth retained in fracture lines become nonvital, provided that their periodontal condition remained normal, they could safely be retained.

Cameron and Ponier-Moorthy (1993) also recommended the retention of teeth associated with fracture lines, unless there was an absolute indication to their removal. They noted that nonvitality of teeth near fracture lines was significantly higher after treatment of the fracture by plating than by wiring procedures. They noted that 48% of teeth in the line of fractures were found to be nonvital but asymptomatic. Rix *et al.* (1991) noted in their series of 80 patients after mandibular fracture that there were some periodontal defects and resorption of the teeth adjacent to the old fracture lines.

Children may have many teeth at various stages of development. A fracture affecting the tooth-bearing area thus has the potential to disrupt not only deciduous teeth but also their permanent successors. Fortunately, fractures of the facial bones in children are uncommon, but a displaced fracture has the potential to result in the loss of several teeth adjacent to the fracture line. Similarly, treatment of fractures by osteosynthesis has resulted in disturbance to tooth germs. Hardt and Gottsauner (1993) noted that injuries to the tooth germ could be reduced or avoided if the smallest version of any plating osteosynthesis equipment was used.

Displacement of the teeth by trauma in a growing jaw may result in a poor cosmetic appearance and may require orthodontic treatment. Tonacka *et al.* (1993) followed up 81 cases of maxillofacial fractures in children. They noted that alveolar fractures produced a malocclusion in 25% of these patients. They suggested that a longer period of intermaxillary fixation and follow-up should be routine after dento-alveolar fractures in children.

Treatment options affecting outcome

The diagnosis and treatment of trauma to the teeth or to the dento-alveolar structures should be made as soon as possible. Fracture of the crown of a tooth should be checked to test whether the dentine and the pulp have been involved. If so, those structures must be protected against infection, for example by use of a celluloid crown former filled with calcium hydroxide paste. A slightly displaced or injured tooth should be checked carefully that it is not out of the natural bite (i.e. in traumatic occlusion). A tooth that has been displaced out of its natural position can temporarily be splinted with metal foil to hold it in its proper relationship to adjacent and opposite teeth. Where there is an obvious fracture of the root, the tooth crown should be temporarily splinted and the patient referred to a specialist dental surgeon. Any very loose pieces of tooth should be removed and given to the patient to show to the dental surgeon.

A completely avulsed tooth should be recovered. As soon as possible, it should be cleaned, preferably with saline. An attempt to replace it into its bony socket should be made and metal foil used temporarily to splint it in place. If a reimplantation attempt fails, the tooth should be placed in milk or in the patient's blood and the patient immediately referred to a specialist dental surgeon. Where there is an obvious fracture of the dento-alveolar structures, the bone should be lightly pinched together and the patient very carefully checked to make sure that other teeth and adjacent bone have not also been injured.

Emergency first aid treatment of injuries to the teeth, if incorrectly carried out, may prejudice the eventual outcome. For example, failure to treat an exposed pulp will later result in the whole root canal becoming infected and will make prolonged endodontic treatment inevitable. Failure to splint a tooth in the correct position or to reimplant it will lead to loss of the tooth.

Radiographs are of the utmost importance in the assessment of possible injuries to the teeth. In the multiply-injured patient, the management of an individual fractured tooth may have a very low priority. Nevertheless, it is important to record each injury to a tooth at the earliest opportunity. This should be done when the patient is well enough not only to tolerate radiograph examination of the affected teeth but also to withstand possibly complex dental treatment.

Teeth, or parts of teeth or restorations, may have been lost at the time of injury. Some may have been knocked out or spat out or, in the dazed and unconscious patient, may have been swallowed or inhaled. Apart from a thorough clinical examination of the mouth, pharynx and larynx, it is wise to exclude this possibility by means of chest and abdominal radiography.

Soft tissue radiograph films should be obtained if there are extraoral lacerations, compound lacerations through the lips or cheek, or intraoral lacerations in association with missing or jagged teeth, fillings or other restorations. Foreign bodies, including dental fragments, can then be identified and removed.

Degree of disability

After injury, damaged or missing upper front teeth produce considerable cosmetic disability. Occasionally the loss of an upper premolar or canine tooth may be masked if the patient is fortunate enough to have a long upper lip but the person will often remain very self-conscious about the gap. Women are particularly affected by the loss of any teeth, especially the upper or lower front teeth. Indeed, the cosmetic and resultant psychological disability becomes very great and the patient may refuse to smile in greeting for fear of disclosing a gap or an inadequate restoration of an anterior tooth.

Careful consideration should be given to the type of treatment used to restore any gap in the front teeth. Most dental surgeons will suggest various types of dental bridges. These may be very expensive. In particular they may require that apparently uninjured teeth on either side of the missing one should be cut down to provide a firm base on which to build subsequent crowns as abutments for the bridge. Thus, not only the missing or injured tooth but also the adjacent sound teeth may be involved in such restoration work. Similarly, it may be necessary to use other teeth in the dental arch in order to hold certain retaining devices, for example, for a partial upper denture. It is recommended that a full description of immediate and subsequent treatment should be included in a report obtained from the attending dental surgeon, who should also be asked to produce an exact sketch or photograph of all the teeth affected by restorative measures following the injury.

Posterior teeth, when lost through injury, may not produce an obvious cosmetic defect. Nevertheless, their absence may severely affect the patient's ability to chew and to benefit from restorative measures. In addition, there may be other long-term effects such as temporomandibular joint dysfunction.

In addition to injuries to the natural teeth, any injuries to pre-existing restorations must be carefully charted and a record of previous work obtained from the patient's dental surgeon.

Risk of future complications

Delayed complications following injury to the teeth may result in a lifetime of repeated examinations and of necessary replacement of any post-traumatic restorations. It should be noted that the replacement of a missing tooth or the carrying out of restorative measures on a damaged tooth is not the end of the problem, for any crown or bridge may not last longer than about 10 years; it may last a much shorter time than this, depending upon eating habits and other factors.

Modern techniques of treatment for fractures of the jaws are increasingly reliant on internal fixation using miniplates as osteosyntheses. Unless extreme accuracy is achieved at the time of the reduction of a fracture, imperfections of the occlusion may result. Such imperfections, typically those of one or more prematurities of occlusal contact, may in turn produce further damage to the teeth involved. This may result in a loss of vitality in the long term and in periodontal problems and pain as soon as the patient attempts to chew. Adjustments of minor degrees of prematurity of contact will resolve the difficulty in most patients. Unfortunately, in a few cases, especially those in which the patient has remained unconscious for many weeks, natural adjustments to the occlusion cannot take place and more gross occlusal problems may result. It is therefore useful for the maxillofacial surgeon who is treating the injured jaws to record whether intermaxillary fixation has been used, whether internal or external skeletal fixation was employed, and whether teeth were lost or even slightly displaced at the time of the injury. In this way, any future likelihood of occlusal problems can be identified and treatment commenced.

Any tooth that has been damaged in an accident or an injury may die months or even years later. In those circumstances it can be difficult to ascribe to the accident the eventual loss of vitality of a tooth. However, in the absence of another recorded cause, it is more likely than not that the injury was the reason for the loss of vitality. If this occurs, more complicated treatment may then be necessary, including root filling treatment. Amongst other long-term problems that become evident in previously injured teeth are internal (i.e. at the root canal) or external resorption of the root following trauma. This can occur years after the injury and may be only slowly progressive. Another problem is that some teeth may be affected by the cementum of the root slowly becoming indistinguishable from the surrounding socket bone and becoming ankylosed.

Long-term prognosis

The long-term prognosis of accidental injury to teeth is poor. Amongst the factors that require to be taken into account are the patient's oral hygiene, the periodontal condition at the time of the accident, and, subsequently, whether the patient is physically able to comply with any recommended hygiene measures. The person's financial status and diet, and the status of every tooth in the arch prior to the accident are also important in determining the eventual outcome. Whether a mouth guard was worn is also important if it was a sports related injury.

Any injured teeth should subsequently be subjected to regular and routine medical examination and tests of vitality with repeated radiograph examinations to assess the periapical state.

Reports made for medicolegal purposes after injury to the mouth and teeth benefit greatly from an unbiased statement of the patient's pre-accident oral and dental status. Since it is likely that many patients will have received some form of previous dental treatment, then a good record may well be available. In addition to the dental records, radiographs, plaster models and photographs may each contribute to a fair assessment of the preaccident status. These records can then be compared with postaccident records and thus any associated costs of restoration of a damaged mouth can be assessed. The various methods of recording dental restorations, gaps in the occlusion and other detailed information differ between countries. It is recommended that for the purposes of a medicolegal report the WHO classification should be used, together with accurate diagnosis of each tooth surface restored. Intraoral radiographs submitted for report purposes must be dated and mounted and labelled so that the nondental professional can see their precise location in the mouth.

References

Andreasen JD, editor. (1970) *Traumatic injuries to the teeth.* Copenhagen: Munksgaard.

Berger S, Dittta Pape H. (1992) Teeth in the fracture lines. *Int J Oral Maxillofac Surg* **21**: 145–46.

Bollam F, Wanneumacher M. (1974) Individually functional mouthguard for contact sports. *Quintessence Int* **5**(1): 34.

Cameron HA, Ponier-Moorthy A. (1993) Fate of teeth in fracture lines. *Int J Oral Maxillofac Surg* **22**: 97–101.

Cathcart JF. (1968) Practical preventive dentistry: the use of mouth protectors in contact sports. *Dent Dig* **58**: 348.

Hardt M, Gottsauner G. (1993) Treatment of mandibular fractures in children. *J Craniomaxillofac Surg* **21**: 214–19.

Jarvinen S. (1980) On causes of traumatic dental injuries with special reference to sports accidents in a sample of Finnish children. *Acta Odont Scand* **38**: 151.

Jones JJ. (1979) Wisconsin Interscholastic Athletic Association. In: Andreason JO, editor. *Traumatic injuries to the teeth.* Copenhagen: Munksgaard, 442.

Lees GH, Gaskell PH (1976) Injuries to the mouth and teeth in an undergraduate population. *Br Dent J* **140**: 107–108.

Lie LH, Lucht U. (1977) Ridesportsulykker 1. Under sogdes of en myterpopulation med saeligt lenblic pa ulykkesfrekvensen. *Ugeskr Laeger* **134**: 1687.

Nicholas NK. (1976) Mouthguards in sport (Letter). *N Z Med J* **84**: 31.

Rix L, Stevenson ARL, Ponier-Moorthy A. (1991) Analysis of 80 cases of mandibular fractures treated with miniplate osteosynthesis. *Int J Oral Maxillofac Surg* **20**: 337–41.

Tonacka N, Usheides N, Suzuki K, *et al.* (1993) Maxillofacial fractures in children. *J Craniofac Surg* **21**: 289–93.

33

Soft tissue injuries of the face and mouth

Richard F Edlich, Nguyen D Nguyen, Raymond F Morgan

Introduction

The human face defines our identity and, when injured, it adversely affects our self image. In addition to the aesthetic appearance, our society places a premium on the function of the face. When either are damaged, legal action is frequently taken against those responsible (Schultz, 1988). Facial wounds are among the most frequently encountered injuries. Wounds of the face may be divided into two basic groups: injuries to the soft tissues and injuries to the bone. This chapter focuses on soft tissue injuries of the face. The goals of treatment are first to care for all injuries that are an immediate threat to life, and secondly, to repair wounds so that there is an optimal return of function and restoration of appearance.

Because facial injuries may be associated with serious injuries to other sites, emergency treatment of the life-threatening conditions must take precedence over the management of facial injuries. Active bleeding from soft tissue wounds of the face should be treated immediately by a pressure dressing. Because a carefully applied dressing will usually arrest bleeding, shock is not a frequent consequence of haemorrhage from facial trauma. Before applying the dressing, all kinked or twisted flaps of tissue should be returned to their original positions to prevent further vascular compromise. Bleeding from the oral cavity that cannot be controlled by pressure can obstruct the airway. In such patients, a patent airway can be maintained,

usually by suctioning blood from the mouth using a Yankauer tonsil sucker. The patient should be transported immobilized and secured to a backboard. Aspiration can be prevented by turning the patient and the backboard as a unit so that the patient is lying on his or her side.

Reconstructive surgery of facial soft tissue injuries requires an understanding of the mechanism of injury, the anatomy of each specific site, an assessment of the aesthetic and functional deformity, and selection of the appropriate techniques for repair. We will discuss the techniques to measure the outcome of soft tissue injuries to the face by examining the relevant information required by a medical report, the use of photography for medicolegal purposes, and the method of evaluating permanent impairment of the face secondary to facial injuries. Finally, we will explore the nearly unavoidable consequence of soft tissue injuries – scarring – by examining its pathogenesis and management options.

Mechanism of injury

The outcome of injury can be predicted by applying the concepts of power, work, and force that were first appreciated in the seventeenth century. There are three mechanical forces that can lead to soft tissue injury: shear, tension and compression. The divided edges of a wound are more susceptible to infection than unwounded tissue (Edlich *et al.*, 1982). The magnitude of this enfeebled resistance varies with the mechanism of injury. In approximately 80% of soft tissue injuries, a force that is shearing in nature is applied to tissue by a piece of glass, a metal edge, or a knife (Figure 33.1). The resultant linear wound exhibits considerable resistance to the development of infection, with the infective dose being 10^6 bacteria per gram of tissue or greater (Edlich *et al.*, 1988).

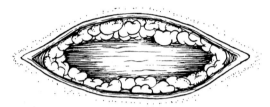

Figure 33.1. Linear laceration cause by shear forces.

When a wound is caused by the collision of two bodies, the mechanisms of injury are predominantly compression and/or tension. In each case, two forces of equal magnitude are applied in opposite directions to the tissues. Unlike shear forces, compression and tension forces act in the same plane. The mechanism of injury is mainly tension when a flat body collides against soft tissue not supported by underlying bone. For impact injuries to soft tissue overlying bone, tissue failure is caused primarily by compressive forces. The energy required to injure tissue as a result of these forces is considerably greater than for shear forces because the energy is distributed over a larger volume of tissue. The amount of energy absorbed by tissue during an impact can be calculated by the following equation:

$$T = MV^2/2$$

Where T = kinetic energy (joules), M = mass of impacting object (kilograms), and V = relative velocity between the impacting object and tissue (metres per second). The extent of compressive or tension injuries will vary with the size (mass) of the object and its velocity when it makes contact. Changes in the relative velocity have a greater influence on the level of kinetic energy than do variations in its mass.

When the mechanism of injury is compression, tissue failure occurs at energy levels of 2.5 J/cm², which is comparable with the energy encountered when a car travelling at 8 km/h strikes a tree (Cardany *et al.*, 1976). In this event, the momentum of the collision causes the victim's head (weighing approximately 4 kg) to hit the dashboard with an area of impact of approximately 8 cm². This absorbed energy disrupts the skin, resulting in a characteristic stellate laceration (Figure 33.2). In addition, the wound edges are damaged and rendered relatively ischaemic. Wounds caused by impact injuries are 100 times more susceptible to infection than wounds caused by shear forces, and immediate antibiotic treatment is indicated to suppress the growth of any bacterial contaminants. Even then, antibiotic efficacy is substantially less than in contaminated wounds caused by shear forces (Edlich *et al.*, 1988).

Although impact injuries with energy levels lower than 2.5 J/cm² do not result in division of the skin, they can result in disruption of its vessels. Vascular injury to the skin is manifest clinically as ecchymosis. Disruption of vessels in the underlying tissue results in a haematoma. Some haematomas will reabsorb, but some may become encapsulated. These usually require surgical treatment as, left untreated, they may result in permanent subcutaneous deformity. When still in the 'currant jelly' stage, a haematoma is best treated by incision and drainage. As further liquefaction occurs, aspiration with a large bore needle (18-gauge or larger) may be possible.

Firearm injuries cause a considerably higher level of energy absorption per unit volume of tissue than blunt injuries. As tissues are struck by a missile, a combination of shear, tension and compressive forces interact to produce a relatively reproducible amount of destruction, the severity of the wound being related to the amount of kinetic energy deposited (Sturdivan *et al.*, 1984).

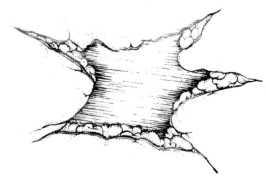

Figure 33.2. Stellate laceration caused by compression of skin overlying a bony structure.

Epidemiology

Hussain *et al.* (1994) provided the largest prospective study of the complete range of craniofacial trauma encountered in an urban university hospital, enabling a greater understanding of the range and magnitude of these injuries. Their survey included diagrams of the whole head divided by grids into 43 zones, according to anatomical differences. Soft tissue injury was recorded in all zones affected, and was classified as contusion, laceration or skin loss. The cases were divided into the following seven categories according to the mechanism of injury: falls, nonfall impacts, assaults, road user crashes, sports, occupational and others.

Of the 1059 craniofacial soft tissue injuries, 508 were due to lacerations and 551 were due to contusions. Of the lacerations, 260 were due to falls, 90 to nonfall impacts, 89 to assaults, 31 to road user crash, 36 to sports, 29 to occupational injuries, and 13 to others. Of the contusions, falls remained the most frequent cause, but to a much lesser degree than lacerations, with 178 such injuries. In nonfall impacts there was a significant decrease in the incidence of contusions compared with that of lacerations. On the other hand, assaults accounted for a dramatic increase in the incidence of contusions compared with lacerations, with 168 of injuries. Of the other causes (road user crash, sports, occupational and other), there were similar frequencies for lacerations and for contusions.

Craniofacial trauma was found to be very common at all ages. The causes were directly related to age, sex and alcohol consumption. Falls accounted for most of the injuries in children and the elderly, whereas interpersonal violence was mainly responsible for those occurring in patients aged between 15 and 50 years, especially in young male adults. Fights occurred mainly between strangers who had consumed excessive amounts of alcohol.

In patients sustaining a soft tissue injury from a fall, most injuries occurred to the front of the head, in a 'T-shape' distribution, involving the forehead, nose, lips and chin. This distribution was also encountered in assaults. The incidence of craniofacial trauma can be greatly reduced by improvements in interior home design, education in alcohol abuse and in handling potentially hostile situations, and by improvements in automotive safety devices and compliance with their use by motor vehicle occupants, and the utilization of full-face helmets by cyclists and motor-cyclists (Hussain *et al.*, 1994).

Clinical assessment, structural pathology and treatment

To understand fully the pathophysiological consequences of disruption of the integrity of the skin, one must appreciate the organization and morphological features of normal skin. The skin is the largest organ of the body; it has three major tissue layers. The outermost layer, the epidermis, is stratified epithelium whose thickness is relatively uniform in all areas of the body (75–100 μm), except on the palms and soles, where it is particularly thick (0.4–0.5 mm). Beneath the epidermis is the dermis, which is composed primarily of a dense fibroelastic connective tissue stroma with collagen and elastic fibres and an extracellular gel called the ground substance. This amorphous gel is composed of acid mucopolysaccharide protein as well as salts, water and glycoproteins. The functions of the ground substance are not known with certainty, but it is believed that it contributes to salt and water balance, serves as a support for other components of the dermis and subcutaneous tissue, and participates in collagen synthesis. The dermal layer encloses an extensive vascular and nerve network as well as special glands and appendages that communicate with the overlying epidermis. The dermis can be subdivided into two parts. Its most superficial portion, the papillary dermis, is moulded against the epidermis and encloses superficial elements of the microcirculation of the skin. It consists of a relatively cellular, loose connective tissue with collagen and elastic fibres that are smaller in diameter and fewer in number than in the underlying reticular dermis. Within the papillary dermis there are dermal elevations that indent the inner surface of the epidermis. Between the dermal papillae, the downward projections of epidermis appear peg-like and are referred to as rete pegs. In the reticular portion of the dermis, the collagen and elastic fibres are thicker and greater in number; here there are fewer cells and less ground substance than in the papillary dermis.

The thickness of the dermis varies from 1 mm to 4 mm in different anatomical regions. It is thickest on the back, followed by the thigh, abdomen, forehead, wrist, scalp, palm and eyelid. Its thickness varies with the individual's age. In the very old the dermis is often atrophic, whereas in the very young it is not fully developed.

The third layer of the skin is the subcutaneous tissue, which is composed of areolar and fatty connective tissue. It shows great regional variation in thickness and adipose content. The subcutaneous layer insulates underlying tissue and protects it from external trauma.

The colour of normal human skin is related to the number, type, size and distribution of the melanosomes. These specialized organelles are products of unicellular glands (melanocytes) that transfer them into the epithelial cells. The concentration of melanosomes varies considerably within an individual and between individuals. The pigmentation or colouring of a patient's skin is an important consideration in reconstructive surgery. Ideally the colour of the reconstructed tissue should be similar (colour match) to that of contiguous tissue. When reconstructing the facial or cervical region, skin taken from the scalp, upper part of the chest, or upper part of the back provides the most satisfactory colour match (Edgerton and Hansen, 1960).

The muscles of facial expression are connected to the overlying skin by superficial. connective tissue strands. During the process of ageing,

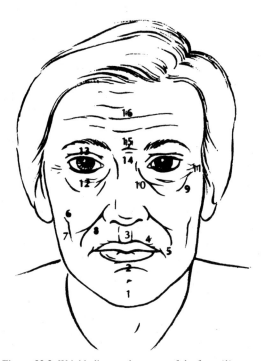

Figure 33.3. Wrinkle lines and grooves of the face: (1) mental fovea; (2) mentolabial groove; (3) philtrum; (4) circumoral striae; (5) oromental groove; (6) buccal fovea; (7) buccomandibular groove; (8) nasolabial groove; (9) orbitozygomatic line; (10) inferior orbital groove; (11) lateral orbital lines; (12) inferior palpebral lines; (13) superior orbital groove; (14) transverse nasal lines; (15) vertical glabellar lines; (16) transverse frontal lines.

natural wrinkle lines appear perpendicularly to the direction of contraction of the underlying muscles of facial expression (Figure 33.3). For example, the wrinkle lines in the perioral region lie perpendicularly to the direction of contraction of the orbicularis oris muscle. It has been recommended that the lines of either excision or incision coincide with these natural wrinkle lines, resulting in a more aesthetically pleasing scar (Cox, 1941; George and Singer, 1993; Kraissl, 1951).

Nose

Lacerations of the nose may be limited to the skin, or they may involve the deeper structures (sparse nasal musculature, cartilaginous framework and nasal mucous membrane). They are repaired by accurate reapproximation of each tissue layer. When the laceration extends through all tissue layers, closure should begin with a marginal suture (5/0 monofilament, nonabsorbable synthetic) that aligns the skin surrounding the entrances of the nasal canals, to prevent malapposition and notching of the alar rim (Figure 33.4a). Traction upon the long, untied ends of the marginal suture approximates the wound and aligns the anterior and posterior margins of the divided tissue layers. The mucous membrane should then be repaired with interrupted 5/0 uncoated, absorbable synthetic sutures with their knots buried in the tissue. The divided edges of the cartilage should then be approximated with interrupted 5/0 braided, absorbable synthetic sutures (Figure 33.4b). The cut edges of the skin, with its adherent musculature, are closed with interrupted 5/0 monofilament, nonabsorbable synthetic sutures (Figure 33.4c). During wound repair, linear lacerations of the alar rim may shorten and result in notching of the rim. A Z-plasty at the alar rim will correct this deformity.

In any nasal injury, the nasal septum must be inspected for haematoma formation. Packing the nose with gauze soaked in a vasoconstrictive agent (4% cocaine) limits nasal bleeding and facilitates examination. If a nasal haematoma is detected, it must be evacuated. An untreated septal haematoma will typically absorb and destroy the septal cartilage, especially if it is infected, resulting in septal perforation and/or a saddle-nose deformity. If the cartilaginous framework of the nose is repositioned accurately, packing of the nose is unnecessary, and should be avoided if possible. Nasal packing may obstruct drainage from the overlying wound and

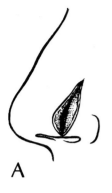
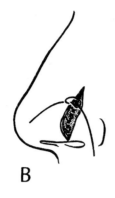

A

B

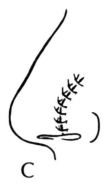

C

Figure 33.4. (a) Placement of initial epidermal marginal sutures prevents malapposition and notching of the alar rim; (b) the divided edges of the nasal cartilages are approximated with interrupted 5/0 braided absorbable sutures; (c) the skin edges are closed with interrupted 5/0 monofilament nonabsorbable synthetic sutures.

precipitate bleeding and separation of the mucous membrane upon removal.

When there is avulsion of components of the nose, it is best to restore the architecture with the avulsed specimen. If the avulsed tissue is not recovered or not suitable for replantation, the technique of reconstruction will depend on the magnitude and depth of injury. Skin loss is best replaced by full thickness skin grafts using post-auricular skin as the donor site. Oval or round defects can be converted into angular defects conforming to the contours of the nasal skin. Segmentalization of the defect will disguise the deformity. Immobilization of the graft with a pressure (stent) dressing for four days is advised.

Full thickness loss of nasal alar tissue can be replaced by a composite graft from the ear margin. This graft contains skin for covering, cartilage for support, and skin for the lining. A favourite donor site is the superior part of the auricle. The secondary defect is closed by direct approximation. Notching of the helical rim is avoided by performing a Z-plasty. When using a composite graft, one should attempt to increase the raw surface available for revascularization. The contact surface may be enlarged by turning down a hinge flap at the edge of the defect, provided that the skin is well vascularized. The composite graft will survive if no part of it is more than 1.0–2.5 cm from a blood supply. The skin on one side of the graft is approximated to the nasal lining with interrupted 5/0 uncoated, absorbable synthetic sutures; interrupted 5/0 monofilament, nonabsorbable synthetic sutures are used to appose the skin on the other side. Vaseline-impregnated gauze packing of the vestibular portion of the nasal canal beneath the composite graft forms a satisfactory internal splint. Postoperative iced compresses for 48–72 hours help graft survival.

For most large defects of the nose, flap tissue will provide the best reconstructive result. Donor sites include the nose itself, the adjacent cheek and forehead, or other parts of the head and neck. The choice of tissue will depend on the requirements for reconstruction. The colour and consistency of flap tissue from these sites matches that of nasal skin. The thickness of flap tissue is sufficient to avoid the depression encountered occasionally when a skin graft is used to repair the defect.

When the defect is small, local flap tissue can be used to cover it. Even though the skin over the nose in younger patients is relatively inelastic, some shifting of the skin in the normal nose is possible in order to close small defects. In the older patient, nasal skin can be easily rotated or advanced to cover defects up to 2 cm wide. Incisions are made at the junction of the nose with the surrounding structures and adjacent to the defect, with a base maintained on the appropriate side. The tissue can be advanced across the nose or rotated and advanced toward the tip.

The nasolabial cheek flap is useful, especially in older individuals, to provide skin coverage of the nose. In males, the nasolabial fold separates the hair-bearing area of the upper lip from the nonhair-bearing area of the cheek. When a defect in the nose is being repaired with a nasolabial flap in males, it should be taken from above the nasolabial fold in the nonhair-bearing area. In ideal circumstances, the size of the nasolabial flap may be as much as 3 cm wide and 10 cm long with relative safety. The cheek skin is undermined to facilitate closure of the donor site. After the nasolabial flap is raised, the donor site is closed by direct approximation. Closure of the donor site advances the base of the flap closer to the nose. The nasolabial flaps are usually based superiorly for reconstruction of the columella, nasal floor, alae and nasal dorsum. Inferiorly based flaps are useful for coverage of either the nasal floor or alae. The flaps should be kept thin, and consist only of skin and subdermal fat.

When there is loss of the cartilaginous framework and overlying skin, the use of forehead flaps to replace most of the nasal surface is the most efficient solution. They have the same advantage as nasolabial flaps, but provide a greater quantity of tissue. The types of forehead flaps that are used for nasal reconstruction are the midline flaps with donor sites that can be closed primarily, and the vertically orientated flaps (e.g. up-and-down flap, scalping flap). The nose is best designed to be oversize, with trimming undertaken as a secondary procedure.

Lips

The technique of closure will depend largely on the type of lip wound. There are essentially two types of wound: laceration and avulsion. Superficial lacerations involve the skin and subcutaneous tissue. Deep lacerations may extend through the muscle and underlying mucosa. Bleeding may be profuse if the labial arteries are involved. Clamping the cut ends of the vessels with a haemostat and tying them with ligatures will control bleeding. Each tissue layer must be meticulously reapproximated. The vermilion-cutaneous and the vermilion-mucosal margins are important anatomical landmarks that must be apposed by key stitches to prevent the development of a 'step-off' deformity that is difficult to correct at a later date.

Repair of a laceration through the lip requires a three-layered closure (Figure 33.5a). Using skin hooks, traction is applied to align the anterior and posterior borders of the laceration. Closure of the wound is begun first at the vermilion-skin junction with a 6/0 monofilament, nonabsorbable synthetic suture. The orbicularis oris muscle is then repaired with interrupted 4/0 braided, synthetic absorbable sutures (Figure 33.5b). The vermilion-mucous membrane junction is approximated with a 5/0 uncoated, synthetic absorbable suture. This suture ligature is constructed so that its knot is buried in the subcutaneous tissue. The divided edges of the mucous membrane and vermilion are then closed using interrupted 5/0 uncoated, absorbable synthetic sutures with a buried knot construction. The skin edges of the laceration are usually jagged and irregular, but can be fitted together as the pieces of a jigsaw puzzle, using interrupted 6/0 monofilament, nonabsorbable synthetic sutures with their knots formed on the surface of the skin (Figure 33.5c). During healing, a linear wound of the lip may undergo contraction, resulting in notching of the lip. The deformity can be corrected by a Z-plasty revision of the linear scar.

Tissue loss from the lip usually involves either the skin surface or all tissue layers. Defects involving all tissue layers can be further classified by their location into median and lateral defects,

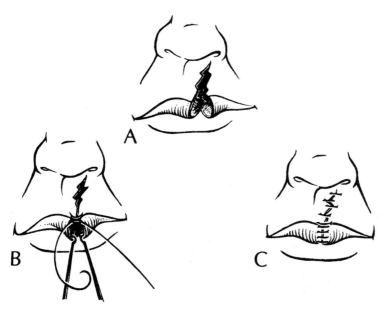

Figure 33.5. (a) Full thickness laceration of the upper lip; **(b)** using skin hooks, traction is applied to align the anterior and posterior borders of the laceration; closure of the wound first at the vermilion-skin junction with a 6/0 monofilament nonabsorbable synthetic suture; **(c)** the divided edges of the skin are approximated by interrupted 6/0 monofilament nonabsorbable synthetic sutures.

and complete loss of lip. Tissue loss at the commissure is a distinct entity that deserves special consideration. In planning reconstruction of the lip, the following principles should be followed.

1. If the avulsed tissue is available, replantation using microsurgical techniques is the optimal method of reconstruction.
2. If the avulsed tissue specimen is either not recovered or not amenable to replantation, the lip defect should be reconstructed with inner-vated muscle-containing tissue with inner and outer epithelial linings.
3. The remaining portion of the injured lip should be considered first for the reconstruction of the defect. If there is not sufficient contiguous lip tissue, tissue from the opposite lip can be used to fill the defect.
4. If sufficient lip tissue from the opposite lip is not available, flaps can be rotated from the sides of the defect.
5. Distant flaps shrink and curl due to the absence of muscle and should be avoided.
6. When the patient's condition precludes a pro-longed procedure to reconstruct large tissue defects, mucous membrane must be sutured to skin and the definitive procedure postponed until the patient's condition improves.

When there is significant skin loss from the upper or the lower lip, the entire aesthetic unit should be resurfaced with a full thickness pattern graft from either the retroauricular or the supraclavicular regions, or a split thickness (0.356 mm) skin graft from the scalp. Small defects in the mucous membrane can be closed with transposition flaps. For larger defects, skin grafts are required on the labial surface alone, allowing the alveolar surface to re-epithelialize spontaneously. Nonhair-bearing skin should be used for intraoral grafts whenever possible. The contraction encountered in skin grafts in the oral cavity during the first three to six months can be limited by moulds or prostheses.

Median or lateral defects of up to one-third of either lip can be closed without unduly constricting the mouth. The technique of approximation of the wound edges is similar to that employed in the repair of vertical lacerations of the lip.

When the avulsion involves the central half of the upper lip, the Abbé flap alone is the procedure of choice, since the scars of the flap simulate the philtral margins and the lip commissures are not altered. The Abbé flap consists of a full thickness flap, pedicled on the labial vessels, taken from the lower lip to fill a similarly shaped defect of the upper lip. In the design of the Abbé flap, it is made approximately half the width of the defect to be filled so that both lips share in the reduction. The base of the flap should be placed so that, after closure of the donor defect, the pedicle will be opposite the upper lip defect. The blood supply of the Abbé flap is from the inferior labial vessels. The apex of the defect will be excised for better simulation of the philtrum. The flap is incised and rotated into the defect. Transposition and insetting of the flap with closure of each tissue layer (mucous membrane, orbicularis oris muscle, skin) closes the defect in the upper lip. A layered closure of the donor site results in a vertical scar. The flap is divided at 10–14 days with readjustment of the vermilion borders. Within 6–12 months, motor and sensory functions return to normal. When more than half of the upper lip is avulsed, the Abbé flap must be combined with the advancement of lateral lip segments toward the midline. This is facilitated by excising either a Bürow's triangle from each nasolabial angle, or by perialar crescentic excisions.

In moderate size lateral defects of the upper lip, the Estlander operation is a valuable reconstructive procedure. Like the Abbé flap, this uses a triangu-lar flap based on the labial artery. The flap is outlined, with the labial artery being preserved in the vermilion of the pedicle. Closure of the donor site and flap incisions cause a shortened, rounded commissure that requires secondary revision. Reconstruction of the commissure can be accom-plished four to six weeks after the initial proce-dure, with a vermilion flap for the upper lip part of the commissure and a mucosal and muscle flap being used to reconstruct the lower lip portion. Zisser (1975) reported a modification in the design of the flap that eliminated the need for this secondary procedure at the commissure. For com-plete loss of the upper lip, lateral cheek flaps may be combined with an Abbé flap to reconstruct the upper lip. Advancement of the lateral cheek flaps is facilitated by either perialar or Bürow's triangular excisions (Webster, 1960).

The operative procedures previously described for the reconstruction of the upper lip are applica-ble to defects of the lower lip. However, care must be taken to supply either supporting tissue or suspensory tissue to counteract the effects of gravity that tend to pull down the lip and results in drooling. Small-size defects involving less than one-third of the lower lip can be repaired either by a triangular wedge excision of the inferior part of the defect and closure, or by the Hagedorn rectangular flap technique (Andrews, 1964). A 'step' bilateral rectangular flap advancement is an approach designed on the line of the chin crease to mask the scars (Andrews, 1964).

In the case of large median loss of the lower lip, a modification of the Bernard operation can be used to repair the defect (Fries, 1973). Advancement of the lateral cheek flaps is facilitated by excision of Bürow's triangles. The oral mucosa is preserved in the area of excision of the Bürow's triangles and is used to restore the vermilion border of the advancement quadrilateral cheek flaps. In larger lateral defects of the lower lip, an Estlander flap is a valuable technique of reconstruction. Nasolabial flaps and lateral rotation cheek flaps are alternative approaches.

Reconstruction of total loss of the lower lip can be accomplished by rectangular advancement flaps created by excising Bürow's triangles from the nasolabial region and perimentum, and preserving the oral mucosa. Mucosal incisions are made at the level of the skin incision inferiorly, but at a higher level superiorly. The cheek flaps are advanced medially and sutured together. The superior borders of the cheek flaps are denuded of epithelium along the site of the future free margin of the lower lip. The mucosal flaps are incised, and then folded over the cheek flaps to form the vermilion.

Innervated lower lip reconstruction has also been performed using neurovascular local cheek flaps. Myocutaneous flaps of orbicularis oris have subsequently been separated from the surrounding facial musculature, with minimal mucosal separation, and have been effective in achieving innervated lower lip reconstruction. When restoration of the muscular function of the lower lip is not possible, some function may be restored, either by a fascia lata sling or by rotating down a nasolabial flap. Extensive loss of the commissure of the mouth has been treated by the Estlander procedure in reverse.

Cheeks

Lacerations of the cheek are of great concern because they may be associated with injury to the parotid duct. Injury to the duct should be suspected if clear fluid is seen emerging from a wound in the cheek. The injury can be readily identified by passing a small silicone catheter into the duct opening (Figure 33.6a). After the distal divided end is identified, the catheter is passed into the proximal end of the duct as far as possible. The divided ends are then approximated over the silicone catheter, using 6/0 monofilament, nonabsorbable synthetic sutures (Figure 33.6b). The silicone catheter should be sutured to the oral mucosa to prevent it from being dislodged (Figure 33.6c). The catheter is removed after 7 days. When the duct is injured in its proximal portion, the divided distal end may be sutured to the cheek mucosa, creating a new ostium. If the parotid duct

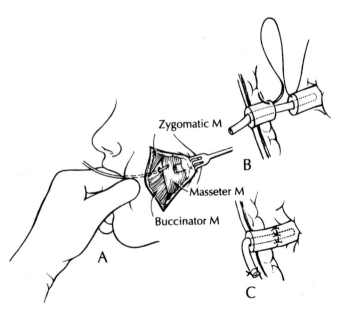

Figure 33.6. (a) The injury to the parotid duct can readily be identified by passing a small silicone catheter into the opening of the parotid duct; **(b)** the divided ends of the duct are then approximated over the silicone catheter, using 6/0 monofilament, nonabsorbable synthetic sutures; **(c)** the silicone catheter is sutured to the oral mucosa to prevent it from being dislodged.

is ligated, the gland eventually atrophies and function ceases. Division of the submandibular glands and ducts does not require repair; they will drain through a fistula that usually develops after injury to the floor of the mouth.

Lacerations of the cheek should be reapproximated with interrupted 5/0 monofilament, nonabsorbable synthetic sutures in a manner similar to that of putting together a jigsaw puzzle. In resurfacing skin loss of the cheek, the defect should be converted into one that conforms to the aesthetic unit of the face. When possible, large skin defects should be replaced by transposition flaps rather than a skin graft. This is especially important in the male, since the skin graft is hairless, making it very apparent in a heavily bearded individual. Transposition flaps from the neck and preauricular area are used to resurface large skin defects of the cheek.

Severe trauma may result in through-and-through defects of the cheeks. Repair requires an inner lining and external covering. When the lip commissure has been lost in continuity with a cheek defect, it is advisable to reconstruct the commissure first, before repair of the cheek defect. Large full thickness defects of the cheek can be repaired with forehead flaps, cervical and pectoral flaps, and myocutaneous flaps. Recent advances in microvascular surgery have led to the successful use of large, free flaps for reconstruction of the cheek.

Measurement of outcome

When soft tissue injuries of the face occur, legal action is frequently taken against the party responsible. This process involves the legal profession, the medical profession, and usually the insurance industry. The treating physician must provide accurate, specific information regarding injury and treatment, which can be facilitated by keeping careful records. This documentation can be enhanced by photographs of facial injury. These photographs may cause an emotional rather than intellectual reaction from the lay community; consequently attorneys often exercise caution in their use. Establishment of validity of claim and awarding of damages are based partly on the initial temporary disfigurement, but the results of treatment and the permanency of the patient's injuries are subsequently more important factors (Schultz, 1988).

In Schultz's review (1988) of 3000 consecutive patients with facial injuries who were treated over a 25-year period, several practical conclusions were drawn regarding involvement of medical personal in subsequent personal injury litigation. First, the treating physician became involved in personal injury litigation in approximately 31% of patients. This involvement took the form of any or all of the following: narrative medical report to attorneys, subpoena of medical records, discovery deposition, evidence deposition, and court testimony. Secondly, the average interval between injury and the surgeon's awareness of litigation was in excess of six months. The longest intervals involved children, probably because of the extended statute of limitations in these cases. Thirdly, the most common cause of facial injury involving the physician in personal injury litigation was the automobile accident (86%). Finally, the prototype patient was the young unmarried woman injured as a front seat passenger in the car of a friend.

Medical report

The treating physician is usually first made aware of personal injury litigation by the patient's attorney in a letter requesting a detailed medical report. This letter will often contain a comment to the effect that, in the event of settlement, the physician's outstanding bill will be protected. In response to this letter, the physician should respond likewise by letter, requesting proper written authorization (if not already received) to release this information and advising the attorney of what type of report he is prepared to provide, as well as what fee he expects for such preparation.

The report should identify the patient accurately. It should state exactly when and where the patient was first seen and how the physician was contacted (e.g. by the emergency department, another physician, etc.). A brief statement should be included about how the patient allegedly sustained the injury. If the physician's responsibility was for care of the facial injuries alone, remarks should be confined to these injuries, unless previous or other concomitant injuries directly bear on the deposition of the facial injuries. The injuries should be accurately located on the face with appropriate quantitative measurements. Laboratory or radiographic findings related to or influencing treatment of the facial injuries should be mentioned to clarify the treatment and prognosis.

The treatment and hospital course should be summarized. When operations are performed it is preferable to include the operative report, rather than a narrative discussion of the surgery. Any complications encountered during surgery or post-operatively should be indicated. The patient's conditions at the time of hospital discharge should be discussed (Schultz, 1988). The dates or frequency of the patient's follow-up care should be provided.

The permanence and location of the scar or the deformity (functional or cosmetic) is important. Statements regarding permanence must be particularly explicit, as they relate to anticipated additional surgery (i.e. will the condition still be present, improve or become worse after completion of all revisions and reconstructive procedures?). Specific functional handicaps such as a decrease in the range of movement and the presence of abnormal neurological signs such as paraesthesia, sensory loss, or loss of motor function, should also be recorded. For such purposes, the American Medical Association (1984) has published a text on evaluating permanent impairment. A grading scale is given for each aspect of function of the skin. Physicians are urged to be familiar with this book so they may communicate about the permanent impairment of scars with consistency and agreement.

Evaluation of permanent impairment

The face and its structural components serve multiple functions in humans. The portal for deglutition is the mouth and lips. Disturbances in function can result in drooling or the inability to contain fluid or food while eating. The lips and mouth also serve in vocal articulation. The nose and mouth are the portals of entry for respiration. Impairment can be the result of scar formation and contracture of the lips, or loss of tissue.

The skin of the face has various functions, including body covering, resistance to trauma, sensory perception, and regulation of temperature. In addition the face has a unique role in communication. No other part of the body serves as specific a function for personal identity and for expression of thought and emotion. Facial expressions are an integral part of normal living and communication.

In evaluating permanent impairment from a disorder of the face, functional capacity and structural integrity are considered. In this section, impairment is limited to abnormalities in structural integrity only, rather than loss of function. Loss of structural integrity can result from cutaneous

disfigurement, such as that due to abnormal pigmentation or scars, or from loss of supporting structures, such as loss of soft tissue, bone or cartilage of the facial skeleton. In the AMA's *Guides to the evaluation of permanent impairment* (1984), it outlined four specific classes of impairment of the face.

- *Class 1* Impairment of the whole person, 0–5%: a patient belongs in class 1 when the facial abnormality is limited to a disorder of the cutaneous structures such as a visible scar or abnormal pigmentation.
- *Class 2* Impairment of the whole person, 5–10%: a patient belongs in class 2 when there is loss of supporting structures of the face with or without cutaneous disorder.
- *Class 3* Impairment of the whole person, 10–15%: a patient belongs in class 3 when there is absence of a normal structural area of the face (e.g. nose, eye, etc.).
- *Class 4* Impairment of the whole person, 15–35%: a patient belongs in class 4 when facial disfigurement is so severe that it precludes social acceptance.

Disfigurement of the face can result from many causes, particularly burns, accidental injuries, surgery and infection. Even though the effects upon an individual can very tremendously, the AMA recommends that total disfigurement of the face after treatment is completed should be deemed 15–35% impairment of the whole person. Facial disfigurement can be considered total if it is severe and grossly deforming of face and features, and if it involves the entire area between the brow line and the upper lip on both sides. Severe disfigurement above the brow line should be deemed at a maximum 1% impairment of the whole person. If it extends to below the upper lip, it may be deemed 8% impairment of the whole person. On the basis of the above guidelines, reasonable impairment values can be placed on other facial disfigurements (American Medical Association, 1984).

Because a principal purpose for rating impairment has to do with disability rating for workers' compensation programmes, disability insurance, or social security disability payments, a major concern is how the ratings will be used for administrative or legal purposes. The permanent rating should be understood as an assessment of health status that is made in accordance with established, accepted medical criteria. Each administrative or legal system that uses permanent impairment as a basis for disability rating should define its own process for translating the rating into an estimate of the degree to which the individual's capacity to meet personal, social, or occupational demands is limited by the impairment (American Medical Association, 1984).

Claiming compensation

While the treating physician receives frequent requests for reports on patients seeking compensation for personal injuries and related losses, formal training in the preparation of medical reports is seldom provided. Generally, the requisite knowledge and skill are acquired informally, through experience gained in responding to requests for such reports and in receiving advice from experienced colleagues. While a common core of clinical injury is the most frequently and extensively reported upon, other aspects are dealt with less adequately. Information is regularly reported on the nature of injuries resulting from accidents and the effects of treatment, and of any persistent symptoms and physical signs. Patients therefore appear to be well served with regard to the information and advice needed to reach conclusions about general damages for pain and suffering and the requirement for future medical or surgical treatment. The major clinical theme that is perhaps not adequately recorded is the description of previous medical history. Even the absence of a pre-accident medical complaint should be recorded. In addition, less frequent and incomprehensive coverage is given to the functional consequences of injury, any resulting social and vocational handicaps, and any need for rehabilitation services. This information is very important because it allows the insurer or courts to reach fair and valid conclusions about such matters as the reasonableness of complaints, how far the accident was responsible for conditions found on examination, and the likely effect of injury on the patient's potential to earn a living and resume pre-accident domestic and leisure pursuits (Cornes and Aitken, 1992).

Deposition

As the process of litigation develops, the physician may be subpoenaed for a discovery deposition. Upon receipt of the subpoena, it is advisable to contact the attorney who requested the medical report. The time, location and fees payable should be discussed. The most appropriate place for the deposition is the physician's office where the patient's records are kept. The physician should respond only to specific questions. He should remember that terminology used in his original medical report will be compared with his deposition (Schultz, 1988).

Court testimony

The treating physician may be subpoenaed to testify. There should be mutual understanding between the physician and the attorney regarding the fees payable for the time spent in delivering the court testimony. As several years may have elapsed since the treating physician last saw the patient, preparation for testimony should include a re-examination of the patient as well as a pretrial conference with the attorney. When describing facial injuries and their location, it is best to point them out on the patient, a model, a drawing or a picture, rather than attempting to refer to one's own face during the explanation. If the decision has been made to use photographs of the patient, they should be of the highest quality, or their admissibility as evidence will more than likely be questioned by the opposing attorney (Schultz, 1988). Because photography plays such a key role, standardization in photography of the face is essential for proper medicolegal documentation.

Photography

Standards for photography differ in the emergency department (ED) or operating room (OR) setting, as well as the clinic setting. In the ED and OR, the situation may be a life-threatening condition and does not leave time or reason properly to compose an optimal photograph as would a clinic setting. In addition, the ED and the OR do not usually have the proper space or equipment to take ideal photographs. Despite such restrictions, there are a few guidelines that may be helpful in obtaining a better photographic composition (Cordell *et al.*, 1980).

1. Take many shots from several different angles and from varying distances.
2. Compose the picture in the way you would normally look at that anatomical area.
3. Use a back drop and remove extraneous objects. Remove all instruments because these may reflect the light source and cause poor pictures.

4. Clean blood, stains and soap from the area to be photographed.
5. Fill the frame with the subject.
6. Remove other light sources that could alter the finished colour of the slide or photograph.
7. Place all objects in the same focal plane.
8. The best pictures tell a story.
9. Consider the value of the photograph. Will the photograph document the patient's problem or treatment? Will the photograph be of educational value?

The standard views of the face are frontal, oblique, lateral and nasal basal. A close-up view is added for small irregular lesions. The keystone of positional consistency is the 'Frankfort plane' in which the horizontal plane traverses the top of the tragus and the infraorbital rim (Figure 33.7). The Frankfort plane is utilized for all frontal and lateral views, keeping that plane horizontal. The frontal view covers the entire circumference of the head down to the sternal heads of the clavicles, with the camera lens at eye level. The oblique view (or three-quarter oblique view) uses the same boundaries as above except that the nasal tip is now aligned with the outline of the contralateral cheek. The lateral view is known as the profile view. Leaving a space between the nasal tip and the edge of the photograph is allowable in order to show the full outline of the face. The nasal basal view requires the patient to place the gnathion horizontally with the tragus and the nasal tip at the interbrow area. The important information for the close-up view is that one needs to demonstrate the relationship of the lesion or scar to other structures of the face such as the scalp, neck, cheek or nose.

The view does not need to be any closer than from the eyebrows to the lower lip (Tardy *et al.*, 1980). These views are to be rigorously adhered to and are not subject to change.

With all the standards above, it is no wonder that errors occasionally occur and purposeful misrepresentations are easily made. Lack of adherence to the proper equipment can change the size of facial features and lesions. Shadowing for the purpose of artistry is beautiful, but should be avoided for scientific purpose; a shadowed scar is worthless. Underemphasizing or overemphasizing a lesion is also undesirable. The lesion should be presented in a photograph as it appears in real life. The patient's position can also distort the size of facial features as well as cause unwanted shadowing (Tardy *et al.*, 1980).

Biology of wound repair

The discussion of soft tissue injury of the face is not complete without considering the ultimate unavoidable result of this injury: healing and scarring. The plastic surgeon can achieve wound closure with minimum deformity and dysfunction by following surgical principles that are based on the biology of wound repair. Repair is the response of living tissues to injury and is the keystone on which plastic surgery is founded. Many plastic surgeons have not grappled fully with the concepts of the biology of wound repair and do not appreciate that wound healing processes can now effectively be altered to reduce the pathophysiological consequences of the injury.

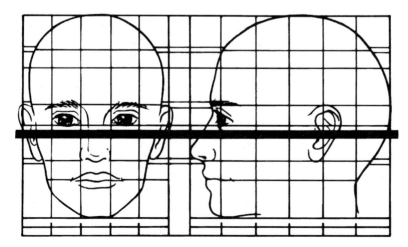

Figure 33.7. 'Frankfort' plane of the standard views of the face.

The repair of skin wounds represents a highly dynamic, integrated series of cellular, physiological and biochemical events. Although these processes of repair of skin wounds occur concomitantly, examining all the processes simultaneously can be confusing. For the purposes of discussion, several natural components of wound healing will be reviewed separately.

Inflammation

It is almost axiomatic that injury is followed by inflammation that can be characterized by vascular and cellular responses designed to protect the body against alien substances, and to dispose of dead and dying tissue preparatory to the repair process. In either a surgical or a traumatic assault on the body that results in disruption of the skin, there is a physical interruption of the blood vessels, leading to immediate haemorrhage. The body's response to the injury is basically the same regardless of the cause. The most significant element of this response is seen in the local vasculature. The immediate response of the small vessels is vasoconstriction, which lasts for 5–10 minutes and limits blood loss.

Almost immediately after the injury, leucocytes 'stick' to the endothelium of the injured vessels. At the same time, red blood cells adhere to each other and form rouleaux, which tend to plug the cut ends of capillaries. Because platelet thrombi do not form until later, this occlusion can be reversed. Coagulation is initiated by agglutinated platelets that adhere first to the subendothelial collagen of the cut ends of the injured vessels. Within minutes, fibrinogen is converted to fibrin, which then forms a mesh at the vessel opening. The fibrin screen aggregates more platelets and their developing pseudopods contract the fibrin mesh to form a firmer plug, sealing the ends of the blood vessels.

The fluids that escape from the vessels, combined with migrating leucocytes, constitute an inflammatory exudate. The magnitude of this increase in vascular permeability can be correlated with the duration of exposure of the wound (Edlich *et al.*, 1973). Closure of the wound within one hour after injury appears to reduce vascular permeability. If the wound is left open for three hours, there is a dramatic increase in vascular permeability that results in the development of a relatively thick inflammatory exudate on the wound surface. This exaggerated inflammatory response to prolonged exposure (longer than three hours) limits the therapeutic value of antibiotics. This fibrinous coagulum forms a protective cover around bacteria on the surface of the wound and prevents antibiotics administered systemically or topically from contacting them. Similarly, this developing inflammatory exudate accounts for the diminished effectiveness of delayed antibiotic treatment. Moreover, it is the reason for the success of preoperative antibiotics in the prevention of infection. In the absence of the inflammatory exudate, the antibiotic can gain access to the bacteria and prevent the subsequent development of wound infection.

Paradoxically, the fibrinous wound coagulum that limits the effectiveness of antibiotics is an important factor in the open wound's defences against infection (Edlich *et al.*, 1969). This coagulum serves as a plug in the transected ends of lymphatics in the wound, thereby becoming an obstacle to the invasion of bacteria, and, in part, enhancing the resistance of an open wound to systemic sepsis, while the fibrinous coagulum prevents the lymphatic invasion of bacteria, the underlying wound gradually gains sufficient resistance to infection to permit an uncomplicated closure. The reparative process of the open wound, associated with the developing resistance to infection, is characterized by the appearance of capillary buds and young fibrous tissue, referred to as granulation tissue. On or after the fourth postoperative day, the margins of an open wound without devitalized tissue can be approximated with minimum risk of infection.

Virtually any condition that contributes to a decrease in the delivery of white blood cells to an area of bacterial contamination will promote the development of infection. These conditions are usually caused by a diminution in blood flow, as may be found in vasocclusive states, in hypovolaemic shock, and after the use of vasopressors. The infection-potentiating effects of tissue ischaemia are documented with local anaesthetic agents containing epinephrine (Stevenson *et al.*, 1975). This drug is a potent vasoconstrictor that limits the clearance of local anaesthetic agents from the tissue, thereby prolonging the duration of anaesthesia. This beneficial effect of epinephrine is, however, associated with damage to the local wound defences. The infection-potentiating effect of this powerful vasoconstrictor is proportional to its concentration and results from its vasoactivity. This damage to the tissue defences argues against the use of epinephrine in heavily contaminated wounds.

Epithelialization

After an incision, the divided parts of the epithelium are closed by cellular migration and mitosis. Within hours of injury the peri-incisional epithelium reacts by thickening and begins to migrate across the incisional gap as two long sheets of epithelium, one moving along each side of the entire length of the wound. The normal rate of mitosis increases from about 7% to 30% at the margin of the wound (Hell and Cruickshank, 1963). The maximum activity is seen just a short distance (a few cell widths) back from the incision. The two thickening advancing surface epithelial sheets invert by growing down in the upper part of the incision. This downward growth of epithelial cells bridges the wound and each epithelial surface unites with the other across the incision. Such epithelial union most commonly occurs at the level of the reticular dermis, creating an epithelium-lined furrow along the entire length of the incision.

The time that this epithelial bridge takes to become complete depends on the technique of closure. With slight eversion of the coapted skin edges, epithelial bridging occurs within 18–24 hours. End-to-end approximation of the skin edges results in an additional 12-hour delay in the formation of an epithelial bridge. If the wound edges are inverted, epithelial bridging is complete 72 hours after closure. Even after the incision is bridged by epithelium, some growth occurs further down in the dermal breach, forming epithelial spurs. Short secondary epithelial spurs invade laterally and downward from the sides of the simple inversion of epithelium.

This epithelial bridge forms a protective barrier against the invasion of bacteria into the wound. Before its formation, the wound is susceptible to surface infection by bacterial contamination. Experimental studies performed in our laboratory have demonstrated that, as they heal, sutured wounds are susceptible to infection by surface contamination during the first 48 hours after wound closure (Schauerhamer *et al.*, 1971). Such surface contamination on the third postoperative day was shown not to produce gross infection in the sutured wound. This susceptibility to infection during the early postoperative period confirms the apparent value of dressings to protect the sutured wound from surface contamination.

Cell division is seen consistently in the advancing tongue of migrating epithelium, indicating that migration and mitosis occur concurrently at the leading edge of the epithelium. Cells at the surface of the tongue of advancing epithelium do not differentiate into keratinized and cornified cells until either migration slows down or epithelial union of the advancing epithelium occurs. At some distance back from the incision, the cells continue their usual progression towards the surface of the epithelium.

Once the epithelial cells bridge the gap, they begin to acquire some of the structural features of the adjacent uninjured epithelium. They become columnar in shape, commence mitosis, and migrate upward towards the surface of the epithelium, with the development of keratin in the uppermost epithelial cells. By 10–15 days, the invasive epithelium begins to resorb. Until the twentieth day, the inversion of the epithelium is distinguishable microscopically. Thereafter it becomes less obvious as the epithelial surface becomes level.

The organization of scar epithelium has little resemblance to that of uninjured skin. Normally, epithelium is bound tightly to the underlying dermis through its undulating basement membrane and epidermal appendages. Unlike normal skin, scar epithelium is relatively atrophic, and lacks rete pegs and epidermal appendages. Because the junction between scar epithelium and underlying dermis has limited surface contact, it is prone to shear forces that result in epidermal-dermal disjunction.

Downgrowth of epithelial cells occurs not only at the incision but also at any interruption of the skin, such as suture tracts (Ordman and Gillman, 1966). In the presence of percutaneous sutures, epithelial cells migrate downward, forming a perisutural cuff. Within this connective tissue milieu the epithelial cells undergo cellular differentiation, eventually ending in keratinization, which induces an intense inflammatory reaction and scar formation. If the percutaneous sutures are removed before the eighth postoperative day, the invasive spurs of epithelium regress, leaving no discernible deformity. After that time the suture track's reaction to the foreign body becomes so intense that permanent deformity results (i.e. needle puncture scars), which will be a constant and unnecessary reminder to the plastic surgeon and the patient of the operative intervention.

Crikelair (1958) enumerated factors that predispose to the development of suture scars. The anatomical location of the skin was an important factor. The skin of the eyelids, the palms of the hands and the soles of the feet seldom showed suture puncture scars. By comparison, the skin of the back, chest, upper part of the arms and lower extremities was shown to be more likely to develop suture puncture tracks. Patients with an inherent tendency to keloid formation were prone to suture puncture scars. Of the variable factors under the control of the plastic surgeon, the length of time the skin suture remained in place was the most important determinant. The size of either the suture needle or the suture was not significant. Surprisingly, the inherent skin tension or the tightness of the tied sutural loop did not predispose to the development of sutural scars.

Dermal repair

The fibroblasts within the dermis, which have a full complement of metabolic pathways, synthesize collagen, elastin and ground substance. Collagen is the principal component of the scar tissue in the dermis and accounts for the tensile strength of the normal and repaired skin. In the uninjured skin, the collagen fibres are unbranched and extremely long structures (Thacker *et al.*, 1975). Because there are no known anatomical linkages between the collagen fibres, it is assumed that the elastic fibres are so interlaced with them to restore the collagen network to its normal position after a mechanical load has been removed from the skin. In the relaxed skin dermis, the fibres appear randomly in convoluting intertwining coils. As a load is applied to the skin, the fibres become aligned until eventually most are lying parallel to the direction of maximum skin stretch. After the fibres have become uncoiled and orientated the further elastic property of skin resembles that of collagen.

From the plastic surgeon's point of view, the rate of gain of strength of the wound is a key determinant of many decisions, including when the sutures can be removed, the level of patient activity, and the selection of the incision. The answers to these questions are found in the results of bioengineering studies of wound strength. Even though collagen fibres are evident on the third day after injury, a skin wound has negligible tensile strength (Levenson *et al.*, 1965). During the first eight days after closure, the wound is held together by blood vessels crossing the wound, epithelialization, and a fibrinous coagulum. If the percutaneous sutures are removed at this time, the wound may be disrupted easily unless supported by dermal sutures and/or skin closure tapes. Over the next 13 days (8–21 days after injury) there is a rapid gain in strength, which continues at a relatively rapid and constant rate for four months and at a slower rate for one year. The strength of repaired skin incisions never reaches that of uninjured skin. Adamsons and Kahan (1970) demonstrated that rabbit skin wounds closed with a continuous 4/0 silk suture regained only 40% of the strength of unwounded tissue 120 days after wounding. In the dog, Van Winkle and associates (1975) noted that skin wounds approximated by different percutaneous sutures developed 70% of their normal strength by 120 days. Consequently, the skin wound remains a relatively brittle structure that is capable of absorbing much less energy than normal skin.

Through the years, imaginative biologists have suggested methods to accelerate healing. To date, this avenue of research has resulted in important findings on the repair of dehisced and resutured wounds. Incised wounds allowed to heal for short periods, then dehisced and immediately resutured, developed strength at a significantly faster rate than the primary wound (Botsford, 1941). Experiments in animals demonstrated that the strength gained in secondary wound healing correlated with the rate of collagen synthesis at the time of dehiscence rather than the collagen content of the wound (Madden and Smith, 1970). It is interesting to note that excision of the wound edges and reapproximation of the debrided edges eliminated this acceleration of healing (Dunphy and Jackson, 1962). Such debridement of the edges of a dehisced wound is therefore clearly an error in surgical judgement. The benefits of secondary wound healing can be realized in patients requiring surgical intervention soon after the first procedure. Those with wounds exhibiting gross malapposition of the skin edges should be returned immediately to the operating theatre to reapproximate these edges. The development of complications, such as ischaemia of the wound edges or haematoma, also warrants re-exploration. When performed between the first and fourth week after injury, the secondary wound exhibits a greater breaking strength than the first. This accelerated healing is associated with enhanced resistance to infection (Edlich *et al.*, 1969).

Scar remodelling

During healing, scar remodelling occurs with progressive changes in its configuration. As the scar matures, it contracts in all dimensions. The collagen becomes more dense, the fibroblast population decreases, and many vascular channels are obliterated. As the collagen becomes more dense and the vascular supply reduced, the mature scar becomes flatter, thinner and paler, making it less conspicuous and more aesthetically pleasing. Because these changes usually evolve over 12 months, it is best to wait at least one year before making the decision about whether surgical revision is really necessary. Consequently, experienced plastic surgeons consider the biological processes of remodelling of scars to be their allies in improving the scar's appearance. Patients will unknowingly attribute these pleasing changes in the appearance of their scars to the initial surgery; which is a misconception that reinforces their confidence in their plastic surgeons.

Remodelling occurs by a process of resorption that occurs concomitantly with synthesis. In most scars, a balance is reached between the production of collagen by fibroblasts and degradation by epidermal collagenase. The rate of collagen synthesis and degradation is high for about six months and then diminishes greatly. When the rate of collagen synthesis remains greater than degradation for extended periods, hypertrophic scars, or keloids, develop. The mechanisms for controlling remodelling are still poorly understood. Clinical observations in humans suggest that the biomechanical properties of the skin play an important role at the site of surgical incision or excision.

Biomechanical properties

The ultimate appearance and function of a scar can be predicted by the static and dynamic skin tensions of the surrounding skin (Thacker *et al.*, 1975). The static skin tensions are the forces that stretch the skin over the underlying bony framework when the body remains motionless. These inherent forces are dependent partly on the natural characteristics of dermal collagen fibres and partially on the pattern in which they are woven. The clinical evidence of these tensions is the retraction of wound edges, permitting visualization of the underlying tissue.

Static skin forces differ considerably in their magnitude and direction within the same person and between individuals. Large differences are noted between various anatomical sites. The skin in one region may be relatively taut; in others it is lax. In one human volunteer, the static skin tensions were fivefold greater in the extremities than in the abdominal skin. In some regions of the body there is a directional orientation of static skin tensions. This was first appreciated by Dupuytren in 1834 when he examined a suicide victim who sustained three self-inflicted puncture wounds made by an awl. He noted that the wounds assumed an elliptical shape similar to the shape of skin wounds caused by a knife. He concluded that skin tensions in the long axis of the defect were substantially greater than in its short axis, which distorted the wound accordingly.

In 1861, Langer (translated 1978) published a more comprehensive study on the biomechanical properties of human skin. His observations were made by inserting an awl 2.0 mm in diameter to a depth of 2.5 mm into the skin of cadavers, which were lying in the normal anatomical position. As Dupuytren reported (1834), the circular defect was drawn into an ellipse. By drawing lines between the major axes of the ellipses, Langer identified the direction in which the tension predominated. These static lines of maximum skin tensions are known as 'Langer's lines'. In 1892, 31 years later, Kocher (1907) advocated that surgical incisions should follow Langer's lines. For nearly 100 years, surgeons referred to Langer's lines as the most appropriate guides for incisions that would heal with minimum scarring. It is now realized that the charts of Langer's lines appearing in textbooks and articles have little practical application because they are erroneous in most cases and do not consider the highly important effect of the dynamic skin tensions on a healing scar.

The static skin tensions continually pull on the wound edges, resulting in the development of a visible scar. The width of this scar is proportional to the magnitude of the skin tensions (Wray, 1983). Incisions made in skin subjected to strong skin tensions usually heal with wide, unattractive scars. In contrast, narrow, fine scars usually result from the repair of incisions made in skin with weak, static skin tensions.

Dynamic skin tensions also have considerable impact on static skin tensions and on the magnitude and extent of scar formation. These changing tensions are caused by a combination of forces that are associated with either joint movement or muscle contraction. In the face, the dynamic skin tensions are perpendicular to natural skin wrinkles and parallel to the direction of contraction of the underlying muscles. The clinical significance of dynamic tensions is apparent in skin of changing dimensions, where elasticity is needed for normal function. In general, a linear scar intersecting the wrinkle lines or lying parallel to the dynamic skin tensions can result in a serious contracture because the scar does not stretch or recoil like uninjured skin.

Planning incisions

In planning incisions, the plastic surgeon's primary responsibility is to identify a site through which the operative procedure can be completed successfully and safely. The plan must also allow adequate skin coverage of the surgical defect. If a variety of plans can achieve the same result, the plastic surgeon's selection should be based on the resultant cosmetic and physical deformity. Without sacrificing the goals of the procedure, the incision should be placed so that the healing scar is the most aesthetically pleasing. Hiding the scar within hairbearing skin or within the hidden recesses of the body (nose or oral cavity) is the best approach to minimizing deformity.

Unfortunately, incisions cannot always be placed in such hidden positions, and the choice of the site where the scar will be as inconspicuous as possible must be made. It is now generally recognized that the most aesthetically pleasing scar occurs when the long axis of the scar is in the direction of maximum skin tension.

The directional orientation of incisions should be parallel to the natural wrinkles or perpendicular to the dynamic skin tensions. Clinical observation of the wound after the incision is made provides a reliable method of predicting the appearance of the healing scar after closure. The degree to which the divided skin edges retract provides a rough estimate of the magnitude of static skin tensions. Wounds with marked retraction of the edges are subjected to strong static skin tensions and heal with wide scars. When there is minimum separation of the wound edges, repair will be accomplished with fine scars. When treating a patient with a gaping wound with marked retraction of its edges, it is best to warn the patient that the wound may heal with a wide scar, which may require revisional surgery 12 or more months after injury if the patient so desires. This information should be shared with the patient and the family so that they can appropriately credit the aesthetic result to the biology of wound repair.

Unfortunately, an accidental injury does not gain the benefit of this preplanning and may result in a laceration in which the long axis is parallel to the dynamic skin tensions and perpendicular to the natural wrinkle lines. This directional orientation of the wound predisposes to repair by a wide, unattractive scar. In such cases, it is imperative to warn the patient of the impending development; referral to a plastic surgeon for follow-up examination and treatment is recommended. Failure to anticipate these developments may make the patient think the cause of the unattractive scar is proximal to the needle holder rather than distal to it. At a later date (beyond 12 months) the scar can be revised by either a W- or Z-plasty so that the orientation of a portion of the wound becomes perpendicular to the dynamic skin tensions. The success of these scar revisions is also related to the increase in the length of the perimeter of the wound, accounting for lower skin tensions per unit length of wound.

This same inverse relationship between the length of the wound perimeter and the magnitude of the static skin tension accounts for the excellent aesthetic results encountered after closure of uneven, jagged-edged lacerations. In such wounds, the perimeter of the wound is considerably longer than that in the linear incision. Consequently, the magnitude of static tensions per unit length of a jagged-edged wound is less than that for a linear laceration. Plastic surgeons have learned that meticulous reapproximation of the jagged edges of the wound yields a gratifying result with a narrow scar. Plastic surgeons, unaware of the biomechanical principles involved in wound repair, may elect to convert the jagged wound edges into a linear wound. This decision adds insult to the injury. This ill-conceived debridement eliminates the potential benefits of the long wound perimeter and leaves a lenticular-shaped defect that is considerably wider than the initial wound.

Reapproximation of the edges of the debrided wound will require greater closing forces than would have been needed before debridement, and lead to the development of a wide, unattractive scar. Faced with this physical deformity, the patient may seek the advice of a plastic surgeon. Twelve or more months after the injury, the plastic surgeon may elect to revise the scar by either a W- or Z-plasty. The revised incision, the shape of which is reminiscent of the original laceration, will usually heal with a narrower scar.

There are certain similarities between the healing of skin wounds and that of other organ systems, as well as individual differences peculiar to the organ involved. In general, the return of prewounding strength is inversely proportional to the tensile strength of the unwounded tissue. The modern plastic surgeon must welcome objective data regarding the biology of repair of each organ system that will allow the selection of the most appropriate closure technique. Influencing decisions are data on the normal strength of the unwounded tissue, the rate with which wounds gain in strength, the strength of the closure technique, the rate at which the closure technique loses strength in the tissues, and the interactions between the closure technique and the tissues.

Acknowledgement

Supported by a generous gift from Michael L Blumenfeld, DDS, Brookville, NY.

References

Adamsons RJ, Kahan SA. (1970) The rate of healing of incised wounds of different tissues in rabbits. *Surg Gynecol Obstet* **130**: 837–46.

American Medical Association. (1984) *Guides to the evaluation of permanent impairment*. Chicago: AMA.

Andrews EB. (1964) Repair of lower lip defects by the Hagedorn rectangular flap method. *Plast Reconstr Surg* **34**: 27–33.

Botsford TW. (1941) The tensile strength of sutured skin wounds during healing. *Surg Gynecol Obstet* **72**: 690–97.

Cardany CR, Rodeheaver GT, Thacker JG, *et al.* (1976) The crush injury: a high risk wound. *J Am Coll Emerg Physicians* **5**: 965–70.

Cordell W, Zollman W, Karlson H. (1980) A photographic system for the emergency department. *Ann Emerg Med* **9**: 210–14.

Cornes P, Aitken RCB. (1992) Medical reports on persons claiming compensation for personal injury. *J R Soc Med* **85**: 329–33.

Cox HT. (1941) The cleavage lines of the skin. *Br J Surg* **29**: 234–40.

Crikelair GF. (1958) Skin suture marks. *Am J Surg* **96**: 631–38.

Dunphy JE, Jackson DS. (1962) Practical applications of experimental studies in the care of the primarily closed wound. *Am J Surg* **104**: 273–81.

Dupuytren JF. (1834) *Traité théorique et pratique des blessure par armes de querre*, vol. 1. Paris: Baillère.

Edgerton MT, Hansen FC. (1960) Matching facial color with split thickness skin grafts from adjacent areas. *Plast Reconstr Surg* **25**: 455–64.

Edlich RF, Rodeheaver GT, Morgan RF, *et al.* (1988) Principles of emergency wound management. *Ann Emerg Med* **17**: 1284.

Edlich RF, Rodeheaver GT, Thacker JG. (1982) Technical factors in the prevention of infections. In: Simmons RL,

Howard RJ, editors. *Surgical infectious diseases*. New York: Appleton-Century-Crofts, 449–72.

Edlich RF, Rogers W, Kasper G, *et al.* (1969) Studies in the management of the contaminated wound: I. Optimal time for closure of contaminated open wounds: II. Comparison of the resistance to infection of open and closed wounds during healing. *Am J Surg* **117**: 323–29.

Edlich RF, Smith QT, Edgerton MT. (1973) Resistance of the surgical wound to antimicrobial prophylaxis and its mechanisms of development. *Am J Surg* **126**: 583–91.

Fries R. (1973) Advantages of a basic concept in lip reconstruction after tumor resection. *J Maxillofac Surg* **1**: 13–18.

George RM, Singer R. (1993) The lines and grooves of the face: a suggested nomenclature. *Plast Reconstr Surg* **92**: 540–42.

Hell EA, Cruickshank CND. (1963) The effect of injury on the uptake of H^3-thymidine by guinea pig epidermis. *Exp Cell Res* **31**: 128–39.

Hussain K, Wijetunge DB, Grubnic S, *et al.* (1994) A comprehensive analysis of craniofacial trauma. *J Trauma* **36**: 34–37.

Kocher T. (1907) *Circurgishe Operationslehr.* Jena, Germany: G. Fisher.

Kraissl CJ. (1951) Selection of appropriate lines for elective surgical incisions. *Plast Reconstr Surg* **8**: 1–8.

Langer K. (1978) On the anatomy and physiology of the skin: I. The cleavability of the cutis. *Br J Plast Surg* **31**: 3–8.

Levenson SM, Geever EF, Crowley LV, *et al.* (1965) The healing of rat skin wounds. *Ann Surg* **161**: 293–308.

Madden JW, Smith HC. (1970) The rate of collagen synthesis and deposition in dehisced and resutured wounds. *Surg Gynecol Obstet* **130**: 487–93.

Ordman LJ, Gillman T. (1966) Studies in the healing of cutaneous wounds: III. A critical comparison in the pig of the healing of surgical incisions closed with sutures or adhesive tape based on tensile strength and clinical and histological criteria. *Arch Surg* **93**: 911–28.

Schauerhamer RA, Edlich RF, Panek P, *et al.* (1971) Studies in the management of the contaminated wound: VII. Susceptibility of surgical wounds to postoperative surface contamination. *Am J Surg* **122**: 74–77.

Schultz RC, editor. (1988) Medicolegal sequelae. In: *Facial injuries*, 3rd edition. Chicago: Year Book, 657–68.

Stevenson TR, Rodeheaver GT, Golden GT, *et al.* (1975) Damage to tissue defenses by vasoconstrictors. *J Am Coll Emerg Physicians* **4**: 532–35.

Sturdivan LM, Sacco WJ, Edgerton MT, *et al.* (1984) Firearm injuries: medicolegal considerations. In: Wolcott BW, Rund DA, editors. *Emergency medicine annual*. Norwalk, CT: Appleton-Century- Crofts, 125–68.

Tardy ME, Thomas JR, Przekop H. (1980) Uniform photographic documentation in facial plastic surgery. *Otolaryngol Clin North Am* **13**: 367–81.

Thacker JG, Iachetta FA, Allaire PE, *et al.* (1975) Biomechanical properties – their influence on planning surgical excisions. In: Krizek TJ, Hoopes PE, editors. *Symposium on basic science in plastic surgery*, vol. 15. St Louis, O: Mosby, 72–79.

Van Winkle W, Hastings JC, Barker E, *et al.* (1975) Effect of suture materials on healing skin wounds. *Surg Gynecol Obstet* **140**: 7–12.

Webster JP. (1960) Crescentic peri-alar cheek excision for upper lip advancement with a short history of upper lip repair. *Plast Reconstr Surg* **25**: 434–64.

Wray CR. (1983) Force required for wound closure and scar appearance. *Plast Reconstr Surg* **72**: 380–82.

Zisser G. (1975) A contribution to the primary reconstruction of the upper lip and labial commissure following tumour excision. *J Maxillofac Surg* **3**: 211–17.

Section V

Spinal trauma

34

Spinal cord trauma

B P Gardner, P Teddy

Introduction

The medical expert's report is pivotal in the settlement of claims for compensation following spinal cord injury. The court is unlikely to approve an item claimed without implicit or explicit medical support. The initial medical report must be comprehensive and thorough. The purpose of this chapter is to help the medical expert to construct a report that incorporates all the relevant aspects so that the rest of the legal team of experts can be set on the right path from the outset (Bedbrook, 1981; Grundey and Swain, 1993; Guttman, 1976; Hardy and Elson, 1976; Illis, 1988, 1992, 1993; Vinken *et al.*, 1992). Nursing, physiotherapy, occupational therapy, psychology, housing, employment and special equipment needs should be identified and quantified by appropriate experts who have to hand the initial medical report. A case conference will clarify any uncertainties before the schedule of expenses is prepared.

Cases prepared in this way result in the minimum of legal expense because an appropriate and cohesive case is prepared with the minimum of correspondence. The plaintiff's compensation comes at the earliest possible time after the prognosis has become clear. This enables the person to restart his or her life at the earliest opportunity. There is no place for the excessive delays that still occur today in the settlement of claims.

Definitions

A spinal cord injury is complete if there is no somatic motor or sensory function below the level of the injury. If the arms are spared, the patient has paraplegia, or tetraplegia if they are involved (Bedbrook, 1981; Grundy and Swain, 1993). The level of injury is the lowest intact spinal cord segment (Bedbrook, 1981). If there is residual function several segments below this then the injury is incomplete and the patient has either paraparesis or tetraparesis. The use of the terms quadriplegia and quadriparesis should be avoided.

Epidemiology

The incidence of traumatic spinal cord injury varies in different countries and series between 10 and 50 per million population each year (Bedbrook, 1981; Grundy and Swain, 1993; Guttman, 1976; Hardy and Elson, 1976; Illis, 1988, 1992, 1993; Smart and Sanders, 1976; Stover and Fine, 1986, 1987; Vinken *et al.*, 1992). The figure in the UK is towards the lower end of this range. Only a minority result in legal claims because negligence with causation by another party usually cannot be established. Nontraumatic cases seldom give rise to legal claims.

Clinical assessment

Liability: negligence and causation

Medical experts are seldom involved in these issues. Occasionally they are required to advise regarding the extent to which different negligent incidents have caused the consequent disability, for example, in multiple vehicle accidents or where there was inappropriate handling at the scene of injury.

Victims may have contributed to their injury, for example, by not wearing a seat belt. In the latter a 25% reduction is usually applied but there is room for medical argument based on the nature of the injuries sustained and the pattern of the accident. An understanding of the mechanism of spine and spinal cord injury is important.

Medical negligence is the major area where expert advice is crucial. There is considerable variation in opinion regarding the correct management of spinal cord trauma. Provided that the particular treatment selected is reasonable and is carried out competently and with an acceptable degree of care then negligence will not be proven.

Missed fractures are an important area of medical negligence (Ravichandran and Silver, 1982). Common sites include the cervicodorsal junction and spinal fractures below the major spinal fracture site. Simple basic principles are sometimes overlooked. Accurate radiological evaluation may not be possible immediately after the accident. If there are reasonable grounds for believing that the patient has sustained an unstable spinal injury, then appropriate steps must be taken to immobilize the spine until such time as the diagnosis can be confirmed or refuted.

Causation is often a major uncertainty. Negligent treatment of a patient with an established complete spinal cord injury results in much less harm than in a person whose injury is incomplete.

Complications such as pressure sores can usually be avoided with good care.

Quantum

To assist lawyers and experts to understand the relevant medical issues it is advisable to divide the consequences of spinal cord injury into categories. In each of the latter, acute and chronic aspects should be considered.

Associated injuries

These play an important part in the quantum consequences of spinal cord damage. Amongst the more important are the following:

Brain

Successful rehabilitation following spinal cord injury is dependent on the total involvement of the disabled person. Impairment of personality, memory, concentration and intellect can profoundly alter outcome. Good executive function is of particular importance in enabling the spinal cord-injured person to lead a safe and well integrated life. Relatively minor degrees of higher cerebral impairment can interact with the other problems associated with spinal cord injury, making employment much more difficult.

Limb joints and bones

Spinal cord-damaged persons are more dependent on their arms than they were prior to the injury. Joint damage, and to a lesser extent long bone fractures, can severely impair transfers and wheelchair skills. Contractures are frequently very disabling. Because the arm joints, especially the shoulders, are put under stress by the routine activities of wheelchair life, problems commence in them at an earlier age. The onset is accelerated by damage sustained at the time of injury.

Peripheral nerve injuries, especially brachial plexus

Peripheral nerve and brachial plexus injuries occasionally occur in association with the spinal cord injury. Paraplegics require both arms for most activities. The affected arm cannot cope so well with transfers and wheelchair control. The functional impact can be reduced by trick movements that can take years to develop.

Chest and abdominal

Chest and abdominal injuries, although life threatening at the time of the original event, are seldom important in quantum terms as they do not often result in an increased requirement for care or equipment.

Neurology

The level, degree of completeness and pattern of the spinal cord injury are of central importance in determining outcome and prognosis (Bedbrook, 1981; Grundy and Swain, 1993; Guttman, 1976; Hardy and Elson, 1976; Illis, 1988, 1992, 1993; Vinken *et al.*, 1992; Volle *et al.*, 1992). There is no level of neurological disability, including ventilator dependency, that is incompatible with life in the community (Carter, 1979; Whiteneck *et al.*, 1989).

Incomplete injuries are associated with a longer expectation of life. Preserved sensation enables the paralysed person to become aware of complications as they arise below the level of injury. Complete spinal cord-injured persons also learn to recognize signals coming from the paralysed and denervated parts of the body, but these are less precise. It is not just pressure sores but also other complications such as intra-abdominal events and long bone fractures that are recognized in this way. When there is useful motor, as well as sensory, function below the level of injury then life expectation is further improved.

Every neurological level in the cervical region is of vital importance.

Patients with complete lesions at C3 and above usually require a greater or lesser degree of ventilatory support, such as intermittent positive pressure ventilation and phrenic nerve pacing (Carter, 1979; Whiteneck *et al.*, 1989). Less widely used techniques include intercosto-phrenic nerve anastomosis and artificial ventilation by mouth.

C4 level patients can almost always breathe independently but are otherwise almost totally dependent. Electric wheelchair mobility and control of the environment via the Possum and other systems is achievable using retained head and neck control.

C5 level patients have good shoulder control as well as elbow flexion. With aids, such as feeding straps, limited function is possible. Assistance is required with every activity.

C6 level patients have good wrist dorsiflexion. Elbow extension is achieved by means of trick movements. By locking the elbow, transfers are sometimes possible. Wrist dorsiflexion is associated with passive tenodesis of the fingers and the thumb. Upper limb reconstructive procedures can be of great benefit at this level of injury. Active elbow extension can be achieved by the Moberg posterior deltoid to triceps transfer procedure. A stronger and more active key grip can be achieved by tendon transfers around the wrist, such as insertion of the extensor carpi radialis longus into flexor digitorum profundus and the brachioradialis into flexor pollucis longus. These procedures do not usually increase transfer capability but they do improve upper limb control and so lead to an improved quality of life (Ainsley *et al.*, 1985; Moberg, 1978). When these upper limb reconstructive procedures are carried out, the upper limb is immobilized for six weeks in plaster for elbow reconstruction and three weeks for wrist procedures. An electric wheelchair and increased care are required temporarily.

C7 and C8 level patients lack fine intrinsic hand muscle control but have sufficient upper limb function to achieve a degree of independence in transfers and activities of daily living.

Upper thoracic, T2–T6, level patients lack the abdominal and lower paraspinal muscle control that is essential to achieve good truncal balance. Backwheel balance control and transfers are impaired as a result. Spontaneous spasms are likely to cause problems in transfers. Ambulation in long leg calipers is difficult. Braces that stabilize the upper body, such as the reciprocating and hip guidance orthoses, are usually required if ambulation is to be achieved.

Lower thoracic, T7–T12, patients have greater abdominal and paraspinal muscle control and hence better truncal balance. Higher kerbs can be negotiated because better backwheel balance is achieved.

L1 level patients frequently achieve ambulation, although this is seldom of functional benefit. The good quadriceps control of midlumbar levels usually allows functional ambulation in younger patients.

Longer term neurological consequences

In recent years it has become clear that the incidence of tertiary spinal cord change is much more common than had previously been recognized. These changes continue to develop throughout the life of the spinal cord-injured person. The most important is the spinal cord syrinx. In a recent study at Stoke Mandeville Hospital of 153 patients whose spinal cord injury occurred more than 20 years ago, the overall incidence of syrinx formation was 20%. The longer the patient has been injured the more likely the development of a syrinx becomes.

The previously quoted incidence of syrinx formation of 2% and 4% was largely based on clinically diagnosis. It is now clear that the incidence of syrinx is much greater than this because the majority do not have diagnostic clinical features.

The aetiology and management of syrinx remains controversial (Birbhamer *et al.*, 1993; Cho *et al.*, 1994; Honan and Williams, 1993; Squier and Lehr, 1994) and is discussed in Chapter 36. Surgery is not usually required; continued review is essential. If a person has a spinal cord syrinx it is necessary to alter the lifestyle to avoid those abrupt stresses, strains and other events that could cause serious spinal cord deterioration. Falling out of a wheelchair, for example, can be associated with the loss of use of a hand or an arm.

A patient with a spinal cord syrinx needs a greater degree of care assistance at an earlier stage because of the need to avoid the risks associated with deterioration, such as falls during transfers.

Spine

Following the acute event, spinal problems are not usually a major difficulty (Bedbrook, 1981; Grundy and Swain, 1993; Guttman, 1976; Hardy and Elson, 1976). Arthritis may occur at an earlier stage in the intact spinal joints above and below the injured segment. This can give rise to increased spinal pain and stiffness in later years. This contributes to the greater dependence that occurs with ageing. Deformities such as gibbus are seldom functionally important.

Long spinal fixation can be very disabling. A young person with paraplegia and a long fixation is usually totally independent in the younger years but, when older, the loss of truncal mobility cannot be so readily compensated for by increased movement in the hips. This brings forward the stage at which that person's dependence increases. Long fixations in the cervical region prevent tetraplegic patients from looking around themselves, making driving a car more difficult.

Around 10% of spinal-injured patients have fractures at multiple levels. Those below the level of the main fracture are important if they cause neurological damage or scoliosis.

Progressive skeletal deformity is a particular problem in children. Regular careful review of their spinal position is required until skeletal maturity. Whereas gibbus does not significantly increase disability, scoliosis can be a particular problem. Sitting posture, the pattern of pressure on the ischial areas, and transfers are impaired.

Pain

Musculoskeletal and neurogenic pains are common following spinal cord injury. They can be intractably disabling. Treatment is frequently difficult (Balazy, 1992; Burnham *et al.*, 1993; Fenollosa *et al.*, 1993; Mariano, 1992; Richards, 1992; Sie *et al.*, 1992; Summers *et al.*, 1991; Umlauf, 1992). Sometimes the pain makes it necessary for patients to shift from one position to another or to lie down at intervals during the day. Employment can be difficult for this reason and also because of the effect on concentration of the pain itself and of associated medication. A careful description of the manner in which the pain affects the patient is essential.

Urinary tract

Lower urinary tract

Bladder sensation and control are impaired. The precise pattern of bladder management varies with the individual (Barnes *et al.*, 1993; Bickel *et al.*, 1991; Brindley, 1993a,b, 1995; Brindley *et al.*, 1986; Chancellor *et al.*, 1993a,b; Chao *et al.*, 1993a,b; Decter and Bauer, 1993; Fanciullacci *et al.*, 1988; Gardner *et al.*, 1984, 1985a, 1986a; Gerridzen *et al.*, 1992; Hollander and Diokno, 1993; Jackson and DeVivo, 1992; Levy and Resnick, 1993; Lindan *et al.*, 1987; Madersbacher and Oberwalder, 1987; Menon and Tan, 1992; Parsons and Fitzpatrick, 1991; Perkash *et al.*, 1992; Sauerwein *et al.*, 1990; Schwartz *et al.*, 1994; Stover *et al.*, 1989; Timoney and Shaw, 1990; Trop and Bennett, 1992; Van-Kerrebroeck *et al.*, 1993; Wyndaele, 1987, 1992; Yadav *et al.*, 1993).

All methods of bladder care are associated with events that can be distressing and inconvenient. With intermittent self-catheterization, there is incontinence. Toilets are frequently inaccessible. With automatic drainage, the urinary sheath occasionally comes off, causing the patient to become soaked (Perkash *et al.*, 1992). Minor penile problems prevent application of the sheath, forcing the patient to remain in bed or to insert an indwelling catheter.

When partial control remains, there is often a degree of urgency and frequency that seriously impairs the male patient's quality of life, for example by forcing him to plan his journey according to the location of accessible toilets.

Bladder management for females is particularly difficult (Jackson and DeVivo, 1992; Lindan *et al.*, 1987; Timoney and Shaw, 1990; Trop and Bennett, 1992). There are no satisfactory external collecting appliances. The risk of incontinence and the awareness that there may be a smell of urine impairs self-confidence and femininity.

A variety of urological procedures exist that benefit certain groups of patients. The more commonly used include augmentation cystoplasty, distal urethral sphincterotomy, the artificial urinary sphincter and the Brindley sacral anterior root stimulator (Brindley, 1993a,b, 1995; Brindley *et al.*, 1986; Chancellor *et al.*, 1993a,b; Hollander and Diokno, 1993; Sauerwein *et al.*, 1990; Schwartz *et al.*, 1994). The latter is of particular benefit in females.

Many patients elect to have an indwelling suprapubic or urethral catheter. Although this is associated with an increased risk to life because of the inevitable infection, the quality of life is often improved. Indwelling bladder catheter-associated problems include bladder stones, intravesical bladder changes, urethral discharges and the problems associated with catheter blockage, especially autonomic dysreflexia (Chao *et al.*, 1993b; Trop and Bennett, 1992).

Upper urinary tract

Continued vigilance of the upper urinary tract is required throughout the life of the paralysed person (Gardner *et al.*, 1984, 1985a, 1986a; Gerridzen *et al.*, 1992; Parsons and Fitzpatrick, 1991). Asymptomatic problems such as calculi and dilatation can occur. The pattern of review that is required varies with the individual. An annual evaluation will usually suffice to ensure early diagnosis and treatment before problems arise. Improved urological techniques, such as percutaneous and whole body lithotripsy, have reduced the morbidity of upper tract stones (Gardner *et al.*, 1985a).

Bowels

Upper gastrointestinal problems are seldom significant. Faecal evacuation is usually a major problem. Most patients require suppositories or digital stimulation. Some require aperients. A disciplined pattern of bowel control is essential. Episodes of incontinence occur and can be very distressing. They are minimized by attention to discipline and the avoidance of precipitating factors such as hot curries and similar foods.

Most paraplegics are able to manage their bowels by transferring on to the toilet, followed by suppository insertion or digital evacuation. The rectum needs to be checked after bowel emptying to ensure that no faeces remain.

Most tetraplegics need a greater or lesser degree of assistance. Bowel evacuation whilst seated on a shower chair over the toilet and followed by a shower at the end of evacuation is a commonly adopted pattern. After the shower the patient is dried. The top half is then dressed whilst still sitting on the shower chair, and the bottom half after transfer on to the bed.

Bowel problems are common in chronic spinal cord injury (Banwell *et al.*, 1993; Binnie *et al.*, 1988, 1991; Carone *et al.*, 1993; MacDonagh *et al.*, 1990; Stone *et al.*, 1990; Varma *et al.*, 1986). Faecal evacuation can take a progressively longer time. Aperients become less effective. If it takes several hours to evacuate the bowel, then employment is difficult to maintain.

Joints

The wear and tear on upper limb joints is increased. As paraplegic patients become older, episodes of upper limb joint pain and stiffness occur with increasing frequency. Extra help is needed at these times.

Heterotopic ossification can occur in the early stage following injury (Banovac *et al.*, 1993; Colachis and Clinchot, 1993; Colachis *et al.*, 1993; Daud *et al.*, 1993). Hip mobility can be severely impaired. Transfers and activities of daily living become more difficult. The ossification process eventually becomes quiescent. Surgery is rarely required; it should only be undertaken after ascertaining that there is no residual bony activity. There is a small place for radiotherapy immediately following excision.

Contractures interfere with independent living, effective mobility and transfers. They give rise to pain and disability. In tetraplegia, contractures of the shoulders, elbows and wrists are a particular problem. In paraplegia, lower limb contractures frequently prevent ambulation and interfere with transfers.

Spasms

Spasms and spasticity are the usual accompaniments of spinal cord injury. They are sometimes helpful but more usually a hindrance. They cause embarrassment when out of doors. They can be dangerous if they occur abruptly during a transfer or when driving. The sleep of both the paralysed person and the partner is disturbed. They throw the legs out of position in bed.

The treatment of spasms includes eradication of any precipitating cause (particularly intravesical- and bowel-related), good physiotherapy (including standing), systemic drugs such as baclofen, dantrolene and diazepam, and, in rare circumstances, operative intervention such as the insertion of an intrathecal baclofen infusion system (Bohannon, 1993; Eltorai and Montroy, 1990; Ochs *et al.*, 1989; Sindou *et al.*, 1991; Teddy *et al.*, 1992).

The systemic medication for spasticity has adverse effects. Baclofen causes drowsiness and interferes with concentration. This has implications for employment. The intrathecal drug delivery systems have potential complications that can be serious (Teddy *et al.*, 1992). Tubing dislodgement and kinking occurs, necessitating revision. Pump replacement is sometimes necessary, in particular with the battery-driven types.

Respiratory

Permanent ventilator-dependent patients can live safely in the community provided that they have sufficient care (Carter, 1979, 1993; Lee *et al.*, 1989; Whiteneck *et al.*, 1989). A trained carer must be at hand at all times. Alarms to summon help immediately are required. With a portable ventilator, supplemented where appropriate by a phrenic pacemaker and other systems, free movement out of doors, including aircraft travel, can readily be achieved.

Mid and low cervical-injured patients have good diaphragmatic control but no intercostal or abdominal muscle function. Their cough is weak and may need to be assisted (Derrickson *et al.*, 1992; Jaeger *et al.*, 1993). Physiotherapy may be required during chest infections. Respiratory functional impairment is the most important increased risk to life in tetraplegic patients. Carers need to be carefully instructed in the relief of choking, the assisted cough, postural drainage of the chest and clearance of secretions (Arnold *et al.*, 1992; Clough *et al.*, 1986; Gardner *et al.*, 1985b, 1986b; Goldman *et al.*, 1986; Pentland, 1993). Midthoracic-injured paraplegic patients lack a good cough because their abdominal muscle control is absent. They require help with chest infections in their older years.

Cardiovascular

Postural hypotension in the seated position is a common problem in the early stage following spinal cord injury. It is seldom disabling thereafter, although tetraplegic patients may require occasional assistance with being tilted back when hypotension occurs (Engelke *et al.*, 1994; Groomes and Huang, 1991).

The blood pressure in tetraplegics is usually reduced. This is protective in life expectancy terms (Cardus *et al.*, 1992; Krum *et al.*, 1992).

Autonomic dysreflexia is a serious potential problem in all patients with injuries at T6 level and above (Braddom and Rocco, 1991; Mathias, 1991; Mathias *et al.*, 1983). It can be precipitated by any stimulus arising below the level of injury, most commonly from the bladder and the bowels. Some events, such as rectal electrostimulated semen emission and vibrator-induced ejaculation, are particularly virulent stimuli.

During autonomic dysreflexic episodes, the arterial blood pressure can rise to dangerously high levels; cardiac dysrhythmias can occur. Patients describe that their heads are bursting open with pain. The sweating may be so profuse that a change of clothes or bedding is necessary.

Because those with tetraplegia cannot deal with the factors that precipitate autonomic dysreflexia, care support needs to be available to ensure that, should such an attack occur, it is dealt with promptly and safely.

In spite of immobility and leg dependency, deep venous thromboses and pulmonary emboli are uncommon, except in the early stage following spinal cord injury. Anticoagulation is rarely required following the acute stage (Green *et al.*, 1992; Weingarden, 1992).

Peripheral oedema and superficial skin changes are common. Careful attention must to be paid to the feet so that cellulitis and other complications are avoided. Chiropody is sometimes helpful.'

Skin

Immobility and loss of sensation contribute to the risk of pressure sores (Bar, 1991; Dover *et al.*, 1992; Ferguson-Pell *et al.*, 1980; Fuhrer *et al.*, 1993a; Gilsdorf *et al.*, 1990; Henderson *et al.*, 1994; Hobson, 1992; Hobson and Tooms, 1992; Odderson *et al.*, 1991; Richardson and Meyer, 1982; Rochon *et al.*, 1993; Rodriguez and Garber, 1994; Rogers, 1978; Shields and Cook, 1992; Sprigle *et al.*, 1990; Swarts *et al.*, 1988; Vidal and Sarrias, 1991). Careful discipline and good care will largely prevent their development. The insensitive skin must be inspected both morning and evening. The minor red marks and skin abrasions that occur during transfers are best treated by rest in bed until the skin has returned to normal. This can interfere with employment as well as the quality of life. When these people are confined to bed in this way, extra care is required.

With ageing, the skin and its underlying tissues become less resilient and the risk of pressure sores increases. Patients may go for many years without a pressure sore and then develop one that is serious.

During the acute stage following injury, turning in bed is necessary two hourly. In the later stages, such frequent turning is rarely required. Prone lying is an excellent way of maintaining the hips, minimizing spasticity and preventing pressure sores. Paraplegic patients are usually able to turn in bed independently in their younger years. They require increasing help as they get older. Various aids such as monkey poles are helpful. Those with tetraplegia usually require assistance from one or more persons. The required time gap between turns in bed at night depends on the individual. It decreases with ageing. Whether one or two persons are required for turns depends on the patient. In Europe, including the UK, European regulations must be applied. These frequently mean that two people are required for activities, turns or transfers, when, prior to the EEC rulings, one person sufficed.

The selection of an appropriate bed is important. This will change during the lifetime of the person concerned. Variable height beds help carers by making transfers easier. Hoists are required for very disabled patients. The ability to elevate the head of the bed is useful. Rotating beds are seldom popular. Most patients prefer double beds with double mattresses that they can share with partners. Beds that appear normal are preferred to beds which, although functional, retain a hospital ambience. An appropriate mattress will increase the time gap between turns and hence reduce the burden on the carers. Many different types are available. Some permit the patient to remain in one position for long periods. Unfortunately, these can also make turns more difficult.

Many different types of cushions are available. One appropriate for the individual must be selected. A spare cushion should always be to hand in case the main one is damaged. In the prevention of pressure sores, it is not just the cushion and its characteristics that are important but the whole posture and seating status of the person (Gilsdorf *et al.*, 1990; Henderson *et al.*, 1994; Hobson, 1992; Odderson *et al.*, 1991; Sprigle *et al.*, 1990). The Jay Back may also be required to correct posture.

The Jay Protector enables patients to go up and down steps on their bottoms and to travel more safely in vehicles when other methods for buttock support are not available.

Sexual function

Sexuality is severely impaired following spinal cord injury. A spinal cord-injured man sometimes feels incomplete because not only is normal sexual intercourse impossible but also because he cannot be a full husband, father and breadwinner, or be involved in masculine activities (Alexander, 1991; Alexander *et al.*, 1993; Schuler, 1982). Although many approaches are available to achieve an erection, including implants, intracavernosal injections and external aids, the spontaneity, sensation and orgasm of normal intercourse are lost (Bodner *et al.*, 1987, 1992; Heller *et al.*, 1992; Kimoto and Iwatsubo, 1994).

Fertility in these men is severely impaired (Blockmans and Steeno, 1988; Brindley, 1986; Brindley *et al.*, 1989; Francois and Maury, 1987; Seager and Halstead, 1993). Obtaining semen is the first problem. Methods for achieving this include the penile vibrator, rectal electrostimulated semen emission, vas cannulation, microepididymal sperm aspiration and the hypogastric plexus stimulator. The second and more important problem is oligoasthenospermia. It is usually necessary for the services of a fertility centre to be used if parenthood is to be achieved. These include preparation of the semen followed by various treatments of the female partner to increase her fertility (Elliot *et al.*, 1991; Leeton *et al.*, 1991; Macourt *et al.*, 1991). Women can lose their self-respect. Wearing attractive clothes such as skirts is limited by the leg-bag and the wheelchair. Urinary incontinence produces the sense of always being surrounded by a smell of urine (Charlifue *et al.*, 1992; Sipski, 1991).

Female intercourse is possible but passive. Orgasm does not occur except in women with lower levels of injury. Fertility is usually unimpaired (Baker *et al.*, 1992; Berard, 1989; Creighton, 1989; Cross *et al.*, 1922; Hughes *et al.*, 1991; Letcher and Goldfine, 1986; Sipski and Alexander, 1993; Verduyn, 1986; Wanner *et al.*, 1987; Young, 1994).

Both male and female spinal cord-injured persons are unable to be parents in the full sense. They cannot take their children out to the park or play with them as previously. Relationships and marriages are under greater stress following spinal cord injury (Crewe and Krause, 1988, 1992; Kreuter *et al.*, 1994; Peters *et al.*, 1992; Urey and Henggeler, 1987). For those who are not married at the time of injury, the prospects are reduced for developing a firm, lasting relationship. This is particularly the case for young women.

Mobility

The wheelchair must be carefully selected. A spare is always required. Different wheelchairs are necessary for different purposes. For example, a sports wheelchair, a lightweight wheelchair and an electric wheelchair for outdoor use may all be required by the same person for use at different times. The pattern of wheelchair requirement varies with the individual. It also changes with age. A young tetraplegic patient can cope with a lightweight wheelchair indoors on level surfaces and up shallow steps. In the older years, an electric wheelchair is required indoors instead. The range and type of wheelchairs that are available is enormous and constantly changing. Before the appropriate wheelchair for an individual can be selected it should both be seen and evaluated in a practical setting. The most sophisticated wheelchairs, such as the Permobil, allow control of the environment using the infrared signalling system that is built into this wheelchair. These chairs can also accommodate portable ventilators. They also offer a stand-up or a reclining facility.

The wheelchair must be integrated with an appropriate car for satisfactory mobility out of doors. Either the patient must be able to get the wheelchair in and out of the car or get into the vehicle whilst still seated in the wheelchair. The selection of the appropriate vehicle and its controls sometimes requires assessment in a specialized centre. The individual characteristics of the patient must be considered. Tall people have a restricted range of vehicle that they can use whilst seated in an electric wheelchair. One adjunct that assists transfers in and out of the car is the swivel seat. Car mileage is usually increased. Car telephones are important; if the car breaks down then the paraplegic person cannot easily get to a local telephone. The car must be well-maintained as the paralysed person is so dependent on it. Many spinal cord-injured persons have not passed their driving test. It is mandatory that they do so. In general, those who are tetraplegic at the level of C5 and below are able to drive; those at C5 usually require joy-stick control. Some who are tetraplegic at C6 and those at C7 and below can usually cope with vehicles with hand controls, automatic transmission, servo assisted brakes and power-assisted steering.

Ambulation is seldom a functional form of mobility for those with paraplegia or tetraplegia. It does convey dignity and is a form of exercise; it is helpful for these reasons. For persons with poor truncal balance, such as those with low tetraplegia and higher thoracic paraplegia, the reciprocating or hip guidance orthoses, which provide truncal support, are necessary. With lower levels of thoracic and upper lumbar injury, the knee-ankle-foot orthoses suffice. Those with good quadriceps control usually cope with ankle-foot orthoses alone (Bajd *et al.*, 1989; Barbenel and Paul, 1992; Granat *et al.*, 1993; Jaeger *et al.*, 1989). The majority of spinal cord-injured patients cease to use their walking devices even though they have successfully learned to ambulate in them. Few regret having mastered the technique.

Public transport, such as overground and underground trains, and buses are difficult or impossible. Air travel is usually feasible. There are a number of recreational mobility devices, such as the three-wheeler bicycle and the motorized quadbike, which some individuals need. Children can be placed at the back of the three-wheeler bicycle. Men involved in country pursuits need the quadbike for mobility over rough ground. A portable ramp is useful when visiting friends or other places where ramped access is not available.

Transfers

This refers to the way in which a paralysed person moves from one position to another. Nearly all paraplegic persons become independent in level transfers. Most achieve the more difficult ones, such as from the easy chair into the wheelchair, and out of the bath. The most difficult transfers, such as getting from the floor into the wheelchair, and from the floor into the upright position having fallen in calipers, are achieved by only the most able. There is great individual variation between paraplegic people in their capability with transfers. The factors associated with reduced ability include increasing age, poor truncal balance, spasticity, spasms, obesity, and upper limb problems such as muscle strains, nerve injury and joint contractures. Those with a low arm to trunk length ratio, for example in achondroplasia, seldom achieve transfers. A few with low-level tetraplegia become totally independent in transfers, usually with the aid of a sliding board, but most require help.

The minimum pattern of help required by each individual is best determined following a course of rehabilitation in a spinal cord injury unit (Bromley, 1991; Cull and Hardy, 1977; Curtis, 1985; Ford and Duckworth, 1987; Nixon, 1985; Yarkony *et al.*, 1992a,b). Hoists are important aids. Portable hoists are versatile, but ceiling mounted hoists take up less room. Strengthening of the ceiling is required with the latter; EEC regulations apply.

Activities of daily living

This refers to the normal activities of daily life that the able bodied take for granted (Bates *et al.*, 1993; Curtin, 1994; Frieden and Cole, 1985; Garber, 1985; Hurlburt and Ottenbacher, 1992; Noreau *et al.*, 1993; Sargant and Braun, 1986). The simplest way of determining how each spinal cord-injured person deals with normal daily life is to take them through a typical day and find out how they cope with each different aspect. In general, those with paraplegia are independent, whilst those with tetraplegia are partially dependent, usually in lower half activities such as washing, dressing and personal hygiene. Obesity, poor truncal balance, increasing age, upper limb musculoskeletal problems, spasms, spasticity and short arms all reduce activities of daily living ability (Flett, 1992; Krajnik and Bridle, 1992; Marino *et al.*, 1993; Seeger *et al.*, 1989).

Higher level tetraplegics benefit substantially from environmental control systems (Anson, 1991; Efthimiou *et al.*, 1981; Gardner *et al.*, 1985c; McDonald *et al.*, 1989; Woods and Jones, 1990). Provided the person can control voluntarily, in an accurate and predictable manner, a single muscle, then that person can control his or her environment, such as opening and closing curtains and using the telephone. An expert is required to advise each individual regarding which system is most appropriate. The optimum application is best determined at a home visit. A system should usually be in the bedroom, the living room and the study.

Most paraplegic and tetraplegic persons benefit from a remote control door opener. If a person with paraplegia is sitting in an easy chair and someone calls at the house, there is not time to transfer into a wheelchair to go and open the door.

Paraplegic people are usually able to manage the shower seat. Those with higher levels of paraplegia and low tetraplegia find the shower chair system most helpful, as described above. Most of those with paraplegia can manage a normal bath whilst they are young. This becomes more difficult with ageing; a bath board may then help. Eventually, a specialized bath may be required to relieve the carer.

Psychology

The effects of sudden paralysis, potential double incontinence, impotence, infertility, loss of relationships and all the other manifestations of spinal cord damage, insinuate into every facet of the person's life. The impact can be devastating. In spite of this, depression is not a major consequence of spinal cord injury. Most paraplegic and tetraplegic persons who have been through a spinal cord injury unit have learned to minimize the effects of their disabilities. They seldom concentrate on what they cannot do. It takes careful questioning to elicit the various ways in which the quality of their lives has been irretrievably altered by their condition. It is essential that such an understanding is achieved if the true impact of their condition is to be understood (Bach and Tilton, 1994; Chase and King, 1990; Clayton and Chubon, 1994; Craig *et al.*, 1994; Curcoll, 1992; Cushman and Hassett, 1992; DeVivo *et al.*, 1991; Elliott *et al.*, 1991; Fuhrer *et al.*, 1992; Fuhrer *et al.*, 1993b; Fullerton *et al.*, 1981; Geller and Greydanus, 1979; Gerhart *et al.*, 1992; Glass, 1992; Hammell, 1992; Judd and Brown, 1992a,b; Kennedy and Marsh, 1993; Krause, 1992a; Perez and Pilsecker, 1994; Richards, 1982; Richards *et al.*, 1991; Stambrook *et al.*, 1991; Stewart and Rossier, 1978; Tate *et al.*, 1994a,b; Trieschmann, 1992; Zager and Marquette, 1981).

The risk of suicide is not much greater in the spinal cord-injured population compared with the able-bodied.

Counselling may be helpful at various stages. It is usually resisted although it is often valuable when eventually accepted.

Family

The enormous impact of paralysis on the family, including parents, siblings, spouses and children, must be considered. Relationships can be destroyed. The old age of parents can be shattered by paralysis in their children. The ability of the spinal cord-injured person to be a true father, wife, husband or mother is severely impaired (Abrams, 1981; Buck and Hohmann, 1981; DeVivo and Richards, 1992; Oliver *et al.*, 1987; Steinglass *et al.*, 1982; Van-Asbeck *et al.*, 1994; Whiteneck *et al.*, 1992a). Careful questioning will elicit the precise manner in which the family has been affected. The adverse effects rebound on the patient who sometimes feels guilty for the suffering caused.

The view that family members should look after their spinal cord-injured relative is no longer widely accepted. It is better for normal relationships to be retained. This will increase the likelihood of preserving the integrity of the family. In particular, a wife should remain a wife, mother and lover, rather than become a nurse and a carer.

Home

The accommodation that a person has at the time of injury is seldom suitable for life in a wheelchair. A housing expert will advise on detail, but the medical specialist needs to point out those housing alterations that are reasonable and necessary as a result of the injury. The precise requirements depend on the person concerned and the pattern of the disability (Adaptations of housing, 1978; Design of housing, 1978; Goldsmith, 1976; How new homes, 1986; Wheelchair housing, 1975).

People with incomplete paraplegia who can ambulate and cope with stairs in their younger years find this increasingly difficult as they grow older. Many eventually become wheelchair dependent. Those with tetraplegia and complete paraplegia are safest in ground floor wheelchair-accessible accommodation from the outset. Amongst the many housing aspects that must be considered are the following:

1. A covered way for the car and between the car and the front door, together with adequate space to get in and out;
2. Appropriate, usually ramped, access to the house;
3. Doorways and corridors of sufficient width to accommodate the wheelchair base and turning circle;
4. Adequate storage space to avoid equipment cluttering up corridors and living space;
5. A bedroom of sufficient size for easy wheelchair mobility and with storage space for catheters, urinary sheaths and other personal equipment;
6. An en-suite toilet and bathroom, because the spinal cord-injured person usually needs to get to and from the bathroom and toilet whilst seated in the wheelchair in a state of undress;
7. Appropriate hoists for intermittent use when unwell in the younger years and regular use when older;
8. A second toilet and bathroom, as spinal cord-injured patients take a considerable time to empty their bowels;

9. Carer accommodation, for those with tetraplegia, and paraplegia in the last years of their lives; the regular recruitment of satisfactory carers cannot be overemphasised; their accommodation must be comfortable and attractive to help to ensure this;
10. Paraplegic and tetraplegic persons are less able to maintain their body temperature; in tetraplegia, temperature control is further compromised by altered sympathetic nervous control and central heating is advised in all cases; because tetraplegics can become overheated in hot weather, at least one room in the house should have air conditioning;
11. Spinal cord-injured persons are more vulnerable to the destructive elements in society; household alarms are recommended;
12. Wear and tear on carpets and skirting boards is increased by the wheelchair.

Recreation

A careful history should be taken to determine the recreational activities enjoyed before the injury and those that are now possible (Guttman, 1976b; Yerxa and Locker, 1990). A home computer system is often helpful. Those with high tetraplegia benefit from page turners. Although some with paraplegia and tetraplegia enjoy wheelchair sports the majority are no more interested in sport than the rest of the population. Access to places of public enjoyment such as theatres and cinemas is difficult or impossible.

Because the range of recreational opportunities is limited and employment often precluded, it is essential that regular holidays are taken to maintain morale and family relationships. Holidays are usually more expensive as the cheaper hotels are inaccessible to wheelchairs. Extra help is required on holiday.

A regular visit from an occupational therapist is helpful in bringing the person up to date with modern developments in aids, equipment and recreational activities. Disabled clubs and societies will provide appropriate information.

Employment

The opportunities for employment are greatly reduced following spinal cord injury. Retraining centres exist and the disablement resettlement officer can also advise. Many universities have facilities where spinal cord-injured persons can study, although there is a great divide between obtaining a qualification and achieving employment. In general, the wheelchair dependent are overlooked when there is competition for employment (Athanasou and Murphy, 1993; Crisp, 1992; Fallon, 1979; Golding, 1976; Hammel *et al.*, 1992; Kanellos, 1985; Kantor *et al.*, 1993; Krause, 1992b; Noreau and Shephard, 1992; Taricco *et al.*, 1992; Trieschmann, 1980, 1988). Those who had physical outdoor manual employment prior to injury, in particular those with poor academic backgrounds, are at a great disadvantage and usually remain unemployed. Academically capable patients, and those who succeed in retraining clerically, have better prospects but still face many problems. It takes longer to get up and make ready in the morning. At work, the car must be under cover and with access from it to the workplace. The latter must be wheelchair accessible. Getting from one floor to another and from one building to another is difficult or impossible. There must be facilities to allow for episodes of incontinence. Employers have to accept that complications such as red skin marks and urinary tract infections will result in time off work. Drugs such as baclofen interfere with concentration and mental agility.

Although many paraplegic and some tetraplegic persons achieve some form of employment, compared with the able-bodied, it is more likely to be part- than full-time, be intermittent rather than continuous, and involve early retirement. The employment expert will advise not only regarding the ability of the individual concerned but also the relevant opportunities available in the locality.

Medical care

Following the acute stage after spinal cord injury, complications can arise, such as pressure sores and urinary tract infections. Some can be treated successfully at home. If the patient is confined to bed then a carer should be at hand to assist. When hospitalization is required, this should be prompt and in a spinal unit.

An annual comprehensive review in a spinal cord injury unit is required. This should include upper urinary tract assessment, magnetic resonance imaging and a comprehensive clinical, occupational therapy, physiotherapy and general review.

Ageing

Some of the effects of ageing have been considered above. It is essential that these are taken into account when arriving at a prognosis (Eisenberg and Saltz, 1991; Whiteneck *et al.*, 1992b, 1993). There is no stereotypic pattern for ageing. Some people are intrinsically more able than others. Others have the effects of ageing brought forward by problems such as contractures.

Care attendant needs

Low level paraplegic individuals are usually independent when they are young, apart from needing help with domestic activities, shopping, certain obstacles out of doors, gardening, do-it-yourself work and home maintenance. They usually require stand-by assistance when ambulating in calipers or similar devices.

Those with midlevel paraplegia require additional assistance with getting into and out of the standing frame, out of the bath, in and out of the car, and lifting the wheelchair in and out of the car. Spasticity, spasms, intrinsic ability, obesity, truncal balance and age are all important.

Some with low level tetraplegia are almost independent. The majority require some assistance. For example, they can use a spoon for eating but not cut up meat. They can drive a car but not transfer into it or lift their wheelchair in and out independently. Because tetraplegic persons can suffer from autonomic dysreflexia or choke on food, someone should always at hand to deal with an emergency should the need arise. Notwithstanding this, many live on their own for substantial periods of time. This is a reflection of the inadequacy of resources available in the community, rather than the particular needs of the tetraplegic person.

As mentioned above, in general it is not appropriate for family members to be involved in the physical and personal care of their relations. Nevertheless, they frequently choose to do so and provide extremely good care. The optimum pattern of care for tetraplegic individuals usually involves two full-time carers. Each works for three-and-a-half days a week. They live in an annexe to the main house with their own separate lounge, toilet and bathroom. An overlap is required for those activities requiring two carers.

The pattern and type of physiotherapy required depends on the individual. In general, carers can carry out the straightforward physiotherapy activities of joint ranges of motion and assisting patients into the standing frame. More specialized physiotherapy tasks, such as the assisted cough, often require a chartered physiotherapist.

Expectation of life

The expectation of life of a spinal cord-injured person is reduced. Although some experts state that the expectation of life of those with paraplegia is normal, there is no evidence to support this view (Burke *et al.*, 1960; Burney *et al.*, 1983; Charlifue and Gerhart, 1991; Cox, 1972; Cutler and Ederer, 1958; Daverat *et al.*, 1989; De Vivo and Stover, 1995; DeVivo *et al.*, 1987, 1989, 1992a,b, 1993; Dietrick and Russi, 1958; Draus *et al.*, 1979; Ducharme *et al.*, 1981; Freed *et al.*, 1966; Frisbie and Kache, 1983; Geisler *et al.*, 1977, 1983; Griffin *et al.*, 1985; Hackler, 1977; Hardy, 1976; Kiwerski *et al.*, 1981; Kraus and Crewe, 1987; Kraus and Kjorsvig, 1992; Le and Price, 1982; Mesard *et al.*, 1978; Minaire *et al.*, 1983; Nyquist and Bors, 1967; Ravichandran and Silver, 1982b; Samsa *et al.*, 1993; Sneddon and Bedbrook, 1982; Tribe, 1963; Webb *et al.*, 1984). An assessment of expectation of life is an essential component of any report because it determines the appropriate multiplier for the claim.

The assessment of the life expectancy of any spinal cord-injured person cannot be deduced simply by referral to life expectancy tables, such as those of Geisler *et al.*, (1977) and DeVivo *et al.* (1987, 1992a). These are an important guide but factors relating to the individual must also be carefully considered. In considering life expectancy the following should be taken into account:

1. Date of injury;
2. Age at injury;
3. Present age;
4. Years since injury;
5. Level and completeness of injury;
6. Statistics of life expectancy for the country concerned;
7. Factors relating to the sex, class and environment;
8. Published literature on the subject; most are not based on known deaths but on predicted deaths using standard mortality ratios; for example, a standardized mortality ratio of two implies that the mortality rate of persons with spinal cord injuries in that strata is twice the rate of the general population of comparable age, sex and race; when the ratio is multiplied by 100 a percentage figure is obtained;
9. Family history;
10. History to date in relation to known causes of death in spinal cord-injured patients; the major causes of death in the spinal cord-injured are renal, cardiovascular and respiratory disease;
11. Medication history;
12. Reliability in attending follow-up appointments; asymptomatic complications can be detected early and treated appropriately through such follow-up visits;
13. Pattern of care.

The expectation of life of the spinal cord-injured person continues to improve. Newer techniques that have assisted the diagnosis and treatment of life-threatening complications include magnetic resonance imaging scans for spinal syrinx detection, the Brindley stimulator, newer and more effective antibiotics, percutaneous and whole body lithotripsy devices to shatter kidney and bladder stones without recourse to major surgery, computerized and other drug delivery systems for the

Table 34.1. Headings for a comprehensive report on spinal cord injury care

---

Liability
   Seat belt
   Alcohol
   Medical/other negligence
Quantum
1. Associated injuries
       Brain
       Limb joints/bones
       Peripheral nerves/brachial plexus
       Chest/abdominal
2. Neurology: level, completeness: syrinx
3. Spine: deformities, arthritis
4. Pain
5. Bladder: upper and lower urinary tract
6. Bowels
7. Joints: heterotopic ossification
8. Spasms/spasticity
9. Respiratory
10. Cardiovascular: hypotension, autonomic dysreflexia
11. Skin: turns in bed, mattress, cushion, bed, shower chair, bath
12. Sexual function: fertility, intercourse, sexuality
13. Mobility: wheelchair, car, orthoses, recreational mobility, ramps
14. Transfers: hoists
15. Activities of daily living: environmental control systems
16. Psychology: counselling
17. Family
18. Home
19. Recreation: holidays
20. Employment
21. Medical care: inpatient and outpatient
22. Ageing
23. Care attendant needs
24. Physiotherapy needs
25. Occupational therapy needs
26. Equipment
27. Expectation of life

---

eradication of intractable spasticity, the artificial urinary sphincter and other urological operative advances, and improvements in intensive care and anaesthesia. There was also further development in the spinal cord injury service in the UK during the 1980s when two completely new units were established in Odstock and Stanmore. Recently, the specialty of spinal injuries has been established to enable physicians and surgeons to be trained specifically in this area of medicine.

Conclusion

The preparation of a quantum report for a spinal cord-injured person is critically dependent on a careful understanding of that particular individual including his past history, current situation and future aspirations. Although many experts are involved in the preparation of quantum reports, the medical evidence is of central importance. To ensure that no key areas are omitted, doctors are advised to apply a check similar to that shown in Table 34.1.

References

Abrams KS. (1981) The impact on marriages of adult-onset paraplegia. *Paraplegia* **19**: 253–59.

Adaptations of housing for people who are physically handicapped. (1978) (Circular 59/78.): Department of the Environment.

Ainsley J, Voorhees C Drake E. (1985) Reconstructive hand surgery for quadriplegic persons. *Am J Occup Ther* **39**: 715–21.

Alexander CJ. (1991) Psychological assessment and treatment of sexual dysfunctions following spinal cord injury. *J Am Paraplegia Soc* **14**: 127–31.

Alexander CJ, Sipski ML, Findley TW, *et al.* (1993) Sexual activities, desire, and satisfaction in males pre- and post-spinal cord injury. *Arch Sex Behav* **22**: 217–28.

Anson D. (1991) Using the HeadMaster with Macintosh, Apple II, and MS-DOS computers. *Am J Occup Ther* **45**: 889–97.

Arnold PB, McVey PP, Farrell WJ, *et al.* (1992) Functional electric stimulation: its efficacy and safety in improving pulmonary function and musculoskeletal fitness. *Arch Phys Med Rehabil* **73**: 665–68.

Athanasou JA, Murphy GC. (1993) Employment rates for compensatable spinal injuries in Australia. *Int J Rehabil Res* **16**: 151–56.

Bach JR, Tilton MC. (1994) Life satisfaction and well-being measures in ventilator assisted individuals with traumatic tetraplegia. *Arch Phys Med Rehabil*, **75**: 626–32.

Bajd T, Kralj A, Turk R, *et al.* (1989) Use of functional electrical stimulation in the rehabilitation of patients with incomplete spinal cord injuries. *J Biomed Eng* **11**: 96–102.

Baker ER, Cardenas DD, Benedetti TJ (1992) Risks associated with pregnancy in spinal cord-injured women. *Obstet Gynecol* **80**: 425–28.

Balazy TE. (1992) Clinical management of chronic pain in spinal cord injury. *Clin J Pain* **8**: 102–10.

Banovac K, Gonzalez F, Wade N, *et al.* (1993) Intravenous disodium etidronate therapy in spinal cord injury patients with heterotopic ossification. *Paraplegia* **31**: 660–66.

Banwell JG, Creasey GH, Aggarwal AM, *et al.* (1993) Management of the neurogenic bowel in patients with spinal cord injury. *Urol Clin North Am* **20**: 517–26.

Bar CA. (1991) Evaluation of cushions using dynamic pressure measurement. *Prosthet Orthot Int* **15**: 232–40.

Barbenel JC, Paul JP. (1992) Bioengineering developments for paraplegic patients. *Paraplegia* **30**: 61–64.

Barnes DG, Shaw PJ, Timoney AG, *et al.* (1993) Management of the neuropathic bladder by suprapubic catheterisation. *Br J Urol* **72**: 169–72.

Bates PS, Spencer JC, Young ME, *et al.* (1993) Assistive technology and the newly disabled adult: adaptation to wheelchair use. *Am J Occup Ther* **47**: 1014–21.

Bedbrook G, Editor: (1981) *The care and management of spinal cord injuries.* Springer-Verlag.

Berard EJ. (1989) The sexuality of spinal cord injured women: physiology and pathophysiology. A review. *Paraplegia* **27**: 99–112.

Bickel A, Culkin DJ, Wheeler JS. (1991) Bladder cancer in spinal cord injury patients. *J Urol* **146**: 1240–42.

Binnie NR, Creasey GH, Edmond P, *et al.* (1988) The action of cisapride on the chronic constipation of paraplegia. *Paraplegia* **26**: 151–58.

Binnie NR, Smith AN, Creasey GH, *et al.* (1991) Constipation associated with chronic spinal cord injury: the effect of pelvic parasympathetic stimulation by the Brindley stimulator. *Paraplegia* **29**: 463–69.

Birbamer G, Buchberger W, Felber S, *et al.* (1993) Spontaneous collapse of post-traumatic syringomyelia: serial magnetic resonance imaging. *Eur Neurol* **33**: 378–81.

Blockmans D, Steeno O. (1988) Physostigmine as a treatment for anejaculation with paraplegic men. *Andrologia* **20**: 311–13.

Bodner DR, *et al.* (1987) The application of intracavernous injection of vasoactive medications for erection in men with spinal cord injury. *J Urol* **138**: 310–11.

Bodner DR, Leffler B, Frost F. (1992) The role of intra-cavernous injection of vasoactive medications for the restoration of erection in spinal cord injured males: a three year follow-up. *Paraplegia* **30**: 118–20.

Bohannon RW. (1993) Tilt table standing for reducing spasticity after spinal cord injury. *Arch Phys Med Rehabil* **74**: 1121–22.

Braddom RL, Rocco JF. (1991) Autonomic dysreflexia. A survey of current treatment. *Am J Phys Med Rehabil* **70**: 234–41.

Brindley GS. (1986) Sexual and reproductive problems of paraplegic men. *Oxf Rev Reprod Biol* **8**: 214–22.

Brindley GS. (1993a) Physiological considerations in the use of sacral anterior root stimulators. *Neurourol Urodyn.*, 12(5), 485–86.

Brindley, GS. (1993b) History of the sacral anterior root stimulator, 1969–1982. *Neurourol Urodynamics* **12**: 481–83.

Brindley GS. (1995) The first 500 sacral anterior root stimulators: implant failures and their repair. *Paraplegia* **33**: 5–10.

Brindley GS, Polkey CE, Rushton DN, et al. (1986) Sacral anterior root stimulators for bladder control in paraplegia: the first 50 cases. *J Neurol Neurosurg Psychiatry* **49**: 1104–14.

Brindley GS, et al. (1989) Hypogastric plexus stimulators for obtaining semen from paraplegic men. *Br J Urol* **64**: 72–77.

Bromley I. (1991) *Tetraplegia and paraplegia: a guide for physiotherapists*, 4th edition. Edinburgh: Churchill Livingstone.

Buck FM, Hohmann GW. (1981) Personality, behavior, values, and family relations of children of fathers with spinal cord injury. *Arch Phys Med Rehabil*, **62**: 432–38.

Burke MH, Hicks AF, Robbins M, et al. (1960) Survival of patients with injuries to the spinal cord. *JAMA* **172**: 121–24.

Burney RE, Maio RF, Maynard F, et al. (1993) Incidence, characteristics and outcome of spinal cord injury at trauma centers in North America. *Arch Surg* **123**: 596–99.

Burnham RS, May L, Nelson E, et al. (1993) Shoulder pain in wheelchair athletes. The role of muscle imbalance. *Am J Sports Med* **21**: 238–42.

Cardus D, Ribas-Cardus F, McTaggart WG. (1992) Coronary risk in spinal cord injury: assessment following a multivariate approach. *Arch Phys Med Rehabil* **73**: 930–33.

Carone R, Vercelli D, Bertapelle P. (1993) Effects of cisapride on anorectal and vesicourethral function in spinal cord injured patients. *Paraplegia* **31**: 125–27.

Carter RE. (1979) Experience with high tetraplegics. *Paraplegia* **17**: 140–46.

Carter RE. (1993) Experience with ventilator dependent patients. *Paraplegia* **31**: 150–53.

Chancellor MB, Erhard MJ, Strup S, et al. (1993a) Bladder augmentation using the stomach in spinal cord injured patients with impaired renal function. *Arch Phys Med Rehabil* **74**: 1222–24.

Chancellor MB, Karasick S, Strup S, et al. (1993b) Transurethral balloon dilation of the external urinary sphincter: effectiveness in spinal cord-injured men with detrusor-external urethral sphincter dyssynergia. *Radiology* **187**: 557–60.

Chao R, Clowers D, Mayo ME. (1993a) Fate of upper urinary tracts in patients with indwelling catheters after spinal cord injury. *Urology* **42**: 259–62.

Chao R, Mayo ME, Bejany DE, et al. (1993b) Bladder neck closure with continent augmentation or suprapubic catheter in patients with neurogenic bladders. *J Am Paraplegia Soc* **16**: 18–22.

Charlifue SW, Gerhart KA. (1991) Behavioral and demographic predictors of suicide after traumatic spinal cord injury. *Arch Phys Med Rehabil*, **72**: 488–92.

Charlifue SW, Gerhart KA, Menter RR, et al. (1992) Sexual issues of women with spinal cord injuries. *Paraplegia* **30**: 192–99.

Chase BW, King KF. (1990) Psychosocial adjustment of persons with spinal cord injury. *Int J Rehabil Res* **13**: 325–27.

Cho KH, Iwasaki Y, Imamura H, et al. (1994) Experimental model of post-traumatic syringomyelia: the role of adhesive arachnoiditis in syrinx formation. *J Neurosurg* **80**: 133–39.

Clayton KS, Chubon RA. (1994) Factors associated with the quality of life of long-term spinal cord injured persons. *Arch Phys Med Rehabil* **75**: 633–38.

Clough P, Lindenauer D, Hayes M, et al. (1986) Guidelines for routine respiratory care of patients with spinal cord injury. A clinical report. *Phys Ther* **66**: 1395–402.

Colachis SC, Clinchot DM. (1993) The association between deep venous thrombosis and heterotopic ossification in patients with acute traumatic spinal cord injury. *Paraplegia* **31**: 507–12.

Colachis SC, Clinchot DM, Venesy D. (1993) Neurovascular complications of heterotopic ossification following spinal cord injury. *Paraplegia* **31**: 51–57.

Cox DR. (1972) Regression models and life tables. *JR Stat Soc* **34(B)**: 187–220.

Craig AR, Hancock KM, Dickson HG. (1994) Spinal cord injury: a search for determinants of depression two years after the event. *Br J Clin Psychol* **33**: 221–30.

Creighton C. (1989) Pregnancy and quadriplegia: an occupational therapy home program. *Am J Occup Ther* **43**: 44–46.

Crewe NM, Krause JS. (1988) Marital relationships and spinal cord injury. *Arch Phys Med Rehabil* **69**: 435–38.

Crewe NM, Krause JS. (1992) Marital status and adjustment to spinal cord injury. *J Am Paraplegia Soc* **15**: 14–18.

Crisp R. (1992) Vocational decision making by sixty spinal cord injury patients. *Paraplegia* **30**: 420–24.

Cross LL, Meythaler JM, Tuel SM, et al. (1992) Pregnancy, labor and delivery post spinal cord injury. *Paraplegia* **30**: 890–902.

Cull JG, Hardy RE. (1977) *Physical medicine and rehabilitation approaches in spinal cord injury*. Springfield, Ill: Charles C. Thomas.

Curcoll ML. (1992) Psychological approach to the rehabilitation of the spinal cord injured: the contribution of relaxation techniques. *Paraplegia* **30**: 425–27.

Curtin M. (1994) Development of a tetraplegic hand assessment and splinting protocol. *Paraplegia* **32**: 159–69.

Curtis KA. (1985) Physical therapist role satisfaction in the treatment of the spinal cord-injured person. *Phys Ther* **65**: 197–200.

Cushman LA, Hassett J. (1992) Spinal cord injury: 10 and 15 years after. *Paraplegia* **30**: 690–96.

Cutler SJ, Ederer F. (1958) Maximum utilization of the life table method in analyzing survival. *J Chronic Dis* **8**: 699–712.

Daud O, Sett P, Burr RG, et al. (1993) The relationship of heterotopic ossification to passive movements in paraplegic patients. *Disabil Rehabil* **15**: 114–18.

Daverat P, Gagnon M, Dartigues JF, et al. (1989) Initial factors predicting survival in patients with a spinal cord injury. *J Neurol Neurosurg Psychiatry* **52**: 403–406.

Decter RM, Bauer SB. (1993) Urologic management of spinal cord injury in children. *Urol Clin North Am* **20**: 475–83.

Derrickson J, Ciesla N, Simpson N, *et al.* (1992) A comparison of two breathing exercise programs for patients with quadriplegia. *Phys Ther* **72**: 763–69.

Design of housing for the convenience of disabled people. (1978) (British Standard Code of Practice 5619.)

DeVivo MJ, Richards JS. (1992) Community reintegration and quality of life following spinal cord injury. *Paraplegia* **30**: 108–12.

DeVivo MJ, Stover SL. (In press) Long-term survival and causes of death. In: Stover SL, editors. *Spinal cord injury: critical outcome from the model system.* Aspen.

DeVivo MJ, Kartus PL, Stover SL, *et al.* (1987) Seven-year survival following spinal cord injury. *Arch Neurol* **44**: 872–75.

DeVivo MJ, Karus PL, Stover SL, *et al.* (1989) Cause of death for patients with spinal cord injuries. *Arch Intern Med* **149**: 1761–66.

DeVivo MJ, Black KJ, Richards JS, *et al.* (1991) Suicide following spinal cord injury. *Paraplegia* **29**: 620–27.

DeVivo MJ, Stover SL, Black KJ. (1992a) Prognostic factors for 12-year survival after spinal cord injury. *Arch Phys Med Rehabil* **73**: 156–62.

DeVivo MJ, Rutt RD, Black KJ, *et al.* (1992b) Trends in spinal cord injury demographics and treatment outcomes between 1973 and 1986. *Arch Phys Med Rehabil* **73**: 424–30.

DeVivo MJ, Black KJ, Stover SL. (1993) Causes of death during the first 12 years after spinal cord injury. *Arch Phys Med Rehabil* **74**: 248–54.

Dietrick RB, Russi S. (1958) Tabulation and review of autopsy findings in fifty five paraplegics. *JAMA* **166**: 41–44.

Dover H, Pickard W, Swain I, *et al.* (1992) The effectiveness of a pressure clinic in preventing pressure sores. *Paraplegia* **30**: 267–72.

Draus JF, Franti CE, Borhani NO, *et al.* (1979) Survival with an acute spinal cord injury. *J Chronic Dis* **32**: 269–83.

Ducharme SH, Freed MM, Oates C, *et al.* (1981) The role of self-destruction in spinal cord injury mortality. *Model Syst SCI Dig* **2**(4): 29–38.

Efthimiou J, Gordon WA, Sell GH, *et al.* (1981) Electronic assistive devices: their impact on the quality of life of high level quadriplegic persons. *Arch Phys Med Rehabil* **62**: 131–34.

Eisenberg MG, Saltz CC. (1991) Quality of life among aging spinal cord injured persons: long term rehabilitation outcomes. *Paraplegia* **29**: 514–20.

Elliot S, Szasz G, Zouves C. (1991) The combined use of vibrostimulation and *in vitro* fertilization: successful pregnancy outcome from a retrograde specimen obtained from a spinal cord-injured male. *J In Vitro Fertil Embryo Transf* **8**: 348–52.

Elliott TR, Herrick SM, Patti AM, *et al.* (1991) Assertiveness, social support, and psychological adjustment following spinal cord injury. *Behav Res Ther* **29**: 485–93.

Eltorai I, Montroy R. (1990) Muscle release in the management of spasticity in spinal cord injury. *Paraplegia* **28**: 433–40.

Engelke KA, Shea JD, Doerr DF, *et al.* (1994) Autonomic functions and orthostatic responses 24th after acute intense exercise in paraplegic subjects. *Am J Physiol* **266**: R1189–96.

Fallon B. (1979) *Able to work.*: Spinal Injuries Association.

Fanciullacci F, Zanollo A, Sandri S, *et al.* (1988) The neuropathic bladder in children with spinal cord injury. *Paraplegia* **26**: 83–86.

Fenollosa P, Pallares J, Cervera J, *et al.* (1993) Chronic pain in the spinal cord injured: statistical approach and pharmacological treatment. Paraplegia, 31(11), 722–29.

Ferguson-Pell MW, Wilkie IC, Reswick JB, *et al.* (1980) Pressure sore prevention for the wheelchair-bound spinal injury patient. *Paraplegia* **18**: 42–51.

Flett PJ. (1992) The rehabilitation of children with spinal cord injury. *J Paediatr Child Health* **28**: 141–64.

Ford JR, Duckworth B. (1987) *Physical management for the quadriplegic patient*, 2nd edition. Philadelphia, PA: Davis.

Francois N, Maury M. (1987) Sexual aspects in paraplegic patients. *Paraplegia* **25**: 289–92.

Freed MM, Bakst HJ, Barrie DL. (1966) Life expectancy, survival rates, and causes of death in civilian patients with spinal cord trauma. *Arch Phys Med Rehabil* **47**: 457–63.

Frieden L, Cole JA. (1985) Independence: the ultimate goal of rehabilitation for spinal cord-injured persons. *Am J Occup Ther* **39**: 734–39.

Frisbie JH, Kache A. (1983) Increasing survival and changing causes of death in myelopathy patients. *J Am Paraplegia Soc* **6**: 51–56.

Fuhrer MJ, Rintala DH, Hart KA, *et al.* (1992) Relationship of life satisfaction to impairment, disability, and handicap among persons with spinal cord injury living in the community. *Arch Phys Med Rehabil* **73**: 552–57.

Fuhrer KJ, Garber SL, Rintala DH, *et al.* (1993a) Pressure ulcers in community-resident persons with spinal cord injury: prevalence and risk factors. *Arch Phys Med Rehabil* **74**: 1172–77.

Fuhrer MJ, Rintala DH, Hart KA, *et al.* (1993b) Depressive symptomatology in persons with spinal cord injury who reside in the community. *Arch Phys Med Rehabil* **74**: 255–60.

Fullerton DT, Harvey RF, Klein MH, *et al.* (1981) Psychiatric disorders in patients with spinal cord injuries. *Arch Gen Psychiatry* **38**: 1369–71.

Garber SL. (1985) New perspectives for the occupational therapist in the treatment of spinal cord-injured individuals. *Am J Occup Ther* **39**: 703–704.

Gardner BP, Parsons KF, Machin DG, *et al.* (1984) The role of urodynamics in the management of spinal cord injured patients. *Paraplegia* **22**: 157–61.

Gardner BP, Parsons KF, Soni BM, *et al.* (1985a) The management of upper urinary tract calculi in spinal cord damaged patients. *Paraplegia* **23**: 371–78.

Gardner BP, Theocleous F, Watt JW, *et al.* (1985b) Ventilation or dignified death for patients with high tetraplegia? *Br Med J (Clin Res)* **291**: 1620–22.

Gardner BP, Jefocate RM, Dyke RG, *et al.* (1985c) Microcomputer aids: appropriate allocation of a valuable resource. *Br J Health Care Comput* **2**:.

Gardner BP, Parsons KF, Machin DG, *et al.* (1986a) The urological management of spinal cord damaged patients: a clinical algorithm. *Paraplegia* **24**: 138–47.

Gardner BP, Watt JWH, Krishnan KR. (1986b) The artificial ventilation of spinal cord injured patients: a retrospective study of 44 cases. *Paraplegia* **24**: 208–20.

Geisler WO, Jousse AT, Wynne-Jones M. (1977) Survival in traumatic transverse myelitis. *Paraplegia* **14**: 262–75.

Geisler WO, Jousse AT, Wynne-Jones M, *et al.* (1983) Survival in traumatic spinal cord injury. *Paraplegia* **21**: 364–73.

Geller B, Greydanus DE. (1979) Psychological management of acute paraplegia in adolescence. *Pediatrics* **63**: 562–64.

Gerhart KA, Johnson RL, Whiteneck GG. (1992) Health and psychosocial issues of individuals with incomplete and resolving spinal cord injuries. *Paraplegia* **30**: 282–87.

Gerridzen RG, Thijssen AM, Dehoux E. (1992) Risk factors for upper tract deterioration in chronic spinal cord injury patients. *J Urol* **147**: 416–18.

Gilsdorf P, Patterson R, Fisher S, *et al.* (1990) Sitting forces and wheelchair mechanics. *J Rehabil Res Dev* **27**: 239–46.

Glass CA. (1992) Applying functional analysis to psychological rehabilitation following spinal cord injury. *J Am Paraplegia Soc* **15**: 187–93.

Golding, C. (1976) *Employment of tetraplegics*.: National Fund for Research into Crippling Diseases.

Goldman JM, Rose LS, Williams SJ, *et al.* (1986) Effect of abdominal binders on breathing in tetraplegic patients. *Thorax* **41**: 940–45.

Goldsmith S. (1976) *Designing for the disabled*, 3rd edition. London: RIBA Publications Limited.

Granat MH, Ferguson AC, Andrews BJ, *et al.* (1993) The role of functional electrical stimulation in the rehabilitation of patients with incomplete spinal cord injury – observed benefits during gait studies. *Paraplegia* **31**: 207–15.

Green D, Hull RD, Mammen EF, *et al.* (1992) Deep vein thrombosis in spinal cord injury. Summary and recommendations. *Chest* **102** (6 suppl): 633S–35S.

Griffin MR, O'Fallon WM, Opitz JL, *et al.* (1985) Mortality, survival and prevalence: traumatic spinal cord injury in Olmsted County, Minnesota, 1935–1981. *J Chronic Dis* **38**: 643–53.

Groomes TE, Huang CT. (1991) Orthostatic hypotension after spinal cord injury, treatment with fludrocortisone and ergotamine. *Arch Phys Med Rehabil* **72**: 56–58.

Grundy D, Swain A, editors. (1993) *ABC of spinal cord injury*. London: British Medical Journal.

Guttmann L. (1976a) *Spinal cord injuries: comprehensive management and research*. Oxford: Blackwell.

Guttmann L. (1976b) *Textbook of sport for the disabled*. New York: John Wiley.

Hackler RH. (1977) A 25 year prospective mortality study in the spinal cord injured patient: comparison with the long-term living paraplegic. *J Urol* **117**: 486–88.

Hammel JM, Van-der-Loos HF, Perkash I. (1992) Evaluation of a vocational robot with a quadriplegic employee. *Arch Phys Med Rehabil* **73**: 683–93.

Hammell KR. (1992) Psychological and sociological theories concerning adjustment to traumatic spinal cord injury: the implications for rehabilitation. *Paraplegia* **30**: 317–26.

Hardy AG. (1976) Survival periods in traumatic tetraplegia. *Paraplegia* **14**: 41–46.

Hardy AG, Elson R. (1976) *Practical management of spinal injuries*.: Churchill Livingstone.

Heller L, Keren O, Aloni R, *et al.* (1992) An open trial of vacuum penile tumescence: constriction therapy for neurological impotence. *Paraplegia* **30**: 550–53.

Henderson JL, Price SH, Brandstater ME, *et al.* (1994) Efficacy of three measures to relieve pressure in seated persons with spinal cord injury. *Arch Phys Med Rehabil* **75**: 535–39.

Hobson, D.A. (1992) Comparative effects of posture on pressure and shear at the body–seat interface. *J Rehabil Res Dev* **29**: 21–31.

Hobson DA, Tooms RE. (1992) Seated lumbar/pelvic alignment. A comparison between spinal cord-injured and non-injured groups. *Spine* **17**: 293–98.

Hollander JB, Diokno AC. (1993) Urinary diversion and reconstruction in the patient with spinal cord injury. *Urol Clin North Am* **20**: 465–74.

Honan WP, Williams B. (1993) Sensory loss in syringomyelia: not necessarily dissociated. *J R Soc Med* **86**: 519–20.

How new homes can be made better for all age groups. (1986) The Prince of Wales Advisory Group on Disability and the National House-Building Council.

Hughes SJ, *et al.* (1991) Management of the pregnant woman with spinal cord injuries. *Br J Obstet Gynaecol* **98**: 513–18.

Hurlburt M, Ottenbacher KJ. (1992) An examination of direct selection typing rate and accuracy for persons with high-level spinal cord injury using QWERTY and default on-screen keyboards. *J Rehabil Res Dev* **29**: 54–63.

Illis LS, editor. (1988) *Spinal cord dysfunction. Vol. 1: Assessment.* Oxford: Oxford University Press.

Illis LS, editor. (1992) *Spinal cord dysfunction. Vol. 2: Intervention and treatment.* Oxford: Oxford University Press.

Illis LS. editor. (1993) *Spinal cord dysfunction. Vol. 3: Functional stimulation.* Oxford: Oxford University Press.

Jackson AB, DeVivo M. (1992) Urological long-term follow-up in women with spinal cord injuries. *Arch Phys Med Rehabil* **73**: 1029–35.

Jaeger RJ, Yarkony GM, Roth EJ. (1989) Rehabilitation technology for standing and walking after spinal cord injury. *Am J Phys Med Rehabil* **68**: 128–33.

Jaeger RJ, Turba RM, Yarkony GM, *et al.* (1993) Cough in spinal cord injured patients: comparison of three methods to produce cough. *Arch Phys Med Rehabil* **74**: 1358–61.

Judd FK, Brown DJ. (1992a) Psychiatric consultation in a spinal injuries unit. *Aust N Z J Psychiatry* **26**: 218–22.

Judd FK, Brown DJ. (1992b) Suicide following acute traumatic spinal cord injury. *Paraplegia* **30**: 173–77.

Kanellos MC. (1985) Enhancing vocational outcomes of spinal cord-injured persons: the occupational therapist's role. *Am J Occup Ther* **39**: 726–33.

Kantor C, Andrews BJ, Marsolais EB, *et al.* (1993) Report on a conference on motor prostheses for workplace mobility of paraplegic patients in North America. *Paraplegia* **31**: 439–56.

Kennedy P, Marsh NJ. (1993) Effectiveness of the use of humour in the rehabilitation of people with SCI: a pilot study. *J Am Paraplegia Soc* **16**: 215–18.

Kimoto Y, Iwatsubo E. (1994) Penile prostheses for the management of the neuropathic bladder and sexual dysfunction in spinal cord injury patients: long term follow up. *Paraplegia* **32**: 336–39.

Kiwerski J, Weiss M, Chrostowska T. (1981) Analysis of mortality of patients after cervical spine trauma. *Paraplegia* **19**: 347–51.

Krajnik SR, Bridle MJ. (1992) Hand splinting in quadriplegia: current practice. *Am J Occup Ther* **46**: 149–56.

Kraus JS, Crewe NM. (1987) Prediction of long-term survival of persons with spinal cord injury: an 11-year prospective study. *Rehabil Psychol* **32**: 205–13.

Kraus JS, Kjorsvig JM. (1992) Mortality after spinal cord injury: a four-year prospective study. *Arch Phys Med Rehabil* **73**: 558–63.

Krause JS. (1992a) Longitudinal changes in adjustment after spinal cord injury: a 15 year study. *Arch Phys Med Rehabil* **73**: 564–68.

Krause JS. (1992b) Employment after spinal cord injury. *Arch Phys Med Rehabil* **73**: 163–69.

Kreuter M, Sullivan M, Siosteen A. (1994) Sexual adjustment after spinal cord injury (SCI) focusing on partner experiences. *Paraplegia* **32**: 225–35.

Krum H, Howes LG, Brown DJ, et al. (1992) Risk factors for cardiovascular disease in chronic spinal cord injury patients. *Paraplegia* **30**: 381–88.

Le CT, Price M. (1982) Survival from spinal cord injury. *J Chronic Dis* **35**: 487–92.

Lee MY, Kirk PM, Yarkony GM. (1989) Rehabilitation of quadriplegic patients with phrenic nerve pacers. *Arch Phys Med Rehabil* **70**: 549–52.

Leeton J, Yates C, Rawicki B. (1991) Successful pregnancy using donor oocytes fertilized *in vitro* by spermatozoa obtained by electro-ejaculation from a quadriplegic husband. *Hum Reprod* **6**: 384–85.

Letcher JC, Goldfine LJ. (1986) Management of a pregnant paraplegic patient in a rehabilitation center. *Arch Phys Med Rehabil* **67**: 477–78.

Levy DA, Resnick MI. (1993) Management of urinary stones in the patient with spinal cord injury. *Urol Clin North Am* **20**: 435–42.

Lindan R, Leffler EJ, Bodner D. (1987) Urological problems in the management of quadriplegic women. *Paraplegia* **25**: 381–85.

MacDonagh RP, Sun WM, Smallwood R, et al. (1990) Control of defaecation in patients with spinal injuries by stimulation of sacral anterior nerve roots. *Br Med J* **300**: 1494–97.

Macourt D, Engel S, Jones RF, et al. (1991) Pregnancy of gamete intrafallopian transfer (GIFT) with sperm aspirated from the vaso-epididymal junction of spinal injured man: case report. *Paraplegia* **29**: 550–53.

Madersbacher G, Oberwalder M. (1987) The elderly para- and tetraplegic: special aspects of the urological care. *Paraplegia* **25**: 318–23.

Mariano AJ. (1992) Chronic pain and spinal cord injury. *Clin J Pain* **8**: 87–92.

Marino RJ, Huang M, Knight P, et al. (1993) Assessing selfcare status in quadriplegia: comparison of the quadriplegia index of function (QIF) and the functional independence measure (FIM). *Paraplegia* **31**: 225–33.

Mathias CJ. (1991) Role of sympathetic efferent nerves in blood pressure regulation and in hypertension. *Hypertension* **18** (5 suppl): III22–30.

Mathias CJ, et al. (1983) Clinical manifestations of malfunctioning sympathetic mechanisms in tetraplegia. *J Auton Nerv Syst* **7**: 303–12.

McDonald DW, Boyle MA, Schumann TL. (1989) Environmental control unit utilization by high-level spinal cord injured patients. *Arch Phys Med Rehabil* **70**: 621–23.

Menon EB, Tan ES. (1992) Bladder training in patients with spinal cord injury. *Urology* **40**: 425–29.

Mesard L, Carmody A, Mannarino E, et al. (1978) Survival after spinal cord trauma. *Arch Neurol* **35**: 78–83.

Minaire P, Demolin P, Bourret J, et al. (1983) Life expectancy following spinal cord injury: a ten-year survey in the Rhone-Alpes region, France, 1969–1980. *Paraplegia* **21**: 11–15.

Moberg E. (1978) *The upper limb in tetraplegia: a new approach to surgical rehabilitation*. Berlin: Georg Thieme.

Nixon V. (1985) *Spinal cord injury: a guide to functional outcomes in physical therapy management*. London: Heinemann.

Noreau L, Shephard RJ. (1992) Return to work after spinal cord injury: the potential contribution of physical fitness. *Paraplegia* **30**: 563–72.

Noreau L, Shephard RJ, Simard C, et al. (1993) Relationship of impairment and functional ability to habitual activity and fitness following spinal cord injury. *Int J Rehabil Res* **16**: 265–75.

Nyquist RH, Bors E. (1967) Mortality and survival in traumatic myelopathy during nineteen years, from 1946 to 1965. *Paraplegia* **5**: 22–48.

Ochs G, Struppler A, Meyerson BA, et al. (1989) Intrathecal Baclofen for long-term treatment of spasticity: a multi-centre study. *J Neurol Neurosurg Psychiatry* **52**: 933–39.

Odderson IR, Jaffe KM, Sleicher CA, et al. (1991) Gel wheelchair cushions: a potential cold weather hazard. *Arch Phys Med Rehabil* **72**: 1017–20.

Oliver M, et al. editors. (1987) *Personal and social implications of spinal cord injury: a retrospective study*. London: Thames Polytechnic.

Parsons KF, Fitzpatrick JM, editors. (1991) *Practical urology in spinal cord injury*. Berlin: Springer-Verlag.

Pentland B. (1993) Quadriplegia and cardiorespiratory fitness. *Lancet* **341**: 413–14.

Perez M, Pilsecker C. (1994) Group psychotherapy with spinal cord injured substance abusers. *Paraplegia* **32**: 188–92.

Perkash I, Kabalin JN, Lennon S, et al. (1992) Use of penile prostheses to maintain external condom catheter drainage in spinal cord injury patients. *Paraplegia* **30**: 327–32.

Peters LC, Stambrook M, Moore AD, et al. (1992) Differential effects of spinal cord injury and head injury on marital adjustment. *Brain Inj* **6**: 461–67.

Ravichandran G, Silver JR. (1982a) Missed injuries of the spinal cord. *Br Med J* **284**: 953–56.

Ravichandran G, Silver JR. (1982b) Survival following traumatic tetraplegia. *Paraplegia* **20**: 264–69.

Richards JS. (1992) Chronic pain and spinal cord injury: review and comment. *Clin J Pain* **8**: 119–22.

Richards B. (1982) A social and psychological study of 166 spinal cord injured patients from Queensland. *Paraplegia* **20**: 90–96.

Richards JS, Osuna FJ, Jaworski TM, *et al.* (1991) The effectiveness of different methods of defining traumatic brain injury in predicting post-discharge adjustment in a spinal cord injury population. *Arch Phys Med Rehabil* **72**: 275–79.

Richardson RP, Meyer PR. (1982) Prevalence and incidence of pressure sores in acute spinal cord injuries. *Paraplegia* **20**: 235–47.

Rochon PA, Beaudet MP, McGlinchey-Berroth R, *et al.* (1993) Risk assessment for pressure ulcers: an adaptation of the National Pressure Ulcer Advisory Panel risk factors to spinal cord injured patients. *J Am Paraplegia Soc* **16**: 169–77.

Rodriguez GP, Garber SL. (1994) Prospective study of pressure ulcer risk in spinal cord injury patients. *Paraplegia* **32**: 150–58.

Rogers EC. (1978) Nursing management in relation to beds used with the National Spinal Injuries Centre for the prevention of pressure sores. *Paraplegia* **16**: 147–53.

Samsa GP, Patrick CH, Feussner JR. (1993) Long-term survival of veterans with traumatic spinal cord injury. *Ann Neurol* **50**: 909–14.

Sargant C, Braun MA. (1986) Occupational therapy management of the acute spinal cord-injured patient. *Am J Occup Ther* **40**: 333–37.

Sauerwein D, Ingunza W, Fischer J, *et al.* (1990) Extradural implantation of sacral anterior root stimulators. *J Neurol Neurosurg Psychiatry* **53**: 681–84.

Schuler M. (1982) Sexual counselling for the spinal cord injured: a review of five programs. *J Sex Marital Ther* **8**: 241–52.

Schwartz SL, Kennelly MJ, McGuire EJ, *et al.* (1994) Incontinent ileovesicostomy urinary diversion in the treatment of lower urinary tract dysfunction. *J Urol* **152**: 99–102.

Seager SW, Halstead LS. (1993) Fertility options and success after spinal cord injury. *Urol Clin North Am* **20**: 543–48.

Seeger BR, Law D, Creswell JE, *et al.* (1989) Functional electrical stimulation for upper limb strengthening in traumatic quadriplegia. *Arch Phys Med Rehabil* **70**: 663–67.

Shields RK, Cook TM. (1992) Lumbar support thickness: effect on seated buttock pressure in individuals with and without spinal cord injury. *Phys Ther* **72**: 218–26.

Sie IH, Waters RL, Adkins RH, *et al.* (1992) Upper extremity pain in the post-rehabilitation spinal cord injured patient. *Arch Phys Med Rehabil* **73**: 44–48.

Sindou M, Abbott R, Keravel Y, editors. (1991) Neurosurgery for spasticity: a multidisciplinary approach. Berlin: Springer-Verlag.

Sipski ML. (1991) The impact of spinal cord injury on female sexuality, menstruation and pregnancy: a review of the literature. *J Am Paraplegia Soc* **14**: 122–26.

Sipski ML, Alexander CJ. (1993) Sexual activities, response and satisfaction in women pre- and post-spinal cord injury. *Arch Phys Med Rehabil* **74**: 1025–29.

Smart CN, Sanders CR. (1976) *The costs of motor vehicle related SCI*. Washington, DC: Insurance Institute for Highway Safety.

Sneddon DG, Bedbrook G. (1982) Survival following traumatic tetraplegia. *Paraplegia* **20**: 201–207.

Sprigle SH, Faisant TE, Chung KC. (1990) Clinical evaluation of custom-contoured cushions for the spinal cord injured. *Arch Phys Med Rehabil* **71**: 655–58.

Squier MV, Lehr RP. (1994) Post-traumatic syringomyelia. *J Neurol Neurosurg Psychiatry* **57**: 1095–98.

Stambrook M, Moore AD, Peters LC, *et al.* (1991) Head injury and spinal cord injury: differential effects on psychosocial functioning. *J Clin Exp Neuropsychol* **13**: 521–30.

Steinglass P, Temple S, Lisman SA, *et al.* (1982) Coping with spinal cord injury: the family perspective. *Gen Hosp Psychiatry* **4**: 259–64.

Stewart TD, Rossier AB. (1978) Psychological considerations in the adjustment to spinal cord injury. *Rehabil Lit* **39**: 75–80.

Stone JM, Wolfe VA, Nino-Murcia M, *et al.* (1990) Colostomy as treatment for complications of spinal cord injury. *Arch Phys Med Rehabil* **71**: 514–18.

Stover SL, Fine PR. (1986) *Spinal cord injury: the facts and figures*. Birmingham, AL: The University of Alabama at Birmingham.

Stover SL, Fine PR. (1987) The epidemiology and economics of spinal cord injury. *Paraplegia* **25**: 225–28.

Stover SL, Lloyd LK, Waites KB, *et al.* (1989) Urinary tract infection in spinal cord injury. *Arch Phys Med Rehabil* **70**: 47–54.

Summers JD, Rapoff MA, Varghese G, *et al.* (1991) Psychosocial factors in chronic spinal cord injury pain. *Pain* **47**: 183–89.

Swarts AE, Krouskop TA, Smith DR. (1988) Tissue pressure management in the vocational setting. *Arch Phys Med Rehabil* **69**: 97–100.

Taricco M, Colombo C, Adone R, *et al.* (1992) The social and vocational outcome of spinal cord injury patients. *Paraplegia* **30**: 214–19.

Tate D, Forchheimer M, Maynard F, *et al.* (1994a) Predicting depression and psychological distress in persons with spinal cord injury based on indicators of handicap. *Am J Phys Med Rehabil* **73**: 175–83.

Tate DG, Stiers W, Daugherty J, *et al.* (1994b) The effects of insurance benefits coverage on functional and psychological outcomes after spinal cord injury. *Arch Phys Med Rehabil* **75**: 407–14.

Teddy P, Jamous A, Gardner B, *et al.* (1992) Complications of intrathecal Baclofen delivery. *B. J Neurosurg* **6**: 115–18.

Timoney AG, Shaw PJ. (1990) Urological outcome in female patients with spinal cord injury: the effectiveness of intermittent catheterisation. *Paraplegia* **28**: 556–63.

Tribe CR. (1963) Causes of death in the early and late stages of paraplegia. *Paraplegia* **1**: 19–47.

Trieschmann RB. (1980) The psychological, social, and vocational adjustment to spinal cord injury. *Annu Rev Rehabil* **1**: 304–18.

Trieschmann RB. (1988) *Spinal cord injuries: psychological, social and vocational adjustment*. New York: Demos.

Trieschmann RB. (1992) Psychosocial research in spinal cord injury: the state of the art. *Paraplegia* **30**: 58–60.

Trop CS, Bennett CJ. (1992) Complications from long-term indwelling Foley catheters in female patients with neurogenic bladders. *Semin Urol* **10**: 115–20.

Umlauf RL. (1992) Psychological interventions for chronic pain following spinal cord injury. *Clin J Pain* **8**: 111–18.

Urey JR, Henggeler S. (1987) Marital adjustment following spinal cord injury. *Arch Phys Med Rehabil* **68**: 69–74.

Van-Asbeck FW, Raadsen H, van-de-Loo ML. (1994) Social implications for persons 5–10 years after spinal cord injury. *Paraplegia* **32**: 330–35.

Van-Kerrebroeck PE, Koldewijn EL, Scherpenhuizen S, *et al.* (1993) The morbidity due to lower urinary tract function in spinal cord injury patients. *Paraplegia* **31**: 320–29.

Varma JS, Binnie N, Smith AN, *et al.* (1986) Differential effects of sacral anterior root stimulation on anal sphincter and colorectal motility in spinally injured man. *Br J Surg* **73**: 478–82.

Verduyn WH. (1986) Spinal cord injured women, pregnancy and delivery. *Paraplegia* **24**: 231–40.

Vidal J, Sarrias M. (1991) An analysis of the diverse factors concerned with the development of pressure sores in spinal cord injured patients. *Paraplegia* **29**: 261–67.

Vinken P, Bruyn GW, Frankel HL, editors. (1992) *Handbook of clinical neurology Spinal cord trauma.* (Revised Series 17): Elsevier Science.

Volle E, Assheuer J, Hedde JP, *et al.* (1992) Radicular avulsion resulting from spinal injury: assessment of diagnostic modalities. *Neuroradiology* **34**: 235–40.

Wanner MB, Rageth CJ, Zach GA. (1987) Pregnancy and autonomic hyperreflexia in patients with spinal cord lesions. *Paraplegia* **25**: 482–90.

Webb DR, Fitzpatrick JM, O'Flynn JD. (1984) A 15-year follow-up of 406 consecutive spinal cord injuries. *Br J Urol* **56**: 614–17.

Weingarden SI. (1992) Deep venous thrombosis in spinal cord injury. Overview of the problem. *Chest* **102**(6 suppl): 636S–39S.

Wheelchair housing. (1975) (Department of the Environment Housing Development Directorate Occasional Paper 2/75).

Whiteneck GG, *et al.* (1989) *The management of high quadriplegia.* New York: Demos.

Whiteneck GG, Charlifue SW, Gerhart KA, *et al.* (1992a) Quantifying handicap: a new measure of long-term rehabilitation outcomes. *Arch Phys Med Rehabil* **73**: 519–26.

Whiteneck GG, Charlifue SW, Frankel HL, *et al.* (1992b) Mortality, morbidity and psychological outcomes of persons spinal cord injured more than 20 years ago. *Paraplegia* **30**: 617–30.

Whiteneck GG, *et al.* (1993) *Aging with spinal cord injury.* New York: Demos.

Woods BM, Jones RD. (1990) Environmental control systems in a spinal injuries unit: a review of 10 years' experience. *Int Disabil Stud* **12**: 137–40.

Wyndaele JJ. (1987) Urology in spinal cord injured patients. *Paraplegia* **25**: 267–69.

Wyndaele JJ. (1992) Neurourology in spinal cord injured patients. *Paraplegia* **30**: 50–53.

Yadav A, Vaidyanathan S, Panigrahi D. (1993) Clean intermittent catheterisation for the neuropathic bladder. *Paraplegia* **31**: 380–83.

Yarkony GM, Roth EJ, Cybulski G, *et al.* (1992a) Neuromuscular stimulation in spinal cord injury. I: Restoration of functional movement of the extremities. *Arch Phys Med Rehabil* **73**: 78–86.

Yarkony GM, Roth EJ, Cybulski GR, *et al.* (1992b) Neuromuscular stimulation in spinal cord injury. II: Prevention of secondary complications. *Arch Phys Med Rehabil* **73**: 195–200.

Yerxa EJ, Locker SB. (1990) Quality of time use by adults with spinal cord injuries. *Am J Occup Ther* **44**: 318–26.

Young BK. (1994) Pregnancy in women with paraplegia. *Adv Neurol* **64**: 209–14.

Zager RP, Marquette CH. (1981) Development considerations in children and early adolescents with spinal cord injury. *Arch Phys Med Rehabil* **62**: 427–31.

35

Vertebral fractures

Peter J A Hutchinson, Robert Macfarlane

Introduction

Most publications reviewing the management of vertebral injury are retrospective, and direct comparison of prognosis in different series is difficult because the inclusion criteria vary substantially. In addition, many studies rely heavily on anecdotal data. It is therefore hardly surprising that the reported outcomes of treatment appear inconsistent. Because of this, no attempt will be made to compare the results of conservative treatment with those of surgical intervention, to contrast the relative merits of different surgical techniques, or to evaluate the various types of instrumentation available to treat any single condition.

The overall incidence of spinal cord injury in all types of vertebral fractures and dislocations is approximately 14%, whilst 17% of traumatic spinal cord injuries have no overt radiological evidence of vertebral injury (Riggins and Kraus, 1977). The assessment of neural injury is discussed in Chapter 34.

Definitions

A *stable* injury is one in which normal movements will not result in further displacement of the vertebrae. In an *unstable* injury, further changes in alignment may occur. The concept of the 'three column' spine, as proposed by Holdsworth (1970) and refined by Denis (1983), is widely accepted as a means of assessing stability. The anterior column is formed by the anterior longitudinal ligament, the anterior annulus fibrosus of the intervertebral disc, and the anterior part of the vertebral body. The middle column is formed by the posterior longitudinal ligament, the posterior annulus fibrosus, and the posterior wall of the vertebral body. The posterior column is formed by the posterior arch, the supraspinous and interspinous ligaments, and the ligamentum flavum. Disruption of two of the columns renders the spine unstable.

In a *teardrop fracture*, axial compression breaks off the anteroinferior corner of a vertebral body.

Kyphosis is an abnormal posteriorly-directed sagittal plane curvature of the spine. This is generally measured by the Cobb angle (Cobb, 1948). In the cervical or lumbar spine, 5° or more, and in the thoracic spine, 40° or more, of fixed kyphotic deformity is considered abnormal (White *et al.*, 1977).

A *burst fracture* is when there is a failure of both the anterior and middle columns of the spine, usually under axial loading.

Spondylolisthesis is anterior subluxation of one vertebral body on another (usually L5 on S1, or L4 on L5). This can be graded as: I = <25% of the width of the vertebral body; II = 25–50%; III = 50–75%; IV = 75% – complete. The cause may be congenital, degenerative, traumatic or pathological.

Mechanisms of injury

Other injuries frequently accompany spinal trauma, afflicting 47% of individuals in one series (Saboe *et al.*, 1991). Indirect (non-penetrating) vertebral injury results from one of several mechanisms:

1. *Avulsion fractures* Muscle tension may be sufficient to avulse the transverse or spinous processes of vertebrae. Although, by themselves, these fractures are of little consequence, they may indicate serious related injury, such as renal trauma.
2. *Hyperextension* This is common in the cervical region, but rare in the thoracolumbar spine. The anterior ligaments and disc may be disrupted, or the neural arch may fracture.
3. *Flexion* This is the most common injury. Usually the posterior elements remain intact, and the vertebral body is crushed into a wedge. If the posterior ligaments are torn, then subluxation may occur and the injury becomes unstable.
4. *Axial compression* This results from a vertical force applied to a straight segment of the spine. The disc is disrupted and the vertebral body may 'burst', driving bone or disc fragments back into the spinal canal (retropulsion).
5. *Flexion with posterior distraction* Unlike a pure compressive lesion, this injury is unstable because the posterior elements are disrupted. The most common mechanism is a lap seat-belt injury. Occasionally, a horizontal fracture of the vertebral body and neural arch results, and is known as a Chance fracture (Chance, 1948).
6. *Flexion with rotation* This leads to tearing of the ligaments, and may cause one or both facet joints to dislocate, or the facets to fracture. The consequence is fracture and/or dislocation of the vertebra.
7. *Horizontal translation* The vertebra is displaced either anteroposteriorly or laterally in relation to its neighbour, creating an unstable spine with a high risk of associated neural injury.

Cervical spine injury

A detailed review of the literature on the biomechanics of cervical spine injury following road traffic accidents can be found in Huele *et al.* (1981). Most upper cervical spinal injuries are the result of blows to the head (Benzel *et al.*, 1994). As many as 25–40% of individuals who sustain high cervical trauma in motor vehicle accidents die as a result of their injuries (Hadley *et al.*, 1986). Soft tissue injury to the neck ('whiplash') is considered in Chapter 37.

Atlas burst fractures (Jefferson fractures)

Fractures of the first cervical vertebra represent 7% of all acute cervical spine fractures (Hadley *et al.*, 1988b). The atlas is well protected by soft tissues; the majority of injuries are therefore blunt. The usual mechanism is axial loading. Because of the sloping face of the articular facets, the lateral masses are forced apart, the bony ring is disrupted, and the transverse ligament may be torn. The latter is particularly likely to occur if the degree of spread is 7 mm or greater; this significantly increases the likelihood of instability (Kesterson *et al.*, 1991). Atlas fractures are accompanied by fractures of the odontoid in 24% of patients (Kesterson *et al.*, 1991).

Kesterson *et al.* (1991) reviewed the outcome of 17 Jefferson fractures, of which four were unstable and were managed operatively. Neck pain was the presenting complaint in each patient, all of whom experienced improvement in their pain following treatment. Despite occiput–C2 wiring and bone grafting in three patients, there was no significant complaint of restriction of neck movement at one year of follow-up. In a series of 32 isolated C1 fractures managed by external fixation for 8–16 weeks, there was no evidence of nonunion or instability at follow-up (Hadley *et al.*, 1988b); the incidence of neck pain was 10% (median follow-up 40 months).

Odontoid fractures

Fractures of the dens have been classified into three groups by Anderson and D'Alonzo (1974): type I, oblique avulsion of the upper part of the odontoid; type II, fracture occurring at the junction of the dens with the body of C2; type III, the fracture extends from the base of the dens down through the body of the axis. Type I fractures are rare, and require simple immobilization and symptomatic treatment only. Type II fractures have the highest rate of non-union because the transverse ligament may become interposed between the bone fragments. Hadley *et al.* (1985, 1986) found that

67% of fractures with a displacement of more than 6 mm failed to unite, compared with 10% of those with displacement of less than 4 mm. There was no correlation between age and the rate of union. In contrast, type III fractures have a 96% chance of fusion following closed reduction and halo vest fixation (Anderson and D'Alonzo, 1974; Montesano *et al.*, 1991).

Reviewing the results of 23 anterior paired screw fixations of dens fractures, the overall rate of fracture union was 92%, with an average resolution time of 5.5 months (Etter *et al.*, 1991). Delayed union was likely if a significant anterior fracture gap was evident.

Lower cervical spine injuries (C3–7)

Cadaveric studies have shown that horizontal subluxation of more than 3.5 mm or more than 11° of angulation of one vertebral body relative to the next indicates ligamentous instability (White *et al.*, 1975). Comminuted fractures of the vertebral body treated by closed reduction and immobilization in a halo for three months will result in spontaneous fusion at the injured segment in 36–66% of patients (White *et al.*, 1976). Ripa *et al.* (1991) reported the treatment results of 92 patients who underwent anterior cervical decompression, grafting and plating for single level trauma (52% for three column injury, 22% for two column injury, and most of the remainder for posterior ligament rupture with disc prolapse or vertebral body fracture). The fusion rate was 99%, occurring at an average of 3.2 months. The incidence of screw loosening was 4%.

Fehlings *et al.* (1994) treated 44 patients with cervical instability (42 were the result of trauma) by lateral mass plating without bone grafts. A solid fusion was obtained in 93% at six months. Progression of kyphosis necessitating further surgery was observed in 5%. The incidence of screw loosening in this series was also 4%. Watts *et al.* (1993) reported the results of sublaminar wiring for unstable cervical spine injuries in 34 patients; there were no cases of wire breakage.

Multiple fractures

Certain types of injury are likely to occur in conjunction with others. Around 44–77% of atlas fractures are accompanied by C2 fractures (Hadley *et al.*, 1988b; Ryan and Henderson, 1992).

Although the majority of odontoid and hangman's fractures (a fracture of the pedicles of C2) are isolated, 15% of the former and 9% of the latter are associated with atlas fractures (Ryan and Henderson, 1992). Multiple noncontiguous fractures can be anticipated in 9% of patients with C1–2 fractures (Ryan and Henderson, 1992).

Unilateral facet dislocations

In Beatson's series (1963), 13 of 14 patients with unilateral facet dislocations that remained unreduced had minimal or no symptoms. However, this is not the experience of others, who found that 70% of unilateral facet dislocations allowed to heal without reduction developed disabling neck pain, most of which required surgery (Rorabeck *et al.*, 1987). In a retrospective review of 36 patients with unilateral facet dislocation or fracture dislocation, 54% of those managed by traction and immobilization alone underwent spontaneous fusion, but only 36% achieved anatomical alignment, and 42% had complaints of pain or stiffness (Beyer *et al.*, 1991). In contrast, only 10% of those treated surgically by posterior fusion had significant long-term chronic pain or stiffness.

Cervical disc disruption

In a retrospective MRI analysis of 78 patients with acute cervical cord injury, Flanders *et al.* (1990) detected evidence of associated disc herniation in 51%, predominately at the C5/6 (40%) and C6/7 (23%) levels. The presence of a herniated disc fragment did not by itself indicate a higher incidence of neurological injury, although residual cord compression following reduction was associated with a poorer outcome. The sensitivity of non-contrasted CT in detecting disc prolapse was poor, failing to delineate 40% of cases of herniation which were readily apparent on MRI.

Raynor (1977) investigated 20 patients with moderate or severe neurological deficit after cervical spine injury; twelve had significant fractures of a cervical vertebra, and nine had disc protrusions. Of eight treated surgically, 50% experienced significant improvement in motor power. Of 68 patients with subluxation or dislocation of a cervical facet, six (9%) had an associated large disc prolapse (Eismont *et al.*, 1991). Reduction of the facet dislocation without prior discectomy may result in neurological deterioration (Berrington *et al.*, 1993; Eismont *et al.*, 1991).

Pre-injury cervical canal diameter and neurological outcome

Several studies have demonstrated a link between congenital or acquired cervical canal stenosis and a predisposition to spinal cord injury after trauma (Eismont *et al.*, 1984; Ladd and Scranton, 1986; Matsuura *et al.*, 1989). However, a more recent study of 33 patients with unilateral or bilateral facet fractures or dislocations concluded that the degree of vertebral trauma and the severity of the initial neurological deficit were the major prognostic indicators, and that there was no correlation between the preinjury canal diameter or the canal ratio (the ratio of the sagittal diameter of the spinal canal to the sagittal midbody diameter of the vertebra) and outcome (Lintner *et al.*, 1993). Other groups have also failed to correlate pre-existing spinal stenosis or degenerative spondylosis with the severity of neurological injury (Flanders *et al.*, 1990).

Delayed/missed diagnosis

Gerrelts *et al.* (1991) reviewed a total of 1331 patients with suspected cervical spine injury after blunt trauma. The diagnosis of injury was made during the initial radiological evaluation in 91.8% of patients. Delayed diagnosis in the remainder was largely the result of incomplete imaging. In this series, the sensitivity of plain radiographs (with five views: anteroposterior (AP), lateral, odontoid, coned–down C1–2, and swimmer's view) was 85.2%, and the sensitivity of CT was 97.2%. Davis *et al.* (1993) also concluded that delayed or missed diagnosis, which occurred in 4.6% of 740 cervical spine injuries, was largely the result of failure to obtain adequate plain radiographs. Their practice was to obtain a standard series of three views: AP, lateral (to include C7/T1), and odontoid. The consequence of delayed diagnosis is neurological deterioration in around 10–29% of patients, compared with 1.5% risk of deterioration for those diagnosed on initial evaluation (Davis *et al.*, 1993; Reid *et al.*, 1987).

Cervical spinal movement

Della Torre and Rinonapoli (1992) managed 27 patients with displaced cervical spine injuries (13 C1/2; 14 C3–7) by halocast immobilization, and reported that, ultimately, spinal movement was full in 63%, whilst 'slight reduction' was evident in 29%. The remaining 8% had lost more than 50% of cervical movement.

Halifax clamp posterior cervical fusion

Aldrich *et al.* (1993) reported recently the results in 50 consecutive patients of posterior cervical fusion using Halifax interlaminar clamps, the majority for post-traumatic instability. Follow-up time averaged 21 months. Surgical failure occurred in 10% of patients, and was most common at the atlantoaxial level due to screw loosening (18% failure rate), although none of the failures occurred in patients with trauma.

Complications of halo vests

In a prospective study of 102 patients randomized to 6 lb/in^2 or 8 lb/in^2 of pin torque and immobilized for around 10 weeks, the incidence of pin loosening was 20% and 26% respectively. The infection rates were 7.3% and 13% in the two groups (Rizzollo *et al.*, 1993). At three months of follow-up, 12% of patients complained of 'severe' pin scars and 25% of severe pin pain. 'Moderate' scars or pain afflicted 40% and 21% of patients respectively. Longer follow-up data are not available. Other complications of halo vests include pressure sores under the jacket (11%), nerve injury (2%), dysphagia (2%), and dural penetration (1%) (Garfin *et al.*, 1986; Glaser *et al* 1986).

Thoracolumbar spine injury

Considerable controversy exists regarding whether such injuries should be managed conservatively or operatively. This is beyond the remit of this chapter, and will not be discussed further.

In a review of 371 patients, Frankel *et al.* (1969) noted that the risk of neurological deterioration with postural reduction and recumbancy was 0.5%. Cantor *et al.* (1993) managed 18 neurologically intact adults with burst fractures (T10–L2) but without evidence of posterior column disruption (defined as a kyphosis of <30°, <50% anterior loss of vertebral height, and no widening of interspinous distance or evidence of facet disruption) by early mobilization in an extension brace. At an average follow-up of 19 months, 77% were able to resume an 'active' lifestyle without any limitations, and 83% rated their pain as 'very little' or 'none' and were not taking analgesics. Overall, 95% of patients were able to return to their previous level of activity with very few restrictions. There was no progression of the average initial kyphosis of 19°, and follow-up CT scans in eight patients demonstrated a minimum 50% resorption of the initial degree of canal compromise.

In a similar study of 41 adults with fractures between T11 and L5 who were managed nonoperatively and followed for an average of two years, 49% had an excellent outcome relative to pain and function; 17% were good, 22% fair and 12% poor (Mumford *et al.*, 1993). Overall, 63% had no restriction in their work, 23% were working but not to their previous level, and 15% were unable to work; 9.7% as a result of back pain. Unlike the study by Cantor *et al.* (1993), serial radiographs documented significant progression of the kyphus by an average of 8% over two years. This was predominantly in patients sustaining injuries between T11 and L2. Further angulation was small after the first year, suggesting that stabilization of the deformity had occurred. This and other studies have shown that neither the degree of kyphus nor loss of vertebral body height correlate with symptoms at follow-up (Aglietti *et al.*, 1983; Cantor *et al.*, 1993).

Some degree of chronic back pain is common after injuries that have been managed conservatively. Mumford *et al.* (1993) reported that this affected 76% of patients, but was severe enough to prevent work in only 9.7%. A similar nine-year follow-up by Aglietti *et al.* (1983) indicated that 81% returned to their previous employment and 14% to other types of work. Weinstein *et al.* (1988) followed patients for over 20 years and noted pain in 90%, although the majority (63%) rated this as 'very little'. Nicholl (1949) reported residual pain in 59% of his patients. Burke (1973) indicated that the incidence of chronic pain was higher after operative than after non-operative management.

Cammisa *et al.*, (1989) reported that 37% of burst lumbar fractures managed operatively were found to have a dural tear at surgery. Although this was associated with an increased risk of neurological deficit, it was not followed by a significant likelihood of developing a false meningocoele.

Post-traumatic kyphosis

A detailed account of the biomechanics of posttraumatic kyphotic deformities can be found in White *et al.* (1977). Comparative studies of three different methods of posterior instrumentation and fusion for unstable fractures of the thoracic and lumbar spine (Harrington rods, Luque rods and pedicular screws) indicate that all three techniques fail to maintain vertebral alignment, particularly in the sagittal plane (Sasso and Cotler, 1993). Esses *et al.* (1990) compared the results of patients randomized to anterior decompression with instrumentation and posterior distraction with pedicle screw fixation for burst fractures of the thoracolumbar and lumbar spine. Although there was no significant difference in the degree of reduction of kyphosis, anterior decompression was significantly better at reducing canal compromise.

Doubt exists about whether or not surgical correction of deformity results in an improvement of symptoms. Nicoll (1949) found no correlation between the two, although more recent series have disputed this (Soreff *et al.*, 1982). Soreff *et al.*, (1982) compared 20 unstable fractures of the thoracolumbar spine managed conservatively with 18 stabilized surgically, and concluded that the incidence of residual deformity was significantly less in the surgical group (7° versus 28° residual kyphosis respectively), although the initial degree at injury was the same (20° and 18°).

Failure to correct and stabilize an acute posttraumatic kyphus increases the likelihood that the deformity will progress; this in turn may cause disabling pain or progressive neurological deficit (Malcolm *et al.*, 1981; White *et al.*, 1977). The main factors that contribute to the progression of a kyphus are failure of the anterior elements under compression (the load on the vertebral body is increased because of the moment arm created by the angulation, and is particularly likely to occur if loss of vertebral height is greater than 50%), and failure of the posterior elements, which are subjected to an increased tensile load. Malcolm *et al.* (1981) reviewed 48 patients with symptomatic post-traumatic kyphosis of the thoracic or lumbar spine; pain (94%), progressive kyphosis (39%) and neurological deficit (27%) were the major indications for intervention. Fusion was achieved by anterior, posterior or combined approaches. Pain was abolished in 67% and improved in a further 31%, despite only a 'meagre' reduction in deformity. Jodoin *et al.* (1989) reviewed the records of 16 patients who underwent anterior and/or posterior surgery to correct post-traumatic kyphosis. After a mean follow-up of 38 months, there was an average loss of correction of 3.5°. Roberson and Whiteside (1985) treated 34 late post-traumatic thoracolumbar kyphoses by anterior or posterior or combined fusion, and achieved a stable fusion with halt of progression in 33. Pain relief was good in 70% and fair in a further 15%.

Thoracic disc prolapse

Thoracic disc prolapse is uncommon, accounting for 0.15–0.8% of disc protrusions, but many cases are precipitated by a fall or other trauma (Simeone and Rashbaum, 1988). Prolapse may be acute or chronic, leading to radicular pain, long tract signs, or paraparesis. Conservative therapy is generally inappropriate, except in cases without neurological deficit. An anterior or lateral approach is reported to alleviate symptoms in 61–75% of patients (Patterson and Arbit, 1978), compared with only 32% after laminectomy (Perot and Munro, 1969).

Burst fractures

These result from failure of the vertebral body under an axial load. Fracture of anterior and middle columns may cause the posterior wall of the vertebral body to be retropulsed into the spinal canal. The main problems with this type of injury are kyphosis and encroachment on the spinal canal. Laminar fractures are a common association, occurring in 59% of patients in one series (Mumford *et al.*, 1993).

A group of 20 patients with burst fractures of L2 – L5 and not associated with neurological impairment were managed conservatively. Despite an average canal compromise of 40%, there were no patients who developed late cauda equina compression over a mean follow-up period of 3.9 years (Chan *et al.*, 1993). The risk of increase in the kyphotic deformity was small, with no patient progressing by more than 6°. All patients in employment returned to full-time work. Only 5% of these patients found it necessary to take analgesics for back pain.

A burst fracture of L5 is an uncommon injury (2.2% of thoracolumbar fractures; Finn and Stauffer, 1992). Mick *et al.* (1993) reported the outcome of a non-randomized study of 11 patients, five of whom had neurological deficit, comparing non-operative with operative treatment. The two groups are not directly comparable because those subjected to surgery had a greater degree of compromise to the spinal canal. At an average follow-up of 29 months, 60% of the non-operated group (*n* = 5) were free of pain and working full-time, 20% had mild limitation of function, and 20% had persistent severe back or leg pain. In the operated group (*n* = 6), who were managed by decompression and pedicle screw fixation, 17% were pain-free, 67% had mild pain or limitation of function but were working full-time, and 17% had moderate pain and limitation of function. Non-operative treatment was associated with a loss of lumbar lordosis (flat back) on postoperative radiographs. In contrast, Finn and Stauffer (1992) managed seven patients conservatively by immobilization for six to eight weeks in a body jacket and found no early or late loss of lumbar lordosis. After a mean follow-up of three years, all still suffered with occasional backache, two had persistent radiculopathy, and two showed radiological evidence of degeneration in the lumbar spine.

Chronic pain after thoracolumbar fractures

Bohlman *et al.* (1994) treated chronic pain in 44 patients with thoracolumbar fractures (four of which were pathological) by anterior decompression and grafting an average of 4.5 years after injury. Pain was present in the back and legs in 38, in the legs in five, and in both the back and the groin in one. The indication for anterior decompression was persistent pain with evidence of residual neural compression. Symptoms were abolished in 67% of patients, and improved in a further 26%.

Lumbar disc prolapse

Approximately 26% of patients with lumbar spondylosis have a previous history of trauma (Weinstein *et al.*, 1977). However, it can be difficult at times to prove causation since nontraumatic back pain has a high prevalence in the general population. Scandanavian studies indicate that 53% of those engaged in light work and 64% of heavy labourers will at some time experience significant low back pain (Hult, 1954). Back pain after trauma is discussed in Chapter 38.

Most cases of sciatica will resolve spontaneously. Within one month, 60–74% will be symptom-free, rising to 85% at three months (Long, 1987). Weber (1983) conducted a randomized prospective trial comparing operative with nonoperative therapy for lumbar disc prolapse. At one year, 92% of operated patients and 60% of those managed conservatively had improved substantially. However, there was no significant difference between the two groups at four and 10 years. Caspar *et al.* (1991) reported recently the results of 299 microdiscectomies. Good or excellent results were achieved in 74% of patients, with 89% returning to their previous occupation.

Spondylolisthesis

Dickman *et al.* (1992) undertook transpedicular screw/rod fixation in 29 patients with spondylolisthesis and an additional 75 patients with other pathologies. Spondylolistheses were fused *in situ* for acute instability or chronic pain, with no attempt at reduction. Of the whole group, 89% of those with neurological deficit showed some improvement. Although the osseous fusion rate was 96%, only 21% of patients had near or complete resolution of back pain, 59% had moderate intermittent back pain but were able to work, and 20% remained incapacitated by severe pain. Instrument failure (loosening/breakage) ultimately occurred in 17%, of which half were symptomatic and required revision.

Sacral and coccygeal injury

Fewer than 5% of sacral fractures occur in isolation. Pelvic fractures involve the sacrum in 45% of patients (Levine, 1992). Neurological deficit occurs in 6% of alar fractures, in 28% of those involving the foraminae, and in 57% of those with sacral canal encroachment (Denis *et al.*, 1988). Roy-Camille *et al.* (1985) reported on the treatment of 13 patients with transverse fractures of the upper sacrum. Of 11 patients available for follow-up, all but one showed some recovery of peripheral nerve involvement, but only one patient regained cauda equina neurological function. However, the results for peripheral nerve recovery in this series may be unduly optimistic. The prognosis for recovery of foot drop in another series of 16 patients was poor in 75% of cases (Patterson and Morton, 1961). This is in line with the results of an autopsy study of severe pelvic injuries, in which nerve root avulsions were identified in 40% (Huittinen, 1976). None of the 10 patients followed up long term by Patterson and Morton (1961) attained full neurological recovery, although seven returned to heavy work with little disability.

Coccydynia

This is defined as pain in and around the coccyx. It occurs typically when sitting, or rising from the sitting position. Wray *et al.* (1991) conducted a five-year trial of treatment in 120 patients and concluded that physiotherapy was of little benefit, but that 60% of patients responded to infiltration of the region with steroid and local anaesthetic. Manipulation of the coccyx combined with injection brought relief in 85% of patients. Coccygectomy was undertaken in 19%, with a success rate of 91%. Although a number of patients had evidence of lumbar disc disease, this was not significant in the aetiology of the pain. Only three of 50 patients subjected to a comprehensive psychological assessment exhibited abnormal personality traits.

Chronic donor site pain from iliac crest bone grafting

Fernyhough *et al.* (1992) evaluated by questionnaire 151 patients in whom bone was harvested from the iliac crest for spinal fusion. The most common complications were chronic pain, hypaesthesia, dysaesthesia or anaesthesia over the donor site. However, many other complications have also been described, including visceral injury and lumbar hernia (Kurz *et al.* 1989). The authors concluded that the incidence of chronic donor site pain 1–10 years after surgery was 18% in spinal trauma but 39% when bone was harvested for spinal reconstruction. Typically, the pain was exacerbated by cold/damp weather or local pressure. Whether the incision was vertical or oblique made no difference to the incidence of long-term sequelae. The treatment and prognosis of this condition was not discussed.

Paediatric spinal injury

Vertebral column injury is relatively uncommon in children, with those under 12 years accounting for less than 3–5% of spinal cord trauma victims (Hadley *et al.*, 1988a; Ruge *et al.*, 1988). The most common mechanism of injury is simple wedge compression (approximately 40%) (Evans and Bethem, 1989). The changing anatomy and biomechanics of the vertebral column during development makes certain areas of the paediatric spine more vulnerable than others at different ages. The immature spine is more mobile because of ligamentous laxity, underdevelopment of the cervical musculature, incomplete ossification of the vertebrae, wedge-shaped vertebral bodies, and shallow horizontally-directed facet joints (Henrys *et al.*, 1977). Four distinct patterns of injury occur in children, namely fracture only, fracture with subluxation, subluxation only, and spinal cord injury without radiological abnormality (Hadley *et al.*, 1988a).

The cervical spine accounts for 75% of injuries between infancy and the age of eight years, and 60% of those occurring in the 8–14 year age group. Beyond this, the pattern of injury parallels the adult population (Menezes and Osenbach, 1994). The reason for this is the combination of a relatively large head on top of a hypermobile cartilaginous spine with lax ligaments. Injuries under the age of eight years tend to be avulsions, epiphyseal separations or fractures of the growth plate, rather than true fractures (Menezes and Osenbach, 1994).

In children under the age of eight years, 50% of the cervical fractures occur between the occiput and C2 (Hadley *et al.*, 1988a). However, after this age, the spine behaves in an 'adult-type' way, and lower cervical injuries predominate. In a series of 24 patients aged between four and 18 years, 71% of injuries were below C2 (Evans and Bethem, 1989).

Most paediatric spinal injuries can be managed non-operatively. In one series of 122 patients, only 16% required primary surgery (Hadley *et al.*, 1988a). The indications for surgery included non-reducible or markedly unstable injuries, significant subluxation, spinal cord compression with incomplete spinal cord injury, and injuries that remained unstable after conservative management. Of 22 such cervical spinal injuries treated conservatively, 14% developed kyphotic deformity at an average follow-up of 16 months, but none developed pain (Evans and Bethem, 1989). Most of the late sequelae developed in patients with wedge compression fractures.

McGrory and Klassen (1994) reviewed 42 children aged 1–15 years who underwent arthrodesis for traumatic instability of the cervical spine a minimum of seven years previously. There was no change in stability, deformity or the fusion mass during follow-up, but a significant increase in osteoarthritic changes in unfused segments was observed in 29% of these patients. Other complications included spontaneous extension of the fusion in 38%, pain or dysaesthesia at the donor site in

14%, and incomplete fusion in 2%. There was no significant difference in outcome between groups below or above the age of 10 years. Outcome was not dependent upon whether the injury involved the upper or the lower cervical spine. An extension of the fusion occurred more frequently after upper cervical injury, and when subluxation or dislocation had occurred.

Progressive post-traumatic spinal deformity is very common in children, particularly those who are rendered paraplegic by their injuries. The exception are those children who are near the end of their growth period. The major contributing factors to deformity are destruction of the growth centres, ischaemic necrosis of the epiphyseal growth plates, paralysis of the postural muscles below the level of injury, and secondary changes in the vertebral bodies due to deficient growth on the concave and excessive growth on the convex sides of a developing curve. The incidence of progressive spinal deformity in children with long-term follow-up exceeds 90% (Bradford, 1987).

References

Aglietti P, DiMuria GV, Taylor T. (1983) Conservative treatment of thoracic and lumbar vertebral fractures. *Ital J Orthop Traumatol* (Suppl): 83–87.

Aldrich EF, Weber PB, Crow WN (1993) Halifax interlaminar clamp for posterior cervical fusion: a long-term follow-up review. *J Neurosurg* **78**: 702–708.

Anderson LD, D'Alonzo RT (1974) Fractures of the odontoid process of the axis. *J Bone Joint Surg Am* **56A**: 1663–74.

Beatson TR. (1963) Fractures and dislocations of the cervical spine. *J Bone Joint Surg Br* **45B**: 21–35.

Benzel EC, Hart BL, Ball PA, Baldwin NG, Orrison WW, Espinosa M. (1994) Fractures of the C-2 vertebral body. *J Neurosurg* **81**: 206–12.

Berrington NR, van Standen JF, Willers JG, van der Westhuizen J. (1993) Cervical intervertebral disc prolapse associated with traumatic facet dislocations. *Surg Neurol* **40**: 395–99.

Beyer CA, Cabanela ME, Berquist TH. (1991) Unilateral facet dislocations and fracture-dislocations of the cervical spine. *J Bone Joint Surg Br* **73B**: 977–81.

Bohlman HH, Kirkpatrick JS, Delamarter RB, Leventhal M. (1994) Anterior decompression for late pain and paralysis after fractures of the thoracolumbar spine. *Clin Orthop Rel Res* **300**: 24–29.

Bradford DS. (1987) Deformities of the thoracic and lumbar spine secondary to spinal injury In: Bradford DS, Lonstein JE, Moe JH, Ogilvie JW, Winter RB, editor. *Moe's textbook of scoliosis and other spinal deformities* 2nd edition. Philadelphia: Saunders, 435–63.

Burke DC. (1973) Pain in paraplegia. *Paraplegia* **10**: 297–313.

Cammisa FP, Eismont FJ, Green BA. (1989) Dural laceration occurring with burst fractures and associated lumbar fractures. *J Bone Joint Surg Am* **71A**: 1044–52.

Cantor JB, Lebwohl NH, Garvey T, Eismont FJ. (1993) Nonoperative management of stable thoracolumbar burst fractures with early ambulation and bracing. *Spine* **18**: 971–76.

Caspar W, Campbell B, Barbier DD, Kretschmmer R, Gotfried Y. (1991) The Caspar microsurgical discectomy and comparison with a conventional standard lumbar disc procedure. *Neurosurgery* **28**: 78–87.

Chan DPK, Seng NK, Kaan KT. (1993) Nonoperative treatment of burst fractures of the lumbar spine (L2–5) without neurologic deficits. *Spine* **18**: 320–25.

Chance GQ. (1948) Note on a type of flexion fracture of the spine. *Br J Radiol* **21**: 452–53.

Cobb JR. (1948) Outline for the study of scoliosis In: JW Edwards. *Instructional course lectures: the American Academy of Orthopedic Surgeons*, vol. 5. Michigan: Ann Arbor, 261–75.

Davis JW, Phreaner DL, Hoyt DB, Mackersie RC. (1993) The etiology of missed cervical spine injuries. *J Trauma* **34**: 342–46.

Della Torre P, Rinonapoli E. (1992) Halo-cast treatment of fractures and dislocations of the cervical spine. *Int Orthop* **16**: 227–31.

Denis F. (1983) The three column spine and its significance in the classification of acute thoracolumbar spinal injuries. *Spine* **8**: 817–31.

Denis F, Davis S, Comfort T. (1988) Sacral fractures: an important problem. Retrospective analysis of 236 cases. *Clin Orthop Rel Res* **227**: 67–81.

Dickman CA, Fessler RG, MacMillan M, Haid RW. (1992) Transpedicular screw-rod fixation of the lumbar spine: operative technique and outcome in 104 cases. *J Neurosurg* **77**: 860–70.

Eismont FJ, Clifford S, Goldberg M, Green B. (1984) Cervical sagittal spinal canal size in spine injury. *Spine* **9**: 663–66.

Eismont FJ, Arena MJ, Green BA. (1991) Extrusion of an intervertebral disc associated with traumatic subluxation or dislocation of cervical facets. *J Bone Joint Surg Am* **73A**: 1555–60.

Esses SI, Botsford DJ, Kostuik JP. (1990) Evaluation of surgical treatment for burst fractures. *Spine* **15**: 667–73.

Etter C, Coscia M, Jaberg H, Aebi M. (1991) Direct anterior fixation of dens fractures with a cannulated screw system. *Spine* **16**: S25–S31.

Evans DL, Bethem D. (1989) Cervical spine injuries in children. *J Pediatr Orthop* **9**: 563–68.

Fehlings MG, Cooper PR, Errico TJ. (1994) Posterior plates in the management of cervical instability: long-term results in 44 patients. *J Neurosurg* **81**: 341–49.

Fernyhough JC, Schimandle JJ, Weigel MC, Edwards CC, Levine AM. (1992) Chronic donor site pain complicating bone graft harvesting from the posterior iliac crest for spinal fusion. *Spine* **17**: 1474–80.

Finn CA, Stauffer ES. (1992) Burst fracture of the fifth lumbar vertebra. *J Bone Joint Surg Am* **74A**: 398–403.

Flanders AE, Schaefer DM, Doan HT, Mishkin MM, Gonzalez CF, Northrup BE. (1990) Acute cervical spine trauma: correlation of MR imaging findings with degree of neurological deficit. *Radiology* **177**: 25–33.

Frankel HL, Hancock DO, Hyslop G, *et al.* (1969) The value of postural reduction in the initial management of closed injuries of the spine with paraplegia and tetraplegia: Part I. *Paraplegia* **7**: 179–92.

Garfin SR, Botte MJ, Waters RL, Nickel VL. (1986) Complications in the use of the halo fixation device. *J Bone Joint Surg Am* **68A**: 320–25.

Gerrelts BD, Petersen EU, Mabry J, Petersen SR. (1991) Delayed diagnosis of cervical spine injuries. *J Trauma* **31**: 1622–26.

Glaser JA, Whitehill R, Stamp WG, Jane JA. (1986) Complications associated with the halo-vest. A review of 245 cases. *J Neurosurg* **65**: 762–69.

Hadley MN, Browner C, Sonntag VKH. (1985) Axis fractures: a comprehensive review of management and treatment in 107 cases. *Neurosurgery* **17**: 281–90.

Hadley MN, Sonntag VKH, Grahm TW, Masferrer R, Browner C. (1986) Axis fractures resulting from motor vehicle accidents. The need for occupant restraints. *Spine* **11**: 861–64.

Hadley MN, Zabramski JM, Browner CM, Rekate H, Sonntag VKH. (1988a) Pediatric spinal trauma. Review of 122 cases of spinal cord and vertebral column injuries. *J Neurosurg* **68**: 18–24.

Hadley MN, Dickman CA, Browner CM, Sonntag VKH. (1988b) Acute traumatic atlas fractures: management and long-term outcome. *Neurosurgery* **23**: 31–35.

Henrys P, Lyne ED, Lifton C, Salciccioli G. (1977) Clinical review of cervical spine injuries in children. *Clin Orthop Rel Res* **129**: 172–76.

Holdsworth F. (1970) Fractures, dislocations, and fracture-dislocations of the spine. *J Bone Joint Surg Am* **52A**: 1534–51.

Huele DF, O'Day J, Mendelsohn RA. (1981) Cervical injuries suffered in automobile crashes. *J Neurosurg* **54**: 316–22.

Huittinen V-M. (1976) Lumbosacral nerve injury in fracture of the pelvis. *Acta Chir Scand* **Suppl 429**: 7–43.

Hult L. (1954) The Munkfors investigation. *Acta Orthop Scand* **suppl 16**: 5–76.

Jodoin A, Gillet P, Dupuis PR, Maurais G. (1989) Surgical treatment of post-traumatic kyphosis: a report of 16 cases. *Can J Surg* **32**: 36–42.

Kesterson L, Benzel E, Orrison W, Coleman J. (1991) Evaluation and treatment of atlas burst fractures (Jefferson fractures). *J Neurosurg* **75**: 213–20.

Kurz LT, Garfin SR, Booth RE. (1989) Harvesting autologous iliac bone grafts: a review of complications and techniques. *Spine* **14**: 1324–31.

Ladd AL, Scranton PE. (1986) Congenital cervical stenosis presenting as transient quadriplegia in athletes: report of two cases. *J Bone Joint Surg Am* **68A**: 1371–74.

Levine AM. (1992) Lumbar and sacral spine trauma. In: Browner BD, Jupiter JB, Levine AM, Trafton PG, editors. *Skeletal trauma. Fractures, dislocations, ligamentous injuries*. Philadelphia PA: Saunders, 805–48.

Lintner DM, Knight RQ, Cullen JP. (1993) The neurologic sequelae of cervical spine facet injuries. The role of canal diameter. *Spine* **18**: 725–29.

Long DM. (1987) Nonsurgical therapy for low back pain and sciatica. *Clin Neurosurg* **35**: 351–59.

Malcolm BW, Bradford DS, Winter RB, Chou SN. (1981) Post-traumatic kyphosis. A review of forty-eight surgically treated patients. *J Bone Joint Surg Am* **63A**: 891–99.

Matsuura P, Waters RL, Adkins RH, Rothman S, Gurbani N, Sie I. (1989) Comparison of computerized tomography parameters of the cervical spine in normal control subjects and spinal cord-injured patients. *J Bone Joint Surg Am* **71A**: 183–88.

McGrory BJ, Klassen RA. (1994) Arthrodesis of the cervical spine for fractures and dislocations in children and adolescents. A long-term follow-up study. *J Bone Joint Surg Am* **76A**: 1606–16.

Menezes AH, Osenbach RK. (1994) Spinal cord injury In: Cheek WR, editor. *Pediatric neurosurgery: surgery of the developing nervous system*, 3rd edition. Philadelphia PA: Saunders, 320–43.

Mick CA, Carl A, Sachs B, Hresko MT, Pfeifer BA. (1993) Burst fractures of the fifth lumbar vertebra. *Spine* **18**: 1878–84.

Montesano PX, Anderson PA, Schlehr F, Thalgott JS, Lowrey G. (1991) Odontoid fractures treated by anterior odontoid screw fixation. *Spine* **11**: S33–S37.

Mumford J, Weinstein JN, Spratt KF, Goel VK. (1993) Thoracolumbar burst fractures. The clinical efficacy and outcome of nonoperative management. *Spine* **18**: 955–70.

Nicholl EA. (1949) Fractures of the dorsolumbar spine. *J Bone Joint Surg Br* **31B**: 376–94.

Patterson FP, Morton KS. (1961) Neurologic complications of fractures and dislocations of the pelvis. *Surg Gynecol Obstet* **112**: 702–706.

Patterson RH Jr, Arbit E. (1978) A surgical approach through the pedicle to protruded thoracic discs. *J Neurosurg* **48**: 768–72.

Perot PL Jr, Munro DD. (1969) Transthoracic removal of midline thoracic disc protrusions causing spinal cord compression. *J Neurosurg* **31**: 452–58.

Raynor RB. (1977) Cervical cord compression secondary to acute disc protrusion in trauma. Incidence and response to decompression. *Spine* **2**: 39–43.

Reid DC, Henderson R, Saboe L, Miller JDR. (1987) Etiology and clinical course of missed spine fractures. *J Trauma* **27**: 980–86.

Riggins RS, Kaus JF. (1977) The risk of neurologic damage with fractures of the vertebrae. *J Trauma* **17**: 126–33.

Ripa DR, Kowall MG, Meyer PR, Rusin JJ. (1991) Series of ninety-two traumatic cervical spine injuries stabilized with anterior ASIF plate fusion technique. *Spine* **16**: S46–S55.

Rizzolo SJ, Piazza MR, Cotler JM, Hume EL, Cautilli G, O'Neill DK. (1993) The effect of torque pressure on halo pin complication rates. A prospective study. *Spine* **18**: 2163–66.

Roberson JR, Whitesides TE. (1985) Surgical reconstruction of late post-traumatic thoracolumbar kyphosis. *Spine* **10**: 307–12.

Rorabeck CH, Rock MG, Hawkins RJ, Bourne RB. (1987) Unilateral facet dislocation of the cervical spine. An analysis of the results of treatment in 26 patients. *Spine* **12**: 23–27.

Roy-Camille R, Saillant G, Gagna G, Mazel C. (1985) Transverse fracture of the upper sacrum. Suicidal jumpers fracture. *Spine* **10**: 838–45.

Ruge JR, Sinson GP, McLone DG, Cerullo LJ. (1988) Pediatric spinal injury: the very young. *J Neurosurg* **68**: 25–30.

Ryan MD, Henderson JJ. (1992) The epidemiology of fractures and fracture-dislocations of the cervical spine. *Injury* **23**: 38–40.

Saboe LA, Reid DC, Davis LA, Warren SA, Grace MG. (1991) Spine trauma and associated injuies. *J Trauma* **31**: 43–48.

Sasso RC, Cotler HB. (1993) Posterior instrumentation and fusion for unstable fractures and fracture-dislocations of the thoracic and lumbar spine. A comparative study of three fixation devices in 70 patients. *Spine* **18**: 450–60.

Simeone FA, Rashbaum R. (1988) Transthoracic disc excision In: Schmidek H, Sweet W, editors. *Operative neurosurgical Techniques*, 2nd edition. Orlando: Grune & Stratton, 1367–74.

Soreff J, Axdorph G, Bylund P, Odeen I, Olerud S. (1982) Treatment of patients with unstable fractures of the thoracic and lumbar spine: a follow-up study of surgical and conservative treatment. *Acta Orthop Scand* **53**: 369–81.

Watts C, Smith H, Knoller N. (1993) Risks and cost-effectiveness of sublaminar wiring in posterior fusion of the cervical spine. *Surg Neurol* **40**: 457–60.

Weber H. (1983) Lumbar disc herniation: a controlled prospective study with 10 years of observation. *Spine* **8**: 131–40.

Weinstein JN, Collatto P, Lehman TR. (1988) Thoracolurban 'burst' fractures treated conservatively. A Long-term follow-up. *Spine* **13**: 33–38.

Weinstein PR, Ehni G, Wilson CB. (1977) Clinical features of lumbar spondylosis and stenosis. In: Weinstein PR, Ehni G, Wilson CB, editors. *Lumbar spondylosis: diagnosis, management, and surgical treatment*. Chicago: Year Book, 115–33.

White AA, Johnson RM, Panjabi MM, Southwick WO. (1975) Biomechanical analysis of clinical stability in the cervical spine. *Clin Orthop Rel Res* **109**: 85–96.

White AA, Southwick WO, Panjabi MM. (1976) Clinical instability in the lower cervical spine. A review of past and current concepts. *Spine* **1**: 15–27.

White AA, Panjabi MM, Thomas CL. (1977) The clinical biomechanics of kyphotic deformities. *Clin Orthop Rel Res* **128**: 8–17.

Wray CC, Easom S, Hopkinson J. (1991) Coccydinia. Aetiology and treatment. *J Bone Joint Surg Br* **73B**: 335–38.

36

Post-traumatic syringomyelia

Spiros Sgouros, the late Bernard Williams

Introduction

Syringomyelia is a condition characterized by longitudinal cavities extending over several segments within the spinal cord. It is not a disease, but a process that may be associated with a variety of other pathologies, such as hindbrain herniation, spinal tumours, or traumatic paraplegia. In all circumstances there seems to be a functional obstruction in the subarachnoid space, which creates a pressure differential. If the cavities spread upwards they may destroy not only neurological function in the arms but eventually affect the lower brain stem, producing respiratory paralysis and death.

Epidemiology

The incidence of post-traumatic syringomyelia is around 1–3% of all patients with paraplegia (Barnett and Jousse, 1976; Rossier et al., 1985). Why so few patients develop syringomyelia following spinal cord injury is not known. There is a male predominance and a relatively young mean age. This is characteristic of paraplegia in general. From a total of 583 patients treated in the Syringomyelia Clinic of Birmingham, UK, between 1973–1992, 43 had post-traumatic syringomyelia. Of these, 35 (81.4%) were males. The mean age at diagnosis was 33.7 years (range 17–58). Regarding the anatomical level of the injury, 17.5% had cervical, 52.5% upper thoracic, 22.5% lower thoracic, and 7.5% lumbar spinal fractures. Complete paraplegia was present in 28 patients (65.1%).

The time between injury and symptomatic presentation may vary from a few months to 30 years. An average interval of 6.8 years has been observed in our patients. It is clear that no patient is safe from the possibility of syringomyelia after complete or partial paraplegia. It may strike after any time, at any level of injury, with any degree of severity, with or without a primary cyst, and with no difference between the sexes.

Structural pathology

Pathogenesis

These patients had normal spinal cords before the injuries. As a result of trauma, cord contusion leads to oedema, blood effusion and subsequent liquefaction. In a proportion of patients this progresses to cavity formation (Kakulas, 1984). On MRI, almost 50% of cord-injured patients show a small cyst opposite the fracture site. This may be called a 'primary cyst' (Figure 36.1). When there is a lengthy syringomyelia, a similar cyst may be seen communicating with an upward- or downward-running syrinx (Figure 36.2). The primary cyst is commonly separated from the syringomyelia cavity by an intact septum. There may be more than one primary cyst; the presence of three is not uncommon. The primary cysts differ from syringomyelia because the syrinx may go flat above and below the injury site following treatment, while the primary cysts may remain unchanged. The presence of primary cysts may support the theory of cavity formation shortly after the injury (Williams, 1992).

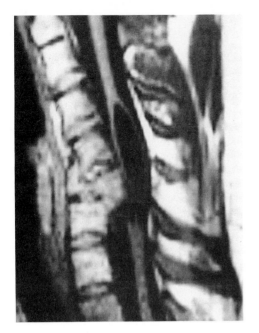

Figure 36.1. A large primary cyst in a complete paraplegic starting opposite a fracture of the C6 vertebra. This probably does not deserve to be called syringomyelia (compared with Figure 36.2). Nevertheless, a cyst of this size threatens the cord function for one-and-a-half vertebrae above the fracture and looks as though it may be life-threatening. Surgery deflated this cyst but with no observable neurological improvement. Note that the top one-third of the cord shown in this illustration is normal.

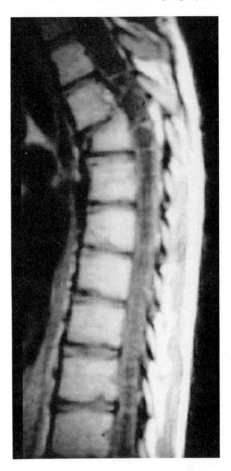

Figure 36.2. A fracture of T4 vertebra with a segmented syrinx cavity running downwards and a suggestion of one or more primary cysts. The upward cavity extending out of sight at the top of the picture is shown in Figure 36.3.

Syrinx cavities are much bigger than primary cysts and contain cerebrospinal fluid (CSF). The absence of a cavity opposite the spinal fracture in some patients, while cavities exist above and below, indicates that there may be other mechanisms contributing to cavity formation. Meningeal fibrosis may cause syringomyelia in the absence of primary cord injury. Examples include meningitis (particularly tuberculous meningitis), chemical insults such as antibiotics or myodil (Pantopaque), epidural abscess, Pott's disease or idiopathic meningeal fibrosis (Williams, 1992). There is thus some way in which fluid is forced to enter the cord.

Evolution of syringomyelia

As the acute injury settles, inflammation is followed by adhesions in the subarachnoid space and gliosis within the cord (Kakulas, 1984). Obstruction of the CSF pathways may be compounded by narrowing of the bony canal due to the spinal fracture. All these factors contribute to obstruction of the subarachnoid space opposite the fracture site, and may lead to dissociation of pressures on either side of the block (Williams, 1992).

Fluid may enter the cord at the fracture site. At operation, the cord is usually thin-walled and fluid can sometimes be seen oozing through its wall. The spinal cord is not waterproof. Potential spaces along the vessels of the cord have been described by Virchow and Robin (Williams, 1992).

Every time a Valsalva manoeuvre takes place (e.g. coughing, straining), pressure from the chest and abdominal cavities is transmitted to the spinal canal through the valveless venous plexus around the vertebral bodies. Large swings of pressure may move up to 12 ml of CSF. Normally, pressures are equalized readily between the top and bottom of the spine, with a half-life of less than 0.1 s. In the presence of a partial subarachnoid block, fluid is forced upwards past the obstruction more efficiently than it can run down again. This leads to a collapsed theca below the block. This is the 'suck' mechanism (Williams, 1992).

Fluid that has entered the cord cavity moves in response to the pressure changes that have been described. Syrinx fluid may move more readily than the CSF in the subarachnoid space, which finds some resistance from the arachnoid strands, the dentate ligaments, the vessels, and the nerve roots that connect the cord to the dura. The movement of the syrinx fluid can be violent enough to extend the excavation of the cavity both cranially and caudally. This is the 'slosh' mechanism (Williams, 1992).

Although these mechanisms account for the evolution of syrinx, there are nevertheless some observations awaiting explanation, in particular the formation of septations within the syrinx cavity (Figure 36.3), and why adjacent cavities can be under different pressures despite their apparent communication. The excavation of new cavities alongside old ones that have apparently healed usually represents a failure of drainage (Williams, 1992).

Clinical assessment

Presentation

The clinical presentation of syringomyelia following spinal cord injury is variable. The location of symptoms may be correlated with radiological examination. The most important features are those that ascend; a descending syrinx is rarely diagnosed. Cases of incomplete paraplegia which deteriorate may be associated with syringomyelia affecting the fracture site, although the significance of the syrinx may be doubtful. The symptoms can be grouped into those of pain, sensory and motor loss, and disordered autonomic function. They can be strikingly unilateral even though the syrinx occupies the central part of the cord.

Bulbar features

Ascending syringomyelia may cut into the lowermost part of the medulla. Such a syrinx comprises the ascending form of syringobulbia. The most common symptom is spreading numbness of the face. Swallowing and phonation may also be affected, followed by vision, hearing and finally respiratory function.

Symptoms below the established level of paraplegia

Following incomplete paraplegia, deterioration of motor and sensory function can be observed as well as new autonomic dysfunction. In complete paraplegia, an improvement of leg spasms could imply a downward extension of the syrinx, so also could an alteration of sweating patterns and impairment of other autonomic functions such as bladder and bowel control or sexual function. New contralateral symptoms in a patient who has had drainage treatment for a deteriorating syrinx and has been stable for a while may imply the excavation of a new cavity alongside the previous one.

Pain is common in post-traumatic syringomyelia. A paraplegic patient complaining of severe pain has syringomyelia until proven otherwise (Williams, 1992). It is frequently precipitated by straining and

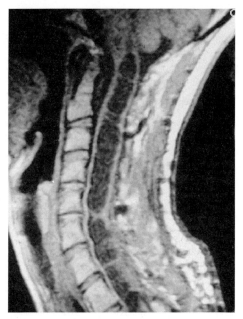

Figure 36.3. Severe syringomyelia cavity spreading up to the top of the spinal cord. Same patient as Figure 36.2. Note the transverse septations. A syrinx of this size is compatible with total paralysis and death. The patient was astonishingly well with severe sensory changes but almost normal motor function. Surgery for such a patient is mandatory.

associated with progression of neurological deficit. Although pain is commonly experienced at the level of the deficit, it can affect sites above or below that level, and may be confused with chest or abdominal pathology. Not infrequently it is soon replaced by dysaesthetic sensory loss.

The degree of sensory loss can also be variable. Usually it is unilateral and tends to involve the upper limb early, progressing by an increase in the density of the deficit more often than by anatomical extension. The classic description of dissociated sensory loss (loss of pain and temperature sensation with preserved light touch and proprioception) is not always present. It can even be variable throughout the course of the day, and is related presumably to a variable state of filling of the syrinx.

The motor loss follows a similar pattern to the sensory loss. Unilateral involvement of one upper limb, not infrequently associated with a sudden strain and associated pain, is seen commonly. An ascending syrinx may first affect the inferior part of the cervical enlargement. The small muscles of the hand become weak, and wasting of the first dorsal interosseous muscle may be an early finding. As with all the other features, any level can be affected first without necessarily following an anatomical pattern. Thus, the triceps or the shoulder musculature could be affected before the hand. In patients with advanced disease it is not uncommon to find a claw deformity in the hand with wasting of the forearm and arm musculature. In a similar fashion, the loss of the arm tendon reflexes can be observed (Dworkin and Staas, 1985; Umbach and Heilporn, 1991). Asymmetry is not uncommon and certain reflexes may be spared unexpectedly.

A variety of autonomic disturbances can be seen in post-traumatic syringomyelia (Barnett and Jousse, 1976). Gross disturbance of sweating occurs (Stanworth, 1983). Dry skin or hyperidrosis can be observed, usually symmetrically in the lower half of the body, although the upper limbs may be affected in an asymmetrical distribution with facial involvement at times. Occasionally, unequal pupils may be the only feature.

Radiology

Radiological studies include plain radiographs and MRI scanning. Plain films often show post-traumatic kyphosis and associated narrowing of the spinal canal.

Prior to the advent of MRI, postmyelography CT scanning was the investigation of choice for such patients. The entry of contrast into the syrinx is not usually immediate, and it may be necessary to repeat the CT scan some hours later. MRI is excellent for delineation of the syringomyelic cavity and septa (Figure 36.2). Detailed anatomy and an estimate of tension within the cavity can be assessed, as can the relationship between the syrinx and any primary cord cyst (Quencer, 1988). Information relating to CSF circulation is useful, both for assessing the results of treatment and for following patients over time.

Treatment

In some patients the need for treatment is obvious at presentation.

The patient with a sudden onset of symptoms, possibly related to straining, and with radiological evidence of a syrinx extending over a number of segments, demands treatment. Similarly, a tense syrinx occupying the cervical cord, even if asymptomatic, merits surgical treatment. On the other hand, the patient with a small, single-level cavity and with no symptoms relating to it can be watched.

The difficult group of patients are those with unremarkable symptoms and whose syrinx is not progressing, or is of moderate fullness. When, in addition, the paraplegia is incomplete, a decision for or against surgery can be difficult. The risk of allowing further deterioration to occur by not intervening surgically is evident. It is not uncommon for a patient who has what appears to be a stable syrinx to develop rapid clinical deterioration after a number of years. However, as there is a complication rate associated with any operative procedure, it is often difficult to justify surgery in stable patients. As the natural history of syringomyelia can be variable, it is recommended to err towards early surgical treatment, as it is likely that untreated patients will deteriorate. In general, we believe that early surgery offers better long-term results (Williams, 1994c).

The surgical procedures have evolved over the years. The use of syringosubarachnoid and syringopleural shunts has been recommended. Early results were encouraging (Barbaro, 1991; Bleasel *et al.*, 1991; Edgar and Quail, 1994; Lesoin *et al.*, 1986; Lyons *et al.*, 1987; Padovani *et al.*, 1989; Peerless and Durward, 1982; Rossier *et al.*, 1985; Shannon *et al.*, 1981; Umbach and Heilporn, 1991;

Williams and Page, 1987), but long-term effectiveness has been questioned (Sgouros and Williams, 1995; Williams, 1994a). As clinical observation gradually improved our understanding of the filling mechanism, the philosophy of the primary treatment moved towards decompressive laminectomy and the formation of a surgical meningocoele. Drainage procedures have little place in the management of syringomyelia; they have a variety of associated problems. Infection of the drain has been reported, as well as mechanical failure (Sgouros and Williams, 1995). The drain functions for some time, the cord collapses around it, and the draining holes become occluded by gliotic tissue. Subsequently, the syrinx reaccumulates if the filling mechanism has not been addressed surgically. A proportion of patients continue to deteriorate despite drainage. Of 19 patients treated with a syringopleural shunt at the Syringomyelia Clinic, 15 improved initially, but seven of these patients subsequently deteriorated. Three patients remained stable and one deteriorated in the immediate postoperative period. Three drains became dislodged and migrated, requiring further surgery, whereas three other drains were found to be blocked at reoperation. Of the four patients treated with syringosubarachnoid shunts, two deteriorated postoperatively.

The present treatment in this clinic is decompressive laminectomy, opening of the subarachnoid pathways past the fracture site, and the formation of a surgical meningocoele (Sgouros and Williams, 1996). A wide laminectomy is performed, centred on the fracture site and extending over up to five laminae, depending on the extent of the meningeal fibrosis. The dura is opened and the subarachnoid adhesions are divided. An artificial meningocoele is created by leaving the dura open (Williams, 1994b). The subarachnoid space may be kept patent by using temporary stents, which are removed in the early postoperative period. The filling mechanism of the syrinx is disabled as the partial subarachnoid block is bypassed through the meningocoele (Figure 36.4).

Of the eight patients treated surgically by decompressive laminectomy in this clinic during the last three years, seven have remained clinically stable or improved at a minimum follow-up of one year. In comparison, seven of the 19 patients treated primarily with syringopleural shunt in the early 1980s deteriorated clinically following an immediate postoperative improvement. Of these, four deteriorated within the first year and the other three at between two and six years. Similarly, of

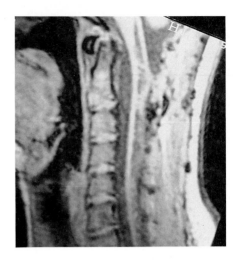

Figure 36.4. Same patient as Figures 36.2 and 36.3. This is the postoperative result, which shows good deflation of the syrinx. It seems probable that the prognosis has been improved by this surgery but the progression of the neurological deficits related to gliosis (scarring of the cord tissues) over the next 20 years or so is unpredictable. Note that on this image the cavity goes up into the skull.

four patients treated with syringosubarachnoid shunts, two deteriorated clinically, both within a year of surgery. The results of a cumulative series reported from the literature are shown in Table 36.1 (Barbaro, 1991).

Comparisons between drainage procedures performed in previous years and decompressive surgery performed in recent years is difficult because of the differences in follow-up periods.

Cord transection is an effective alternative for patients with complete paraplegia (Barnett and Jousse, 1976; Shannon *et al.*, 1981; Williams, 1992). In the 1980s at the Syringomyelia Clinic, eight patients were treated with cord transection in association with the insertion of a syringopleural shunt. All of them improved and there have been no late relapses (Sgouros and Williams, 1995). Omental graft transposition has been recommended but, in our experience, offers no advantage over decompressive laminectomy. It is associated with considerable morbidity, and hence has been abandoned.

Complications

The surgical complication rate is low for post-traumatic syringomyelia. Wound infection, meningitis, urinary tract infection and thromboembolic

Table 36.1. Results of surgery for post-traumatic syringomyelia

Series	Outcome		
	Improved	*Unchanged*	*Worse*
Barbaro *et al.* (1984) (*n* = 6)	3	2	1
Barnett *et al.* (1973) (*n* = 7)	4	2	1
Edgar (1976) (*n* = 6)	5	1	0
Peerless and Durward (1983) (*n* = 26)	12	8	6
Tator and Briceno (1988) (*n* = 11)	6	2	3
Williams and Page (1987) (*n* = 10)	3	5	2
Total (%) (*n* = 66)	33 (50)	20 (30)	13 (20)

(Adapted from Barbaro, 1991)

complications have all been observed. Of the 43 patients treated at the Syringomyelia Clinic, one suffered a wound infection, one developed a CSF leak from the laminectomy wound, two developed meningitis and there was one urinary tract infection. Two cases of postoperative confusion were associated with pneumocephalus seen on cranial CT scan. No perioperative mortality was recorded.

Measurement of outcome

Following successful treatment, many symptoms improve with a varying pattern. It should be noted that most surgical treatment modalities are associated with good early results, although the long-term effectiveness can vary (Williams, 1992).

Paraplegia is a severe disability. Nevertheless, it is possible for people with paraplegia to retain their independence. Ascending syringomyelia has the capacity to damage sensation and motor function of the arms. The effects of operation do not reverse the cord damage. Even after apparently successful surgery, the following problems may result.

Loss of pain sensitivity is not of great consequence on its own but it leads to other problems, particularly if the motor system is intact and the patient uses the arms energetically. Trophic changes may supervene in skin or joints. Skin lesions include a propensity to multiple burns, and there is tendency to self-mutilation affecting the intellectually challenged, including nail biting and picking at sores or callosities. The fingers may become coarsely thickened and painless hands may be damaged by a wheelchair. Damage to joints that have lost pain sensation may be severe (neuropathic or Charcot joints); about half are painful. The process of destruction proceeds rapidly once it

has started. In the shoulder, the head of the humerus may rapidly absorb. The process is more than impairment of painful impulses and the body attacks and dissolves its own joint. The elbow tends to become overgrown with massive osteophytes and limitation of movement is common. Of 583 patients with syringomyelia treated in our clinic, 35 have Charcot joints (6%) (Table 36.2). Two of these patients belong in the post-traumatic group. The mean age at presentation of this condition is about 20 years after the first clinical manifestations of syringomyelia.

In addition, these patients have an increased risk of developing cervical spondylosis, which is possibly related to increased use of their arms as a result of the paraplegia.

All the sufferers of post-traumatic syringomyelia treated in the Syringomyelia Clinic were asked to score their performance in a variety of aspects relevant to activities of daily living and to assess the effect of surgery. The questionnaire used was a modification of the scale of the Japanese Orthopedic Association (1975) for cervical myelopathy. The mean time from injury to surgery in this group was 9.8 years (range 1–33), and the mean length of

Table 36.2. Thirty-eight Charcot's joints in 35 patients from a database of 583 cases of syringomyelia

	Hindbrain-related	*Nonhindbrain-related*
Neck	2	0
Shoulder	21	1
Elbows	6	2
Wrists	1	0
Fingers	2	0
Legs	3	0
Total	35	3

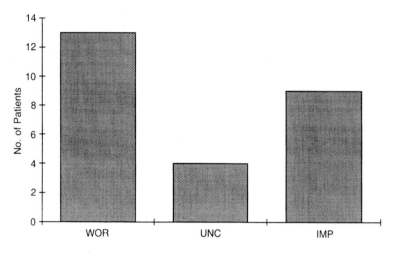

26 Patients

Figure 36.5. Diagram showing the overall outcome of patients with post-traumatic syringomyelia, irrespective of the treatment modalities employed. A significant proportion of patients (50%) deteriorated over the years despite treatment. All these patients had radiological improvement of the syrinx on MRI, although for some more than one operation proved necessary. With recent improvements in the understanding of the condition that proportion may improve. WOR, worse; UNC, unchanged; IMP, improved.

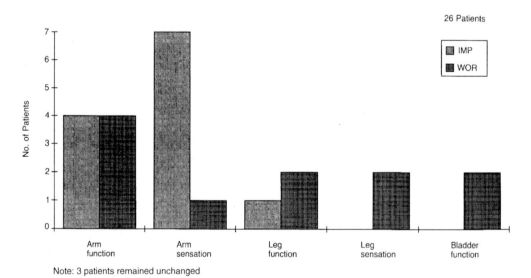

Note: 3 patients remained unchanged

Figure 36.6. Diagram showing long-term changes in arm and leg function and sensation as well as bladder function in patients with post-traumatic syringomyelia, irrespective of the treatment modalities employed. Although in some patients arm function and sensation improved with treatment, all other aspects deteriorated, but not significantly. All these patients had improved radiological appearances on MRI. (Changes in leg function and sensation would not be expected in view of the paraplegia.) It should be noted that the improvement in arm sensation and motor function was observed in patients that were of good grade at presentation. IMP, improved; WOR, worse.

follow-up postoperatively was 7.3 years (18 months – 33.5 years). Thirty-six questionnaires were delivered, and 26 patients responded (72%). Of these, 34.6% reported overall improvement after surgery, in comparison with 15.4% who reported no change and 50% who reported deterioration. It is of interest that all these patients had radiological improvement even though more than one operation proved necessary in some cases. The results are shown in Figure 36.5. Similarly, Figure 36.6 shows the effect of surgery on a variety of functional aspects, including limb motor and sensory function, as well as bladder function.

Prognosis

If untreated, syringomyelia follows a progressive course. The cavity may extend both proximally and distally as the tension of the fluid within it continues to increase. Eventually it may affect the upper cervical cord, disrupting respiration and leading to death (Williams, 1994c).

Postmortem studies have shown that a chronic syrinx provokes gliosis in the cavity walls and the surrounding cord (Foo *et al.*, 1989; Sgouros and Williams, 1995). A drain inserted in the syrinx may become encased by gliotic tissue (Sgouros and Williams, 1995). Even though surgical treatment may lead to radiological collapse of the syrinx cavity, often this is not associated with clinical improvement. Gliosis inside the cord may lead to progressive loss of function, even after successful surgery (Williams, 1994c).

Most post-traumatic syringomyelia occurs in either complete or badly damaged patients with paraplegia. Clearly, the development of syringomyelia worsens almost all aspects of paraplegia or quadriplegia. Quality of life, morbidity and mortality are all affected adversely. Whiteneck observed that the problems of paraplegic patients markedly exceeded those of the normal population at all ages, and for quadriplegics the outlook was worse than for paraplegics by a factor of 1.4 (Whiteneck *et al.*, 1992). A similar multiplier might be applied for patients with post-traumatic syringomyelia, depending upon the extent of the problems.

References

Barbaro NM. (1991) Surgery for primarily spinal syringomyelia. In: Batzdorf U, editor. *Syringomyelia concept in diagnosis and treatment.* Baltimore MD: Williams & Wilkins, 183–98.

Barbaro NM, Wilson CB, Gutin PH, Edwards MSB. (1984) Surgical treatment of syringomyelia. Favorable results with syringoperitoneal shunting. *J Neurosurg* **61**: 513–38.

Barnett HJM, Jousse AT. (1976) Post-traumatic syringomyelia (cystic myelopathy). In: Vinken PJ, Bruyn GW, editors. *Handbook of clinical neurology*, vol. 26. Amsterdam: North-Holland, 113–57.

Barnett HJM, Foster JB, Hudgson P, editors. (1973) *Syringomyelia.* (Major problems in neurology, vol. 1.) London: Saunders.

Dworkin GE, Staas WE. (1985) Post-traumatic syringomyelia. *Arch Phys Med Rehabil* **66**: 329–31.

Edgar RE. (1976) Surgical management of spinal cord cysts. *Paraplegia* **14**: 21–27.

Edgar RW, Quail P. (1994) Progressive post-traumatic cystic and non-cystic myelopathy. *Br J Neurosurg* **8**: 7–22.

Foo D, Bignami A, Rosie AB. (1989) A case of post-traumatic syringomyelia. Neuropathological findings after 1 year of cystic drainage. *Paraplegia* **27**: 63–69.

Japanese Orthopedic Association. (1975) Criteria on the evaluation of the treatment of cervical spondylotic myelopathy. *J Jpn Orthop Assoc* **49**: addendum 12.

Kakulas B. (1984) Pathology of spinal injuries. *Cent Nerv Syst Trauma* **1**: 117–29.

Lesoin F, Petit H, Thomas CE, Viaud C, Beleriaux D, Jomin M. (1986) Use of the syringoperitoneal shunt in the treatment of syringomyelia. *Surg Neurol* **25**: 131–36.

Lyons BM, Brown DJ, Calvert JM, Woodward JM, Wriedt CH. (1987) The diagnosis and management of post-traumatic syringomyelia. *Paraplegia* **25**: 340–50.

Padovani R, Cavalo M, Gaist G. (1989) Surgical treatment of syringomyelia: favourable results with syringosubarachnoid shunting. *Surg Neurol* **32**: 173–80.

Peerless SJ, Durward QJ. (1983) Management of syringomyelia: a pathophysiological approach. *Clin Neurosurg* **30**: 531–76.

Quencer RM. (1988) The injured spinal cord: evaluation with magnetic resonance and intraoperative sonography. *Radiol Clin North Am* **26**: 1025–45.

Rossier AB, Foo D, Shillito J, Dyro FM. (1985) Post-traumatic cervical syringomyelia. *Brain* **108**: 439–61.

Sgouros S, Williams B. (1995) A critical appraisal of drainage in syringomyelia. *J Neurosurg* **82**: 1–10.

Sgouros S, Williams B. (1996) Management and outcome of posttraumatic syringomyelia. *J Neurosurg* **85**: 197–205.

Shannon N, Symon L, Logue V, Cull D, Kang J, Kendall B. (1981) Clinical features, investigation and treatment of post-traumatic syringomyelia. *J Neurol Neurosurg Psychiatry* **44**: 35–42.

Stanworth P. (1982) The significance of hyperidrosis in patients with post-traumatic syringomyelia. *Paraplegia* **20**: 282–87.

Tator CH, Briceno C. (1988) Treatment of syringomyelia with a syringosubarachnoid shunt. *Can J Neurol Sci* **15**: 48–57.

Umbach I, Heilporn A. (1991) Post-spinal cord injury syringomyelia. *Paraplegia* **29**: 219–21.

Whiteneck GG, Charlifue SW, Frankel HL, *et al.* (1992) Mortality, morbidity, and psychosocial outcomes of persons spinal cord injured more than 20 years ago. *Paraplegia* **30**: 617–30.

Williams B. (1994a) Pathogenesis of post-traumatic syringomyelia [letter]. *Br J Neurosurg* **8**: 114–15.

Williams B. (1994b) Non-hindbrain related and post traumatic syringomyelia. In: Schmidek HH, Sweet WH, editors. *Operative neurosurgical techniques*, 3rd edition. Philadelphia PA: Saunders, 2119–38.

Williams B. (1994c) Syringomyelia. In: Swash M, Wilden J, editors. *Outcomes in neurological and neurosurgical disorders*. Cambridge: Cambridge University Press, (in press).

Williams B, Page N. (1987) Surgical treatment of syringomyelia with syringopleural shunting. *Br J Neurosurg* 31: 63–80.

37

Whiplash injuries

Randolph W Evans

Introduction

One of the most controversial topics in this volume is whiplash injuries. Controversy persists among both clinicians (Evans *et al.*, 1994) and the general public about the nature of the injury, the cause of persistent symptoms, prognosis, medico-legal aspects, and treatment.

Even the term 'whiplash' is controversial. Yates and Smith (1994) argue:

> The term 'whiplash' is not a diagnosis. It is hardly a medical term. . . . As judged by current case reports in the legal literature, the term 'whiplash' is a most convenient legal peg on which to hang one's case, as the word seems to be synonymous with a generous financial settlement. . . . The term 'whiplash' should be removed from the medical dictionary.

However, the term seems to be well established in both the medical and lay vocabularies. It is interesting to note that, in some other languages, the term used for this injury is a literal translation of whiplash: 'latigazo' in Spanish (in Mexico and Chile); 'chicotada' in Portuguese; 'colpo di frusta' in Italian; and 'pisksnartskada' in Swedish. Other descriptive terms include 'coup du lapin' in French, which means 'rabbit's blow' and, in German, 'schleudertrauma', meaning 'slinging trauma' (Evans, 1995a).

This chapter will review definitions, epidemiology, pathology, symptoms and signs, radiographic findings, prognosis and treatment.

Definitions

The time of first use of the term 'whiplash' is not entirely certain. An American orthopaedist, Crowe (1964), reports being the first to introduce the term in a presentation in 1928. However, the first use of the term that I can find is in a 1945 article by another American orthopaedist, Davis (1945). During the 1950s, the term became widely used.

Whiplash refers to the hyperextension followed by flexion of the neck that occurs to an occupant of a motor vehicle that is hit from behind by another vehicle. Some clinicians also use the term to describe other types of collisions in which the neck is subjected to different sequences and combinations of flexion, extension and lateral motion. Other terms commonly used include cervical sprain, cervical myofascial pain syndrome, acceleration–deceleration injury, and hyperextension injury.

Whiplash is a descriptive term for the mechanism of injury. When dealing with the sequelae of the injury, it is best to be as specific as possible when describing the cause (i.e. neck pain due to myofascial injury, headache of the muscle contraction type with greater occipital neuralgia, etc.).

Epidemiology

Whiplash injuries are common and occur world-wide. According to an estimate of the National Safety Council (1995), there were 11 200 000 motor vehicle accidents in the USA in 1994 including 2 600 000 rear-end collisions. Although there is no agency collecting precise data of whiplash injuries per year in the USA, a rather rough estimate is of more than 1 000 000 (O'Neill *et al.*, 1972). According to a survey of clinicians in the USA, the following specialists see the following number of patients with whiplash injuries per month: family practitioners, 3.2; neurologists, 10.3; neurosurgeons, 7.0; and orthopaedists, 9.9 (Evans *et al.*, 1994).

Rear-end collisions are responsible for about 85% of all whiplash injuries (Deans *et al.*, 1986). The incidence decreases as crash severity increases. There is an 82% incidence of whiplash injuries in collisions in which the car is not towed away versus a 66% incidence in accidents in which it is towed (Kahane, 1982). In a low velocity rear-end collision, the occupants of the vehicle that is struck are more likely to develop neck pain than the occupants of the other vehicle, who sustain a flexion-type injury (McNab, 1964; Severy *et al.*, 1955). Neck pain develops in 56% of persons involved in a front or side impact accident (Deans *et al.*, 1986).

Various safety devices may decrease the incidence of whiplash injuries. Seventy-three per cent of occupants wearing seatbelts develop neck pain compared with 53% of those not wearing seatbelts (Deans *et al.*, 1987). The proper use of head restraints can reduce the incidence of neck pain in rear-end collisions by 24% (Morris, 1989; Nygren, 1984). Unfortunately, many people are not aware of how to set the proper height of a restraint. About 75% of adjustable restraints are left in the down position (Kahane, 1982). If the adjustable head restraint is set too low, it can act as a fulcrum and result in a more severe hyperextension injury. Cars equipped with centre, high mounted stop lamps are 17% less likely to be struck in the rear while braking than those without such a lamp (Kahane, 1989).

Women have persistent neck pain more often than men, especially in the 20–40-year age group, by a ratio of 7 : 3 (Balla, 1980; Hohl, 1974; Pearce, 1989). The greater susceptibility of women to whiplash injuries may be due to a narrower neck with less muscle mass supporting a head of roughly the same volume (Kahane, 1982).

Decreased width of the cervical spinal canal, a risk factor for persistent symptoms, is more common in women (Pettersson *et al.*, 1995).

Debates about organicity

After an acute whiplash injury, complaints of neck pain and headaches are well recognized by the medical profession. However, when patients have persistent complaints, the argument is made that sprains should heal within a few weeks and there must be another reason that patients continue to report pain. Non-organic explanations advanced for persistent complaints include emotional problems (Neck injury and the mind, 1991); a culturally conditioned and legally sanctioned illness, a man made disease (Awerbuch, 1992; Mills and Horne, 1986) and a result of social and peer copying (Livingston, 1993); secondary gain and malingering; and demanding an explanation outside the realm of organic psychiatry and neurology (Pearce, 1994).

A recent study which retrospectively examined the incidence of chronic symptoms after rear-end motor vehicle accidents in Lithuania where few people are covered by insurance also challenged the organicity of chronic complaints (Schrader *et al.*, 1996). Chronic pain and headaches were no more common in 202 accident victims than controls. The authors conclude that expectation of disability, a family history, and attribution of pre-existing symptoms to the trauma may be more important determinants for those who develop chronic symptoms. Although the results are intriguing, the study has significant sources of bias. Though the study methodology yields a representative sample of individuals who called the police following an accident, persons at risk for late whiplash syndrome may be included in the study sample at very low rates. If a particular kind of motor vehicle accident-related injury or the combination of biological vulnerability and the right kind of injury are necessary to produce the syndrome, the study may be severely underpowered. Background rates of head and neck pain may obscure a characteristic syndrome with overlapping but distinct clinical features. In addition, only 22% of the study population were women. Since most studies report that women are twice as likely as men to have chronic complaints, the small percentage of women may also bias the outcome.

Doubts about the organicity of the late symptoms of whiplash injury are very similar to those doubts about the postconcussion syndrome, both now and in the late nineteenth century (Evans, 1994). Although the case for organicity is not quite as compelling as the one for the postconcussion syndrome (Evans, 1992a; 1996a), as will be reviewed, the pathology, psychological factors (Neck injuries and the mind, 1991), prognostic studies, and persistent complaints after the settlement of litigation all support an organic explanation for the persistence of such complaints.

Pathology

Animal and human studies have demonstrated structural damage from whiplash-type injuries (Barnsley *et al.*, 1994). In different species of monkeys, experimentally caused acceleration/extension injuries have revealed a variety of lesions: muscle tears, avulsion and haemorrhages; rupture of the anterior longitudinal and other cervical ligaments, especially between C4 and C7; avulsions of discs from vertebral bodies and disc herniations; retropharyngeal haematoma; intralaryngeal and oesophageal haemorrhage; cervical sympathetic nerve damage associated with damage to the longus colli; nerve root injury; cervical spinal cord contusions and haemorrhages; cerebral concussion; and gross haemorrhages and contusions over the surface of the cerebral hemispheres, brain stem and cerebellum (McNab, 1964; Ommaya *et al.*, 1968; Wickstrom *et al.*, 1967).

Human studies have revealed similar injuries (Barnsley *et al.*, 1993). An MRI study of selected patients carried out within four months of a whiplash injury has revealed: ruptures of the anterior longitudinal ligament; horizontal avulsion, separation of the disc, and occult fractures of the horizontal end plate; acute posterolateral cervical disc herniations; focal muscular injury of the longus colli muscle; posterior interspinous ligament injury; and prevertebral fluid collections (Davis *et al.*, 1991). Autopsy series have demonstrated clefts in the cartilage plates of the intervertebral discs, posterior disc herniation through a damaged annulus fibrosis, and haemarthrosis in facet joints (Taylor and Kakulas, 1991; Taylor and Twoney, 1993).

Symptoms and signs

Table 37.1 lists the sequelae of whiplash injuries. These include neck and back injuries, headaches

Table 37.1. Sequelae of whiplash injuries

Neck and back injuries
  Myofascial
  Fractures and dislocations
  Disc herniation
  Spinal cord compression
  Spondylosis
  Radiculopathy
  Facet joint
  Increased development of spondylosis
Headache
  Muscle contraction type
  Greater occipital neuralgia
  Temporomandibular joint injury
  Migraine
  Third occipital
Dizziness
  Vestibular dysfunction
  Brain stem dysfunction
  Cervical origin
  Barré syndrome
  Hyperventilation syndrome
Paraesthesias
  Trigger points
  Thoracic outlet syndrome
  Brachial plexus injury
  Cervical radiculopathy
  Facet joint
  Carpal tunnel syndrome
  Ulnar neuropathy at the elbow
Weakness
  Radiculopathy
  Brachial plexopathy
  Entrapment neuropathy
  Reflex inhibition of muscle contraction by painful
    cutaneous stimulation
Cognitive, somatic and psychological sequelae
  Memory, attention and concentration impairment
  Nervousness and irritability
  Sleep disturbance
  Fatiguability
  Depression
  Personality change
  Compensation neurosis
Visual symptoms
  Convergence insufficiency
  Oculomotor palsies
  Abnormalities of smooth pursuit and saccades
  Horner's syndrome
  Vitreous detachment
Rare sequelae
  Torticollis
  Transient global amnesia
  Oesophageal perforation and descending mediastinitis
  Hypoglossal nerve palsy
  Cervical epidural haematoma
  Vertebral artery dissection

Modified from: Evans RW. (1992b) Some observations on whiplash injuries. *Neurol Clin* **10**: 981, with permission.

dizziness and paraesthesias, and cognitive, somatic, psychological and rare sequelae (Evans, 1992b; 1996b). When the symptoms are persistent, an argument is frequently made that these patients are just having subjective complaints that are common in the general population and are not due to the whiplash injury. Although the symptoms are common in the general population, patients with whiplash injuries have the following symptoms at the following ratios compared with a control population: neck pain 8:1; paraesthesia 16:1; neck and back pain 32:1; and occipital headache 11:1 (Bannister and Gargan, 1993).

Neck pain

Most neck pain is due to a cervical sprain, which is a myofascial injury (Fricton, 1993). Cervical disc herniations, cervical spine fractures and dislocations are uncommon. Facet joint injury may also be an important source of pain in 54% of patients with chronic neck pain (Barnsley, 1995; Bogduk, 1996).

Headaches

Headaches following whiplash injuries are usually of the muscle contraction type. Occipital neuralgia or referred pain from trigger points from suboccipital muscles can produce a pattern of pain radiating variably over the occipital, temporal, frontal and retro-orbital distribution (Graff-Radford *et al.*, 1986). Headache may be referred from the C2-3 facet joint that is innervated by the third occipital nerve, third occipital headache (Bogduk, 1986). Using third occipital nerve blocks to diagnose the condition, the prevalence of this type of headache among patients with persistent headaches after whiplash injury was 38% (Lord *et al.*, 1994). Whiplash trauma can also injure the temporomandibular joint and cause jaw pain, often associated with headache (Brooke and Lapointe, 1993). Occasionally, whiplash injuries can precipitate new but recurring attacks of common, classic and basilar migraines (Weiss *et al.*, 1991).

Dizziness

In one study of 262 patients who had persistent neck pain and headaches for four months or longer after an injury, other symptoms were reported as

follows: vertigo 50%; floating sensations 35%; tinnitus 14%; and hearing impairment 5% (Oosterveld *et al.*, 1991). Post-traumatic dysfunction of the vestibular apparatus, brain stem, cervical sympathetics, and cervical proprioceptive system, and vertebral insufficiency, have all been postulated as causing dizziness (Chester, 1991). Hyperventilation syndrome can also occur in patients with pain, producing dizziness and paraesthesias periorally and/or of the extremities. This can be bilateral or unilateral (Evans, 1995).

Paraesthesias

In one study, 33% of patients with symptoms but no objective findings complained of acute paraesthesias and 37% reported paraesthesias after a mean follow-up of 19.7 months (Norris and Watt, 1983). Paraesthesias can be caused by trigger points, brachial plexopathy, facet joint disease, entrapment neuropathies, cervical radiculopathy, spinal cord compression, and hyperventilation syndrome.

Entrapment neuropathies can occur from several mechanisms. Carpal tunnel syndrome can be caused by acute hyperextension of the wrist on the steering wheel (Haas *et al.*, 1981; Labal, 1991). If the patient has a cervical radiculopathy or a neurogenic thoracic outlet syndrome from the injury, a double crush syndrome resulting in carpal tunnel syndrome or cubital tunnel syndrome could ensue (Swensen, 1994).

The thoracic outlet syndrome is commonly caused by whiplash injuries (Capistrant, 1977). It occurs four times more often in women than in men (Pollack 1989). The diagnosis of thoracic outlet syndrome can be controversial, since at least 85% of cases are due to the nonspecific neurogenic or so-called 'disputed' type. This is a diagnosis of exclusion (Wilbourn, 1990). The nonspecific type may actually be a myofascial pain syndrome, with referred pain from the anterior neck muscles such as the anterior scalene or from the shoulder area from the pectoralis minor (Hong and Simons, 1993), and not due to neural or vascular compression.

Weakness

Complaints of weakness can be due to cervical radiculopathy, brachial plexopathy, and entrapment neuropathy. However, most patients have only subjective complaints of weakness with no objective findings on physical or electromyographic examination. At times, some clinicians will note this complaint and a finding of a give-way type of weakness on examination as a sign of hysteria or malingering. Although this explanation is appropriate for a small minority of patients, for most, the weakness may be due to reflex inhibition of muscle contraction by painful cutaneous stimulation (Aniss *et al.*, 1988; Wickstrom *et al.*, 1967).

Psychological symptoms and factors

A variety of psychological symptoms have been described after whiplash injuries. A study of selected patients with chronic symptoms reported the following percentages: 67% neurovegetative disturbances (nausea, vomiting, sweating, tremor, hypersensitivity, nervousness and irritability); 50% cognitive disturbances; 44% sleep disturbances; 40% fatiguability; 38% disturbances of vision; 37% symptoms of depression; 85% headache; 100% neck pain; 72% vertigo; and 60% brachialgia (Kischka *et al.*, 1991). However, these symptoms are also common in the general population and among other patient groups without a history of injury, including those with chronic pain, depression, neurosis, histrionic personalities and anxiety. Post-traumatic stress disorder is common after motor vehicle accidents (Mayou *et al.*, 1993) and can be an explanation for psychological symptoms in some patients with whiplash injuries. A number of studies suggest that the psychological symptoms are a consequence of persistent pain and impairment and that pre morbid personality is not predictive of outcome. Thirty-two symptomatic women who had whiplash injuries 1–84 months previously were compared with controls (Lee *et al.*, 1993). Ratings of depression and anxiety were greater in patients than in controls, and patients reported more cold-induced pain during a cold pressor test. Radanov and co-workers have performed three prospective studies based on random samples of patients with whiplash injuries. They had the following findings:

1. Psychosocial factors, negative affectivity, and personality traits were not significant in predicting the duration of symptoms (Radanov *et al.*, 1991);
2. Disabled and non disabled groups at six months did not differ with respect to psychosocial stress, negative affectivity and personality traits as assessed at baseline (Radanov *et al.*, 1993a);

3. Improvement in well-being was associated with recovery from somatic symptoms (Radanov *et al.*, 1994a).

Thus, contrary to prevailing wisdom, Radanov and co-workers' studies suggests that:

> ... (1) the disposition of patients' personality traits does not primarily influence the course of recovery from common whiplash; (2) psychological and cognitive problems of patients with common whiplash may rather be seen as correlates of somatic symptoms; and (3) injury-related psychological and cognitive difficulties can initiate a vicious circle, which may explain the secondary neurotic reaction ... (Radanov *et al.*, 1993a).

Cognitive impairment

Cognitive impairment due to a whiplash injury but without direct head trauma, is a controversial topic. Deficits in tests of attention, concentration, cognitive flexibility, and memory have been described (Aniss *et al.*, 1988; Ettlin *et al.*, 1992; Yarnell and Rossie, 1988). However, a prospective study of a random sample demonstrated delayed recovery of complex attentional functioning, which may be related to adverse the effects of medication (Radanov *et al.*, 1993b).

The same research group performed a second 2-year prospective study of 117 non-selected subjects after whiplash injuries (Di Stefano and Radanov, 1995). Testing was performed at baseline, 6 months, and 2 years. Twenty-one subjects were symptomatic at 2 years. Using matched controls from asymptomatic subjects, symptomatic subjects were impaired on tasks of divided attention (Number Connection Test, Paced Auditory Serial Addition Task, and Trail Making Test Part B) but had no impairment on memory tests. The attention deficits were not explained by medications or pain intensity. The authors do not believe that cerebral injury accounts for the problems in selective aspects of attentional functioning which may explain the patients' cognitive complaints and cause adaptational problems in daily life.

Other sequelae

Interscapular and low back pain are frequent complaints after whiplash injuries and are reported in 20% and 35% of patients, respectively (Hohl, 1974). One prospective study reported a 25% incidence of persistent back pain after a mean follow-up of two years (Hildingsson and Toulanen, 1990). In my experience, the most common cause of low back pain following a whiplash injury is myofascial pain, although other causes such as fractures and disc disease can also be present. As with cervical spine disease, without an examination with; for example, MRI just before the accident, it is difficult to tell for certain what lumbar spine abnormalities may have been pre-existing. As with the cervical spine, asymptomatic lumbar disc disease, including herniations, are common in the general population (Jensen *et al.*, 1994).

Visual symptoms, especially blurred vision, are often reported and are usually due to convergence insufficiency, although oculomotor palsies can occasionally occur (Burke *et al.*, 1992). Rarely, whiplash injuries can precipitate torticollis of onset within six days of the trauma (Truong *et al.*, 1991). Other rare sequelae include transient global amnesia (Fisher, 1982), oesophageal perforation (Stringer *et al.*, 1980), descending mediastinitis (Totstein *et al.*, 1986), hypoglossal nerve palsy (Dukes and Bannerjee, 1993), cervical epidural haematoma (Dougall *et al.*, 1995) and extracranial vertebral dissection (Hinse *et al.*, 1991).

Radiographic findings

Radiologically evident cervical spine disease is often asymptomatic

Because asymptomatic radiographic findings are common, it is frequently difficult to determine what findings are new after a whiplash injury and what findings were pre-existing, unless prior films from shortly before the accident are available. Cervical spondylosis and degenerative disc disease occur with increasing frequency with advancing age and are often asymptomatic (Friedenberg and Miller, 1963; Irvine *et al.*, 1965).

Cervical disc protrusions are also not uncommon in the general population and are often asymptomatic. A study of 100 patients without symptoms of cervical spine disease found that protrusions occurred in 20% of those who were 45–54 years of age and in 57% of those older than 64 years (Teresi *et al.*, 1987). Posterolateral protrusions were seen in 9%. Spinal cord impingement was noted in 16% of patients of 45–64 years of age and in 26% of those over the age of 64. Spinal cord compression solely as a result of disc

protrusion with a reduction of spinal cord area of up to 16% was reported in 7% of these patients.

Trauma may accelerate the development of cervical spine disease

There is evidence to suggest that trauma and whiplash injuries can accelerate the development of cervical spondylosis with degenerative disc disease. People with a history of a serious head or neck injury and miners under the age of 40 have an increased incidence of spondylosis (Irvine *et al.*, 1965). Most studies have reported that whiplash injuries can accelerate the development of cervical spondylosis with degenerative disc disease (Gargan and Bannister, 1990; Hohl, 1974), although one recent retrospective study did not show a relationship (Parmar and Raymakers, 1993). A surgical series provides additional evidence that whiplash injury many cause structural changes predisposing to premature degenerative disc disease (Hamer *et al.*, 1993). The incidence of cervical disc disruption following whiplash injuries was twice that of a control population. The mean age at operation of those patients with a previous whiplash injury was significantly lower than in those patients without a previous injury.

Prognosis

Prognostic studies

Studies on the prognosis after whiplash injuries are difficult to compare because of multiple methodological differences, including the selection criteria of patients, prospective and retrospective designs, patient attrition rates, duration of follow-up, and treatments used (Evans, 1992c; Barnsley *et al.*, 1994a). Although most patients may have only soft tissue injuries, imaging studies other than plain spine radiography have not been routinely performed. The measurement of outcome is based entirely upon patients' complaints of neck pain, headache, paraesthesias, back pain, etc. Objective measures of pain are not available.

Neck pain and headaches

Neck pain and headaches commonly occur after whiplash injuries and may persist in significant numbers of patients, as many studies have

Table 37.2. Percentage of patients with persistence of neck pain and headaches after a whiplash injury

	1 week	1 month	2 months	3 months	6 months	1 year	2 years	10 years
Neck pain (%)	92[a] 88[b]	64[c]	63[d]	38[a] 51[c]	25[a] 43[c]	19[a] 26[c]	29[b,e] 44[f]	74[g]
Headaches (%)	54[b] 57[a]	82[h]		35[a] 73[h]	26[a]	21[a]	9[e] 37[f]	33[g]

a. Radanov *et al.*, 1994b
b. Hildingsson and Toolanen 1990
c. Deans *et al.*, 1987
d. Greenfield and Ilfeld 1977
e. Maimaris *et al.*, 1988
f. Norris and Watt 1983
g. Gargan and Bannister 1990
h. Balla and Karnaghan 1987

Modified from: Evans RW. (1992c) Whiplash syndrome. In: Evans RW, Baskin DS, Yatsu FM, (editors). *Prognosis of Neurological Disorders.* New York: Oxford University Press, with permission.

documented (Table 37.2). After a motor vehicle accident, 62% of patients presenting to the emergency room complain of neck pain (Deans *et al.*, 1986). The onset of neck pain occurs within six hours in 65%, within 24 hours in 28%, and within 72 hours in the remaining 7% of patients (Deans *et al.*, 1987; Greenfield and Ilfeld, 1977). In a prospective study of 180 patients who were seen within four weeks of injury, 82% complained of headaches that were occipitally located in 46%, generalized in 34%, and in other locations in 20% (Balla and Karnaghan, 1987). Fifty per cent of patients had headache present more than half of the time.

Many studies have reported persistence of neck pain and headaches in significant numbers of patients. A well-designed prospective study reported the following percentages of patients with complaints of neck pain and headaches, respectively, at various times after the injury: 92%, 57% – 1 week; 38%, 35% – 3 months; 25%, 26% – 6 months; 19%, 21% – 1 year (Radanov *et al.*, 1994). Two years after injury, neck pain has been variously reported in 29% (Maimaris *et al.*, 1988; Hildingsson and Toolanen, 1990) and 44% of patients (Deans, 1987). In two different studies with a mean time after the accident of 10 years and 13.5 years, neck pain was still present in 74% (Gargan and Bannister, 1990) and 86% (Robinson and Cassar-Pullicino, 1993) of subjects, respectively. Symptoms present two years after injury were still present 10 years after the injury (Gargan and Bannister, 1990).

Headaches have been reported as long-lasting in the following percentages of patients in different studies: two years, 9% (Maimaris *et al.*, 1988); 37% (Norris and Watt, 1983) and 33% (Gargan and Bannister, 1990).

Prognostic variables

The ages of the patients and their occupational categories appear to be important variables. The majority of patients who develop the chronic whiplash syndrome are between the ages of 21 and 50 (Balla, 1980). Older age is prognostically significant of persistent symptoms at various times after the injury, including six months (Radanov *et al.*, 1994b), two years (Maimaris *et al.*, 1988), and 10 years (Gargan and Bannister, 1990). Although one study reported that patients in upper middle compared to lower and higher occupational categories have an increased incidence of symptoms persisting for longer than 6 months (Balla, 1980), another found no relationship between persisting symptoms and the type of vocational activity (Radanov *et al.*, 1994b).

Sturzenegger and colleagues (1994) recently reported on the relationship between accident mechanisms and initial findings: 'Three features of accident mechanisms were associated with more severe symptoms: an unprepared occupant; rear-end collision, with or without subsequent frontal impact; and rotated or inclined head position at the moment of impact.' A higher frequency of multiple symptoms, especially of cranial nerve or brain stem dysfunction, was associated with a rear-end collision. Other studies report only a minimal association of a poor prognosis with the speed or severity of the collision and the extent of vehicle damage (Kenna and Murtagh, 1987).

The following are risk factors (Table 37.3) for a less favourable prognosis: interscapular or upper back pain (Greenfield and Ilfeld, 1977; Maimaris *et al.*, 1988); occipital headache (Maimaris *et al.*, 1988); multiple symptoms or paraesthesias at presentation (Gargan and Bannister, 1990; Radanov *et al.*, 1994b); reduced range of movement of the cervical spine (Norris and Watt, 1983); the presence of an objective neurologic deficit (Norris and Watt, 1983; Maimaris *et al.*, 1988); and pre-existing degenerative osteoarthritic changes (Norris and Watt, 1983; Miles *et al.*, 1988). Abnormal cervical spine curves have been variably reported as prognostic (Griffiths *et al.*, 1995) and not prognostic (Maimaris *et al.*, 1988) of a poor outcome. A history of pretraumatic headache, and both the presence and the intensity of neck pain, are all risk factors for persistent headaches at six months after the injury (Robinson and Cassar-Pullicino, 1993). Cervical stenosis is a risk factor for the development of myelopathy after whiplash injuries both with and without cervical spine fractures or dislocations (Epstein *et al.*, 1980). Narrow diameter of the cervical spinal canal is a risk factor for chronic neck pain (Pettersson *et al.*, 1995).

A recent prospective study of 117 patients, 18% with injury-related symptoms at 2 years, were found to have the following risk factors: 'Sympto-

Table 37.3. Risk factors for persistent symptoms

Accident mechanisms
  Inclined or rotated head position
  Unpreparedness for impact
  Car stationary when hit
Occupant's characteristics
  Older age
  Female gender
Symptoms
  Intensity of initial neck pain or headache
  Occipital headache
  Interscapular or upper back pain
  Multiple symptoms or paraesthesias at presentation
Signs
  Reduced range of movement of the cervical spine
  Objective neurological deficit
Radiographic findings
  Pre-existing degenerative osteoarthritic changes
  Abnormal cervical spine curves
  Narrow diameter of cervical spinal canal

matic patients were older, had higher incidence of rotated or inclined head position at the time of impact, had higher prevalence of pretraumatic headache, showed higher intensity of initial neck pain and headache, complained of a greater number of symptoms, had a higher incidence of symptoms of radicular deficit and higher average scores on a multiple symptom analysis, and displayed more degenerative signs (osteoarthroses) on radiograph' (Radanov *et al.*, 1995). Sturzenegger *et al.* (1995) also performed a 12 month follow-up study of 117 consecutive patients. Variables which predicted persistence of symptoms at 1 year are the following: intensity of initial neck pain and headache; rotated or inclined head position at the moment of impact; unpreparedness at the time of impact; and car stationary when hit.

Return to work and long-term disability

A number of researchers have addressed the issue of return to work and long-term disability in both retrospective and prospective studies. In a retrospective study of 102 consecutive patients seen in the emergency department, patients in the good prognostic group (66% of total) had an average time off work of two weeks, with a maximum of 16 weeks (Maimaris *et al.*, 1988). One-third of these patients had no time off at all. In the poorer prognostic group of patients, 20% had no time off work and 9% did not return to work by two years; the average time off work was six weeks. In a series of consecutive medicolegal cases, 79% of patients returned to work by one month, 86% by three months, 91% by six months, and 94% by one year (Pearce, 1989). In a retrospective analysis of over 5000 patients, 26% were not able to return to normal activities at six months (Balla and Karnaghan, 1987).

Radanov and co-workers performed a prospective study to assess psychological risk factors for disability (Radanov *et al.*, 1993a). At six months, 7% of these patients showed partial or complete disability. The disabled and non disabled patients who were still symptomatic at six months did not differ with respect to psychosocial stress, negative affectivity, and personality traits, as initially assessed at baseline. Finally, Nygren (1984) reported that permanent medical disability occurred in 9.6% of patients involved in rear-end collisions and 3.8% of those involved in front or side impact accidents.

Table 37.4. Persistence of neck symptoms after settlement of litigation

Study	No. patients	Selection of patients	Time from injury to settlement	Length of follow-up after settlement	Neck complaints (%)
Gotten, 1956; Memphis, TN	100	Neurosurgery office practice	Not reported	1–26 mo	54 no 'appreciable' symptoms 34 minor symptoms 12 severe symptoms
MacNab, 1964; Toronto, Ontario	145	Orthopaedic office practice	Not reported	2 or more yr	83 most with minor symptoms
Schutt and Dohan, 1968; Newark, NJ	7, all women	Employees of Radio Corporation of America (RCA) plant	Not reported	Follow-up 6–26 mo after injury	71
Hohl, 1974; Los Angeles, CA	102, total not stated	Orthopaedic office practice, patients without cervical degenerative changes	Within 6 mo	4.5 + yr	17
Norris and Watt, 1983; Sheffield, England		Prospective study of consecutive emergency room presentations	After 18 mo	3.5 + yr	62
Symptoms, no signs	14		17.25 ± 11.9 mo	35.8 ± 8.4 mo	50 improved
Symptoms, reduced range of motion	14		15.9 ± 11.2 mo	43.4 ± 9.4 mo	50 no change 64 no change 36 improved
Symptoms, reduced range of cervical movement, and objective neurological loss	8		27.6 ± 6.5 mo	43 ± 10 mo	50 no change 25 improved 25 worse
Maimaris et al., 1988; Leicester, England	10	Retrospective study of consecutive emergency room presentations	Average 9 mo	15–20 mo	100
Robinson and Caesar-Pullicino, 1993; Shropshire, England	21	Retrospective study of orthopaedic office practice	Not reported	Mean follow-up 13.5 yr after injury	86
Parmar and Raymakers, 1993; Leicester, England	100, all in rear-end accidents	Retrospective study of orthopaedic office practice	Not reported	Mean follow-up 8 yr after injury	55 14 significant pain

From: Evans RW. (1992) Whiplash syndrome. In: Evans RW, Baskin DS, Yatsu FM. (editors) *Prognosis of neurological disorders*. New York: Oxford University Press, with permission.

Litigation and symptoms

Clinicians often consider their involvement in the medicolegal system, either as treating clinicians or as experts to be a pain in the neck. Many clinicians believe that impending litigation is the cause of symptoms. In a survey in the USA, the following percentages of different specialty respondents agreed with the statement: 'Litigation factors rather than organic or emotional factors are most responsible for whiplash symptoms': 28.4%, family physicians; 23.2%, neurologists; 52.3%, neurosurgeons; and 46.6%, orthopaedists (Evans *et al.*, 1994). Many clinicians also agreed with the statement: 'Once litigation is settled, symptoms quickly resolve': 37.3%, family physicians; 31.7%, neurologists; 33%, neurosurgeons; and 52%, orthopaedists.

Thus, many clinicians, and certainly the insurance industry and defence attorneys, believe strongly in the concepts of secondary gain and compensation neurosis: impending litigation is a major cause of persistent symptoms which promptly resolve once the litigation is completed (Awerbuch, 1992; Mills and Horne, 1986). Since pain is by definition subjective, the clinician is almost totally dependent upon the word of the patient. Secondary gain, exaggeration and malingering should be considered in all patients with whiplash injuries. Neurotic, histrionic or sociopathic patients may thrive on the attention and endless treatments recommended by clinicians and be encouraged by the plaintiff's legal advisers. However, the literature does not support this position (Evans, 1992b; Mendelson, 1992). Litigants and nonlitigants have similar recovery rates (Pennie and Agambar, 1990). The majority of patients who have persistent symptoms at the time of the settlement of their litigation continue to have symptoms (Table 37.4) and are not cured by the settlement of these claims (Mendelson, 1982). The end of litigation does not signal the end of symptoms for most of these patients who are still symptomatic. If improvement after settlement of litigation does occur, the mean interval between settlement and even mild improvement is 72 weeks (Parmar and Raymakers, 1993).

After whiplash injuries, the rate of litigation is very high: 81% according to one study (Mendelson, 1992). However, the rate of litigation in those patients with severe symptoms can be almost twice those with mild symptoms (Norris and Watt, 1983). The vast majority of patients file claims because they are truly injured and wish for compensation. This is exactly the expected result in a system of tort law. Unfortunately, by becoming involved in litigation, the victim can be further victimized by unsympathetic family members, physicians, employers, agents of insurance companies, and lawyers who each have their own agendas.

Treatment

There are few prospective controlled studies of treatment (Quebec Task Force, 1995). According to one such study, early mobilization of the neck using the Maitland technique followed by local heat and neck exercises produces more rapid improvement after acute injuries than the use of a cervical collar and rest (Mealy *et al.*, 1986) and is as effective as physical therapy performed during the first eight weeks after the injury (McKinney *et al.*, 1989). Cervical traction may be no more effective than exercises alone (Mendelson, 1992). A recent controlled prospective study showed a lack of effect of intra-articular corticosteroids for chronic pain in the cervical zygapophyseal joints (Barnsley *et al.*, 1994b).

In uncontrolled studies, many treatments have been reported as beneficial. Trigger point injections with a variety of agents, including local anaesthetics, corticosteroids, or just dry needling, can be beneficial for acute and chronic myofascial injuries (Fischer, 1993). Subcutaneous sterile water injections may reduce chronic neck and shoulder pain (Byrn *et al.*, 1993). Occipital nerve blocks with local anaesthetic, which can be combined with injectable corticosteroid, may be helpful for post-traumatic muscle contraction-type headaches with occipital neuralgia (Sjaastad, 1990). Transcutaneous electrical nerve stimulators may help to reduce myofascial pain (Graff-Radford *et al.*, 1989).

Invasive treatments are sometimes recommended. Patients with radicular symptoms and signs may respond better to cervical epidural steroid injections than those with neck pain alone (Ferrante *et al.*, 1993). Although complications are uncommon, the data for efficacy are largely anecdotal (Haddox, 1992). Surgery is sometimes inappropriately recommended for bulging discs and spondylosis. Even with appropriate indications, discectomy and anterior cervical fusion may produce unimpressive results in patients with chronic symptoms after whiplash injury (Algers *et al.*, 1993).

A variety of medications are used empirically, including nonsteroidal anti-inflammatory drugs, muscle relaxants and tricyclic antidepressants.

Narcotics, benzodiazepines and barbiturates should be used sparingly because of the potential for addiction. There may be a subgroup of these chronic pain patients who may benefit from opiate analgesia and who do not develop addiction or drug abuse (Ziegler, 1994).

Most clinicians are appropriately sceptical about the effectiveness of treatment for whiplash injuries (Evans *et al.*, 1994). Patients with persistent symptoms undergo an astounding array of treatments that have been poorly studied and are often uncritically provided. Without prospective controlled studies, placebo effects and the natural history of the disorder may be misattributed to an effect of treatment (Turner *et al.*, 1994).

Patients also go 'shopping around' for treatments. According to one estimate, 94% of patients with chronic whiplash symptoms see more than one specialist (Balla, 1980). Patients desperate for pain relief seek treatment from both clinicians and other healers who are unwitting partners in health care (Murray and Rubel, 1992). In the USA, 34% of the adult population uses unconventional therapy yearly (Eisenberg *et al.*, 1993). The litigation process can also generate unnecessary consultations, testing and treatment. Unfortunately, a small minority of plaintiffs and their lawyers attempt to magnify the alleged injury with large bills.

Until more effective treatments are available, a compassionate sympathetic approach by the clinician might result in greater patient satisfaction (Porter, 1989) and reduce unnecessary expenditure resulting from patients' therapeutic quests. Adequately controlled prospective studies of conventional and unconventional treatments are badly needed to find out what really works and to avoid unnecessary expenditure in beleaguered health care systems around the world (Barry, 1992; Carette, 1994; Newman, 1990; Quebec Task Force, 1995). Laboratory and clinical research is required to discover the pathophysiology and the most effective treatments for such chronic pain.

Acknowledgements

I would like to express my appreciation to my children, Elliott, Rochelle and Jonathan Evans for their assistance with manuscript preparation.

References

Algers G, Pettersson K, Hildingsson C, Toolanen G. (1993) Surgery for chronic symptoms after whiplash injury. Follow-up of 20 cases. *Acta Orthop Scand* **64**: 654–56.

Aniss AM, Gandevia SC, Milne RJ. (1988) Changes in perceived heaviness and motor commands produced by cutaneous reflexes in man. *J Physiol* **397**: 113–26.

Awerbuch MS. (1992) Whiplash in Australia: illness or injury? *Med J Aust* **157**: 193–96.

Balla JI. (1980) The late whiplash syndrome. *Aust NZ J Surg* **50**: 610–14.

Balla J, Karnaghan J. (1987) Whiplash headache. *Clin Exp Neurol* **23**: 179–82.

Bannister G, Gargan M. (1993) Prognosis of whiplash injuries: a review of the literature. *Spine* (State of the art reviews) **7**: 557–69.

Barnsley L, Lord S, Bogduk N. (1993) The pathophysiology of whiplash. *Spine* (State of the art reviews) **7**: 329–53.

Barnsley L, Lord S, Bogduk N. (1994a) Whiplash injury. *Pain* **58**: 283–307.

Barnsley L, Lord SM, Wallis BJ, Bogduk N. (1994b) Lack of effect of intraarticular corticosteroids for chronic pain in the cervical zygapophyseal joints. *N Engl J Med* **330**: 1047–50.

Barnsley L, Lord SM, Wallis BJ, Bogduk N. (1995) The prevalence of chronic cervical zygapophyseal joint pain after whiplash. *Spine* **20**: 20–6.

Barry M. (1992) Whiplash injuries. *Br J Rheumatol* **31**: 579–80.

Bogduk N, Marsland A. (1986) On the concept of third occipital headache. *J Neurol Neurosurg Psychiat* **49**: 775–80.

Bogduk N, Lord SM, Schwarzer AC. (1996) Post-traumatic cervical and lumber zygapophyseal joint pain. In: Evans RW, editor. *Neurology and Trauma*. Philadelphia: W.B. Saunders, 363–72.

Brooke RI, Lapointe HJ. (1993) Temporomandibular joint disorders following whiplash. *Spine* (State of the art reviews) **7**: 443–54.

Burke JP, Orton HP, West J, *et al.* (1992) Whiplash and its effect on the visual system. *Graefes Arch Clin Exp Ophthalmol* **230**: 335–39.

Byrn C, Olsson I, Falkheden L, *et al.* (1993) Subcutaneous sterile water injections for chronic neck and shoulder pain following whiplash injuries. *Lancet* **341**: 449–52.

Capistrant TD. (1977) Thoracic outlet syndrome in whiplash injury. *Ann Surg* **185**: 175–78.

Carette S. (1994) Whiplash injury and chronic neck pain. *N Engl J Med* **330**: 1083–84.

Chester JB. (1991) Whiplash, postural control, and the inner ear. *Spine* **16**: 716–20.

Crowe H. (1964) A new diagnostic sign in neck injuries. *Calif Med* **100**: 12–13.

Davis AG. (1945) Injuries of the cervical spine. *JAMA* **127**: 149–56.

Davis SJ, Teresi LM, Bradley WG, *et al.* (1991) Cervical spine hyperextension injuries: MR findings. *Radiology* **180**: 245–51.

Deans GT, McGalliard JN, Rutherford WH. (1986) Incidence and duration of neck pain among patients injured in car accidents. *Br Med J* **292**: 94–95.

Deans GT, McGalliard JN, Kerr M, Rutherford WH. (1987) Neck sprain: a major cause of disability following car accidents. *Injury* **18**: 10–12.

Di Stefano G, Radanov BP. (1995) Course of attention and memory after common whiplash: a two-yearss prospective study with age, education and gender pair-matched patients. *Acta Neurol Scand* **91**: 346–52.

Dougall TW, Kay NRM, Turnbull LW. (1995) Acute cervical epidural haematoma after soft-tissue cervical spine injury. *Injury* **26**: 345–6.

Dukes IK, Bannerjee SK. (1993) Hypoglossal nerve palsy following hyperextension neck injury. *Injury* **24**: 133–34.

Eisenberg DM, Kessler RC, Foster C, *et al.* (1993) Unconventional medicine in the United States. Prevalence, costs, and patterns of use. *N Engl J Med* **328**: 246–52.

Eismont FM, Clifford S, Goldberg M, Green B. (1984) Cervical sagittal spinal canal size and spinal injury. *Spine* **9**: 663–66.

Epstein N, Epstein JA, Benjamin V, Ransohoff J. (1980) Traumatic myelopathy in patients with cervical spinal stenosis without fractures or dislocations – methods of diagnosis, management and prognosis. *Spine* **5**: 489–96.

Ettlin TM, Kischka U, Reichmann S, *et al.* (1992) Cerebral symptoms after whiplash injury of the neck: a prospective clinical and neuropsychological study of whiplash injury. *J Neurol Neurosurg Psychiatry* **55**: 943–48.

Evans RW. (1992a) The postconcussion syndrome and the sequelae of mild head injury. *Neurol Clin* **10**: 815–17.

Evans RW. (1992b) Some observations on whiplash injuries. *Neurol Clin* **10**: 975–97.

Evans RW. (1992c) Whiplash syndrome. In: Evans RW, Baskin DS, Yatsu FM, editors. *Prognosis of Neurological disorders.* New York: Oxford University Press, 621–31.

Evans RW. (1994) The post-concussion syndrome: 130 years of controversy. *Semin Neurol* **14**: 32–39.

Evans RW, Evans RI, Sharp MJ. (1994) The physician survey on the post-concussion and whiplash syndromes. *Headache* **34**: 268–74.

Evans RW. (1995a) Whiplash around the world. *Headache* **35**: 262–63.

Evans RW. (1995b) Neurological manifestations of hyperventilation syndrome. *Semin Neurol* **15**(2): 115–25.

Evans RW. (1996a) The postconcussion syndrome and the sequelae of mild head injury. In: Evans RW, editor. *Neurology and Trauma.* Philadelphia: W.B. Saunders, 91–116.

Evans RW. (1996b) Whiplash injuries. In: Evans RW, editor. *Neurology and Trauma.* Philadelphia: W.B. Saunders, 439–57.

Ferrante FM, Wilson SP, Iacobo C, *et al.* (1993) Clinical classification as a predictor of therapeutic outcome after cervical epidural steroid injection. *Spine* **18**: 730–36.

Fischer AA. (1993) Pain relief: sterile water for whiplash syndrome. *Lancet* **341**: 470.

Fisher CM. (1982) Whiplash amnesia. *Neurology* **32**: 667–68.

Fricton JR. (1993) Myofascial pain and whiplash. *Spine* (State of the art reviews) **7**: 403–22.

Friedenberg ZB, Miller WT. (1963) Degenerative disc disease of the cervical spine. A comparative study of asymptomatic and symptomatic patients. *J Bone Joint Surg Am* **45A**: 1171–78.

Gargan MF, Bannister GC. (1990) Long term prognosis of soft tissue injuries of the neck. *J Bone Joint Surg Br* **72B**: 901–903.

Gotten N. (1956) Survey of 100 cases of whiplash injury after settlement of litigation. *JAMA* **162**: 865–67.

Graff-Radford SB, Jaeger B, Reeves JL. (1986) Myofascial pain may present clinically as occipital neuralgia. *Neurosurgery* **19**: 610–13.

Graff-Radford SB, Reeves JL, Baker RL, *et al.* (1989) Effects of transcutaneous electrical nerve stimulation on myofascial pain and trigger point sensitivity. *Pain* **37**: 1–5.

Greenfield J, Ilfeld FW. (1977) Acute cervical strain: evaluation and short term prognostic factors. *Clin Orthop* **122**: 196–200.

Griffiths HJ, Olson PN, Everson LI, Winemiller M. (1995) Hyperextension strain or 'whiplash' injuries to the cervical spine. *Skeletal Radiol* **24**: 263–66.

Haas DC, Nord SG, Borne MP. (1981) Carpal tunnel syndrome following automobile collisions. *Arch Phys Med Rehabil* **62**: 204–206.

Haddox JD. (1992) Lumbar and cervical epidural steroid therapy. *Anesthesiol Clin North Am* **10**: 179–203.

Hamer AJ, Gargan MF, Bannister GC, Nelson RJ. (1993) Whiplash injury and surgically treated cervical disc disease. *Injury* **24**: 549–50.

Hildingsson C, Toolanen G. (1990) Outcome after soft-tissue injury of the cervical spine. A prospective study of 93 car-accident victims. *Acta Orthop Scand* **61**: 357–59.

Hinse P, Thie A, Lachenmayer L. (1991) Dissection of the extracranial vertebral artery: report of four cases and review of the literature. *J Neurol Neurosurg Psychiat* **54**: 863–69.

Hohl M. (1974) Soft tissue injuries of the neck in automobile accidents: factors influencing prognosis. *J Bone Joint Surg Am* **56A**: 1675–82.

Hong CZ, Simons DG. (1993) Response to treatment for pectoralis minor myofascial pain syndrome after whiplash. *J Musculoskeletal Pain* **1**: 89–129.

Irvine DH, Fisher JB, Newell DJ, *et al.* (1965) Prevalence of cervical spondylosis in a general practice. *Lancet* **i**: 1089–92.

Jensen MC, Brant-Zawadzki MN, Obuchowski N, *et al.* (1994) Magnetic resonance imaging of the lumbar spine in people without back pain. *N Engl J Med* **331**: 69–73.

Kahane CJ. (1982) *An evaluation of head restraints.* (US Department of Transportation, National Highway Traffic Safety Administration Technical Report DOT HS-806–108.) Springfield, VA: National Technical Information Service.

Kahane CJ. (1989) An evaluation of center high mounted stop lamps based on 1987 data. (US Department of Transportation, National Highway Traffic Safety Administration Technical Report 25 DOT HS 807 442.) Springfield, VA: National Technical Information Service.

Kenna C, Murtagh J. (1987) Whiplash. *Austr Fam Phys* **16**: 727.

Kischka U, Ettlin TH, Heim S. (1991) Cerebral symptoms following whiplash injury. *Eur Neurol* **31**: 136–40.

Label LS. (1991) Carpal tunnel syndrome resulting from steering wheel impact. *Muscle Nerve* **14**: 904.

Lee J, Giles K, Drummond PD. (1993) Psychological disturbances and an exaggerated response to pain in patients with whiplash injury. *J Psychosom Res* **37**: 105–10.

Livingston M. (1993) Whiplash injury and peer copying. *J R Soc Med* **86**: 535–36.

Lord SM, Barnsley L, Wallis BJ, Bogduk N. (1994) Third occipital headache: A prevalance study. *J Neurol Neurosurg Psychiat* **57**: 1187–90.

Maimaris C, Barnes MR, Allen MJ. (1988) Whiplash injuries of the neck: a retrospective study. *Injury* **19**: 393–96.

Mayou R, Bryant B, Duthie R. (1993) Psychiatric consequences of road traffic accidents. *Br Med J* **307**: 647–51.

McKinney LA, Dornan JO, Ryan M. (1989) The role of physiotherapy in the management of acute neck sprains following road-traffic accidents. *Arch Emerg Med* **6**: 27–33.

MacNab I. (1964) Acceleration injuries of the cervical spine. *J Bone Joint Surg Am* **46A**: 1797–99.

Mealy K, Brennan H, Fenelon GCC. (1986) Early mobilization of acute whiplash injuries. *Br Med J* **292**: 656–57.

Mendelson G. (1982) Not 'cured by a verdict'. Effect of legal settlement on compensation claimants. *Med J Aust* **2**: 132–34.

Mendelson G. (1992) Compensation and chronic pain. *Pain* **48**: 121–23.

Miles KA, Maimaris C, Finlay D, *et al.* (1988) The incidence and prognostic significance of radiological abnormalities in soft tissue injuries to the cervical spine. *Skeletal Radiol* **17**: 493–96.

Mills H, Horne G. (1986) Whiplash – manmade disease? *N Z Med J* **99**: 373–74.

Morris F. (1989) Do head-restraints protect the neck from whiplash injuries? *Arch Emerg Med* **6**: 17–21.

Murray RH, Rubel AJ. (1992) Physicians and healers – unwitting partners in health care. *N Engl J Med* **326**: 61–64.

National Safety Council. (1995) *Accident facts.* Itasca, IL: NSC.

Neck injury and the mind [editorial]. (1991) *Lancet* **338**: 728–29.

Newman PK. (1990) Whiplash injury. Long term prospective studies are needed and, meanwhile, pragmatic treatment. *Br Med J* **301**: 2–3.

Norris SH, Watt I. (1983) The prognosis of neck injuries resulting from rear-end vehicle collision. *J Bone Joint Surg Br* **65B**: 608–11.

Nygren A. (1984) Injuries to car occupants: some aspects of the interior safety of cars. *Acts Otolaryngol (Stockh)* **395** (suppl): 1–164.

Ommaya AK, Faas F, Yarnell P. (1968) Whiplash injury and brain damage – an experimental study. *JAMA* **204**: 285–89.

O'Neill B, Haddon W, Kelley AB, *et al.* (1972) Automobile head restraints – frequency of neck claims in relation to the presence of head restraints. *Am J Pub Health* **62**: 403.

Oosterveld WJ, Korschot HW, Kingma GG, *et al.* (1991) Electronystagmographic findings following cervical whiplash injuries. *Acta Otolaryngol (Stockh)* **111**: 201–205.

Parmar HV, Raymakers R. (1993) Neck injuries from rear impact road traffic accidents: prognosis in persons seeking compensation. *Injury* **2**: 75–78.

Pearce JMS. (1989) Whiplash injury: a re-appraisal. *J Neurol Neurosurg Psychiatry* **52**: 1329–31.

Pearce JMS. (1994) Polemics of chronic whiplash injury. *Neurology* **44**: 1993–98.

Pennie BH, Agambar LJ. (1990) Whiplash injuries: a trial of early management. *J Bone Joint Surg Br* **72B**: 277–79.

Pettersson K, Karrholm J, Toolanen G, Hildingsson C. (1995) Decreased width of the spinal canal in patients with chronic symptoms after whiplash injury. *Spine* **20**: 1664–67.

Pollack WW. (1980) Surgical anatomy of the thoracic outlet syndrome. *Surg Gynecol Obstet* **150**: 97–103.

Porter KM. (1989) Neck sprains after car accidents. A common cause of long term disability. **298**: 973–74.

Quebec Task Force on Whiplash-Associated Disorders. (1995) Scientific monograph of the Quebec Task Force on whiplash-associated disorders. *Spine* **20**(8S): 1S–73S.

Radanov BP, Di Stefano G, Schnidrig A, Ballinari P. (1991) Role of psychosocial stress in recovery from common whiplash. *Lancet* **338**: 712–15.

Radanov BP, Di Stefano G, Schnidrig A, Sturzenegger M. (1993a) Psychological stress, cognitive performance and disability after common whiplash. *J Psychosom Res* **37**: 1–10.

Radanov BP, Di Stefano G, Schnidrig A, *et al.* (1993b) Cognitive functioning after common whiplash. A follow-up study. *Arch Neurol* **50**: 87–91.

Radanov BP, Sturzenegger M, DiStefano G, Schnidrig A, Alijinovic M. (1993c) Factors influencing recovery from headache after common whiplash. *Br Med J* **307**: 622–55.

Radanov BP, Di Stefano G, Schnidrig A, Sturzenegger M. (1994a) Common whiplash: psychosomatic or somato-psychic? *J Neurol Neurosurg Psychiatry* **57**: 486–90.

Radanov BP, Sturzenegger M, Di Stefano G, Schnidrig A. (1994b) Relationship between early somatic, radiological, cognitive and psychosocial findings and outcome during a one-year follow-up in 117 patients suffering from common whiplash. *Br J Rheumatol* **33**: 442–48.

Radanov BP, Sturzenegger M, Di Stefano G. (1995) Long-term outcome after whiplash injury. A 2-year follow-up considering features of injury mechanism and somatic, radiologic, and psychosocial findings. *Medicine* **74**: 281–97.

Robinson DD, Cassar-Pullicino VN. (1993) Acute neck sprain after road traffic accident: a long-term clinical and radiological review. *Injury* **24**: 79–82.

Schrader H, Obelieniene D, Bovim G, *et al.* (1996) Natural evolution of late whiplash syndrome outside the medicolegal context. *Lancet* **347**: 1207–11.

Severy DM, Mathewson JH, Bechtol CO. (1955) Controlled automobile rear-end collisions, an investigation of related engineering and medical phenomena. *Can Serv Med J* **11**: 727–59.

Schutt CH, Dohan FC. (1968) Neck injury to women in auto accidents: a metropolitan plague. *JAMA* **206**: 2689–92.

Sjaastad O. (1990) The headache of challenge in our time: cervicogenic headache. *Funct Neurol* **5**: 155–58.

Stringer WL, Kelly DL, Johnston FR, *et al.* (1980) Hyperextension injury of the cervical spine with esophageal perforation. *J Neurosurg* **53**: 541–43.

Sturzenegger M, DiStefano G, Radanov BP, Schnidrig A. (1994) Presenting symptoms and signs after whiplash injury: the influence of accident mechanisms. *Neurology* **44**: 688–93.

Swensen RS. (1994) The 'double crush syndrome'. *Neurol Chronicle* **4**(2): 1–6.

Taylor JR, Kakulas BA. (1991) Neck injuries. *Lancet* **338**: 1343.

Taylor JR, Twomey LT. (1993) Acute injuries to cervical joints: an autopsy study of neck sprain. *Spine* **18**: 1115–22.

Teresi LM, Lufkin RB, Reicher MA, *et al.* (1987) Asymptomatic degenerative disc disease and spondylosis of the cervical spine: MR imaging. *Radiology* **164**: 83–88.

Totstein OD, Rhame FS, Molina E, *et al.* (1986) Mediastinitis after whiplash injury. *Can J Surg* **29**: 54–56.

Truong DD, Dubinsky R, Hermanowicz N, *et al.* (1991) Posttraumatic torticollis. *Arch Neurol* **48**: 221–23.

Turner JA, Deyo RA, Loeser JD, *et al.* (1994) The importance of placebo effects in pain treatment and research. *JAMA* **271**: 1609–14.

Weiss HD, Stern BJ, Goldberg J. (1991) Post-traumatic migraine: chronic migraine precipitated by minor head or neck trauma. *Headache* **31**: 451–56.

Wickstrom J, Martinez J, Rodriguez R. (1967) Cervical sprain syndrome and experimental injuries of the head and neck. In: Selzer ML, Gikas PW, Huelke DF, editors. Proceedings of prevention of highway accidents symposium. Ann Arbor, University of Michigan, 182–87.

Wilbourn AJ. (1990) The thoracic outlet syndrome is overdiagnosed. *Arch Neurol* **47**: 328–30.

Yarnell PR, Rossie GV. (1988) Minor whiplash head injury with major debilitation. *Brain Injury* **2**: 255–58.

Yates DAH, Smith MA. (1994) Orthopaedic pain after trauma. In: Wall PD, Melzack R, editors. *Textbook of pain*. Edinburgh: Churchill Livingstone, 417.

Ziegler DK. (1994) Opiate and opioid use in patients with refractory headache. *Cephalgia* **14**: 5–10.

38

Chronic low back pain

Gregg A Ferrero, Sam W Wiesel

Introduction

Low back pain is a common sequel to occupational injury or road traffic accident. Many of these events result in some type of compensation or litigation process. The clinician is not only faced with treating the low back pathology but in providing opinions on the cause of the injury and the prognosis. This chapter will review the epidemiology and long-term prognosis after a back injury, with particular reference to the compensation/litigation situation. Most of the information will come from work place injuries because there is no good data from road traffic accidents.

Epidemiology: prevalence and incidence

To assess accurately the significance of compensation/litigation on low back pain, one must evaluate both the prevalence and the incidence in the general population. Prevalence is the measure of how many individuals at some time in their lives have attacks of low back pain. Incidence, on the other hand, defines how many individuals have back pain during a specified time period.

The exact incidence and prevalence of low back pain are unknown. It has been estimated that annually 2% of the work-force in the USA incurs industrially-related back injuries (Leavitt et al., 1971). Several population studies in Sweden have demonstrated a prevalence of 60–80% (Bauer, 1985). Rowe (1971) reviewed data from a large group of employees at the Eastman Kodak Company just before their retirement and found that at some time during their career 56% of them had suffered from low back pain severe enough to require medical care.

The impact of low back pain in the work place is formidable. Kelsey and Godlen (1988), reported that, for people below the age of 45 years, back symptoms were the most common chronic condition resulting in decreased work capacity and reduced leisure time activities. Over a 10-year period in Sweden (1960–1971), back pain was responsible for 12.5% of all sickness absence days. Of all available workdays, 1% were lost each year because of back complaints (an average of 2.5 days for each working person yearly (Hansson et al., 1985)). In the UK for 1969–1970, Wood and Bradley found that 3.6% of all workdays were lost as a result of low back pain (Cady et al., 1979). In 1974, they reported 1011 days per 1000 working persons were lost each year for this reason (Wood et al., 1980).

The most recent data from the Department of Labor (1982) Injury and Illness Survey demonstrate that in the 18 states surveyed, back injuries made up 23% of all cases in 1983 involving disability. Most (87%) of these were sprains or strains, with 4% dislocations and 2% bruises or contusions. Although lumbosacral sprain is the most common diagnosis made in compensation cases, herniated intervertebral discs, spinal stenosis and spondylolisthesis have also been diagnosed. In addition, Rowe (1971) reported that inflammatory arthritis may be responsible for up to 20% of 'nonspecific' low back pain.

There are no good data reporting the number of back injuries that result in actual litigation. In the USA, neck injuries due to road traffic accidents are more apt to result in litigation than low back problems but, in the work place, low back pain appears to be the single biggest cause of litigation.

Economic impact

The financial resources allocated to compensation for low back pain are enormous. The most reliable estimate that could be obtained showed that, in 1976 in the USA, $14 billion was spent on treatment and compensation for low back injuries. This figure exceeded all other industrial injury payments combined (Bergenudd and Nilsson, 1988). In view of the fact that medical costs, technological advancement and utilization in this area are probably greater than the average for health care (because of the widespread use of costly procedures such as CT scans and MRI), and with the tremendous escalation of compensation costs, this estimate is likely to be significantly lower than the actual cost.

The 'cost distribution' of this money in the USA has been analysed; the results are most interesting (Bigos *et al.*, 1986). When disability lasted for nine months or less, the average total medical cost of a back injury was no different to that associated with any other injury of the same duration. However, as more time elapsed, back injuries became more expensive. Of the total cost of a low back pain, 45% was related to permanent disability payments, 22% to temporary disability payments and 33% for medical bills. The medical bills can be divided as follows – 33% for physician fees, 33% to hospital bills, 7% to drugs, 5% to appliances, 9% to physical therapy and 12% for diagnostic tests.

Another interesting point is that a high percentage of these costs was concentrated in a small number of cases. For one insurance company, 25% of the low back cases accounted for 90% of their total costs. In a different group of patients (in 1971), the total average cost per case was $2197, but the median cost was $404. Although these dollar figures appear modest by today's standards, the relationship between the two figures is relevant. Only 22% of the cases had a total cost above the median. As might be expected, the high cost cases were those that involved hospitalization, surgery and compensation litigation.

Risk factors for low back pain

It would be ideal if risk factors could be used to identify persons at high risk for low back pain, or at risk for prolonged symptoms once injury had occurred. Unfortunately, the complex epidemiology of this problem makes early identification and screening somewhat difficult. Although as many as 65% of patients suffering from low back pain are unaware of any specific causative factor, several risk factors have been identified (Frymoyer and Cats-Baril, 1987).

Low back pain typically begins in young adulthood, and thus affects the most productive years of life for an industrial worker. There is a rising prevalence with age until the fourth and fifth decades, after which there is a levelling off or a decrease. Attacks of low back pain seem to be more common among those who have had back pain before. Buckle and colleagues (1980) found that, among 68 patients, over 70% reported at least one previous episode. Rowe (1971) similarly noted that 85% of these patients had a history of intermittent episodes of low back pain.

Several studies have examined sex differences in relation to the risk of low back injury (Andersson, 1979). Women represent about 40% of the working population but have only 20% of the industrial low back problems. This may be because women are typically employed in less physically demanding jobs. In a review of 31 000 employees from one manufacturer, Bigos and associates (1986) found that women had statistically fewer injuries than men but had an increased risk of making a high cost injury claim. Magora (1970) reported that, in occupations demanding strenuous physical efforts, women had a higher incidence of low back pain than men. Other investigators have reported an equal prevalence of back pain in men and women.

Many investigators have examined the association between various radiographic abnormalities and the occurrence of back pain, usually concluding that no association exists (Gibson, 1988). Rowe (1971) reported that the prevalence of leg-length differences, increased lumbosacral angle, spondylolisthesis, transitional lumbosacral vertebrae, and spina bifida occulta among low back pain patients was not significantly different to that in a control group. In a cohort study of 321 men, Frymoyer and Cats-Baril (1987) found no correlation between back pain and transitional vertebrae, Schmorl's nodes, or the disc vacuum sign. However, when there were traction spurs or disc space narrowing between the fourth and fifth lumbar vertebrae, an increased incidence of severe low back pain was evident.

At least two studies have found low back pain to be more prevalent in cigarette smokers than in nonsmokers (Frymoyer *et al.*, 1983). It is not clear whether this association is a result of increased intradiscal pressure from chronic coughing and straining, or whether nicotine itself has a direct biochemical role in the pathophysiology of back injury.

Finally, poor physical fitness may be a predisposing factor for back pain. Cady and associates (1979), in a prospective study of firefighters, found that the least fit group of employees was 10 times more susceptible to the development of back pain than the most fit group.

Prevention of low back pain

In view of the elusive nature of the aetiology of industrial low back pain, it is not surprising that attempts at prevention in industry have not met with great success. Previous efforts have focused on the careful selection of workers, training in proper lifting techniques, and designing the job to fit the worker.

The goal of careful worker selection is to screen job applicants in the hope of identifying and bypassing those potentially at increased risk of developing low back pain. The most commonly used screening tool is the pre-employment history and physical examination. An analysis of insurance company data from companies utilizing this method showed no significant difference in the incidence of low back injuries in companies that require such examinations from those that did not (Frymoyer and Cats-Baril, 1987). However, another study estimated that 10% of workers who will have job-related low back pain can be identified on a pre-employment medical examination (Frymoyer *et al.*, 1984). In this study, the best predictor was a history of back trouble, especially if it occurred without a significant prior injury. While these observations are of interest, a more common one is that the person seeking employment may not be entirely candid with an examiner about past medical problems.

In summary, pre-employment history and physical examination have not proven very helpful. However, before this time-honoured and apparently logical procedure is abandoned, more facts are needed to determine if the incidence of back pain can be reduced when these assessments are made under carefully controlled conditions.

Radiographs are in wide use as part of routine pre-employment assessment. However, there have been a number of studies, that have shown conclusively that radiograph examinations are of little value in identifying potential back problems (Gibson, 1988). The American Occupational Medical Association (AOMA) has recommended the following guidelines: 'Lumbar spine radiograph examination should not be used as a routine screening procedure for back problems but rather as a spinal diagnostic procedure available to the clinician following to appropriate indications.'

In reviewing the spinal radiograph films of employees who have developed back pain, fewer than 1% show any abnormality that would have been detected on pre-employment radiograph examination. This percentage of abnormal radiographs is not different from radiographic findings in employees who have no back complaints. Individuals with a suspicious history or physical examination should be selected for radiograph evaluation, but the routine use of pre-employment spinal films is neither medically justified nor cost effective and involves unnecessary radiation. Techniques such as biplanar radiography and new dynamic measurements of flexion-extension views may prove to be more sensitive indicators of early spinal dysfunction. Further investigation of these methods will determine their role in the prediction of low back disorders.

One area that offers some promise is the attempt to match the physical characteristics of the job to the physical abilities of the prospective employee. It has been demonstrated that specific strength testing, using a battery of isometric strength measurements, is effective in screening potential employees to reduce the likelihood of back injuries (Chaffin *et al.*, 1978). A worker's susceptibility to back injury increases significantly when the lifting requirements of the job approach or exceed the individual's strength capacity as determined by these tests.

Pre-employment strength testing was not developed to exclude anyone from the work-force, but there is concern that providing these kinds of guidelines for job placement will do just that. There is apprehension in some quarters that, rather than being used to assist in determining the individual's capacity to do the job, the guidelines actually will be used to reject suitable candidates.

The application of such testing has been subjected to very close scrutiny by the legal profession. The possibility for discrimination, particularly against female applicants in the nontraditional work place, must be carefully considered before any testing programme is actually used. Women are now beginning to compete for the more physically demanding jobs that were traditionally held by men. Women have less experience in physically demanding activities and, given the inherent biological differences, the average female is not as physically strong as the average male. Any strength testing programme must be nondiscriminatory and designed to test only for the position under consideration.

Factors affecting the duration of work loss

Once a low back pain episode has occurred, efforts must be concentrated on returning the employee to work as soon as possible and identifying those patients who will require a permanent adjustment of their work duties. Although 90% of patients return to work within six weeks of the onset of their back pain, the importance of an early return to employment cannot be overemphasized. A longer delay in returning to work is clearly associated with a decreased likelihood of ever returning to the work-force. McGill reported that workers with back complaints who are away from work for over six months have only a 50% chance of ever returning to productive employment (McGill, 1968). If they are off work for over one year, this drops to 25%, and, if more than two years, it is almost zero. Accordingly, Frymoyer and Cats-Baril (1987) have hypothesized that intensive rehabilitation early in the course of the episode can prevent long-term disability, and is cost effective.

Although a multivariate model to predict disability from low back pain has not yet been developed, several factors have been shown to affect the duration of absence from work. First is the severity and type of injury. This may be difficult to evaluate because the history provided by the patient may be consciously or unconsciously biased. Patients who are likely to seek compensation will typically identify the onset of a problem as acute rather than chronic. However, most injuries produce few objective physical findings. Because such findings are usually absent, other factors must be considered. Gallagher and associates (1986) concluded that psychological rather than physical factors can be used to predict a return to work among patients with low back pain. Waddell and colleagues (1984) estimated that objective physical impairment accounts for only one-half of the total disability, which can also be affected by such psychological of reactions as emotional distress. Similar conclusions were reached by Deyo and Tsio-Wu (1987), who found that low educational level and low income strongly correlate with work absenteeism.

The role that the secondary gain of compensation plays in the length of disability is an issue that remains unresolved. Sander and Meyers (1986) found that patients injured on duty had a significantly longer period of disability than those injured off duty. Evaluation of the patient seeking compensation may be complicated by malingering or conscious exaggeration, the creation of symptoms, and the subconscious amplification of the injury and the symptoms. The conscious manipulator often arrives at the clinician's clinic with extensive documentation and an above-average command of the medical jargon pertinent to the injury. These patients take a persistently defensive attitude, may be hostile, and may selectively withhold vital information. In contrast, documentation is less important to the subconscious exaggerator, whose defensive attitude is more transient and who rarely and only briefly expresses anger. This individual will not knowingly withhold useful information.

Financial compensation is another factor affecting time off work in industrial low back pain. In the USA, the Federal Government and the individual states have developed their own regulations; compensation payments can amount to as much as 100% of the worker's wage. Increased settlements for compensation claims and increases in the dollar value of such compensation claims are highly correlated with a subsequent increase in the number of claims made for alleged injury. Several investigations have concluded that a higher level of benefits prolonged the duration of back-related work loss (Walsh and Dumitru, 1988). The presence of compensation claims is also associated with a reduced rate of successful rehabilitation, as well as less successful surgical results.

Workers' compensation laws influence diagnostic evaluation, treatment and recovery from injury. Beals (1984) has suggested that, paradoxically, financial compensation may discourage a return to work, that the appeal process may increase disability, that an open claim may inhibit return to work, and that recovering patients may be unable to return to work. Although one study concluded that personal injury litigants do not describe their pain as more severe than non-litigants, other studies have shown that, if a lawyer becomes involved in the claim process, there is a greater probability of chronic pain and disability.

Health care providers may also share responsibility for delaying a return to work and/or escalating costs. Some clinicians are less comfortable in treating low back pain and continue to see the injured worker at unnecessarily frequent intervals. Others may take advantage of any third party fee-for-service payment system by liberally using their own radiograph and physiotherapy facilities, with questionable medical benefit to the patient. This results in a highly variable quality of health care and in unnecessary expenditure of financial resources. Both of these have served as the impetus for the development of standardized approaches to the diagnosis and treatment of industrial low back pain.

The date of the employee's return to work has been widely used to measure the rate of recovery from low back trauma in the industrial environment. This information is often quoted in support of the success or failure of various back pro-grammes, but there are a number of qualifying circumstances to be considered when using these figures. Individual company policy concerning the availability of appropriate work for employees not yet fully recovered is an important limiting factor. The availability of a limited, light duty, or restricted work environment is frequently mentioned as one of the most significant factors in the encouragement of a rapid return to work. Although there is little published information to support this conclusion, a reduction in time lost due to back injuries has been apparent in those situations where job modification permits the employee to return to less than full regular duties. When it is possible to assign the injured employee to a job where he or she is temporarily protected from heavy lifting and repeated bending, the length of time the employee is out of work is markedly reduced. If nothing but heavy physical work is available, the time lost is usually unnecessarily prolonged.

The amount of time away from work may, in itself, have a significant deleterious effect on the worker's capacity ever to return to productive employment. A report on company employees who were off work for six months showed only a 50% probability of their eventually returning to productive employment (Bauer, 1985). When employ-ees were off work for more than a year, the probability of their returning dropped to 25%, and, if they were off for more than two years, they rarely returned to work. Prolonged absenteeism appeared to have a profound adverse psychological effect on these employees. It has been shown that employees who were off work with back problems for three or more months were more emotionally disturbed than those with injury to an extremity or those in a control group who were off work for a similar length of time.

The question of malingering or exaggeration of complaints often arises in conjunction with low back pain because subjective symptoms play such an important part in diagnosis. The authors of a careful study concluded that, when the subjective complaints were out of proportion to the objective physical findings, there was an unconscious exaggeration of symptoms (Bigos *et al.*, 1986). The study also showed that true malingering (the conscious effort by the individual to create symptoms not physiologically present) was a relatively rare occurrence. This is a subject that deserves much more careful investigation because, in some occupational environments, back pain without confirmatory objective findings is often construed by the employer to be malingering.

Another topic to consider is the effect of workers' compensation legislation on the patient with low back pain and on the return to work. In the USA, the object of the original compensation laws was to provide workers with medical care and salary support for injuries that occurred on the job. Although each state and the Federal Government have developed their own unique sets of workers' compensation regulations, in most settings the employee who is hurt on the job has a free choice of physician or treatment facility, while the employer is responsible for the payment of the costs involved. This financial obligation, however, is limited to some extent by the reasonableness and necessity of care provided. The employee's reimbursement for lost time due to the accident varies widely in different jurisdictions. This is usually a percentage of the individual's wages, most often 66.6% of the employee's current pay, with a designated maximum. Current maximum wage reimbursements range from $112 per week in Mississippi to $996 per week in Alaska. In addition, many companies provide supplementary reimbursement, which may increase the injured employee's salary to as much as 100% of the current wage, all of which is tax-free. These relatively large monetary payments have been targeted as the cause of unnecessary prolongation of complaints by employees.

Finally, there is no doubt that much of the unjustified lost time and expense in such cases is due to overutilization of services by certain health care providers. While most health care professionals are dedicated, conscientious individuals, a small minority have abused the workers' compensation system. The fee-for-service reimbursement of these providers has tended to encourage too-frequent clinic visits, the duplication of diagnostic tests and the prolonged use of a variety of unproven treatment modalities. It is hoped that an independent medical monitoring system will help to limit this kind of abuse in the future.

Causality

After the occurrence of an injury, the treating clinician is first asked if it is directly responsible for the patient's subsequent back pain. This assignment of causalties in many patients is very straightforward but sometimes it can be extremely controversial. If there is a question about cause and effect, the clinician must also state the reasons for such an opinion.

In the majority of patients, there is little doubt about the effect of the injury. The patient's history is important. If there is no previous history of back pain and an injury occurs with subsequent immediate discomfort, it is easy to state that the event caused the patient's problem. A variation on the above is when there is a pre-existing condition, such as osteoarthritis of the spine. Again, the patient's history is crucial, as there is usually no question that the osteoarthritis preceded the accident. In these circumstances, the important point is whether the patient had previously been symptomatic from it or not. If the patient denies ever having experienced any discomfort from the spine prior to the accident, the clinician can state that the patient's condition is an aggravation of a pre-existing condition and that the accident is likely to be directly responsible for the patient's pain. On the other hand, if the patient had symptoms from his back prior to the accident, the allocation of causation becomes more difficult. If the patient gives a past history of pain, which is now consistently worse than the preinjury condition, the clinician can ascribe some percentage of the patient's pain to the accident. Unfortunately, as there are no objective

measurements for pain, the percentage contributed by the accident can only be estimated and this is usually questioned.

Finally, the temporal sequence of the occurrence of symptoms can also be difficult. If the pain begins immediately after an accident, there is little doubt about the cause, but difficulties arise when symptoms begin a few days to several weeks later. There are no good guidelines to follow in this situation. If there had never been a history of a problem, objective findings are present and the time interval is relatively short (up to a week) there may be justification for stating that the accident caused the problem. If there are no objective findings and the time frame is longer, then it is usually difficult to attribute the accident to the cause of the patient's symptoms.

Low back impairment ratings

After the causation is settled, the next step, once the patient has reached the maximum medical improvement, is to assign an impairment rating. Any physical injury that occurs must be quantified especially if the patient is unable to return to the previous level of employment or activity. Each patient must be given a permanent partial impairment rating. This is a task that has few satisfactory or accepted guidelines.

In this process it is necessary to make a distinction between physical impairment and physical disability. Physical impairment is an objective anatomical or pathological dysfunction leading to loss of normal body ability. Permanent impairment is an objective assessment of functional abnormality or loss after the acute injury phase and after maximal medical rehabilitation. Physical disability is a measure of reduced capacity to engage in gainful everyday activity as a consequence of some impairment.

The assessment of physical impairment is a medical responsibility. However, the assignment of the more subjective 'disability rating' may best be made by someone independent of the treating clinician. A disability rating is best calculated by administrative, vocational or legal specialists from impairment ratings generated by the clinician.

Guidelines for assigning a percentage impairment rating to a specific back injury are not available. In evaluating an extremity, the injured limb can be compared with the noninjured injured one, but no such comparison can be made for back injuries. The American Medical Association's (AMA) (1984) publication, *Guides to the evaluation of permanent impairment*, is considered to be the best reference in the USA, but the most experienced evaluators will not use it because it designates range of movement as the sole criterion of impairment and does not acknowledge pain as a factor in low back impairment except when associated with a peripheral nerve injury. Chronic low back pain often exists with few or no objective clinical signs; when there are clinical signs, they may be unrelated to the injury or disability in question. In addition, the measurement of spinal movement, even by the most experienced clinician, is highly subjective. The AMA guide is useful in its 'whole person' concept. Each part of the body is considered to represent only a section of the whole; the percentage each part contributes is based on the notion of function. Since the back is important to many functions, it contributes a maximum of 60% of the whole. Therefore, once impairment of the back is estimated, the 'whole person' impairment can be determined easily.

It must be realized that impairment ratings of spinal injuries are primarily subjective estimates based on the history and physical findings. Inevitably, the rating system carries a heavy subjective component. Pain is the chief limiting factor in spinal disease, and there is enormous variation in an individual's response to it. For example, a person with severe osteoarthritis of the spine undoubtedly has some discomfort every day. This is permanent and, in some people, progressive. Should this individual sustain a superimposed back sprain and even be completely immobilized temporarily, the long-term prognosis for recovery from the sprain may be quite good, assuming that this person has not learned to enjoy inactivity during the immobilization period. If this has occurred, the subjective complaints will not drop back to their previous baseline levels.

A different approach to the assignment of a permanent impairment rating is the use of a specific diagnosis as the determining factor (Wiesel *et al.*, 1985). This was attempted by the use of a questionnaire circulated among 75 American members of the International Society for Study of the Lumbar Spine. This questionnaire included 41 specific clinical entities to be rated. Confirming the chaotic rating situation already described, the responses were anything but consistent but, with statistical analysis, a medium range could be defined in most categories. Figures ranged from 0% for complete recovery from an acute low back

sprain to 25% following failed back surgery. If a diagnosis was complicated by emotional problems or drug addiction, it was not unusual for the percentage to increase up to 50% (in actual practice one often finds even higher ratings in situations where there is obvious bias).

An associated problem is in assigning permanent work restrictions to a patient who has already been given a permanent partial impairment rating. In the USA, one of the best permanent work restriction classification systems is defined by the Social Security Administration, and can be modified to conform to the compensation/litigation setting.

- *Very heavy work* is that which involves the lifting or carrying of objects weighing 150 lb or more.
- *Heavy work* involves lifting no more than 100 lb at a time, with frequent lifting or carrying of objects weighing up to 50 lb.
- *Medium work* is defined as involving the lifting of not more than 50 lb at a time, with frequent lifting or carrying of objects weighing up to 25 lb. Workers with 5% or less back-related permanent partial physical impairment can qualify in this category, but not those with higher ratings.
- *Light work* is described as involving lifting of no more than 20 lb at a time, with frequent lifting or carrying of objects weighing up to 10 lb. Applicants with between 10% and 15% permanent partial physical impairment because of a low back problem should be able to do this type of work.
- *Sedentary work* is described as that involving no more than the lifting of 10 lb at a time and the occasional lifting or carrying of articles like docket files, ledgers or small tools. Applicants with 20% or 25% permanent partial physical impairment should be capable of this type of work.

In summary, there is no good objective method for assigning physical impairment ratings to spine problems. Ratings based on a specific diagnosis appear to hold more promise of accuracy than those based solely on the patient's history and physical findings. There is much work to be done in this area. For now, clinicians must strive to make their reports and evaluations reflect, to the highest possible degree, the true state of a patient's impairment, using methods that are organized and reproducible.

References

American Medical Association. (1984) *Guides to the evaluation of permanent Impairment*, 2nd edition. Chicago: AMA.

Andersson GBJ. (1979) Low back pain in industry; epidemiological aspects. *Scand J Rehabil Med* **11**: 163–68.

Bauer W. (1985) Scope of industrial low back pain. In: Wiesel SW, Feffer H, Rothman R, editors. *Industrial low back pain.* Charlottesville, VA: Michie, 1–35.

Beals RK. (1984) Compensation and recovery from injury. *West J Med* **140**: 223–37.

Bergenudd H, Nilsson B. (1988) Back pain in middle age; occupational workload and psychologic factors: an epidemiologic survey. *Spine* **13**: 58–60.

Bigos SJ, Spengler DM, Martin NA, *et al.* (1986) Back injuries in industry: a retrospective study: II. Injury factors. *Spine* **11**: 246–51.

Buckle P, Kember P, Wood A, *et al.* (1980) Factors influencing occupational back pain in Bedfordshire. *Spine* **5**: 245–58.

Cady L, Bischoff D, O'Connell E, *et al.* (1979) Strength and fitness and subsequent back injuries in firefighters. *J Occup Med* **21**: 269–72.

Chaffin DB, Herin GD, Deyserling WM. (1978) Pre-employment strength testing: an updated position. *J Occup Med* **20**: 403.

Department of Labour: Bureau of Labour Statistics. (1982) *Back injuries associated with lifting.* (Bulletin 2144.) Washington DC, US Government.

Deyo RA, Tsio-Wu YJ. (1987) Functional disability due to back pain – a population-based study indicating the importance of socioeconomic factors. *Arthritis Rheum* **30**: 1247–53.

Frymoyer JW, Cats-Baril W. (1987) Predictors of low back pain disability. *Clin Orthop* **221**: 89–98.

Frymoyer JW, Pope MH, Clements JH, *et al.* (1983) Risk factors in low-back pain. *J Bone Joint Surg Am* **65A**: 213–18.

Frymoyer JW, Newberg A, Pope MH, *et al.* (1984) Spine radiographs in patients with low-back pain. *J Bone Joint Surg Am* **66A**: 1048–55.

Gallagher RM, Rauh V, Langelier R, *et al.* (1986) Psychological, but not physical, factors predict return to work in low back pain. *Psychosom Med* **48**: 296.

Gibson ES. (1988) The value of pre-placement screening radiography of the low back. *Occup Med* (State of the Art Reviews) **3**: 91–107.

Hansson T, Bigos S, Beecher P, Wortley M. (1985) The lumbar lordosis in acute and chronic low back pain. *Spine* **10**: 154–55.

Kelsey JL, Godlen AL. (1988) Occupational and workplace factors associated with low back low back pain. *Occup Med* (State of the Art Reviews) **3**: 7–16.

Leavitt S, Johnston T, Breyer R. (1971) The process of recovery: patterns in industrial back injury: Part 1. Cost and other quantitative measures of effort. *Ind Med* **40**: 7–14.

Magora A. (1970) Investigation of the relation between low back pain and occupation: I. Age, sex, community, education and other factors. *Ind Med Surg* **39**: 465–71.

McGill CM. (1968) Industrial back problems – a control program. *J Occup Med* **10**: 174–78.

Rowe ML. (1971) Low back pain disability in industry: updated position. *J Occup Med* **13**: 476–78.

Sander RA, Meyers JE. (1986) The relationship of disability to compensation status in railroad workers. *Spine* **11**: 141–43.

Waddell G, Main CJ, Morris EW, *et al.* (1984) Chronic low-back pain, psychologic distress, and illness behavior. *Spine* **9**: 209–13.

Walsh NE, Dumitru D. (1988) The influence of compensation on recovery from low back pain. *Occup Med* (State of the Art Reviews) **3**: 109–21.

Wiesel SW, Feffer HL, Rothman RH. (1985) *Industrial low back pain: a comprehensive approach.* Charlottesville, VA: Michie.

39

Litigation and the cauda equina

J R W Gleave

Introduction

This book is mainly concerned with the effects of external trauma on the constituent parts of the nervous system and their protective coverings. With the decline of heavy industry, particularly coal mining, the incidence of fractures at the thoracolumbar junction and of the lumbar spine have dropped markedly. Although crush injuries from falling structures, burst fractures from falls into cellars, and fracture dislocations from high-speed road traffic accidents still lead to claims for compensation because of damage to the cauda equina, the bulk of litigation results from what is perceived to be delay in diagnosis of conditions affecting the cauda equina such as infection, neoplasm and, above all, massive central prolapse of an intervertebral disc. Trauma of course does play a part in the genesis of disc degeneration and protrusion but it varies from minor repeated stresses sustained over years to the more obvious episode of a heavy fall, an epileptic fit, unmodified ECT, or such harmless activities as stooping down to pick up one's handbag, a sneeze, or even sexual intercourse.

Members of the legal profession sometimes seem unaware of what the cauda equina is, both in this country and especially in the USA, where to have or to develop 'cauda equina' is considered to be a disease state or syndrome consisting of certain symptoms and signs. A crude analogy would be to say that a patient had 'lungs' when what was meant was pneumonia. Where such basic misunderstanding exists, conferences with solicitors, barristers and attorneys begin on the wrong foot.

The cauda equina and its skeletal coverings with particular reference to the intervertebral discs

The 'cauda equina' is a direct translation of a Hebrew term found in the Talmud in which the termination of the spinal cord is somewhat fancifully likened to a plaited horse's tail (Field and Harrison, 1946). It consists of all the nerve roots from those of the first lumbar downwards.

The lumbar spine consists of five vertebrae connected together by ligaments and separated from each other by the intervertebral discs. The bulky part of each vertebra is termed the body. Incorporated into the back of the body on each side are the pedicles, which, together with the laminae, constitute the neural or vertebral arch. This encloses the vertebral or spinal canal. The sacrum consists of five such vertebrae, the bodies and neural arches of which are fused together to form a single bone. Not infrequently there are anomalies of segmentation at the lumbosacral interval and remnants of intervertebral disc material between the first and second sacral vertebrae or even lower. The dimensions and shape of the spinal canal may be of importance because, if the canal is congenitally narrow or if the apex of the neural arch is acutely angled, then compression of the contents of the canal may occur more easily. The laminae are joined by a fibroelastic ligament, the ligamentum flavum. This may buckle when the disc spaces become narrow with the passage of the years, or may even hypertrophy. Projecting upwards from the pedicle and downwards from the lower part of the lamina are processes that articulate with each other to form a synovial joint. The superior processes of one vertebra embrace the inferior processes of the vertebra above, the joints lying almost in a sagittal plane. The transverse and spinous processes have no bearing on the cauda equina.

The intervertebral discs lie between the bodies of the vertebrae. They have three functions:

- To unite firmly the bodies of the vertebrae;
- To permit some degree of mobility between the vertebrae;
- To absorb loading and torsional stresses to which the spine may be exposed.

The material of the discs is held in position by strong ligaments, the circumferential one at each level being the annulus fibrosus. Incorporated with this in front and behind are the anterior and posterior longitudinal ligaments of the spine. The discs at birth are composed of a material that seems ideally suited for their function but, presumably as the result of wear and tear, their biochemical and physical properties alter and the nuclear material is replaced by fibrocartilage. By midadolescence, this change may be quite advanced and it is of interest that prolapsed intervertebral discs start to occur at around this age. The degenerative change towards fibrocartilage occurs early and more extensively if the back is exposed to much lifting, torsional stress and repeated shocks, such as falling off horses or playing body-contact sports. Under normal circumstances, the fibrocartilage remains confined by the annulus fibrosus.

However, if a lumbar disc is exposed to too much stress, the annulus fibrosus will be weakened or will rupture, and the fibrocartilage of the disc will fragment. A variable amount of disc material will either protrude backwards, centrally, or more usually, centrolaterally, as a hernia, or will be expressed from the disc space as a sequestrated fragment to compromise the intervertebral foramen or the spinal canal.

The spinal cord ends as the conus medullaris opposite the first or second lumbar vertebra. It is continued as a neurologically nonfunctional strand, the filum terminale, as far as the coccyx. The filum terminale is surrounded by the leash of nerve fibres, the cauda equina. These arise from the lower spinal cord and run to the muscles, viscera and glands of the lower abdomen, pelvis and lower limbs, or to the spinal cord carrying information from these structures and also from the joints, the tendons, and the overlying skin of the lower limbs, buttocks and perineum. Both the motor, sensory and autonomic fibres are segmentally arranged and leave or enter the spinal canal through the intervertebral foramina, which lie laterally between contiguous vertebrae. The separate nerve roots of the cauda equina become mixed peripheral nerves in the intervertebral foramen where are also located the spinal ganglia containing the nerve cells that give rise both to the sensory roots and the sensory fibres of the mixed peripheral nerves. A minor and clinically irrelevant detail is that, due to the fact that the dural sac terminates opposite the body of the second sacral vertebra and the spinal canal narrows rapidly throughout the sacrum, the sacral and coccygeal root ganglia lie within the vertebral canal rather than in the intervertebral foramen and the coccygeal ganglia actually lie within the sacral sac itself. Perhaps of potentially greater clinical significance is the fact that the posterior nerve roots are ensheathed by Schwann cells as far as the pia mater of the spinal cord, where they are replaced by oligodendrocytes. The possible significance lies in the fact that nerve fibres ensheathed in Schwann cells seem capable of regeneration if damaged, but this does not seem to occur in nerve fibres whose myelin is provided by oligodendrocytes. The proliferation of Schwann cells after injury is well known; human oligodendrocytes appear to be incapable of such proliferation. In each intervertebral foramen there is a close relation between the nerve roots and the intervertebral disc.

As the nerve roots of the cauda equina peel off or enter sequentially, it will be obvious that those leaving or entering the upper part of the lumbosacral spine will lie laterally to those that are running to the lower part of the lumbosacral spine. Thus, the lowest sacral fibres will lie most centrally. The shape of the spinal canal is such that the anteroposterior diameter is greatest in the midline, and this may protect these fibres to some degree from pressure from in front.

If an intervertebral disc herniates to a sufficient degree or if a significant sequestration of disc material occurs, it will irritate sensitive structures, causing pain and will also compress motor and sensory nerve roots. This will lead to loss of function in those roots. Such a protrusion of disc material is the last stage of the process. Before it occurs there are usually less severe episodes, which may result in back pain alone, back pain with sciatica, or back pain with sciatica plus some neurological deficit. In these individuals, it would seem likely that there has been a tear of part of the annulus fibrosus with weakening of its ligamentous constraint and, to a lesser or greater extent, herniation of disc material beyond the normal contour of the disc, which irritates the pain sensitive structures or compresses the nerve roots. If the spine is rested, the annulus will heal; it is generally accepted that, in 80% of cases of disc protrusion, the symptoms will subside on conservative management. However, the healed annulus is never as strong as the pristine one and further episodes are likely. When there is a sequestrated piece of fibrocartilage in the spinal canal or intervertebral foramen, surgery is usually advised. Although it is quite frequent for discs to protrude centrally, frank prolapse of fragments of disc material occur most frequently laterally or centrolaterally. Hence, only one set of nerve roots is usually involved and the weakness and sensory loss is limited to the appropriate segment of one limb. Rarely, massive central prolapse will occur and will compress all the fibres of the cauda equina passing to or coming from levels below that of the prolapse. Any accurate assessment of the risk of this complication is very difficult, but, of patients seen by neurosurgeons, perhaps 1% will have some evidence of cauda equina compression but only 0.5% will have the full blown syndrome accompanied by paralysis of the sphincters. By 'cauda equina compression' is meant a syndrome with evidence of bilateral nerve root involvement. The actual risk is very small indeed of any patient developing a massive central protrusion with cauda equina compression. Such a massive central prolapse affecting the central fibres of the cauda equina will manifest itself in saddle anaesthesia, painless retention of urine with overflow, loss of normal bowel function and a lax anal sphincter, loss of sexual sensation and function, and, depending upon the level of the lesion, a variable loss of sensation and weakness in the lower limbs.

The cauda equina cannot be considered in total isolation because the first lumbar nerve roots that constitute its uppermost part emerge from and enter the cord opposite the tenth thoracic vertebra. The lumbosacral enlargement of the cord terminating in the conus medullaris gives rise to and receives all the fibres of the cauda equina and lies opposite the eleventh and twelfth thoracic vertebrae and the first lumbar vertebra. Therefore, the cauda equina surrounds this part of the spinal cord. Thus, lesions in this region will produce a clinical picture that is a combination of nerve root and spinal cord damage.

A final anatomical feature that may require consideration is that, occasionally, the main arterial supply for the conus medullaris enters as a branch of one of the lumbar arteries rather than as a branch of one of the intercostal arteries, most frequently T10.

The clinical presentation of cauda equina lesions

The detailed picture depends upon the level, the nature, the size and the severity of the lesion. The general nature of the deficits has already been indicated. The weakness will be of lower motor neurone type, with decreased tone, wasting, fasciculation and depressed or absent tendon reflexes if the segments concerned with such reflexes are involved. The sensory loss will vary from blunting to pin-prick, which seems to be the earliest sign of compression, to complete anaesthesia and loss of proprioception. In the same way as hypoalgesia is the first sensory loss to be noted, so it is the most persistent, and careful examination following even the successful cure of a lateral disc prolapse will often reveal that a minor degree is still present. Unless the lesion is very large, or essentially centrally situated, the autonomic control of bladder, bowel and sexual functions will not be affected. However, if the patient is in considerable pain there may be difficulty with micturition, particularly in the female patient who cannot move from the recumbent position. This must not be mistaken for retention and the differentiation is quite simple: non-neurogenic retention is painful, neurogenic retention is painless.

Back pain, referred pain and radicular pain are usually prominent features of a cauda equina lesion, although they occur earlier and are more prominent in some conditions than others. Thus, an epidural abscess may be extremely painful and may present with exquisite tenderness; a neurofibroma tends to give severe radicular pain early, while an ependymoma of the filum terminale may merely produce diffuse low back pain until it reaches a considerable size. A massive central disc protrusion was unaccompanied by sciatic pain in 5% of our cases (Gleave and Macfarlane, 1990). The cause of pain in these lesions is probably not the result of the pressure on the nerve roots themselves but of irritation of pain-sensitive structures, such as the nerve root sheaths with their nervi nervorum, the anterior aspect of the dura, and the ligaments of the vertebral canal and annulus fibrosus.

Lesions arising centrally within the cauda equina, the most common being the ependymoma of the filum terminale, will affect the central fibres first, and so impotence and disturbance of sphincter control will appear early. Likewise, the sensory loss from such a lesion is usually bilateral, although not necessarily symmetrical, and tends to affect preferentially the saddle area and the perineum. When there is a lesion in the region of the thoracolumbar junction, there is compromise not only of the cauda equina but of the spinal cord itself. This leads to a paradoxical situation with an upper motor neurone type of lesion affecting the distal parts of the lower limbs and a lower motor neurone type of lesion affecting the proximal parts. The features of the lower motor neurone lesion have already been described. An upper motor neurone lesion shows increased tone and increased reflexes, accompanied by clonus. The weakness itself may not be so profound and the wasting will be less. If there is asymmetry of the lesion, there may be some element of dissociated sensory loss.

There is no doubt about the features of the complete cauda equina syndrome. Kostuik (1993) has defined it in the following words:

> Cauda equina syndrome has been described as a complex of symptoms and signs consisting of low back pain, unilateral or bilateral sciatica, motor weakness of the lower extremities, sensory disturbance, and loss of visceral function, namely bowel and bladder functions, together with saddle anaesthesia. Paraplegia or severe paraparesis may be a final outcome.

However, there is a spectrum of cauda equina involvement starting from a monoradicular loss of motor and sensory function and culminating in the complete syndrome as defined by Kostuik. The most common cause of cauda equina compression is a massive central disc protrusion. In a series of 60 patients 33 showed the complete syndrome but 26 did not have retention of urine, although they had bilateral sensory and motor loss; of these, the majority complained only of some difficulty with micturition. A few had no micturition problems at all. The severity of the neurological involvement depends upon three factors:

1. The size of the lesion, and the relative size and shape of the canal;
2. The speed of the development of the lesion so that, for example, the acute development of a massive central disc prolapse will have a far more devastating effect than a very much larger but slowly developing ependymoma of the filum terminale;
3. The nature of the lesion. Thus, an epidural abscess, as well as producing a direct pressure effect, may also cause thrombosis of the blood supply. Fortunately this is rare. Even more rare is the Cytomegalovirus (CMV) cauda equina syndrome associated with AIDS, as is invasion of the cauda equina by metastatic carcinoma.

The type of neurological deficit depends on the differential sensitivity of the fibres of the cauda equina to the pathological processes to which they are subjected. These are compression, contusion, traction, ischaemia and inflammation. Gasser and Erlanger (1929) showed that, in response to local pressure, motor function and the sense of touch were the first modalities to be lost and pain the last. This coincided with fibre size, the potentials from the large fibres being the first to disappear. Lewis and Pochin (1937) found that ischaemia acted in a similar fashion and it was thought for some time that compression exerted its effect by ischaemia. However Ochoa *et al.* (1972) demonstrated in the baboon that the effect was due to mechanical displacement of the axoplasm and dislocation of the myelin.

Actual tearing of the fibres of the cauda equina has been seen during transthecal exploration for the removal of disc fragments. It would appear to be common sense to suppose that the finer fibres are most susceptible to mechanical interruption of this sort. In my clinical experience with prolapsed intervertebral discs, it is the decreased sensation to pin-prick that is the earliest sign to appear and the most likely deficit to remain permanently. Pain is subserved by finer fibres and I would suggest that it is mechanical disruption from traction and compression that plays the largest part in producing the neurological loss noted in lesions due to pressure on the cauda equina. The autonomic fibres concerned with bladder, bowel and sexual function are similarly of smaller size than those subserving motor function, proprioception and epicritic touch. Therefore, in the same way as impaired function of the pain fibres is more likely to be permanent, so is full recovery in the autonomic fibres if they are interrupted. Thus, in 78% of our patients with the full cauda equina syndrome there was some permanent hypoalgesia (Gleave and Macfarlane, 1990). Likewise, although 79% claimed full bladder control, I suspect that urodynamic studies would have revealed abnormalities in all of them as found by Scott (1965). He studied 10 patients in detail and although they had all regained social continence and half appeared to have bladder control indistinguishable from normal, yet sophisticated studies showed abnormalities in all of them. Sexual function was adequate in three of the seven men in the series.

Prognosis for recovery of cauda equina lesions in relation to the type of trauma and treatment

Neither anterior nor posterior nerve roots regenerate if they are divided surgically, as in the operations of anterior and posterior rhizotomy. Similarly, there will not be recovery of the affected area following a severe crush injury to the conus medullaris. On the analogy of peripheral nerves, from clinical experience, and from the experimental work of Delamarter *et al.* (1991) on beagles, it seems likely that the nerve roots of the cauda equina have the capacity for regeneration following crushing injuries provided that the compressing agent is removed. It seems that the chief factor concerned with the regeneration of nerve fibres damaged in continuity is the closeness of the lesion to the parent cell body. If it is too close, the cell body will die and therefore regeneration will not take place. It is also interesting to speculate that large fibres regenerate better than smaller ones. Therefore, regeneration of all the damaged fibres of the cauda equina is by no means inevitable.

Injuries leading to division accompanied by physical separation of the nerve fibres of the cauda equina are rare and the usual pathological processes result in lesions in continuity. These are in theory capable of regeneration if the compressing agent can be removed without the infliction of further damage in the process. Therefore, when dealing with a progressive process such as an abscess or a tumour, the sooner relief is procured, the better the prognosis is likely to be. It is also good surgical sense that, when the lesion is nonprogressive and purely mechanical, the restoration of the normal anatomy by conservative or surgical means, together with the removal of any residual compressing material, should be carried out with due expedition, taking into consideration the general state of the patient and the facilities available for investigation and operation. On a personal note, however, as these conditions are not life threatening, I would rather be operated on by a fresh surgical team in the morning than a tired surgical team in the middle of the night.

There is good evidence that some massive disc prolapses are progressive and, like Shephard (1959), we were able to classify our patients into two groups (Gleave and Macfarlane, 1990). Kostuik *et al.* (1986) also noted two modes of presentation. They found a slightly shorter mean time to surgery in patients with an acute onset of symptoms compared with those who presented with insidiously progressive lesions. Because those with an acute onset probably had the more severe lesion, this gives rise to the paradoxical observation that those who are operated on earlier do slightly worse than those who are operated on rather later. Delamarter's work on beagles has demonstrated that the ultimate recovery is the same whether the compression is relieved after an hour or after a week (Delamarter *et al.*, 1991). If one accepts the development of the retention of urine as the hallmark of the full cauda equina syndrome, then there are numerous reports in the literature (Gleave and Macfarlane, 1990; Kostuik *et al.*, 1986; Jennett, 1956; O'Laoire *et al.*, 1981; Shephard, 1959) which demonstrate that emergency surgery has no bearing on the degree of clinical recovery. It has been proposed concerning the analogy of the known effects of tourniquet compression of peripheral nerves that, if it were possible to operate within six hours of the onset of compression, then a better result might be achieved. However, recent evidence has been produced by Stephenson *et al.* (1994) working on baboons that the compression has to be relieved within one hour if a good result is to be anticipated.

Leaving these considerations aside, a considerable degree of recovery will follow the relief of compression of the cauda equina and it should therefore be undertaken. Whether this assumption is justified in patients in whom the pathology is nonprogressive is impossible to prove. It would be a very brave surgeon who would not attempt to relieve compression and restore the normal anatomy if it were possible. Controlled trials are not ethically justified with the present state of knowledge. There is therefore a general sentiment that any compression should be relieved as soon as possible and this is standard surgical practice. This chapter is not the place to discuss the techniques of management of the various conditions under consideration. I would merely stress the importance of the special investigations such as CT scanning, MRI and, if necessary, myelography, in order to obtain as full a picture of the pathology as possible. With regard to massive central disc protrusions, which are at the present time probably the most common cause of cauda equina compression, I would entirely support Fager (1985) that adequate bony removal is essential in all these patients. I would go further and maintain that, if any difficulty were encountered in an extradural attempt to remove a large fragment, then a transthecal approach should be used. This has proved necessary in only 15% of my patients (nine of 60), but Garfield (personal communication) advocates such an approach in all massive central disc prolapses.

If recovery from the compression is incomplete, there may be permanent weakness, sensory loss and sphincter disturbances. The weakness may be disabling and affect the gait; the main sensory loss is usually in the saddle and perineal areas; there may be permanent loss of bladder and bowel control, together with loss of sexual function. In addition to these losses, painful dysaesthesia, particularly in the perineum, may be a striking phenomenon. Several patients have remarked that it feels as if they were sitting on a hard football the whole time or that the football was situated in the rectum or the vagina.

The lawyer, the neurosurgeon and the cauda equina

There are two categories of clients for whom a lawyer may ask a neurosurgeon for an opinion: straightforward accident/insurance claims, and claims concerning alleged medical negligence.

The first type of case presents no problem. A thorough history must be obtained from the patient, including past illnesses and accidents, social background, educational attainments, and work record. It is also useful to interview a close relative. Copies of the general practitioner's notes and hospital records must be scrutinized and all investigations, especially imaging, must be carefully reviewed. If necessary, the solicitor should be advised to obtain opinions from orthopaedic surgeons, rehabilitation experts, and those specializing in providing aids around the home and facilitating activities of daily living.

The second category is much more time consuming and presents a far greater challenge. An interview and examination of the patient may not be necessary, although sometimes it is very helpful, but, in addition to a very careful review of all the patient's records and investigations as in the first category, it is also necessary to consider most carefully the plaintiff's statement of claim, the defendant's responses, and the opinion of the other experts involved in the case. There are frequently substantial discrepancies between the plaintiff's statement of claim based on the recollection of events, which usually took place two or three years previously, the recollections of the doctors concerning the same events, and what is, or is not, written in the hospital records. The nursing record may sometimes be more helpful than the doctor's notes. It cannot be emphasized too strongly that, in this regard, the keeping of good records is as important as the practice of good medicine, because without them there is no evidence about what standard of care was provided. On the other hand, in those cases in which the records are good, the contemporary account of events must be preferred to later recollections.

Having established, as far as possible, the facts of the case, the surgeon may be expected to give an opinion concerning negligence, causation, liability and what may be termed foreseeability. The surgeon may be asked for an opinion on only one of these issues. I am indebted to Mr Patrick Gaul, of Weightmann Rutherford's for his advice on these matters, but any legal heresies I may express are my own opinions and not his.

Negligence

In the UK, the classic dictum is set out in the case of *Bolam* v *Friern Hospital Management Committee*:

> A doctor is not guilty of negligence if he has acted in accordance with a practice accepted as proper by a responsible body of medical men skilled in that particular art ... putting it the other way around, a man is not negligent if he has acted in accordance with such a practice, merely because there is a body of opinion who would take a contrary view.

Looked at from the plaintiff's viewpoint this allows considerable latitude to doctors. The plaintiff's expert must be able to say that no reasonable practitioner would have acted in the same way.

Another judgment useful to the defence was Lord Denning's opinion in *Hucks* v *Cole*, when he said,

> Another difference lies in the fact that with the best will in the world things do go amiss in surgical operations or medical treatment so a doctor is not to be held negligent simply because something goes wrong.

However, in the same case Lord Justice Sachs gave the opinion that it did constitute negligence knowingly to take risks of great danger when the risk could be easily avoided.

Another important case is that of *Sidaway* v *Board of Governors of Bethlem Royal Hospital*, where by a majority, the House of Lords considered that the Bolam principle should be applied in cases of alleged negligence in providing information and advice relevant to medical treatment. However, there was some dissent here and medical paternalism, though presumably not judicial paternalism, was frowned upon. In a recent judgment in Australia (*Rogers* v *Whitaker*) it was found to be negligent not to have given a patient information that there was a one in 14 000 chance of a complication occurring.

It seems obvious to me that there are some patients to whom the divulging of the full risks of a procedure would be detrimental in the extreme. Perhaps in these situations the nearest responsible relative should be involved.

Causation

It must be shown that the specific acts or omissions complained of as being negligent actually caused the plaintiff damage and loss, or made a material contribution to such damage and loss.

Liability

This encompasses both negligence and causation. Liability implies responsibility for the consequences of an action.

Foreseeability

If the result of a treatment or an operation is totally unforeseeable, then a necessary element of the legal claim has not been proven.

In cases involving the cauda equina, it seems to me to be difficult to defend such errors as: operating at the wrong level (even though there may be extenuating circumstances, such as anomalies of segmentation at the lumbosacral junction): attempting to remove a nonexistent prolapsed intervertebral disc when the patient required a decompressive laminectomy; inflicting damage on the cauda equina by a decompressive operation when the patient had no neurological deficit prior

to the procedure; failing to give sufficient information of the risks involved in the removal of a massive central disc prolapse from a patient in whom, at the time of removal, there was no sphincteric disturbance; or failing to explain fully the risks of neurological damage inherent in such a procedure as a midline myelotomy of the conus medullaris for pain relief. It is becoming increasingly incumbent on the surgeon to explain in detail all the possible risks of adverse effects associated with any procedure, however remote they may appear. The most frequent cause of litigation in cauda equina cases appears to be what the patient perceives to be delay both in the diagnosis and in the treatment of a massive central disc prolapse. The patient thinks that if there had not been this delay, then the resultant condition might have been better. This is a very difficult, if not an insoluble, problem. As Kostuik has defined the condition, the hallmark is retention of urine. Until that occurs, the clinical presentation may differ in no way from a straightforward prolapsed intervertebral disc, which everyone agrees should be treated conservatively with an 80% chance of recovery. By the time retention of urine has been discovered, the compression of the cauda equina has usually been present for several hours, unless the patient was about to empty the bladder when it occurred and presented straight away with overflow incontinence. Even in this unlikely eventuality, it may take some four to six hours to investigate and get the patient on to the operating table. There is some experimental evidence that the relief of the compression within an hour of its onset is beneficial, but I think that to achieve this is quite impossible in the clinical situation. It has been clearly shown that, once retention of urine has occurred, there is no guarantee of a good result, and, furthermore, there is no particular benefit for the patient in treating the condition as an emergency, although it is obviously to the patient's general benefit to be treated expeditiously. I would therefore maintain that such a case would fail with regard to negligence, causation and liability.

On the other hand, if a large central disc protrusion can be removed before the onset of urinary retention, then the results are very much better (Fager, 1985; Gleave and Macfarlane, 1990). The obvious, but apparently unacceptable, answer is to subject everyone with back pain and sciatica, and indeed the occasional patient just with back ache and no sciatica, to an MRI scan to determine the size and position of the prolapsed disc, or whatever other pathology may be revealed, such as an ependymoma of the filum terminale. I suspect that such a proposal would be strongly resisted by a business-led health service, but I would point out that about 5000 MRI scans could be done for the price of one recent settlement.

References

Delamarter RB, Sherman JE, Carr JB. (1991) Cauda equina syndrome: neurologic recovery following immediate, early, or late decompression. *Spine* **16**: 1022–29.

Fager CA. (1985) Ruptured median and paramedian lumbar disk. A review of 243 cases. *Surg Neurol* **23**: 309–23.

Field EJ, Harrison RJ. (1946) Anatomical terms: their origin, and derivation. Cambridge: Heffer, 25.

Gasser US, Erlanger J. (1929) The role of fibre size in the establishment of a nerve block by pressure or cocaine. *Am J Physiol* **lxxxvii**: 581–91.

Gleave JRW, Macfarlane R. (1990) Prognosis for recovery of bladder function following lumbar central disc prolapse. *Br J Neurosurg* **4**: 205–10.

Jennett WB. (1956) A study of 25 cases of compression of the cauda equina by prolapsed intervertebral discs. *J Neurol Neurosurg Psychiatry* **19**: 109–16.

Kostuik JP. (1993) Controversies in cauda equina syndrome and lumbar disc herniation. *Curr Opin Orthop* **4**(11): 125–28.

Kostuik JP, Harrington I, Alexander D, Rand W, Evans D. (1986) Cauda equina syndrome and lumbar disc herniation. *J Bone Joint Surg Am* **68A**: 386–89.

Lewis J, Pochin EG. (1937) Effects of asphyxia and pressure on sensory nerves of man. *Clin Sci* **3**: 141–55.

O'Laoire SA, Crockard HA, Thomas DG. (1981) Prognosis for sphincter recovery after operation for cauda equina compression owing to lumbar disc prolapse. *Br Med J* **282**: 1852–54.

Ochoa J, Fowler TJ, Gilliatt RW. (1972) Anatomical changes in peripheral nerves compressed by a pneumatic tourniquet. *J Anat* **113**: 433–55.

Scott PJ. (1965) Bladder paralysis in cauda equina lesions from disc prolapse. *J Bone Joint Surg Bc* **47B**: 224–35.

Shephard RH. (1959) Diagnosis and prognosis of cauda equina syndrome produced by protrusion of lumbar disk. *Br Med J* **ii**: 1434–39.

Stephenson GC, Myles Gibson R, Sonntag VKH. (1994) Who is to blame for the morbidity of acute cauda equina compression? *J Neurol Neurosurg Psychiatry* **57**: 388.

Section VI

Peripheral nerve injury

40

Brachial plexus injuries

Hanno Millesi

Definition

A brachial plexus lesion involves the cervical segments C5, C6, C7 and C8, and the first thoracic segment (T1) with their corresponding spinal nerves. It can be a complete lesion of all five spinal nerves; in this case the arm is completely paralysed (flail arm). It may involve the spinal nerves C5 and C6 (upper brachial plexus lesion), when movements of the shoulder and of elbow flexion are impaired. If the spinal nerves C5, C6 and C7 are damaged (extended upper brachial plexus lesion), as well as there being a loss of function in the shoulder and elbow joints, the patient is unable to extend the wrist and fingers. If the spinal nerves C8 and T1 are involved, this is a lower brachial plexus lesion. Of course there are irregular patterns and, in rare cases, one can see an intermediate brachial plexus lesion focused mainly on C7. A peripheral nerve lesion, involving the suprascapular, axillary and musculocutaneous nerves may simulate an upper brachial plexus lesion.

According to the amount of damage suffered, the lesion may be irreversible, or, in lesser degrees of damage (see later), there may be a prospect for spontaneous recovery.

Aetiology

Traumatic lesions

The vast majority of brachial plexus lesions are caused by road traffic accidents (224 of 247 patients in our series). Accidents caused by motor cycles predominate (78%). Much less frequently, brachial plexus lesions are caused by car accidents (12%)

and other trauma (10%). In our series we had only three gunshot wounds and one patient who had been stabbed; however, in other countries the percentage of this type of injury is significantly greater.

Brachial plexus injuries occurring to babies during delivery (obstetric brachial plexus lesions) follow a similar pattern to the post-traumatic lesions. For various reasons they form a special entity and are not discussed in this chapter.

Nontraumatic lesions

Actinic brachial plexus lesions

During the treatment of breast cancer or lymphogranuloma, the area of the neck is treated with ionizing irradiation. This has two consequences:

1. The nerves may be damaged directly by the irradiation. In this case, a gradual loss of function occurs after a long delay. The regenerative power is significantly reduced and surgery cannot improve function. Indeed, sometimes the function of segments that are on the verge of developing spontaneous paralysis may be compromised, even by atraumatic surgery, such that paralysis then develops. However, these operations are mainly performed because of unbearable pain; an eventual loss of function may therefore be acceptable.
2. The irradiation may cause fibrosis of the connective tissue in the area of greatest irradiation. The contracting fibrosis causes injury to the brachial plexus, even if the nerves themselves have not been damaged by the irradiation. In this situation, neurolysis offers the prospect of functional improvement.

Mechanism of injury

Indirect lesion

In the vast majority of patients, the damage to the brachial plexus occurs by blunt trauma striking the shoulder, leaving the head free. The plexus is compressed between the clavicle and the first rib and may suffer damage of differing degrees. The head continues to move away from the shoulder, increasing the distance between them. This exposes the brachial plexus to traction. If the amount of traction is sufficient, the rootlets, the weakest point, will give way and avulsion from the spinal cord will result. This may involve all five roots (about 15% of the cases of root lesions) or only some of them. If the traction occurs with a lifted arm, the roots of C8 and T1 are mainly involved. If the arm is in lateral abduction, C7 is subjected to the most traction. If the site of traction is located more laterally, and the head does not move, a traction lesion may occur also at the level of the trunks or the cords, damaging the tissue to a different degree (see later). A traction lesion may also occur in shoulder dislocation or fracture of the humerus, if the arm is distracted from the body. Compression between the clavicle and the first rib and traction are usually the combined mechanisms of injury.

Direct lesion

The brachial plexus may be damaged directly by a clavicular fracture if the bony fragments involve it. The brachial plexus may suffer secondary damage if a pseudoarthrosis or callus develops at the site of the clavicular fracture. The development of callus may also interrupt the spontaneous regeneration of a lesser degree brachial plexus lesion because of continuous pressure.

Any of these events can lead to a closed brachial plexus lesion. In a traction lesion, the subclavian artery and vein are exposed to tension and one or both may rupture. This leads to a huge haematoma, which may also compress the brachial plexus.

Open lesion

An open injury caused, for example, by a gunshot wound or by stabbing, affords special consideration. An open injury is always an indication for emergency surgery. The wound should be closed. With a clean transection of the brachial plexus, an immediate repair by end-to-end coaptation is the treatment of choice. Gunshot wounds have a tendency for spontaneous recovery; only those not showing spontaneous regeneration require surgery. The prognosis is usually good.

Immediate diagnosis and emergency care

If there is an open injury, the wound is explored and closed. In a clean transection of parts of the brachial plexus, a primary coaptation offers the best prospect for good regeneration. Damage to the artery or vein is treated by vascular reconstruction. A decision must be taken whether the brachial plexus should be explored at the same time and an immediate repair attempted. The decision whether to perform a primary repair should be taken by a surgeon who has experience in brachial plexus surgery. This will, to a large extent, depend on the general condition of the patient, because a primary repair of the brachial plexus will lengthen the operative time by several hours. If an experienced surgeon is not available, no attempt should be made even to define the extent of the damage, as this will cause more fibrosis and render secondary repair more difficult. If there is a clavicular fracture, an osteosynthesis should be performed with a plate and screws.

Final diagnosis and early secondary repair

If it is decided to perform early secondary repair, there is sufficient time to try and establish a precise diagnosis. The following questions should be answered:

Is there a chance of spontaneous recovery?

Depending upon the amount of damage (see below), there is a good chance of spontaneous recovery if the continuity of the nerves has been preserved. The evaluation of this prospect is extremely difficult, and can be achieved only by observation of the clinical course. The first clinical sign of recovery is the occurrence of the Tinel Hofmann sign. This indicates that there has been at least one regeneration neuroma formed and that axon sprouts are developing. If the punctum maximum of the Tinel sign moves in a distal direction, it can be concluded that at least some fibres are growing towards the periphery. If the Tinel sign continues to move in a distal direction, one can wait, while the patient undergoes intensive physiotherapy, to determine whether early signs of recovery can be detected in the most proximal muscles. Conservative treatment is continued either until full recovery is achieved or the progress of regeneration stops. In the case of the latter, regeneration develops only in certain territories, while others remain paralysed. In this instance, surgery is indicated. Surgery is also indicated if the Tinel sign stops and does not move on.

Is there a supra- or an infraganglionic lesion?

A supraganglionic lesion means that the rootlets have been avulsed from the spinal cord. There is no proximal stump and, therefore, no neuroma formation or Tinel's sign. On CT myelography, a meningocoele may be visible. On MRI, the rootlets are no longer visible. The diagnosis of a supraganglionic lesion is further supported if there is denervation of the dorsal neck muscles and if sensory nerve conduction remains positive in the presence of complete paralysis. This is due to the fact that in a supraganglionic lesion the neurones for the sensory fibres are still in contact with the cell bodies and, therefore, no Wallerian degeneration occurs distally. Based on these examinations it should be easy to establish the diagnosis of 'root avulsion'. In clinical practice, this is not so, because avulsion may not involve all five roots. If one root is avulsed and another is not, the electrophysiological tests are inconclusive. Even with CT myelography there may be false positive or false negative results. Therefore, the preoperative evaluation will give the surgeon a good idea of what has really happened at the root level but these findings can never be completely relied upon. If management is to be based on the presence or absence of a root avulsion, this can be proved only by surgical exploration.

The localization and extent of the damage

The localization of the lesion in the peripheral segment of the brachial plexus can be established accurately by clinical examination. If the serratus anterior muscle is functioning and the patient can rotate the scapula upwards, the long thoracic nerve must be intact. Since this nerve is the first branch of the spinal nerves C5, C6 and C7, the absence of paralysis of the serratus anterior means that at least one of these three spinal nerves is not avulsed. If there is partial innervation of the pectoralis major muscle, the lesion must be distal to the nn. pectorales mediales or laterales. If the supra- and infraspinatus muscles contract, the suprascapular nerve is intact. Since this nerve leaves the superior trunk at its distal end, the lesion will probably be at the cord level.

Indications for surgery

Surgery for early secondary repair of the brachial plexus is indicated:

1. If root avulsion can be proved for all five roots, early conservative treatment is useless and surgery should be performed as soon as the general condition of the patient allows. Very early operations, a few days after the accident, as suggested by R. Birch (personal communication) have not proved better than surgery during the first few weeks;
2. If a Tinel Hofmann sign occurs and does not proceed in distal direction during the first few weeks;
3. If signs of recovery have occurred but do not progress.

Surgery should be performed as soon as it is evident that spontaneous recovery will not occur, and always within six months of the injury.

Technique of exploration

Approach and positioning

There are two basic ways for the surgical approach:

Approach from the front

The patient is placed in the semisitting position. The surgeon sits in front of the patient and sees them approximately in the same way as anatomical textbooks present dissection. The major disadvantage of this approach is that several structures, particularly the clavicle, hide the important sections of the brachial plexus. In the early years of brachial plexus surgery, transection of the clavicle was an important step to obtain sufficient access.

Approach from a cranial direction

The patient is placed in the supine position with the shoulder slightly elevated by placing a cushion beneath the scapula. The arm is kept fully mobile. The surgeon sits between the head and arm. The clavicle and the external jugular vein are isolated and this gives excellent access to the supra- and infraclavicular fossa. An osteotomy of the clavicle is never necessary. If more peripheral segments of the brachial plexus have to be exposed in the axilla, or if the peripheral nerves in the upper arm have to be identified, the surgeon moves to the angle between the arm and the trunk and has an equally good view of these operative fields. I personally favour this approach. It is true that an osteotomy of the clavicle is not a difficult procedure, especially if the application of the plate for the later osteosynthesis is done before the osteotomy. However, it is not the clavicle alone that is of importance. There are many other structures, such as the omohyoideus muscle, the connective tissue beneath the clavicle (which contains the suprascapular vessels), the subclavius muscle, and the pectoralis minor muscle, which also limit the surgeon's access when the frontal approach is elected. These structures must also be transected if the osteotomy of the clavicle is to be exploited to its full extent. For a later grafting procedure, it makes a big difference whether the nerve grafts lie directly beneath the osteosynthesized clavicle, or whether there are soft tissue structures to cover them.

Skin incision

When I started to do brachial plexus surgery in the mid-1960s, I utilized a Z-like incision, which commenced behind the sternocleidomastoid muscle, followed its course towards the sternoclavicular joint, then followed the clavicle, and, at about the distal extremity of the clavicle, bent again to traverse the pectoralis major muscle. If necessary, the incision was extended along the ventral axillary fold to the arm and followed the midline of the medial aspect of the upper arm as far as necessary.

This incision was utilized by many brachial plexus surgeons in subsequent years; it has two disadvantages.

First, the scar of the cervical segment very often becomes keloid, and produces very poor cosmetic results.

Secondly, the angle of the flap between the incision on the neck and the incision along the clavicle is rather acute. If the flap is lifted to a major extent, its tip frequently becomes ischaemic. In order to deal with this problem, I have modified this approach such that the incision in the neck does not cross the sternoclavicular joint, but runs across the supraclavicular fossa, to meet the horizontal incision along the clavicle at about the junction between the medial and the middle thirds. Since this incision traverses a concave area, this segment is carried out in zig-zag fashion.

In recent years, I have developed a completely different technique for the skin incision. From a study (Eberhard *et al.*, 1993b) of the skin tension during typical movements of head and shoulder in the supraclavicular area, it was established that a scar following the skin tension lines running across the supraclavicular fossa is exposed to minimal mechanical irritation. This incision therefore gives the best looking scars. In addition, this incision has the major advantage that access from a cranial direction to the spinal nerves, especially the lower ones C8 and T1, is much better than with the previously used incision. To have similar access after a sagittal incision, the cranial flap had to be raised very far dorsally.

If the skin is undermined in cranial and lateral directions, the whole supra- and infraclavicular fossa can be exposed. It does, however, not provide good access to the spinal nerves C5 and C6, and it does not provide good access to the peripheral segment of the brachial plexus lateral to the pectoralis minor muscle. If the whole plexus has to be exposed, two additional incisions are necessary. One runs parallel to the first sagittal incision in the neck. This incision follows the skin tension lines, and the skin between the two incisions can be elevated as a flap, so that the access is excellent. The second incision starts from a point corresponding to the coracoid process of the scapula and follows skin tension lines in the direction of the anterior axillary fold. It then follows the margin of the axillary fold to the axilla and continues to the medial aspect of the upper arm, as with the previously used incision. Again, the skin between this and the sagittal incision in the supraclavicular fossa can be undermined and lifted as a flap. It is true that this is perhaps technically a little more demanding. However, the access is more satisfactory, and much better protection is provided for the surgical procedures underneath.

Surgical exploration

The operation starts with the sagittal incision and the undermining of the skin in both directions. In the supraclavicular fossa, the superior trunk and the intermediate trunk are exposed.

The next step is to perform the curved incision, starting at the coracoid process. From this incision, the space between the deltoid and the pectoralis major muscle is entered, and, after transection of the fascia, the individual elements of the brachial plexus are identified. If dense fibrosis is encountered here, we follow the rule that the individual elements should be identified in normal tissue; this means that we lengthen the incision into the upper arm. We then identify the peripheral nerves at this level and follow them in a central direction into the axillary groove, and from here to the area lateral to the pectoralis minor muscle. Only after the anatomical situation is completely clear does the dissection proceed in a central direction towards the infraclavicular fossa. An exploration of this fossa is enhanced by detachment of the clavicular origin of the pectoralis major muscle. The individual structures are identified at this level.

The next step is the isolation of the clavicle, and the subclavius and the omohyoideus muscles. The same is done with the connective tissue and the dorsal periosteal aspect of the clavicle, which is also isolated and a sling placed around it. At this stage, we have a sequence of windows that allow access to the different segments of the brachial plexus. The first is cranial to the omohyoideus muscle; the second is between the omohyoideus muscle and the connective tissue beneath the clavicle; the third is between this connective tissue and the clavicle; the fourth is between the clavicle and subclavius; the fifth is between the subclavius and pectoralis minor muscles; and the sixth is lateral to pectoralis minor.

If the spinal nerves C5 and C6 are involved, a third incision is performed and the skin between these incisions is elevated as a flap. The approach to the inferior trunk and to the roots C8 and T1 is achieved by pulling the clavicle either in a caudal or a cranial direction, and then by approaching these structures supra- or infraclavicularly, according to the situation.

Operative findings

Usually, a degree of fibrosis is met during the exposure, which varies according to the extent of injury. It has already been mentioned that, if there is fibrosis, the best way to isolate the individual structures is to identify them first at a level having no scarring.

When there is root avulsion, a meningocoele may be encountered. If the meningocoele is opened, it is resected, and the communication to the subarachnoid space is closed in a watertight fashion. In such cases, avulsed roots may be encountered. In others, the spinal nerves can be followed to the intervertebral foramina. If the fibrosis is encountered mainly at a level of cords and trunks and the spinal nerves do not show post-traumatic changes, one can assume that the roots have not been avulsed. In a certain percentage of patients, avulsion of the rootlets occurs but the spinal component is not drawn out of the intervertebral canal. Central stimulation of the precentral gyrus and recording along the spinal nerve using the technique recommended by Turkof *et al.* (1989, 1994), helps to exclude this possibility.

The spinal nerve may be ruptured, with the formation of a neuroma at this level. Neuromas are identified, resected until normal tissue is met, and continuity is restored.

The spinal nerves may have suffered a traction injury, but not lost continuity. In this case, microsurgical neurolysis is performed, to try to establish the degree of damage (see later). According to the findings, the damaged part of the nerve is resected or preserved.

Very similar situations can be found at the level of the trunks or cords.

In order to select the proper way of dealing with the problem, the degree of damage has to be identified. The extent of damage to any nerve has been classified by Sunderland (1951) into five degrees.

First degree

There is conduction block without morphological changes. Electrophysiologically, the nerve tissue continues to conduct distal to the lesion because no Wallerian degeneration occurs. After such a lesion, complete spontaneous recovery is possible.

Second degree

In this case, the continuity of the axons is lost, but the other structures of the nerve remain intact. Wallerian degeneration occurs, and conductivity distal to the lesion is lost within a few days. Complete spontaneous recovery is possible.

Theoretically, there is no indication for surgery in first and second degree lesions because a good spontaneous recovery can be expected. However, due to fibrotic changes, the nerve tissue can be exposed to compression and this prevents spontaneous recovery. These secondary changes were not considered by Sunderland. His system can therefore be modified by adding to the description the reactions of the tissues following the injury. The amount of fibrosis is of particular importance (Millesi, 1986a,b).

- *Type-A fibrosis* The epifascicular epineurium becomes fibrotic and the whole nerve is compressed as if in a tight stocking.
- *Type-B fibrosis* The intrafascicular epineurium also becomes fibrotic.
- *Type-C fibrosis* The content of the fascicles of the endoneurium becomes completely fibrotic.

If type-A or type-B fibrosis is combined with a first or second degree lesion (IA, IB, IIA, IIB), spontaneous recovery will be impeded. This is a situation in which neurolysis helps. (Damage of the degree IC or IIC cannot occur because, according to the definition, the endoneurium remains intact with a first or a second degree lesion.)

Third degree

According to the Sunderland classification, this means a loss of continuity of axons and of endoneurial structures, but with an intact perineurium. This lesion can be combined with type-A or type-B fibrosis. However, type-C fibrosis may occasionally occur if the lesion has been very severe, or if a long time has elapsed since the injury. A lesion of type-IIIA and type-IIIB requires neurolysis. If there is a type-C fibrosis, neurolysis is of no benefit and these segments should be resected and replaced by nerve grafts.

Fourth degree

At this level, all structures have lost continuity, except the epineurial connective tissue. A spontaneous recovery is unlikely to occur. This can be further divided into two subtypes. The remaining link between the proximal and distal ends may be invaded by axon sprouts and some of these may even reach the distal stump. This can be classified as damage of degree IV-N ('neuroma'-like). In other cases, the outgrowth of the neuroma is limited and the link between the two stumps consists only of scar tissue (degree IV-S, 'scar'-like). In both situations, resection of the damaged segment and the restoration of continuity by nerve grafts is indicated.

Fifth degree

This means a complete loss of continuity, and surgical restoration is indicated. In the same nerve segment, differing degrees of damage may be combined, especially a combination of degrees III and IV. The different degrees can be differentiated by intraneural microsurgical neurolysis.

The classification of brachial plexus injury is summarized in Table 40.1.

Technique of repair

If continuity of the nerves is preserved, and the structures of the brachial plexus have been compromised only by external compression, then *external neurolysis* is performed and the causes of compression are removed.

If nerve continuity is preserved, but the structures of the brachial plexus show thickening and fibrosis, a longitudinal transection of the tissue outside the epineurium is performed (*paraneuriotomy*) after external neurolysis. Ultimately, this tissue is removed (*paraneuriectomy*). If there is dense fibrosis, the differentiation between the paraneurium and the epineurium is no longer possible because both layers form a single fibrotic sheath, as in fibrosis of type-A. If this occurs, this layer is transected longitudinally (*epifascicular epineuriotomy*), but, if this is not sufficient to achieve adequate decompression, the tissue is removed from all around the nerve (*epifascicular epineuriectomy*). If the fascicles are still compressed, fibrotic tissue between the fascicles is removed (*interfascicular epineuriectomy*). If interfascicular dissection cannot be performed because the fascicular structure has been lost, or if the fascicles present themselves as thick shrunken structures, the whole *segment is resected* until normal tissue is encountered. Continuity is restored by *nerve grafts*.

Table 40.1. Combined evaluation system for extent of brachial plexus injuries

Degree	Continuity	Fibrosis	Prognosis	Surgical procedure
1	Conduction block	None	Spontaneous recovery	None
1A	Conduction block	Fibrosis of epifascicular epineurium	No spontaneous recovery	Epifascicular epineuriotomy
1B	Conduction block	Fibrosis of interfascicular epineurium	No spontaneous recovery	Epifascicular epineuriectomy interfascicular epineuriectomy (partial)
2	Axons interrupted	None	Spontaneous recovery	None
2A	Axons interrupted	Fibrosis of epifascicular epineurium	No spontaneous recovery	Epifascicular epineuriotomy
2B	Axons interrupted	Fibrosis of interfascicular epineurium	No spontaneous recovery	Epifascicular epineuriectomy interfascicular epineuriectomy (partial)
3	Axons interrupted	None	Partial spontaneous recovery	None
3A	Axons interrupted endoneurial structures damaged, perineurium intact	Fibrosis of epifascicular epineurium	No spontaneous recovery	Epifascicular epineuriotomy
3B	Axons interrupted endoneurial structures damaged, perineurium intact	Fibrosis of interfascicular epineurium	No spontaneous recovery	Epifascicular epineuriectomy, interfascicular epineuriectomy (partial)
3C	Axons interrupted, endoneurial structures damaged, perineurium intact	Fibrosis of endoneurium	No spontaneous recovery	Resection plus nerve grafting
4N	Fascicular structures interrupted, continuity preserved by fibrotic connective tissue with ingrowing neuroma	Continuity preserved by fibrotic connective tissue with ingrowing neuroma	No useful spontaneous recovery	Resection plus nerve grafting
4S	Fascicular structures interrupted	Continuity preserved by fibrotic tissues only (no conduction possible)	No spontaneous recovery	Resection plus nerve grafting
S	Complete loss of continuity		No spontaneous recovery	Nerve grafting, nerve transfer

If continuity has been lost, and a neuroma has formed at the proximal stump, resection is performed of both segments until normal nerve tissue is encountered. Continuity is restored by means of *nerve grafts*.

For the restoration of continuity there are two basic options: between the proximal and the distal stumps; and between the proximal stump and a selected peripheral nerve.

If there is a *limited defect* (e.g. within the superior trunk or within a cord), the best technique is to restore continuity between the proximal and the distal stumps after adequate resection.

However, if there is a *long defect*, the simple restoration of continuity includes the danger of diluting the axons, and it increases the danger of irregular outgrowth, which means that nerve fibres for a certain muscle may also reach antagonists and, even after useful recovery, the functional result may be neutralized. In this case, it is preferable to bypass the distal stump and to unite the proximal stump directly with the peripheral nerve to be innervated (e.g. the musculocutaneous or axillary nerves).

In *root avulsion*, continuity cannot be restored. There have been experimental attempts to insert nerve grafts directly into the spinal cord in the hope that axons will grow into a peripheral nerve (Carlstedt *et al.* 1990). The future will show whether or not this will become an established technique. For the moment, the only way to deal with root avulsion in clinical practice is *nerve transfer*; the available sources are:

- Motor branches of the cervical plexus (Brunelli and Monini, 1984);
- The accessory nerve: this nerve can be used distal to the first branch to trapezius thereby avoiding complete denervation of the muscle;
- The hypoglossal nerve;
- The phrenic nerve (I have no personal experience with either hypoglossal or phrenic nerve transfer, because I hesitate to sacrifice them);
- The dorsal scapular nerve;
- The intercostal nerves: Intercostal nerves can be dissected throughout their length and transferred to the upper arm, in order that they may be directly coapted to the stump of the peripheral nerve (e.g. the musculocutaneous nerve). This means, however, that the nerve must be dissected to a level at which the number of motor fibres is much reduced. The alternative, which I prefer; is to transect the intercostal nerve more proximally where it contains many more motor fibres, and connect it via a nerve graft.

- C7 from the contralateral side: Gu *et al.* (1992) suggested the C7 root from the normal side as a source for nerve grafting. This root can be transected easily without significant loss of function. There is some weakness of the extensor muscles of the wrist and fingers and the triceps, and some loss of sensibility on the dorsal radial aspect of the index finger. After some months, patients will adapt to this loss of function. I have carried out this procedure so far in four patients, although follow-up is not yet long enough to draw firm conclusions as far as functional gain is concerned. None of the four patients has complained about any loss of function. However, there is a danger of more significant loss of function if there is a variation in the distribution of fibres. For this reason, I perform the operation in two stages. In the first stage the root C7 is ligated. If, a few days later,

Table 40.2. Nerve transfer in avulsion of all five roots

(a) Surgery:

Donor	Recipient nerve
Accessory nerve	Suprascapular nerve
Motor branch of cervical plexus	Axillary nerve
Motor branch of cervical plexus	Medial and/or lateral pectoral nerve
Sensory branch of cervical plexus	Median nerve
Dorsal scapular nerve	Long thoracic nerve
Intercostal nerve 2	Thoracodorsal nerve
Intercostal nerves 3–5	Musculocutaneous nerve
Intercostal nerves 6, 7	Radial nerve (branches to triceps muscle)

(b) Results: Results for functional recovery of biceps brachii (BB) and triceps brachii (TB). Patients who achieved the functional result of M3 or better are listed as a fraction of the total number. There are also patients who achieved a function of M3 or better after transfer of the triceps muscle to the biceps tendon (TB TF).

No. patients	7
Follow-up (*n*)	7[a]
BB M3 or better	3/7
TB M3 or better	1/4
TB TF	2[b]
Flexion of the elbow joint M3 or better	5/7

[a]Minimum length of follow-up 4 years.
[b]In one patient, useful elbow flexion was achieved by combining the weak force of the biceps (M2+) and the weak force of the triceps (M2+).
BB, biceps brachii; TB, triceps brachii; TB TF, transfer of the triceps muscle to the biceps tendon.

the patient has not experienced a significant loss of function, the anastomosis is performed. This provides the option to decompress the spinal nerve C7 immediately if an unexpected loss of function occurs (Eberhard and Millesi, 1993a).

Tables 40.2–40.8 summarize our strategy for the management of various root injuries, and the results of treatment.

Table 40.3. Avulsion of four roots (C6, C7, C8, T1)

(a) Surgery: Three variations are used:

Donor nerve	Recipient nerve
C5	Lateral cord
Accessory nerve	Suprascapular nerve
Motor branch of cervical plexus	Axillary nerve
Motor branch of cervical plexus	Medial and/or lateral pectoral nerve
Dorsal scapular nerve	Long thoracic nerve
Intercostal nerve 2, 3 or 4	Thoracodorsal nerve
Intercostal nerves 5–7	Radial nerve (branches to triceps muscle)
C5	Posterior cord
Accessory nerve	Suprascapular nerve
Motor branch of cervical plexus	Medial and/or lateral pectoral nerves
Dorsal scapular nerve	Long thoracic nerve
2nd intercostal nerve	Thoracodorsal nerve
Intercostal nerves 3, 4	Median nerve
Accessory nerve	Musculocutaneous nerve
C5	Posterior cord
Accessory nerve	Musculocutaneous nerve
Motor branch of cervical plexus	Suprascapular nerve
Motor branch of cervical plexus	Medial and/or lateral pectoral nerves
Dorsalis scapular nerve	Long thoracic nerve
2nd intercostal nerve	Thoracodorsal nerve
Intercostal nerves 3–7	Median nerve

(b) Results: (For explanation see Table 40.2.)

No. patients	6
Follow-up (*n*)	6[a]
BB M3 or better	3/6
TB M3 or better	2/6
TB TF M3 or better	2
Flexion of the elbow joint M3 or better after TB TF	5/6

[a]Minimum length of follow-up 4 years.

Table 40.4. Avulsion of two or three roots (C7, C8, T1; C8, T1)

(a) Surgery: (For explanation see Table 40.2.)

Avulsion of C7, C8, T1
  C5 Dorsal cord
  C6 Lateral cord

Avulsion C8, T1
  C5 Dorsal cord (suprascapular nerve, axillary nerve)
  C6 Lateral cord (musculocutaneous nerve)
  C7 Dorsal cord and lateral cord (median nerve) (radial nerve)

(b) Results:

No. patients	11
Follow-up (*n*)	11
BB M3 or better	5/10
TB M3 or better	3/10
TB TF	3
Flexion of the elbow joint M3 or better after TB TF	7[a]

[a]In one patient, the transfer of the triceps did not yield a useful result.

Table 40.5. Rupture of three to five roots

Surgery: Restoration of continuity by nerve grafting

Results: (For explanation see Table 40.2.)

No. Patients	6
Follow-up (*n*)	5
BB M3 or better	3/5
TB M3 or better	3/4
TB TF	2
Flexion of the elbow joint M3 or better after TB TF	5/5

Table 40.6. Rupture of one to two roots

Surgery: Restoration of continuity by nerve grafting

Results: (For explanation see Table 40.2.)

No. patients	10
Follow-up (*n*)	9
BB M3 or better	7/9
TB M3 or better	5/7
TB TF	1
Flexion of the elbow joint M3 or better after TB TF	8/9

Table 40.7. Lesion at the level of the superior trunk with loss of continuity, and complete loss of function of the intermediate and inferior trunks

Surgery: Restoration of continuity by nerve grafting

Results: (For explanation see Table 40.2.)

No. patients	5
Follow-up (*n*)	5
BB M3 or better	2/5
TB M3 or better	1/5
TB TF	2
Flexion of the elbow joint M3 or better after TB TF	4/5[a]

[a] In one patient, satisfactory elbow flexion was achieved by transfer of a sufficiently strong triceps brachii. In a second patient, useful function was restored by combining the weak forceps of the biceps brachii (M2+) and the triceps brachii (M2+).

Table 40.8. Lesion at the level of the cords

Surgery: Restoration of continuity by nerve grafting, frequently combined with neurolysis of noninterrupted segments

Results: (For explanation see Table 40.2.)

No. patients	7
Follow-up (*n*)	7
BB M3 or better	6/7
TB M3 or better	4/6
TB TF	1
Flexion of the elbow joint M3 or better after TB TF	7/7

Source of grafts

1. *Free cutaneous nerve grafts* In the majority of patients, free cutaneous nerve grafts will be applied, utilizing the two sural nerves, the medial cutaneous nerve of the arm, and superficial parts of the radial nerve.
2. *Vascularized nerve grafts* If the roots C8 and T1 are avulsed, the ulnar nerve can be used as a vascularized nerve graft. Using the technique described by Terzis (1993), this nerve can be transferred on the superior ulnar collateral artery as a pedicled or a free microvascular graft.
3. *Split nerve grafts* If a transfer of the ulnar nerve as a vascularized trunk graft is not possible or not suitable, the nerve can be split into its fascicle groups, which are the size of cutaneous nerves and survive free grafting very well (Eberhard and Millesi, 1994).

Postoperative care

The patient is immobilized for 10 days in a plaster cast, which includes the head, the trunk and the arm. Thereafter, passive and active mobilization is commenced. Electrotherapy with exponential current of the denervated muscles is advised. By splinting we try to avoid the elongation of muscles, especially of the biceps. The use of a custom-made orthosis is recommended.

Complications

The most important complication of partial brachial lesions is the secondary loss of function that had been originally preserved. This may occur if segments of the brachial plexus have been traumatized but remain functional, and subsequent surgical manipulation then turns the partial lesion into a complete one. Fortunately, this happens only very rarely, but it has to be discussed with the patient preoperatively. A postoperative haematoma or a problem of wound healing does not usually influence the final outcome.

If long nerve grafts have been used, one has to consider the possibility of a block at the distal site of coaptation. This can be recognized if the Tinel sign advances along the graft, but then stops at the distal stump. The distal anastomosis should be explored and resected, and continuity restored by end-to-end neurorrhapy.

A cerebrospinal fistula may occur after the excision of a meningocoele. Usually it closes spontaneously with serial lumbar punctures.

Further reconstructive surgery

The treatment of patients with a brachial plexus lesion should not only include the surgery on the brachial plexus itself and the immediate postoperative care. It should be a global treatment that cares for these patients preoperatively, and which provides them with the opportunity for a change of occupation, and allows them to be reintegrated into society as soon as possible. This is extremely important because, even when there is useful improvement, the extent of recovery will rarely be sufficient to allow these patients to resume their original occupations.

After surgery, the patient should be re-evaluated, in order to plan further reconstructive surgery. This has the aim of making maximum use of any recovered muscle function, and is particularly indicated in those with partial lesions, but it also plays an important role in patients with complete lesions and partial recovery. The following should be considered:

Shoulder joint

Subluxation of the shoulder joint can be neutralized by transferring the horizontal component of the trapezius muscle, including a bony fragment of the acromion, to the surgical neck of the humerus. This operation always gives static support and sometimes also some dynamic improvement.

External rotation

In order to provide external rotation, we perform a rotatory osteotomy of the humerus and simultaneously transfer the pectoralis major muscle, to give it an external rotational action.

Elbow

When there is simultaneous innervation of the biceps and the triceps, the action of these muscles is neutralized. Elbow flexion can be improved if the triceps is transferred to the biceps tendon; both then act as flexors. If the biceps is paralysed but the triceps muscle has developed sufficient strength, the same transfer can be carried out and the triceps will then take over elbow flexion.

In my experience, the triceps has a good, if not better, tendency to reassume sufficient strength compared with the biceps. Therefore, in recent years in patients with root avulsion we have reinnervated both muscles by intercostal nerve transfer, planning a later transfer of the triceps to gain sufficient strength of elbow flexion. The pectoralis major muscle may also be used to replace the biceps for elbow flexion.

In an upper brachial plexus lesion, the common flexor origin can be transferred to the humeral shaft to provide elbow flexion. In an upper brachial plexus (C5, C6 and C7) lesion, tendon transfer is indicated to replace radial nerve function.

If, in a complete brachial plexus lesion, some forearm muscles recover, a primitive grip function may be restored by tendon transfer following arthrodesis of the wrist joint.

Expected results

The results we can expect are far from satisfactory. However, if the original condition of the patient is considered, having a flail arm, which is rather an obstacle, the overall beneficial effect for the patient is enormous. Generally, patients are very happy with the results of brachial plexus surgery. We consider recovery useful if the patient has regained some control of the shoulder joint and if there is flexion of the elbow joint and adduction and external rotation of the upper arm. If, in addition, a primitive gripping function can be restored in the hand, we are very satisfied. Further improvement may be achieved by free muscle grafting to restore finger flexion and extension (Berger *et al.*, 1990; Doi *et al.*, 1993; Terzis, 1993).

References

Berger A, Flory PJ, Schaller E. (1990) Muscle transfers in brachial plexus lesions. *J Reconstr Microsurg* **2**: 113–66.

Breidenbach W, Terzis JK. (1984) The anatomy of free vascularized nerve grafts. *Clin Plast Surg* **11**: 65–71.

Brunelli G, Monini L. (1984) Neurotization of avulsed roots of the brachial plexus by means of anterior nerves of cervical plexus. *Clin Plast Surg* **11**: 149–52.

Carlstedt T, Risling M, Linda H, *et al.* (1990) Regeneration after spinal nerve injury. *Restorative Neurol Neurosci* **1**: 189–95.

Doi K, Sakai K, Thara K, Abe Y, Kaeai S, Kurafuji Y. (1993) Reinnervated free muscle transplantation for extremity reconstruction. *Plast Reconstr Surg* **91**: 872–83.

Eberhard D, Wenger S, Millesi H. (1993a) Uberlegungen zur Verwendung der Wurzel C7 als Axonspender bei Wurzelausrissen des Plexus brachialis der kontralateralen Seite. Presented at the *31st Annual Meeting of the Austrian Society for Plastic, Esthetic and Reconstructive Surgery*. Zell/See, October 14–16, 1993.

Eberhard D, Reihsner R, Millesi H. (1993b) Advantages of sagittal incisions in brachial plexus exposure. Poster presented at *11th Symposium of the International Society of Reconstructive Microsurgery*. Vienna, June 5–8, 1993.

Eberhard D, Millesi H. (1994) Split nerve graft as an alternative to vascularized nerve grafting. Presented at the *4th Annual Meeting of the American Society for Peripheral Nerves*. New York, May, 13–15, 1994. Split nerve grafting. *J Reconstr Microsurg* **12**: 71–6 (1996).

Gu YD, Zang GM, Yan JG, Cheng XM, Chen L. (1992) Seventh cervical root transfer from the lateral healthy side for treatment of the brachial plexus. *J Hand Surg Br* **17B**: 518–21.

Millesi H. (1986a) Das Problem der Defektbehebung peripherer Nerven. Presented at the *9th Meeting of the Deutschsprachige Arbeitsgemeinschaft fur Mikrochirurgie der peripheren Nerven und Gefasse*. Bern, December, 1986.

Millesi H. (1986b) Eingriffe an peripheren Nerven. In: Gschnitzer F, Kern E, Schweiberer L, editors. *Chirurgische Operationslehre*. Munich: Urban & Schwarzenberg, 1–88.

Sunderland S. (1951) A classification of peripheral nerve injuries producing loss of function. *Brain* **74**: 491.

Terzis JK. (1993) Brachial plexus: functional reconstruction by free muscle graft. Presented at *11th Symposium of the Society for Reconstructive Microsurgery*. Vienna, June 5–8, 1993.

Turkof E, Mayr N, Deecke L, Millesi H. (1989) Central stimulation to prove conductivity of spinal motor roots in brachial plexus surgery. Presented at *4th International Congress of the International Federation of Societies for Surgery of the Hand*. Tel-Aviv, 9–14 April, 1989.

Turkof E, Monsivais J, Bellolo H, Millesi H, Mayr N. (1994) Motor evoked potentials is a reliable method to detect intralaminar root avulsions in brachial plexus surgery: an experimental study on goats. Presented at the *4th Annual Scientific Meeting of The American Society For Peripheral Nerves*. New York, May 13–15, 1994.

41

Peripheral nerve injury

AF Stewart Flemming, Nandagudi S Niranjan

Introduction

Peripheral nerve injuries are still common in civilian life, largely as a result of violence and industrial injury. There are two main sequelae following peripheral nerve injuries: inadequate return of motor or sensory function; and a painful state (neuroma in continuity and reflex sympathetic dystrophy). These two sequelae can be avoided or improved by utilizing an appropriate suture technique.

Definitions

The functional unit of a peripheral nerve is a single cell called a neurone.

Anatomy

A nerve fibre is composed of motor, sensory and sympathetic neurones.

Neurones have their bodies located in the ventral horn of the spinal cord for a motor nerve, and in the posterior root ganglion for a sensory nerve. Motor nerve fibres terminate at the neuromuscular junctions of the muscle; the sensory nerve fibres terminate in the skin as free nerve endings or in specialized receptors.

The components of nerve connective tissue (Figure 41.1) are: endoneurium – the fine connective tissue between nerve fibres; perineurium –

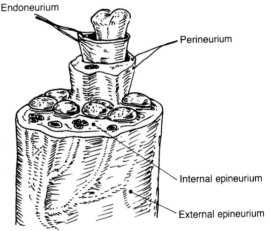

Figure 41.1. Basic composition of the peripheral nerve connective tissue.

the connective tissue that wraps around the fascicles; internal epinenrium – the connective tissue that separates fascicles; and external epineurium – the connective tissue that surrounds the entire nerve.

Fascicular patterns

There are three fascicular patterns: monofascicular (the nerve is composed of a single fascicle), oligofascicular (the nerve contains a few fascicles), polyfascicular (the nerve fibres are arranged in multiple fascicles) (Figure 41.2).

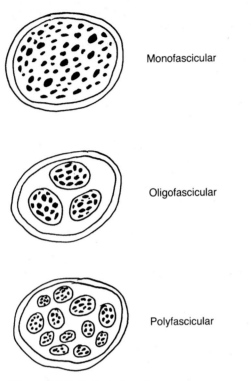

Figure 41.2. Basic fascicular patterns.

Internal topography

The degree of plexus formation that occurs between fascicles decreases as the nerve progresses distally (Figure 41.3).

Blood supply

Peripheral nerves have two distinct blood supplies: segmental (external) and intraneuronal (internal).

Structural pathology

Following injury to a peripheral nerve, the axon swells up, both proximally and distally. In the distal segment this is called Wallerian degeneration. In the proximal nerve stem the degeneration occurs for a variable distance above the site of injury.

The proximal nerve cell body swells up and demonstrates increased metabolic activity for 10–20 days. The rate of axon regeneration is

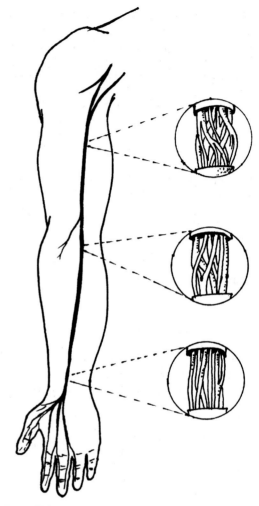

Figure 41.3. Internal topography of the median nerve.

approximately 1–3 mm per day, if and when the severed nerve realigns for repair. The survival and growth of neurones after an injury are dependent upon delicate biochemical mechanisms. A number of neuronotrophic factors have been defined, namely nerve growth factor and neurite promoting factors. Both of these factors are produced by Schwann cells.

Measurement of outcome

Measuring function accurately is not easy in the injured nerve. Modern reviews of the subject (Jerosh-Herold, 1993; Jones, 1989; McAllister and Calder, 1995) reflect the frustration felt by many of the fathers of modern nerve surgery, such as Moberg, Seddon and Sunderland. The simpler the method the less may be inferred from it: but even sophisticated methods of testing may not relate well with hand function. A good history of what the patient can and cannot do is important. Patients may not understand what causes their difficulties and it may be hard to determine how their problems relate to the clinical findings. The inability to manipulate small objects may be due to lack of sweating, lack of sensibility, lack of co-ordination, or a combination of these. Measurements of nerve regrowth, appreciation of different types of sensation, innervation density, localization, stereognosis, proprioception, and functional testing are all important in giving a guide to prognosis. Other tests, such as sudomotor function, wear marks, nerve conduction studies and EMGs also have their place in determining outcome.

Nerve assessment

Nerve assessment may be divided into evidence of nerve regrowth, sensory threshold testing, innervation density testing, and either functional or electronic testing. There is considerable debate in the literature about which tests are the most relevant to practical hand function. A battery of tests done sequentially will provide more information than a test done in isolation. The results will be used to back up or refute the patient's claims of lack of function.

Evidence of nerve regrowth

An advancing Tinel's sign (Hoffman, 1915; Tinel, 1915) is the simplest way of determining nerve regrowth (Sunderland, 1978). It does not relate to the quantity or quality of nerves regrowing, or to final sensory perception. A more powerful Tinel's sign distally than proximally is a favourable sign and suggests that more fibres are regrowing than staying at the site of neurorrhaphy (Henderson, 1948).

Sudomotor function is important to hand function (Harrison, 1974; Moberg, 1958) and its status should always be recorded. Its absence will interfere with the ability to manipulate fine objects and paper. The ninhydrin test (Mobers, 1958; Seddon, 1975) and electrical conductance (Egyed *et al.*, 1980; Richter and Katz, 1943; Smith and

Mott, 1986) can be used where there is doubt, but the plastic pen test and observation are simple tests that will do in most cases. There is wider overlap of autonomic territories than of sensory nerves (Highet, 1942). Sweating only indicates the presence of autonomic fibres, it does not necessarily correlate with nerve recovery (Moberg, 1958). Frequently sensory and autonomic recovery are similar.

The wrinkle test (O'Rain, 1973) is a simple but gross test of innervation. It is most useful in small children and in uncommunicative patients. The hand and finger pulps have a characteristic appearance in long-standing dennervation (Lister, 1993).

In motor palsy there will be typical wasting of the hand and forearm. Increasing strength and muscle bulk are crude signs of recovery; care should be taken not to confuse recovery in one group of muscles with compensatory hypertrophy of others.

Threshold testing

The first sensory modality to return is usually 30 cps vibration sense, followed by moving light touch (Dellon, 1988a; Dellon *et al.*, 1972; Jabaley *et al.*, 1976). The last sensation to recover is 256 cps vibration sense (Dellon, 1988a; Gelberman *et al.*, 1978). Von Frey (1896) hair testing or Semmes–Weinstein fibre testing (Weinstein, 1962) can be used to test the threshold of stimulation of the slowly adapting fibres of the nerve. The tests are inaccurate physically (Levin *et al.*, 1978), but give a measure of nerve recovery if done with care under consistent conditions. Vibrograms (Lundborg *et al.*, 1986) test the rapidly adapting fibres. These tests are subjective and when there is inconsistency in a given test, or between similar types of tests, doubt should be cast upon the results.

Innervation density measurement

Both static and moving two point discrimination 2PD provide a measure of a patient's ability to use the hand but should not be used on their own. Moberg (1962) stated that Weber's (1835) static two-point test correlated best with hand function, but the test needs to be performed carefully (Brand and Hollister, 1992; Callahan, 1984). Dellon has said that static 2PD (1988b) and moving 2PD (1988c) correspond respectively to the number of slow and fast adapting receptors in the skin (1988b). Marsh (1990) has challenged these views and suggested that localization is a better measure if other factors are taken into account. Dellon *et al.* (1974) have suggested that localization recovers early. The clinical experience of those performing nerve surgery is that static 2PD and moving 2PD give a reasonable assessment of spatial discrimination (Burge, 1993), and, in many patients, this correlates reasonably well with hand function (Chassard *et al.*, 1993). Authors differ in what 2PD distance correlates with the ability to manipulate small objects, but less than 8–10 mm is generally accepted. 2PD does not correspond to the cerebral perception of what the hand 'feels' or the normal patterns of use. Some authors suggest that object and texture recognition are the only true tests of nerve function (Wynn Parry, 1987). Sensory re-education improves 2PD (Imai *et al.*, 1991).

Functional testing

Grip strength is helpful in determining the return of gross muscle function, but may be affected by pain (local or general), patient effort, time since surgery, wrist position and age. The dominant hand is not always the strongest (Schmidt and Toews, 1970). Useful checks are the forearm muscle circumference (low if the hand is genuinely not being used), rapid exchange grip (Hildrath *et al.*, 1989) and the differences in strength at different grip widths (Stokes, 1983). Pinch strength is also helpful but key, tip and tripod pinch should be assessed, depending on the problem described by the patient. Other methods are being developed (Trumble *et al.*, 1995), but strength gives no clue about co-ordination and integration of function with sensory feedback. As yet no effective tests for these are available, although those such as the pick-up test (Mobers, 1958), and co-ordination tests (Jebson *et al.*, 1969) come closest. Training and visualizing specific tasks will help to relearn previous behaviour patterns, but these take time and are probably job specific.

Wear marks and the appearance of the pulps (Mobers, 1962) give crude indications of how much the hand is being used. These do not correlate with nerve function but their presence may cast doubt on the patient's assertions and may be used as some evidence of hand function (Moberg, 1958). (NB: a ring will give rise to a

calosity on the palm adjacent to the finger on which the ring is worn).

Localization of touch depends on 'reprogramming' which is assisted by input from intact nerves. Early incorrect localization is replaced quite quickly by more normal responses if sensory retraining is performed (Dellon *et al.*, 1974). Care must be taken when testing, as moving the digit may stimulate proprioceptive impulses or Paccinian corpuscles in uninjured nerves.

Joint position sense may be served by several nerves and is variable in its return. Recovery is rarely perfect and is also dependent on cutaneous sensation (Moberg, 1976). Stereognosis or tactile gnosis is rarely as good as before injury, except in the very young, but can be improved by sensory re-education. People who do fine work are most affected by the loss of these functions, particularly those that do work in which they cannot see their hands. Functional testing, such as the pick-up test (Moberg, 1958), and object identification (Porter, 1966; Seddon, 1972) are useful guides to the progress of nerve recovery, but they can be learned and care should be taken in interpreting them.

Nerve conduction studies and EMGs do not always correlate with function, but give a good indication of nerve regrowth and help to monitor progress. They will show evidence of reinnervation of muscles and define areas of slowed conduction (due to compression or scarring). Intraoperative testing may sometimes be of use in determining how to proceed (van Beek and Heyman, 1991), but one should be aware of the pitfalls of doing so (Dellon, 1991). Sensory scoring and motor power scoring (see Table 41.1) are crude determinants of function but they are some measure of nerve regrowth.

Prognosis

The prognosis of a nerve injury depends on the initial trauma, the nerve, the patient, the repair, and the subsequent treatment. It is important to record sensory and motor function data as accurately as possible in view of the numerous variations in innervation in the hand, both sensory (Botte *et al.*, 1990; Brandsma *et al.*, 1986; Highet, 1942; Kaplan, 1963; McCake and Kleinert, 1990; Meals and Shaner, 1983) and motor (Brandsma *et al.*, 1986; Cannieu, 1896; Riche, 1897; Seradge and Seradge, 1990).

Frequently, the notes are scanty or details have been left out on the basis that it is what is always

Table 41.1. Grading of nerve injury

(a) MRC

	Degree of recovery
MRC grading sensory	
S4	Normal sensibility; 2PD less than 6 mm; tactile gnosis
S3+	Some recovery of 2PD (7–15 mm) within the autonomous area of the nerve
S3	Return of pain and touch with no over-reaction
S2	Return of pain and some touch sensation with no over-reaction
S1	Recovery of deep cutaneous pain
S0	No sensation; Absence of sensibility
MRC grading (motor)	
M5	Full recovery of motor function
M4	All synergic and independent movements possible
M3	All important muscles act against resistance
M2	Return of perceptible contraction in both proximal and distal muscles
M1	Return of perceptible contraction of proximal muscles
M0	No contraction

(b) Sunderland

Sunderland grading	*Terminology*	*Degree of nerve injury*	*Outcome*
1	Neuropraxia	Loss of action of the sodium pump	Complete recovery
		Damage to the Schwann cells without loss of nerve continuity	
2	Axontmesis	Loss of the Schwann cells axon division but outer membranes intact	More or less complete recovery
3	Axontmesis	Loss of fascicular architecture, but inner epineurium intact	Variable recovery
4	Axontmesis	Loss of all of architecture except for outer epineurium	Poor, if any recovery
5	Neurotmesis	Complete division	No recovery without repair
6	Combination of any of the above	Combination of any of the above	Patchy recovery, unpredictable

done. Correspondence with the operating surgeon may be needed. Where details of the injury and operation are not available, a certain amount may be deduced from the patient's history. It is important to realize that the quality of this information is only as reliable as the patient's memory. Well written notes may be a mine of useful information (and protect the writer in case his/her handling of the case is drawn into question).

The pattern of recovery and sequential examinations are important in the early phases. The final outcome may not be apparent until 2–5 years after the last surgical procedure. The prognosis should reflect those problems that will resolve with time and those that are likely to be permanent. Where possible, an expected time to maximum recovery should be given. If this is not possible, this should be stated clearly.

The nerve injury

The degree of injury will determine how the nerve recovers (Steinberg and Koman, 1991). In most patients, this is not within the surgeon's control. Avulsion injuries have a poor prognosis; clean cut nerves have the best (Sullivan, 1985), while in between come a mixture of injuries that combine cut, crush and avulsion, the commonest of which are saw injuries. The extent of the damage seen at operation is important (Kallio and Vastamaki, 1993), but it is rarely recorded; the degree of damage to adjacent tissues may give a clue.

Sunderland grade 1 injuries (neuropraxia) should recover completely. Grade 2 injuries usually undergo complete recovery, but after a longer time. In grade 3 and grade 6 injuries (added by Mackinnon, 1989) the prognosis is uncertain, whilst untreated grades 4 and 5 injuries are unlikely to recover any significant function (Chow and Ng, 1993; Sullivan, 1985). Unfortunately, the external appearance of a nerve is no guide to the Sunderland grading, with the exception of grade 5. Electrical testing may be of help, although even this cannot be performed until at least 72 hours postinjury (Kline and Nulsen, 1972).

Loss of nerve tissue makes the prognosis worse. In a high energy injury, such as a gunshot wound, there will be loss of tissue and adjacent damage (Omer, 1980). The incidence of nerve injury is greater in low velocity injuries (Luce and Griffin, 1978), even though tissue damage is more extensive when there is cavitation and when one would expect more nerve damage. Omer (1974a) has found little difference in the degree of recovery between high velocity bullet injuries and hand gun injuries, although the former may take longer to recover.

The level of the lesion and the time that the regrowing nerve takes to reach its end-organ is likely to affect the degree of reinnervation of the muscles (Kallio and Vastamaki, 1993). The more proximal the lesion, the greater the degree of cross-over in the nerves, whilst distally this is less often the case (Jabaley *et al.*, 1980; Sunderland, 1945). The intrinsic muscles of the hand are most likely to be affected by a delay in regrowth. Gaul (1982) has shown that injuries above the level of the elbow are unlikely to develop small muscle function. A delay in repair reduces the results of motor function (Kallio and Vastamaki, 1993); there is a 1% reduction in potential for every six days of delay (Woodhall and Beehe, 1956). Studies (Gaul, 1982) have shown that muscle function will continue to improve for up to five years following the repair of major nerves. If muscles are not reinnervated within 12–24 months, fibrosis between muscle fibres will dramatically reduce any function despite reinnervation.

The degree of contamination, mechanical or bacterial, will have a bearing on the possibility of infection, wound breakdown, and the amount of scar at the neurorraphy site. This scar may interfere with subsequent nerve growth (Kallio *et al.*, 1993; Sunderland, 1978) as may more proximal compression (Weiss and Taylor, 1944).

In closed injuries in which bone injury or direct blunt trauma has caused nerve dysfunction, it is normal practice to wait and see if there are signs of regrowth. If none has occurred by three to six months, then exploration should be performed. The incidence of nerve injury is higher in dislocations and stretch injuries than from fractures. They occur in some nerves more often than others (radial nerve 60%, ulnar nerve 18%, median nerve 6%). Of these injuries, 83% recover spontaneously (Goodall, 1956; Omer, 1974a, 1986).

The patient

Patient factors include age, general health, pre-existing conditions, the patient's job and recreational activities, co-operation with the treatment regimens, and psychological state.

Age

The age of the patient may affect both the nerve regrowth and the way in which cortical remapping occurs (Steinberg and Koman, 1991). Whilst some primate studies (Almquist *et al.*, 1983) have suggested that the number of neurones regrowing differs little between young and old animals, and that it may be cortical plasticity that changes with age (the ability of the brain to alter the representation of the hand on the cortex and make sense of the incoming messages). As yet little such data is available in humans (Jabaley *et al.*, 1976; Yang *et al.*, 1994).

General health

The patient's general health is important. Diabetes and excessive alcohol consumption will affect the sensory function, as will medications that reduce or impair nerve regrowth or function. The adherence of the nerve repair to the surrounding tissues may cause stretching of the nerve and possibly a reduction in function (Millesi, 1991).

Treatment regimens

Sensory retraining considerably improves the results of nerve repair (Dellon, 1981; Imai *et al.*, 1991; Wynn Parry and Salter, 1976). The degree of effort expended by patients on retraining, the amount that they use the supplied area, their jobs and their hobbies, will contribute to the recovery. Cognitive capacity may also affect functional outcome (Rosen *et al.*, 1994).

Psychological state

The psychological effects of injury, pain, loss of work, loss of self-esteem, and interference with marital and sexual relationships (Grunert *et al.*,

1988a) should not be ignored (Grunert *et al.*, 1988b; Mayou *et al.*, 1993). Enquiries should be made about these problems, as patients may not wish to introduce the subject themselves. Nightmares are common soon after the injury and may disturb sleep, whilst flashbacks may be a sign of early post-traumatic stress disorder. This is not necessarily related to compensation (Grunert *et al.*, 1991). If the psychological aspects are thought to be a significant factor, the patient should be referred to a psychologist for treatment (Grunert *et al.*, 1990; Muss, 1991). Depression may occur late and frequently goes unrecognized; common signs, such as changes in mood, sleep patterns and temperament should be sought from patients and their relatives.

The repair

Important factors in the repair are the time from injury to repair, the degree of ischaemia of the nerve and surrounding tissues, the thoroughness of debridement, the quality of the repair, the need for nerve grafting, and the postoperative management. Birch and Raji (1991) have suggested that 'primary suture is best'. Thorough debridement of all devitalized tissue and foreign material should have been performed to minimize scarring and subsequent nerve entrapment. Lavage should have been sufficient to reduce the risk of bacterial contamination (Gross *et al.*, 1972; Madden *et al.*, 1971).

No difference has been shown between loupe repair and repair using the operating microscope (Marsh and Barton, 1987) given current methods of assessment. There is also debate over whether fascicular repair is better than epineural repair (Brushart *et al.*, 1980; Grabb *et al.*, 1970) (Figure 41.4). It is considered that the better the approximation of fascicles (the less mismatch) the less likely that there will be unsatisfied regrowing neurones (Birch, 1986), particularly when the amount of interfascicular tissue is high (Sunderland, 1991a), although this view has been challenged (Wynn Parry, 1988).

Where there has been loss of nerve tissue, nerve grafting will be needed unless the nerve can be mobilized and repaired without tension. The length of nerve that can be mobilized safely is debatable (Trumble, 1991) and depends upon the site and size of the nerve. Nerve grafts generally do not do as well as primary suture (Chassard *et al.*, 1993).

There are two neurorraphies in a nerve graft and nerve fibres are said to be lost at each. Fewer fibres

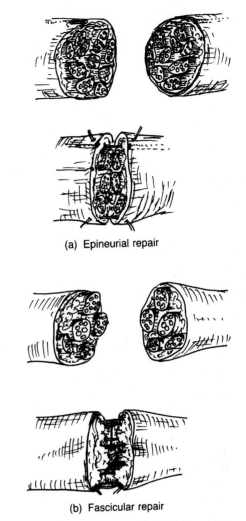

(a) Epineurial repair

(b) Fascicular repair

Figure 41.4. Types of nerve repair: (**a**) Epineural. The epineurium of the divided ends is sutured to restore continuity; (**b**) Fascicular repair. The perineurium of each fascicle is sutured prior to epineural closure.

will therefore reach the skin and muscle receptors. The longer the nerve graft, the poorer the functional motor results (Kallio and Vastamaki, 1993; Kallio *et al.*, 1993; Millesi, 1981; Vastamaki *et al.*, 1993).

Time to repair

Although some animal studies (Forman *et al.*, 1979; McQuarrie *et al.*, 1977) suggested that delay increases the rate of regrowth there is little evidence of this in humans and results seem to be worse after prolonged delay to repairs (Honner *et al.*, 1970;

Poppen *et al.*, 1979). Within reason, the sooner the better seems to be the maxim. The same is true to a lesser extent with nerve grafting, primary grafting being better than leaving the nerve ends tagged and then grafting at a later date, because the length of graft needed is likely to increase.

The nerve injured

There is some evidence to suggest that pure motor or pure sensory nerves regrow better than mixed nerves (Steinberg and Koman, 1991) (although this may be as a result of other feedback), and that certain nerves regrow better (Seddon, 1954; Woodhall and Beehe, 1956). Motor recovery in the radial nerve is said to be better than that in the median or ulnar nerves at similar levels (Omer, 1974b).

Damage to other structures

Injury to other structures has relevance to eventual recovery (Kallio and Vastamaki, 1993), to the scarring around the nerve, to the recovery of other functions, and in terms of the eventual ability of the hand to move. Leclerc *et al.* (1985) have suggested that anastomosis of the ulnar artery improves the results of primary ulnar nerve injuries, but the evidence is slim. An inability to move the digit will decrease the effectiveness of the nerve's recovery (Schlenker *et al.*, 1980). Poor skin and soft tissue cover may cause local tenderness and increase scarring; it will also prejudice the possibility of future surgery.

Postoperative treatment

The place of immobilization is debatable. Some authors suggest that motion can disrupt the neurorraphy (Steinberg and Koman, 1991; Tupper, 1991). Others believe that motion that does not stretch the repair prevents adhesion, and thus reduces entrapment of the nerve. The results of digital nerve repair combined with tendon repair do not appear to be significantly different (Sullivan, 1985) and it is probably safe to commence early movement after the repair. In recent years, experimental work has been done in many areas to improve nerve regrowth with variable success (Zeinowicz *et al.*, 1991).

Sensory re-education and motor retraining are important in the recovery of function (Dellon, 1981; Imai *et al.*, 1991; Wynn Parry and Salter, 1976) and should be started when nerve fibres reach the fingers. Little has been written on motor retraining.

Complications

Complications can be divided into early, intermediate and late for the historical part of the report. For the purposes of prognosis and future treatment, it is probably better to divide them into anatomical, physiological and psychological groups. These include the quality of the repair, wound breakdown and failure of cover, failure of regrowth, disturbed sensation, pain problems, interference with relationships, depression, and posttraumatic stress.

The repair

Complications related to the surgery include incomplete repair, inadequate repair, damage caused during the repair, and disruption of the repair or failed splinting. There may be a failure to recognize the full extent of damage. Dual level lacerations may be missed and damage to other nerves ignored if not actively considered (deep branch of the ulnar nerve, palmar cutaneous branch of the median nerve and radial nerve branches). Iatrogenic damage may occur (medial cutaneous nerve of forearm, palmar cutaneous and radial nerve branches). Careful preoperative documentation is important to avoid the charge that the damage was due to negligent surgery.

The usual signs of compartment syndrome may be masked, but pain out of proportion to the injury should have alerted the surgeon to this problem (Hooper, 1987). It can be very difficult in patients who have difficulty in communicating. It may occur following many different types of injury (Rowland, 1988), but the surgeon should have taken special care if the injury and/or repair was in a site of potential compression, when there was an associated crushing injury, or if there had been prolonged devascularization of all or part of the limb. If doubt still existed, pressure measurements (Matsen *et al.*, 1980; Mubarak *et al.*, 1976; Whitesides *et al.*, 1975) should have been performed.

Later complications of bleeding include infection, scarring, and poor regrowth. Rupture or dehiscence of the repair may occur if it is inadequately protected. The patient may have subjected the repair to excessive strain, but it is important that the surgeon protects the repair. Failure of the repair may also occur with failure of the whole wound (see below).

Wound breakdown

The normal postoperative complications of infection, dehiscence and necrosis may occur, and inadequate cover may expose the nerve to trauma. Poor cover may reduce the blood supply and impair regrowth. Repair of the overlying structures under excessive tension or the use of inadequately vascularized tissue will lead to breakdown and exposure of the nerve repair. Where such conditions exist, re-exploration and flap cover may be needed.

Failure of regrowth

This may vary from no regrowth to impaired function of either motor or sensory modalities. After six to eight weeks, Tinel's signs should start to move from the site of the repair towards the periphery (Jabaley, 1991a). If this has not happened after three months, it is likely that the repair has failed and it should be explored. Failure may be due to disruption of the neurorraphy, damage to the nerve on either side of the neurorraphy, or severe scarring around it.

When the patient complains of inadequate regeneration, one should compare the result with the average figure (see Tables 41.2–41.9 for nerve repair and nerve grafting) and explain the risks and prognosis of neurolysis and nerve grafting. Only after sensory re-education and further time should re-exploration be considered. With poor motor function, EMGs may be helpful in determining prognosis, but the surgeon must decide between redoing the repair and waiting, as further improvement may be seen for up to five years. Dellon suggests that, with sensory retraining, the results at one year will be roughly equivalent to the five-year figure without retraining (Dellon, 1988d). The paradox is that, after five years, the muscles will no longer be functioning and re-repair is worthless.

Where motor function is good and sensation is poor, or vice versa, awake sensory mapping of the nerve (Hakstian, 1968; Jabaley, 1991b) and resection of the appropriate section and nerve grafting around the neuroma may be the only solution. If there is no hope of nerve regrowth, tendon transfers should be performed to replace lost function. Although power may not be increased, function may be dramatically improved. In certain

cases (e.g. high radial nerve repair), when the hope of motor recovery is low, tendon transfers may be done at the time of nerve repair. It is best to perform transfers that cause little loss in case muscle function does return. If the muscles have also been destroyed, the possibility of free, vascularized, innervated muscle transfers should be considered (Kuzon *et al.*, 1988; Manktleow *et al.*, 1984).

When nerve grafts have failed to provide adequate sensation, the options lie between neurolysis with or without wrapping the grafts in a vascularized 'facial' flap (Brunelli *et al.*, 1988), repeating the grafts, doing a free vascularized nerve graft (Briedenbach, 1988), and providing sensation with a sensate flap. The best example of the latter is the Littler neurovascular island flap from ring to thumb. If there is some regrowth, particularly if threshold measurements are high, and there is scarring around the grafts, the first option may be best. If there is no regrowth, it is worth repeating the grafts if the vascular bed is good, and considering a vascularized nerve graft if it is not. It is probable that vascularized nerve grafts only have benefit if the areas that the grafts lie in are avascular (Mani *et al.*, 1992; Merle and Dautel, 1991; Pho *et al.*, 1985). Where previous repair and grafts have failed, this may be due to a defect in regrowth. In this situation the use of a sensate flap may be the best alternative to doing nothing.

Pain problems

Severe postoperative pain is not common following nerve repair, but it may be associated with compartment syndrome or acute nerve compression. This should have been previously recognized and relieved.

Hyperaesthesia is uncommon and may be part of a reflex sympathetic dystrophy (RSD) complex (Kleinert *et al.*, 1973) or occur on its own. It can be extremely difficult to treat. Sometimes all the major nerves to the area may have been stripped out, but extreme hyperaesthesia is present. Pain is probably due to overlapping nerves. Excision of the area and flap cover (Holmberg and Ekerot, 1993) may be the only solution. This is not universally successful and is not recommended by some (Brown and Flynn, 1973).

RSD, or sympathetically maintained pain, is probably more common than is generally recognized (Atkins *et al.*, 1989). There is debate about an agreed definition (Hannington-Kiff, 1987;

Table 41.2. Results of grafting of major nerves

Author	Nerve	Age group	No. pts	S2	S2+	S3	S3+	S4	M2	M3	M4	M5	Nerve gap (cm)
Walton and Finseth, 1977	Median	Adult	8	13.00	0	12.00	63.00	12.00	12.00	0	50.00	0	5–10
Young et al., 1980	Median	Adult	8	0	37.00	38.00	25.00	0	0	0	0	0	>2
		Total (Median; adult)	16										
		Average		6.50	18.50	25.00	44.00	6.00	6.00	0	25.00	0	
		Standard deviation		6.50	18.50	13.00	19.00	6.00	6.00	0	25.00	0	
Brooks, 1955	Median	Mixed	33	21.00	0	69.00	0	0	0	69.00	0	0	>7
Millesi et al., 1976	Median	Mixed	38	3.00	0	60.00	34.00	3.00	7.00	21.00	14.00	46.00	2–20
		Total (Median; Mixed)	71										
		Average		12.00	0	64.50	17.00	1.50	3.50	45.00	7.00	23.00	
		Standard Deviation		9.00	0	4.50	17.00	1.50	3.50	24.00	7.00	23.00	
		Total (Median)	87										
		Average		9.25	9.25	44.75	30.50	3.75	4.75	22.50	16.00	11.50	
		Standard deviation		8.32	16.02	22.02	22.52	4.92	5.07	28.18	20.45	19.92	
Millesi et al., 1976	Ulnar	Mixed	39	0	15.00	65.00	15.00	5.00	8.00	31.00	18.00	31.00	2–20
Hoase et al., 1980	Ulnar	Mixed	26	30.00	5.00	15.00	50.00	0	7.00	45.00	48.00	0	1.5–7.0
Leclerq et al., 1985	Ulnar	Mixed	24	37.00	0	33.00	0	21.00	21.00	25.00	21.00	8.00	?
		Total (Ulnar; mixed)	89										
		Average		22.33	6.67	37.67	21.67	8.67	12.00	33.67	29.00	13.00	
		Standard deviation		16.05	6.24	20.68	20.95	8.96	6.38	8.38	13.49	13.14	
		Total	176										
		Average	25.14	14.86	6.67	41.71	22.71	5.86	7.86	27.29	21.57	12.14	
		Standard Deviation		13.85	6.24	21.74	22.29	7.36	6.71	22.68	18.93	17.36	

The results are shown in percentages. Subaverages and standard deviations are given for adults and mixed age reports, as well as for the final overview of the nerve repairs. This allows comparison of results at different age groups as well as giving an overview.

Table 41.3. Results of repair of high and low radial nerve injuries

Author	Nerve	Age group	Level	No. pts	S2	S2+	S3	S3+	S4	M2	M3	M4	M5
Larsen, 1958	Radial	Mixed	Low	6	0	17.00	0	83.00	0	0	0	0	0
Mailander et al., 1989	Radial			5	0	40.00	40.00	0	20.00	0	0	0	0
			Total	11									
			Average		0	28.50	20.00	41.50	10.00	0	0	0	0
			Standard deviation		0	11.50	20.00	41.50	10.00	0	0	0	0
Larsen, 1958	Radial		High	17	0	35.00	0	59.00	0	6.00	0	76.00	0
Seddon, 1975	Radial			63	0	0	0	0	0	8.00	24.00	54.00	0
Mailander et al., 1989	Radial			2	50.00	0	0	0	0	0	0	100.00	0
			Total	82									
			Average		16.67	11.67	0	19.67	0	4.67	8.00	76.67	0
			Standard deviation		23.57	16.50	0	27.81	0	3.40	11.31	18.79	0
		Total		93									
		Average			10.00	18.40	8.00	28.40	4.00	2.80	4.80	46.00	0
		Standard deviation			20.00	16.86	16.00	35.60	8.00	3.49	9.60	40.28	0
Total				93									
Average				18.60	10.00		8.00	28.40	4.00	2.80	4.80	46.00	0
tandard deviation					20.00		16.00	35.60	8.00	3.49	9.60	40.28	0

The results are shown in percentages. Subaverages and standard deviations are given for mixed age reports, as well as for the final overview of the nerve repairs. This allows comparison of results at different age groups as well as giving an overview.

Table 41.4. Results of repair of high ulnar nerves at different age groups

Author	Nerve	Age group	No. pts	S2	S2+	S3	S3+	S4	M2	M3	M4	M5
Posch and de la Cruz-Saddul, 1980	Ulnar	Adult	11	27.00	9.00	27.00	0	0	54.00	18.00	9.00	0
		Total	11									
		Average		27.00	9.00	27.00	0	0	54.00	18.00	9.00	0
		Standard deviation		0	0	0	0	0	0	0	0	0
Larsen and Posch, 1958	Ulnar	Mixed	18	0	16.00	44.00	44.00	0	0	0	0	0
		Total	18									
		Average		0	16.00	44.00	44.00	0	0	0	0	0
		Standard deviation		0	0	0	0	0	0	0	0	0
Total			29									
Average			14.50	13.50		35.50	22.00	0	27.00	9.00	4.50	0
Standard deviation				13.50		8.50	22.00	0	27.00	9.00	4.50	0

The results are shown in percentages. Subaverages and standard deviations are given for adults and mixed age reports, as well as for the final overview of the nerve repairs. This allows comparison of results at different age groups as well as giving an overview.

Table 41.5. Results of repair of low ulnar nerves at different age groups

Author	Nerve	Age group	No. pts	S2	S2+	S3	S3+	S4	M2	M3	M4	M5
Onne, 1962	Ulnar	Adult	7	0	0	57.00	43.00	0	0	0	0	0
McManamny, 1983	Ulnar		10	0	20.00	0	70.00	10.00	20.00	40.00	0	10.00
Tupper, 1988	Ulnar		9	0	67.00	0	22.00	22.00	22.00	11.00	44.00	0
		Total	26									
		Average		0	29.00	19.00	45.00	10.67	14.00	17.00	14.67	3.33
		Standard deviation		0	28.08	26.87	19.65	8.99	9.93	16.87	20.74	4.71
Onne, 1962	Ulnar	Child	10	0	0	10.00	30.00	60.00	8.00	30.00	30.00	32.00
McManamny, 1983	Ulnar		5	0	0	0	20.00	80.00	0	40.00	60.00	0
		Total	15									
		Average		0	0	5.00	25.00	70.00	4.00	35.00	45.00	16.00
		Standard deviation		0	0	5.00	5.00	10.00	4.00	5.00	15.00	16.00
Sekellarides, 1962	Ulnar	Mixed	39	25.00	15.00	23.00	5.00	0	30.00	6.00	0	0
Flynn and Flynn, 1962	Ulnar		40	50.00	0	13.00	7.00	0	57.00	15.00	18.00	0
Ito et al., 1976	Ulnar		14	0	21.00	29.00	14.00	21.00	28.00	14.00	29.00	21.00
Posche and de la Cruz-Saddul, 1980	Ulnar		20	50.00	0	10.00	30.00	0	55.00	30.00	10.00	0
Leclerq et al., 1985	Ulnar		40	22.50	0	20.00	0	12.50	17.50	35.00	30.00	7.50
Mailander et al., 1989	Ulnar		10	0	0	20.00	0	60.00	10.00	30.00	40.00	10.00
		Total	163									
		Average		24.58	6.00	19.17	9.33	15.58	32.92	21.67	21.17	6.42
		Standard deviation		20.43	8.66	6.26	10.39	21.37	17.62	10.53	13.40	7.64
Total			204									
Average			18.55	13.41		16.55	21.91	24.14	22.50	22.82	23.73	7.32
Standard deviation				19.43		15.89	20.05	27.59	18.45	13.40	19.09	10.15

The results are shown in percentages. Subaverages and standard deviations are given for children, adults and mixed age reports, as well as for the final overview of the nerve repairs. This allows comparison of results at different age groups as well as giving an overview.

Table 41.6. Results of repair of high median nerves at different age groups

Author	Nerve	Age group	No. pts	S2	S2+	S3	S3+	S4	M2	M3	M4	M5
Posch and de la Cruz-Saddul, 1980	Median	Adult	12	8.00	8.00	60.00	17.00	0	16.00	60.00	8.00	0
		Total	12									
		Average		8.00	8.00	60.00	17.00	0	16.00	60.00	8.00	0
		Standard deviation		0	0	0	0	0	0	0	0	0
Larsen and Posche, 1958	Median	Mixed	14	0	8.00	50.00	42.00	0	0	14.00	36.00	0
		Total	14									
		Average		0	8.00	50.00	42.00	0	0	14.00	36.00	0
		Standard deviation		0	0	0	0	0	0	0	0	0
Total			26									
Average			13	4.00		55.00	29.50	0	8.00	37.00	22.00	0
Standard deviation				4.00		5.00	12.50	0	8.00	23.00	14.00	0

The results are shown in percentages. Subaverages and standard deviations are given for adults and mixed age reports, as well as for the final overview of the nerve repairs. This allows comparison of results at different age groups as well as giving an overview.

Table 41.7. Results of repair of low median nerves at different age groups

Author	Nerve	Age group	No. pts	S2	S2+	S3	S3+	S4	M2	M3	M4	M5
Onne, 1962	Median	Adult	17	22.00	18.00	18.00	41.00	0	30.00	23.00	18.00	29.00
Walton and Finseth, 1977	Median		8	13.00	0	12.00	63.00	12.00	12.00	0	50.00	0
Young et al., 1980	Median		8	0	37.00	38.00	25.00	0	7.00	0	57.00	0
McManamny, 1983	Median		14	0	14.00	0	57.00	29.00	7.00	21.00	57.00	14.00
Mailander et al., 1989	Median		10	0	20.00	10.00	10.00	40.00	0	10.00	60.00	30.00
		Total	57									
		Average		7.00	17.80	15.60	39.20	16.20	9.80	10.80	37.00	14.60
		Standard deviation		9.03	11.87	12.61	19.70	15.95	11.07	9.87	23.78	13.20
Onne, 1962	Median	Child	15	0	0	0	27.00	73.00	20.00	13.00	40.00	27.00
McManamny, 1983	Median		6	0	0	0	17.00	83.00	0	16.00	33.00	33.00
Tajima and Imai, 1989	Median		7	0	0	0	43.00	57.00	0	0	0	0
		Total	28									
		Average		0	0	0	29.00	71.00	6.67	9.67	24.33	20.00
		Standard deviation		0	0	0	10.71	10.71	9.43	6.94	17.44	14.35
Brooks, 1955	Median	Mixed	33	21.00	0	69.00	0	0	0	69.00	0	0
Larsen and Posch, 1958	Median		54	0	0	0	0	0	35.00	0	65.00	0
Flynn and Flynn, 1962	Median		40	50.00	0	7.00	10.00	3.00	25.20	38.00	15.00	7.00
Sakallarides, 1962	Median		38	15.00	33.00	13.00	5.00	0	13.00	37.00	11.00	0
Millesi et al., 1976	Median		38	3.00	0	60.00	34.00	3.00	7.00	21.00	14.00	46.00
Ito et al., 1976	Median		8	0	12.00	25.00	12.00	25.00	0	38.00	0	38.00
Posch and de la Cruz-Saddul, 1980	Median		14	7.00	7.00	29.00	57.00	10.00	0	43.00	57.00	0
Tupper, 1988	Median		13	0	54.00	0	36.00	10.00	23.00	0	77.00	0
		Total	238									
		Average		12.00	13.25	25.38	19.25	5.12	12.90	30.75	29.88	11.38
		Standard deviation		16.09	18.69	24.73	19.38	8.16	12.63	21.63	29.17	17.94
		Total	323									
		Average	20.19	8.19		17.56	27.31	20.94	10.76	20.56	31.06	14.00
		Standard deviation		13.24		21.10	20.20	27.14	11.85	19.43	26.06	16.26

Results are shown in percentages. Subaverages and standard deviations are given for children, adults and mixed age reports, as well as for the final overview of the nerve repairs. This allows comparison of results at different age groups as well as giving an overview.

Table 41.8. Results of repair of divided digital nerves

Author	Nerve	Age group	No. pts	S2	S2+	S3	S3+	S4
Poppen et al., 1979	Digital	Adult	48	0	38.00	15.00	42.00	4.00
Young et al., 1981	Digital		23	0	0	34.00	44.00	22.00
Sullivan, 1985	Digital		42	0	0	26.00	50.00	24.00
Tupper, 1988	Digital		109	0	17.00	0	48.00	35.00
Altimissi et al., 1991	Digital		19	0	47.00	26.50	26.50	0
		Total	241					
		Average		0	20.40	20.30	42.10	17.00
		Standard deviation		0	19.29	11.82	8.30	13.08
Poppen et al., 1979	Digital	Child	26	0	4.00	0	58.00	38.00
Young et al., 1981	Digital		9	0	0	0	22.00	78.00
Altimissi et al., 1991	Digital		7	0	0	0	28.50	71.50
		Total	42					
		Average		0	1.33	0	36.17	62.50
		Standard deviation		0	1.89	0	15.66	17.53
Buncke, 1972	Digital	Mixed	18	0	11.00	0	28.00	61.00
Ito et al., 1976	Digital		16	0	12.00	0	88.00	0
Berger et al., 1988	Digital		129	0	9.00	0	91.00	0
Mailander et al., 1989	Digital		107	1.00	8.00	20.00	48.00	23.00
Altimissi et al., 1991	Digital		28	0	18.00	29.00	46.00	7.00
Al-Ghazal et al., 1994	Digital		71	0	9.10	22.80	51.10	17.00
		Total	369					
		Average		0.17	11.18	11.97	58.68	18.00
		Standard deviation		0.37	3.33	12.26	23.01	20.99
Total			652					
Average			46.57	0.07		12.38	47.94	27.18
Standard deviation				0.26		13.02	19.89	25.62

The results are shown in percentages. Subaverages and standard deviations are given for children, adults and mixed age reports, as well as for the final overview of the nerve repairs. This allows comparison of results at different age groups as well as giving an overview.

Table 41.9. Results of grafting of digital nerves

Author	Nerve	Age group	No. pts	S2	S2+	S3	S3+	S4	M2	M3	M4	M5	Nerve gap (cm)
McFarlane and Moyer, 1976	Digital	Adult	17	0	15.00	39.00	46.00	0	0	0	0	0	1.5–3.5
Wilgis and Maxwell, 1979	Digital		11	0	0	0	33.00	67.00	0	0	0	0	1.0–2.5
Rose and Kowalski, 1989	Digital		5	0	20.00	0	20.00	60.00	0	0	0	0	5–8
Rose et al., 1987	Digital		13	0	0	7.00	55.00	38.00	0	0	0	0	4.5
Mackinnon, 1988	Digital		31	6.00	0	0	40.00	54.00	0	0	0	0	1–5
Total			77										
Average				1.20	7.00	9.20	38.80	43.80	0	0	0	0	
Standard deviation				2.40	8.72	15.14	11.86	23.90	0	0	0	0	
Beazley et al., 1984	Digital	Mixed	12	0	42.00	0	58.00	0	0	0	0	0	1–5
Total			12										
Average				0	42.00	0	58.00	0	0	0	0	0	
Standard deviation				0	0	0	0	0	0	0	0	0	
Total			89										
Average			14.83	1.00		7.67	42.00	36.50	0	0	0	0	
Standard deviation				2.24		14.24	12.97	27.25	0	0	0	0	

The results are shown in percentages. Subaverages and standard deviations are given for adults and mixed age reports, as well as for the final overview of the nerve repairs. This allows comparison of results at different age groups as well as giving an overview.

Paice, 1995). Many concentrate on the worst end of the spectrum. Early signs of sweating, swelling, stiffness, pain on motion, vasolability and decreased function should be treated vigorously with increased physiotherapy, Watson stress loading (Watson and Carlson, 1987) and medication to prevent progression. If this does not work, then guanethidine blocks should be given (Hannington-Kiff, 1984) to prevent progression to bony changes and venous pooling with joint changes. By the time joint and bony changes or triple phase bone scans are positive, it may already be too late.

Cold intolerance is relatively common (Morrison *et al.*, 1978). It is not necessarily related to blood flow (Kay, 1985), but may be related to failure of nerve regeneration (Koman *et al.*, 1984). Although it improves with time (Morrison *et al.*, 1978), if unresolved by the end of two years it is unlikely to improve (Porlsen *et al.*, 1995) and the patient may find work in cold conditions to be unsuitable unless the hand can be kept warm with gloves.

Painful neuromas (Herndon *et al.*, 1976; Laborde *et al.*, 1982; Mackinnon and Dellon, 1986) are best identified by nerve blocks (Mackinnon and Dellon, 1987) (occasionally more than one nerve is involved). Initial therapy should be with desensitization and massage. Injections of steroids and long-acting anaesthetics may help in selected patients, and are worth trying (Smith and Gomez, 1970). If this fails, most can be treated by cutting the nerve back, treating it in a variety of ways, and putting it in a safe place (Gorkisch *et al.*, 1984; Herndon and Hess, 1991; Laborde *et al.*, 1982; Robbins, 1986). Some nerves regrow and can be very difficult to treat; burial in bone (Boldney, 1943) or muscle (Dellon and Mackinnon, 1986) may still give rise to problems. The more operations that are done the less the chance of success (Dellon and Mackinnon, 1986). The help of pain physicians should be sought early in the management process to provide a plan of treatment.

Neuroma in continuity can be a problem if there is pain and nerve function is good. External neurolysis may help in certain conditions (Sunderland, 1991b). If it does not, the choice lies between resection and grafting, and conservative management in the hope of spontaneous improvement. If there is improvement, the latter course is the best.

Phantom pain can be troublesome and may be difficult to treat (Nashold and Schieff, 1991). In the lower limb, treatment by central block (Jahangiri *et al.*, 1994) (spinal or epidural) has proved successful and surgery on nerves under this type of anaesthesia is recommended by some (Bach *et al.*, 1988) to reduce the incidence of phantom pain. Little work has been done on the upper limb but it may be that plexus block also offers some protection.

It is tempting to think that patients with persistent pain who cannot be helped are either psychiatrically disturbed or malingering. It is difficult to differentiate cause and effect, although most patients have probably been very distressed by the pain and/or are tired of being told that they are malingering by doctors who cannot find the cause for their symptoms. Sometimes there is evidence of post-traumatic stress disorder (Grunert *et al.*, 1991), which may cloud the clinical picture and result in the patient not putting the maximum effort into anything. It may be worth pointing this out to the patient or the patient's lawyer.

Conclusions

The assessment of peripheral nerve injury is difficult. Anatomical variation, overlap, dual supply and a variety of other changes make accurate assessment almost impossible (McAllister and Calder, 1995). The tests that are currently available are crude. Although they may give a measure of sensibility, power and co-ordination in the hand, they do not always correlate well with hand function (Jerosch-Herold, 1993; Marsh, 1990; Moberg, 1958). Despite these problems, a reasonable understanding of how well the patient can use the hand can be obtained by a careful history, a precise examination and a battery of tests. The changeover time is also a valuable guide to prognosis. Outcome, in terms of the ability to work and return to previous skills and hobbies, will be related not only to the nature of the tasks but also to the individual patient.

References

Al-Ghazal SK, McKiernan M, Khan K, McCann J. (1994) Results of clinical assessment after primary digital nerve repair. *J Hand Surg* **19B**: 255–57.

Almquist EE, Smith OA, Fry L. (1983) Nerve conduction velocity, microscopic and electron microscopic studies comparing repaired adult and baby monkey and median nerves. *J Hand Surg* **8**: 406–10.

Altmissi M, Mancini GB, Azzara A. (1991) Results of primary repair of digital nerves. *J Hand Surg* **16B**: 546–47.

Atkins RM, Duckworth T, Kanis JA. (1989) Algodystrophy following Colles fracture. *J Hand Surg Br* **14B**: 161–64.

Bach S, Noreng MF, Tjellden NU. (1988) Phantom limb pain in amputees during the first 12 months following limb amputation, after peroperative lumbar epidural blockade. *Pain* **33**: 297–301.

Beazley WC, Milek MA, Reiss BH. (1984) Results of nerve grafting in severe soft tissue injury. *Clinical Orthopaedic and Related Research* **188**: 208–12.

Berger A, Mailander P, Schneider W, Becker M. (1988) Sensory recovery by different techniques. *Presented at the 3rd International Symposium on Surgery of the Hand.* Tokyo, Japan.

Birch R. (1986) Lesions of the peripheral nerves: the present position. *J Bone Joint Surg Br* **68B**: 1–8.

Birch R, Raji ARM. (1991) Repair of median and ulnar nerves. Primary suture is best. *J Bone Joint Surg Br* **73B**: 154–57.

Boldney E. (1943) Amputation neuromas in nerves implanted in bone. *Ann Surg* **118**: 1052–57.

Botte MJ, Cohen MS, Lavernia CJ, *et al.* (1990) The dorsal branch of the ulnar nerve: an anatomical study. *J Hand Surg Am* **15A**: 603–607.

Brand PW, Hollister A. (1992) Methods of clinical measurement in the hand. In: *Clinical mechanics of the hand.* St Louis, MO: Mosby, 245–46.

Brandsma JW, Birke JA, Sims DS. (1986) The Martin–Gruber innervated hand. *J Hand Surg Am* **11A**: 536–39.

Breidenbach WC. (1988) Vascularised nerve grafts: a practical approach. *Orthop Clin North Am* **19**: 81–89.

Brooks D. (1955) The place of nerve grafting in orthopedic surgery. *J Bone Joint Surg* **37A**: 299–326.

Brown H, Flynn HE. (1973) Abdominal pedicle flap for hand neuromas and nerve entrapment. *J Bone Joint Surg Am* **55A**: 875.

Brunelli G, Battiston B, Brunelli F. (1988) Free greater omentum transfer in ionising radiation lesion of the brachial plexus. In: Brunelli G, editor. *Textbook of microsurgery.* Milano: Masson, 825–31.

Brushart TM, Tarlov E, Mesulam MM. (1980) A comparison of motor neurone pool organization after epineural and perineural repair in rat sciatic nerves. *Orthop Trans* **4**: 19–20.

Buncke HJ. (1972) Digital nerve repairs. *Surgical Clinics of North America* **52**: 1267–85.

Burge P. (1993) Results of peripheral nerve repair. *Curr Orthop* **7**: 234–38.

Callahan AD. (1984) Sensibility testing: clinical methods. In: Hunter JM, Schneider LH, Mackin EJ, Callahan AD, editors. *Rehabilitation of the hand.* St. Louis: Mosby, 407–31.

Cannieu JMA. (1896) Recherche l'nnervation de l'eminance thenar parle cubital. *J Med Bordeaux*: 377.

Chassard M, Pham E, Comtet JJ. (1993) Two-point discrimination tests versus functional sensory recovery in both median and ulnar nerve complete transections. *J Hand Surg Br* **18B**: 790–96.

Chow SP, Ng C. (1993) Can a digital nerve on one side of the finger be left unrepaired? *J Hand Surg Br* **18B**: 629–30.

Dellon AL. (1981) *Evaluation of sensibility and re-education of sensation in the hand.* Baltimore MD: Williams & Wilkins.

Dellon AL. (1988a) Pattern of sensory recovery. In: *Evaluation of sensibility and re-education of sensation in the hand.* Baltimore MD: Williams & Wilkins, 114–22.

Dellon AL. (1988b) It's academic but not functional. In: *Evaluation of sensibility and re-education of sensation in the hand.* Baltimore MD: Williams & Wilkins, 95–113.

Dellon AL. (1988c) Moving two-point discrimination test. In: *Evaluation of sensibility and re-education of sensation in the hand.* Baltimore MD: Williams & Wilkins, 123–39.

Dellon AL. (1988d) Evaluation of sensibility in the hand. In: *Evaluation of sensibility and re-education of sensation in the hand.* Baltimore MD: Williams & Wilkins, 169–89.

Dellon AL. (1991) Pitfalls in interpreting of electrophysiological testing. In: Gelberman RH, editor. *Operative nerve repair and reconstruction.* Philadelphia: Lippincott, 185–96.

Dellon AL, Mackinnon SE. (1986) Treatment of painful neuromas by neuroma resection and muscle implantation. *Plast Reconstr Surg* **77**: 427–36.

Dellon AL, Curtis RM, Edgerton MT. (1972) Evaluating sensation in the hand following nerve injury. *Johns Hopkins Med J* **130**: 235–43.

Dellon AL, Curtis RM, Edgerton MT. (1974) Evaluation recovery of sensation in the hand following nerve injury. *Plast Reconstr Surg* **53**: 297–305.

Egyed B, Eroy A, VEres T, Manninger J. (1980) Measurement of electrical resistance in after nerve injuries of the hand. *Hand* **6**: 275–81.

Flynn JE, Flynn WF. (1962) Median and ulnar nerve injuries. *Annals of Surgery* **156**: 1002–1009.

Forman DS, Wood DK, DeSilva S. (1979) The rate of regeneration of sensory axons in transected rat sciatic nerve repaired with epineural sutures. *J Neurol Sci* **44**: 55–59.

Gaul JS. (1982) Intrinsic motor recovery – a long term study of ulnar nerve repair. *J Hand Surg* **7**: 502–508.

Gelberman RH, Urbaniak JR, Bright LS, Levin LS. (1978) Digital sensibility following replantation. *J Hand Surg* **8**: 313–19.

Goodall RJ. (1956) Nerve injuries in fresh fractures. *Texas Med* **52**: 93–98.

Gorkisch K, Boese-Landgraf J, Vaubel E. (1984) Treatment and prevention of amputation neuromas in hand surgery. *Plast Reconstr Surg* **73**: 293–96.

Grabb WC, Bement SL, Kaepke GH, *et al.* (1970) Comparison of methods of peripheral nerve suturing in monkeys. *Plast Reconstr Surg* **46**: 31–38.

Gross A, Cutright DE, Bhaskar SN. (1972) Effectiveness of pulsating water jet lavage in treatment of contaminated crushed wounds. *Am J Surg* **124**: 373–77.

Grunert BK, Devine CA, Matloub HS, Sanger SA, Yousif NJ. (1988a) Sexual dysfunction after traumatic hand injury. *Ann Plastic Surg* **21**: 46–48.

Grunert BK, Smith CJ, Devine CA, *et al.* (1988b) Early psychological aspects of severe hand injury. *J Hand Surg Br* **13B**: 177–80.

Grunert BK, Matloub HS, Sanger SA, Yousif NJ. (1990) Treatment of posttraumatic stress disorder after work-related hand trauma. *J Hand Surg Am* **15A**: 511–15.

Grunert BK, Matloub HS, Sanger JR, Yousif NJ, Hettermann S. (1991) Effects of litigation on maintenance of psychological symptoms after severe hand injuries. *J Hand Surg Am* **16A**: 1031–34.

Hakstian RW. (1968) Funicular orientation by direct stimulation. *J Bone Joint Surg Am* **50**: 1178–86.

Hannington-Kiff JG. (1984) Pharmacological target blocks in hand surgery and rehabilitation. *J Hand Surg Br* **9B**: 29–36.

Hannington-Kiff JG. (1987) Reflex sympathetic dystrophy. *J R Soc Med* **80**: 605.

Harrison SH. (1974) The tactile adherence test estimating loss of sensation after nerve injury. *Hand* **6**: 148–49.

Henderson WR. (1948) Clinical assessment of peripheral nerve injuries. Tinel's test. *Lancet* **ii**: 801–805.

Herndon JH, Hess AV. (1991) Neuromas. In: Gelberman RH, editor. *Operative nerve repair and reconstruction*. Philadelphia: Lippincott, 1525–40.

Herndon JH, Eaton RG, Littler JW. (1976) Management of painful neuromas in the hand. *J Bone Joint Surg Am* **58**: 369–73.

Highet WB. (1942) Procaine nerve block in the investigation of peripheral nerve injuries. *J Neurol Psych* **5**: 101–16.

Hildreth DH, Breidenbach WC, Lister GD, Hodges AD. (1989) Detection of submaximal effort by the use of the rapid exchange grip. *J Hand Surg Am* **14A**: 742–45.

Hoase J, Bjerre P, Simesen K. (1980) Median and ulnar nerve transections treated with microsurgical interfascicular cable grafting with autogenous sural nerve. *J Neurosurg* **53**: 73–84.

Hoffman P. (1915) Ueber ein Methode, den Erffolg einer Nervennaht zu beurteilen. *Med Klin* **11**: 359–60.

Holmberg J, Ekerot L. (1993) Post-traumatic neuralgia in the upper extremity treated with extraneural scar excision and flap cover. *J Hand Surg Br* **18B**: 111–14.

Honner R, Fragiadakis EG, Lamb DW. (1970) An investigation of the factors affecting the results of digital nerve division. *Hand* **2**: 21–30.

Hooper G. (1987) Volkmann's ischaemic contracture. In: McFarlane RM, editor. *Unsatisfactory results in hand surgery*. Edinburgh: Churchill Livingstone, 14–23.

Imai H, Tajima T, Natsumi Y. (1991) Successful reeducation of functional sensibility after median nerve repair at the wrist. *J Hand Surg Am* **16A**: 60–65.

Ito T, Hirotani H, Yamamoto K. (1976) Peripheral nerve repairs by the funicular suture technique. *Acta Orthopaedica Scandinavica* **47**: 283–89.

Jabaley ME. (1991a) Modified techniques of nerve repair: epineural splint. In: Gelberman RH, editor. *Operative nerve repair and reconstruction*. Philadelphia: Lippincott, 315–26.

Jabaley ME. (1991b) Electrical nerve stimulation in the awake patient. In: Gelberman RH, editor. *Operative nerve repair and reconstruction*. Philadelphia: Lippincott, 241–57.

Jabaley ME, Burns JE, Orcutt BS, *et al.* (1976) Comparison of histological and functional recovery after peripheral nerve repair. *J Hand Surg* **1**: 119–30.

Jabaley ME, Wallace WH, Heckler FR. (1980) Internal topography of major nerves of the forearm and hand: a current view. *J Hand Surg* **5**: 1–18.

Jahangiri M, Jayatunga AP, Bradley JWP, Dark CH. (1994) Prevention of phantom pain after major limb amputation by epidural infusion of diamorphine, clonidine and bupivacaine.

Ann R Coll Surg Engl **76**: 324–26.

Jebson RH, Taylor N, Trieschmann RB, Trotter MJ, Howard LA. (1969) An objective and standardized test of hand function. *Arch Phys Med Rehabil* **50**: 311–19.

Jerosch-Herold C. (1993) Measuring outcome in median nerve injuries. *J Hand Surg Br* **18B**: 624–28.

Jones LA. (1989) The assessment of hand function: a critical review of techniques. *J Hand Surg Am* **14A**: 221–28.

Kallio PK, Vastamaki M. (1993) An analysis of the results of late reconstruction of 132 median nerves. *J Hand Surg Br* **18B**: 97–105.

Kallio PK, Vastamaki M, Solonen KA. (1993) Late results of secondary microsurgical repair of radial nerve in 33 patients. *J Hand Surg Br* **18B**: 320–22.

Kaplan EB. (1963) Variation of the ulnar nerve at the wrist. *Bull Hosp Joint Dis* **24**: 85–88.

Kay S. (1985) Venous occlusion plethysmography in patients with cold related symptoms after digital salvage procedures. *J Hand Surg Br* **10B**: 151–54.

Kleinert HE, Cole NM, Wayne L, *et al.* (1973) Post-traumatic sympathetic dystrophy. *Orthop Clin North Am* **4**: 917–27.

Kline DG, Nulsen FE. (1972) The neuroma-in-continuity: its preoperative and operative management. *Surg Clin North Am* **52**: 1189–209.

Koman LA, Nunley JA, Goldner JL, Seaber AV, Urbaniak JR. (1984) Isolated cold stress testing in the assessment of symptoms in the upper extremity: preliminary communication. *J Hand Surg Am* **9A**: 305–13.

Kuzon WM, McKee NH, Fish JS, Pynn BR, Rosenblatt JD. (1988) The effect of intra operateive ischaemia on the recovery of contractile function after free muscle transfer. *J Hand Surg Am* **13A**: 263–72.

Laborde KG, Kalisman M, Tsai T. (1982) Results of surgical treatment of painful neuromas of the hand. *J Hand Surg* **7**: 190–93.

Larsen RD, Posch JL. (1958) Nerve injuries in the upper extremity. *Archives of Surgery* **77**: 469–82.

Leclerc DC, Carlier AJ, Khune T, Depierreux L, Lejune GN. (1985) Improvement in the results in 64 ulnar nerve sections associated with arterial repair. *J Hand Surg Am* **10A**(suppl): 997–99.

Levin S, Pearsall G, Ruderman RJ. (1978) Von Frey's method of measuring pressure sensibility in the hand: an engineering analysis of the Weinstien–Semmes aesthesiometer. *J Hand Surg Am* **3A**: 211–16.

Lister G. (1993) Reconstruction (nerves – peripheral). In: *The hand. Diagnosis and indications*. Edinburgh: Churchill Livingstone, 148–49.

Lundborg G, Lie-Stenstorm AK, Sollerman C, *et al.* (1986) Digital vibrogram: a new diagnostic tool for sensory testing in compression neuropathy. *J Hand Surg Am* **11A**: 693–99.

Luce EA, Griffin WO. (1978) Shotgun injuries of the upper extremity. *J Trauma* **18**: 487–92.

McAllister RMR, Calder JS. (1995) Paradoxical clinical consequences of peripheral nerve injury: a review of the anatomical, neurophysiological and psychological mechanisms. *Br J Plast Surg* **48**: 384–95.

McCabe SJ, Kleinert JM. (1990) The nerve of Henlé. *J Hand Surg Am* **15A**: 784–88.

McFarlane RM, Moyer JR. (1976) Digital nerve grafting with the lateral antebrachial cutaneous nerve. *J Hand Surg* **1**: 169–73.

Mackinnon SE. (1988) Results of nerve repair and grafting. In: Mackinnon SE, Dellon AL, editors. *Surgery of the Peripheral Nerve.* New York: Thieme, 115–27.

Mackinnon SE, Dellon AL. (1986) Algorithm for the management of painful neuroma. *Contemp Orthop* **13**: 15–27.

Mackinnon SE, Dellon AL. (1987) Results of treatment of recurrent dorsal radial wrist neuromas. *Ann Plast Surg* **19**: 54–61.

Mackinnon SE. (1989) New directions in nerve surgery. *Ann Surg* **22**: 257–73.

McManamny DS. (1983) Comparison of microscope and loupe magnification: Assistance for the repair of median and ulnar nerves. *British Journal of Plastic Surgery* **36**: 367–72.

Madden J, Edlich RF, Schauerhamer R, Prusak M, Borner J, Wagensteen OH. (1971) Application of principles of fluid dynamics to surgical wound irrigation. *Curr Top Surg Res* **3**: 85–93.

Mailander P, Berger A, Schallter E, Ruhe K. (1989) Results of primary nerve repair in the upper extremity. *Microsurgery* **10**: 147–50.

Mani GV, Shurey C, Green CJ. (1992) Is early vascularisation of nerve grafts necessary? *J Hand Surg Br* **17B**: 536–43.

Manktleow RT, Zucker RM, McKnee NH. (1984) Functioning free muscle transplantation. *J Hand Surg Am* **9A**: 32–39.

Marsh D. (1990) The validation of measures of outcome following suture of divided peripheral nerves supplying the hand. *J Hand Surg Br* **16B**: 25–34.

Marsh D, Barton N. (1987) Does the use of the operating microscope improve the results of peripheral nerve suture? *J Bone Joint Surg Br* **69B**: 625–30.

Matsen FA, Winquist RA, Krugmire RB. (1980) Diagnosis and management of compartment syndrome. *J Bone Joint Surg Am* **62**: 286–91.

Mayou R, Bryant B, Duthie R. (1993) Psychiatric consequences of road traffic accidents. *Br Med J* **307**: 647–51.

McQuarrie IG, Grafstein B, Gershon MD. (1977) Axonal regeneration in rat sciatic nerve. Effect of a conditioning lesion and dcb-AMP. *Brain Res* **132**: 439–53.

Meals RA, Shaner M. (1983) Variations in digital sensory patterns: a study of the ulnar nerve – median palmar communicating branch. *J Hand Surg* **8**: 411–14.

Merle M, Dautel G. (1991) Vascularised nerve grafts. *J Hand Surg Br* **16B**: 483–88.

Millesi H. (1981) Interfasicular nerve grafting. *Orthop Clin North Am* **12**: 287–301.

Millesi H. (1991) Indications and techniques of nerve grafting (mechanical aspects). In: Gelberman RH, editor. *Operative nerve repair and reconstruction.* Philadelphia: Lippincott, 528–29.

Millesi H, Meissl G, Berger A. (1976) Further experience with interfascicular grafting of the median, ulnar and radial nerves. *J Bone Joint Surg* **58A**: 209–18.

Moberg E. (1958) Objective methods for determining the functional value of sensibility in the hand. *J Bone Joint Surg Br* **40B**: 454–66.

Moberg E. (1962) Criticism and study of methods for examining sensibility in the hand. *Neurology* **12**: 8–19.

Moberg E. (1976) Reconstructive hand surgery in tetraplegia, stroke and cerebral palsy: some basic concepts of physiology and neurology. *J Hand Surg* **1**: 29–34.

Morrison W, O'Brien BMcC, MacLeod AM. (1978) Digital replantation and revascularisation: a long term review of one hundred cases. *Hand* **10**: 125–34.

Mubarak SJ, Hargens AR, Owen CA, Garetto LP, Akeson WH. (1976) The wick catheter technique for measurement of intramuscular pressure. A new research and clinical tool. *J Bone Joint Surg Am* **58A**: 1016–20.

Muss D. (1991) *The trauma trap.* London: Doubleday (Transworld Publishers).

Nashold BS, Schieff C. (1991) Phantom and avulsion pain. In: Wynn Parry CB, editor. *Management of pain in the hand and wrist.* Edinburgh: Churchill Livingstone, 146–52.

Omer GE. (1974a) Injuries to the nerves of the upper extremity. *J Bone Joint Surg Am* **56A**: 1615–24.

Omer GE. (1974b) The evaluation of clinical results following peripheral nerve suture. In: Omer GE, Spinner. *Management of peripheral nerve problems.* Philadelphia PA: Saunders, 431–42.

Omer GE. (1980) The evaluation of clinical results following peripheral nerve suture. In: Omer GE, Spinner M, editors. *Management of peripheral nerve problems.* Philadelphia: Saunders, 431–42.

Omer GE. (1986) Acute management of peripheral nerve injuries. *Hand Clin* **2**: 193–206.

Onne L. (1962) Recovery of sensibility and sudomotor activity in the hand after nerve suture. *Acta Chirurgica Scandinavica Supplement* **300**: 1–69.

O'Rain S. (1973) A new and simple test of nerve function in the hand. *Br Med J* **iii**: 615–16.

Paice E. (1995) Reflex sympathetic dystrophy. *Br Med J* **310**: 1645–48.

Pho RWH, Lee YS, Rujiwetpongstorn V, Pang M. (1985) Histological studies of vascularised nerve graft and conventional nerve graft. *J Hand Surg Br* **10B**: 45–48.

Poppen NK, McCarroll HR, Doyle JR, Niebauer JJ. (1979) Recovery of sensibility after suture of digital nerves. *J Hand Surg* **4**: 212–26.

Porter RW. (1966) New test for fingertip sensation. *Br Med J* **ii**: 927–28.

Posche JL, de la Cruz-Saddul F. (1980) Nerve repair in trauma surgery. A ten-year study of 231 peripheral injuries. *Orthopedic Review* **9**: 35–45.

Povlsen B, Nylander G, Nylander E. (1995) Cold induced spasm after digital replantation does not improve with time. A 12 year prospective trial. *J Hand Surg Br* **20B**: 237–39.

Riche P. (1897) Le nerf cubital et les muscles de l'eminance thenar. *Bull Mem Soc Anat Paris* **72**: 251.

Richter CP, Katz TD. (1943) Peripheral nerve injuries determined by the electrical skin resistance method. *JAMA* **122**: 648–53.

Robbins TH. (1986) Nerve capping in the treatment of troublesome neuromata. *Br J Plast Surg* **39**: 239–41.

Rose EH, Kowalski TA, Norris MS. (1989) The reversed venous arterialized nerve graft in digital nerve reconstruction across scarred beds. *Plastic and Reconstructive Surgery* **83**: 593–604.

Rosen B, Lundborg G, Dahlin LB, Holmberg J, Karlson B.

(1994) Nerve repair: correlation of restitution of functional sensibility with specific cognitive capacities. *J Hand Surg Br* **19B**: 452–58.

Rowland SA. (1988) Fasciotomy: the treatment of compartment syndrome. In: Green DP, editor. *Operative hand surgery.* Edinburgh: Churchill Livingstone.

Sakellarides H. (1962) A follow-up study of 172 peripheral nerve injuries in the upper extremity in civilians. *J Bone Joint Surg* **44A**: 140–48.

Schlenker JD, Kleinert HE, Tsai T. (1980) Methods and results of replantation following traumatic amputation of the thumb in sixty-four patients. *J Hand Surg Br* **5**: 63–70.

Schmidt RT, Toews JV. (1970) Grip strength measured by the Jamar dynamometer. *Arch Phys Med Rehabil* **51**: 321–27.

Seddon HJ. (1954) *Peripheral nerve injuries topic.* (MRC Special Report Series 282). London: HMSO.

Seddon HJ. (1972) *Surgical disorders of the peripheral nerves.* Baltimore MD: Williams & Wilkins, 53.

Seddon H. (1975) *Surgical disorders of the peripheral nerves. Clinical phenomena: methods of examination*, 2nd edition. Edinburgh: Churchill Livingstone, 44–47, 303–7.

Seradge H, Seradge E. (1990) Median innervated hypothenar muscle: anomalous branch of median nerve in the carpal tunnel. *J Hand Surg Am* **15A**: 356–59.

Smith JR, Gomez NH. (1970) Local injection therapy of neuromata of the hand with triamcinolone acetonide. A preliminary study of twenty-two patients. *J Bone Joint Surg Am* **52A**: 71–83.

Smith PJ, Mott G. (1986) Sensory threshold and conductance testing in nerve injuries. *J Hand Surg Br* **11B**: 157–62.

Stokes HM. (1983) The seriously injured hand – weakness of grip. *J Occup Med* **25**: 683–84.

Steinberg DR, Koman LA. (1991) Factors affecting the results of peripheral nerve repair. In: Gelberman RH, editor. *Operative nerve repair and reconstruction*. Philadelphia: Lippincott, 349–64.

Sullivan DJ. (1985) Results of digital neurrohaphy in adults. *J Hand Surg Br* **10B**: 41–44.

Sunderland S. (1945) The intraneural topography or the radial, median, and ulnar nerves. *Brain* **68**: 243–98.

Sunderland S. (1978) Regeneration of the axon and associated changes. In: *Nerves and nerve injury*, 2nd edition. Edinburgh: Churchill Livingstone, 121.

Sunderland S. (1991a) End to end nerve repair, (criteria for using group fasicular repair). In: *Nerve injuries and their repair.* Edinburgh: Churchill Livingstone.

Sunderland S. (1991b) Neurolysis, mobilisation, transposition, painful neuromas. In: *Nerve injuries and their repair.* Edinburgh: Churchill Livingstone, 379–93.

Tajima T, Imai H. (1989) Results of median nerve repairs in children. *Microsurgery* **10**: 145–46.

Tinel J. (1915) Le signe du 'formillement' dans les lésion des nerfs périphériques. *Presse Med* **23**: 388–93.

Trumble T. (1991) Overcoming defects in peripheral nerves. In: Gelberman RH, editor. *Operative nerve repair and reconstruction*. Philadelphia: Lippincott, 507–24.

Trumble TE, Khan U, Vanderhoot E, Bach AW. (1995) A technique to quantitate motor recovery following nerve grafting. *J Hand Surg Am* **20A**: 367–72.

Tupper JW. (1991) Fasicular repair. In: Gelberman RH, editor. *Operative nerve repair and reconstruction*. Philadelphia: Lippincott, 295–303.

Tupper JW, Crick JC, Matteck LR. (1988) Fasicular nerve repairs: A comparative study of epineural and fasicular (perineural) techniques. *Orthopedia Clinics of N. America* **19**: 57–69.

Vastamaki M, Kallio PK, Solonen KA. (1993) Late results of secondary microsurgical repair of ulnar nerve injury. *J Hand Surg Br* **18B**: 323–26.

van Beek AL, Heyman P. (1991) Electrophysiological testing. In: Gelberman RH, editor. *Operative nerve repair and reconstruction*. Philadelphia: Lippincott, 171–84.

von Frey M. (1896) Untersuchungen über die Sinnesfunktionen der menschlichen Haut. *Abh Säch Ges (Akad) Wiss* **40**: 175–266.

Walton R, Finseth F. (1977) Nerve grafting in the repair of complicated peripheral nerve trauma. *Journal of Trauma* **17**: 793–6.

Watson HK, Carlson L. (1987) The treatment of reflex sympathetic dystrophy of the hand with an active 'stress loading' program. *J Hand Surg Am* **12A**: 779–85.

Weber E. (1835) Ueber den Tastinn. *Arch Anat Physiol Wissen Med* **1**: 152–59.

Weinstein S. (1962) Tactile sensitivity in the phalanges. *Percept Mot Skills* **14**: 351–54.

Weiss P, Taylor AC. (1944) Impairment of growth and myelination in regenerating nerve fibers subject to constriction. *Proc Soc Exp Biol Med* **55**: 77–86.

Whitesides TE, Haney TC, Morimoto K, Hirada H. (1975) Tissue pressure measurements as a determinant for the need of fasciotomy. *Clin Orthop* **113**: 43–51.

Wilgis EFS, Maxwell GP. (1979) Distal digital nerve grafts: clinical and anatomical studies. *J Hand Surg* **4**: 439–43.

Woodhall B, Beebe GW, editors. (1956) Peripheral nerve regeneration: a follow up study of 3656 World War II injuries. (Veterans Administration monograph.) Washington, DC: US Government Printing Office, 71–201, 241–310.

Wynn Parry CB. (1987) Update on peripheral nerve injuries. *Int Disabil Stud* **10**: 11–20.

Wynn Parry CB. (1988) Update on peripheral nerve injuries. *Int Disabil Stud* **10**: 11–20.

Wynn Parry CB, Salter M. (1976) Sensory re-education after median nerve lesions. *Hand* **8**: 250–57.

Yang TT, Gallen C, Schwartz B, *et al.* (1994) Sensory maps in the human brain. *Nature* **368**: 592–93.

Young VL, Wray RC, Weeks P. (1981) A randomized prospective comparison of fascicular and epineural digital nerve repairss. *Plastic and Reconstructive Surgery* **68**: 89–92.

Young VL, Wray RC, Weeks PM. (1980) The results of nerve grafting in the wrist and hand. *Annals of Plastic Surgery* **5**: 212–15.

Young VL, Wray RC, Weeks PM. (1981) A randomized prospective comparison of fascicular and epineural digital nerve repairs. *Plastic and Reconstructive Surgery* **68**: 89–92.

Zeinowicz RJ, Thomas BA, Kurtz WH, Orgel MG. (1991) A multivariate approach to the treatment of peripheral nerve injury: the role of electromagnetic field therapy. *Plast Reconstr Surg* **87**: 122–30.

42

Traumatic disorders of the sympathetic nervous system

Harold A Wilkinson

Introduction

Traumatic disorders of the sympathetic nervous system include sympathetic interruption or loss of function, such as Horner's syndrome and the dysautonomia of paraplegia, but perhaps the most vexing presentations are those related to sympathetic hyperactivity. Those most commonly occuring are a spectrum of overlapping and intermingled disorders usually involving pain (referred to as 'causalgic'), disturbances of circulation, and dystrophic changes. An occasional case of pathological hyperhidrosis may also occur. In the first group, the disorders nearly always involve the limbs, though occasional facial varieties have been reported, while, in the hyperhidrodic groups, the disorders may be truncal, extremity or gustatory.

Because of the many ways in which these disturbances of function of the sympathetic nervous system may present, their nosology, confirmation and therapy are complex and will be discussed in more detail in this chapter.

Classification

The disorders characterized principally by excessive sweating are termed 'pathological hyperhidrosis'. In addition to those cases following trauma, they also occur idiopathically, congenitally and, at times, familially. Gustatory hyperhidrosis, in which eating triggers diffuse heavy sweating over the face, or over the face, trunk and extremities, is most commonly precipitated by brain stem infarctions, but has also been reported following trauma to the brain stem. Hyperhidrosis over the trunk and lower extremities is an occasional concomitant of spinal cord injury. It usually occurs in paraplegic patients but may occasionally follow partial cervical cord injuries.

The disorders characterized by a combination of pain, circulatory disturbance and dystrophy may occur in a wide variety of presentations, with varying degrees of severity. Unfortunately, there is no uniformity of nomenclature, and the published definitions are often in conflict (see Table 42.1) (Schott, 1986). The vascular changes are usually vasospastic and can often be painful. Pain symptoms are usually referred to as 'causalgic' if there is sympathetically-mediated pain not attributable to tissue destruction from dystrophy or from ischaemic vasospasticity. This type of pain is usually described as a constant burning discomfort with marked hypersensitivity to touch and 'allodynia' (when even a light touch elicits a painful response). Dystrophic changes usually affect joints and skin and can lead to permanent damage to an extremity. Sudek's atrophy (in which the dystrophy is more prominent than the pain), reflex sympathetic dystrophy, and major causalgia (combining severe pain with dystrophic features) are predominantly unilateral but may have some bilateral component. Raynaud's syndrome (peripheral vasospasticity) is predominantly bilateral, but can also be unilateral following a limb injury. These disorders usually affect the extremities, either upper or lower. The painful states are usually maximal distally, but the shoulder/hand syndrome is characterized by pain in the shoulder and distally

Table 42.1 Classification of painful hyperactive sympathetically maintained syndromes

Syndrome[1]	*Severity of component features*[2]		
	Pain[3]	*Dystrophy*	*Vascular*
Major causalgia	+++	+++	+
Reflex sympathetic dystrophy	++/+++	++/+++	0/+
Sudek's atrophy	+	++	0
Minor causalgia	++	0/+	0
Shoulder–hand syndrome	++	0/+	0
Diabetic burning foot syndrome	++	0/+	0/+
Vasospasm post acute arterial occlusion	++	0	+++
Peripheral occlusive vasculopathy	+/++	+	+++
Vasospastic vasculopathy (Raynaud's)	++	0	++/+++
Prinzmetal's angina	++/+++	0	0

[1]Author's choice of terms, since nosology is not standardized or universally accepted.
[2]Graded on a semiquantitated scale of ascending severity; zero to three plus (+++).
[3]Usually 'causalgic': burning and constant with associated hyperpathia and allodynia.

in the arm, with relative sparing of the elbow region. All these disorders were initially considered to occur following injuries to peripheral nerves, but it is now recognized that they can follow even a seemingly trivial injury to an extremity, without involvement of a major peripheral nerve.

It is unclear whether sympathetically-mediated pain is an efferent or an afferent phenomenon, but the distinction has therapeutic implications. Because the bulk of the sympathetic efferent supply to the upper limb is transmitted through the second and third thoracic sympathetic ganglia, extirpation of these two ganglia is usually sufficient to control the peripheral effects of sympathetic hyperactivity. Afferent fibres have been traced from the upper limb into the sympathetic chain from C7 right down to T7 ganglia. Consequently, complete afferent denervation of the upper limb could conceivably require an extensive sympathectomy. Both electrical and mechanical stimulation of the sympathetic chain have been reported to elicit pain and algologists continue to debate the question of an efferent or an afferent basis for sympathetically-dependent pain. However, two observations made by the author argue for an efferent basis. During the course of nearly 1000 electrical stimulations in the vicinity of the sympathetic ganglia (chiefly with 1 ms, 100 Hz stimuli) in conscious human patients, there have been no instances in which distal arm pain has been elicited or in which the patient's spontaneous causalgic pain has been reproduced, although these patients commonly report acute pain or tingling in an intercostal distribution. Secondly, none of these

patients who have undergone sympathectomy for causalgic pain, and in whom pain has persisted despite an effective T2 and T3 sympathectomy, experienced even temporary pain relief when the sympathectomy was extended. Three of the patients subsequently underwent extension of their sympathectomies, and a further eight underwent diagnostic anaesthic blockage of the sympathetic chain at, above or below the area of the lesion, but in none of them was pain relief achieved.

Diagnosis

A 'sympathetically-mediated' or 'sympathetically-maintained' cause is usually readily apparent in those patients who present with classical 'major causalgia' or with the more overt forms of reflex sympathetic dystrophy. In these conditions, the pain is intense, there is marked allodynia and hypersensitivity, and dystrophic changes develop rapidly and are easily identified. There is frequently a vasospastic component with a cool blue extremity (sometimes after an initial period of hyperperfusion), and disorders of sweating are commonly present. However, there are a wide variety of alternative clinical presentations and this at times makes recognition of the aetiology quite difficult, especially in those patients who present with diffuse pain in an extremity, but in whom there is no significant dystrophic change or vasospasticity.

In those patients in whom the aetiology is questionable, an intravenous infusion of phentolamine or guanethidine into the extremity distal to a tourniquet is often used to determine if the condition is sympathetically-mediated. These drugs are considered selectively to block sympathetic hyperactivity, but do not block nociceptor fibre transmissions. Accordingly, if relief is obtained, this is considered to be a strong indicator that the condition has a sympathetic nervous system aetiology. Unfortunately, serious questions have recently been raised about the reliability of the test (Fine *et al.*, 1994; McGlone *et al.*, 1992).

The 'gold standard' for determining whether a condition is of sympathetic origin remains the selective anaesthetic interruption of the sympathetic supply to the involved limb. This is most commonly achieved by stellate ganglion block or selective upper thoracic sympathetic ganglion block for the upper extremity syndromes, and by selective lumbar paravertebral sympathetic blocks for the lower extremity syndromes. As the sympathetic outflow from the stellate ganglion is directed almost exclusively rostrally towards the head and neck, it is theoretically difficult to determine why stellate block influences sympathetic activity in the arm. However, by injecting an anaesthetic labelled with radiopaque contrast material, it can be demonstrated that interruption of sympathetic activity to the arm will occur only if the anaesthetic travels down the paravertebral space to the upper thoracic ganglia. This may occur with anaesthetic volumes as small as 1–2 ml. As most stellate ganglion blocks are performed with volumes ranging between 10 ml and 12 ml, They are likely to prove effective in the majority of patients. These diagnostic blocks are also extremely important therapeutically, as it can be shown that interrupting the sympathetic supply early in the clinical course of a syndrome of sympathetic hyperactivity not uncommonly produces lasting relief and may sometimes reverse it permanently.

Medical treatment

The nonsurgical treatments for syndromes of sympathetically-mediated pain include physiotherapy, pharmacological therapy, psychotherapy and anaesthetic sympathetic block. Not all these therapies are applicable to every syndrome. Additional therapy is usually necessary for the treatment of the other sequelae of the initiating injury, including sympathetically-induced structural changes, such as dystrophic or ischaemic changes in the arms or legs, and the psychosocial aspect of chronic disability.

The noninvasive therapy of these disorders is mainly aimed at controlling pain and improving function. Physiotherapy programmes (exercise, massage, thermal therapy, ultrasound, diathermy) attempt to lessen pain and maintain the range of movement and flexibility in affected joints. Lessening the stiffness in these joints may help to reduce pain on movement. 'Contact desensitization' techniques attempt to reduce painful awareness from the hypersensitive areas by the periodic application of excessive tactile, or even slightly painful, cutaneous stimuli. The application of astringents or electrophoresis may help to reduce pathological hyperhidrosis, but large areas of involvement may limit the usefulness of astringents (which may be irritating), and electrophoresis is generally applicable only to the flat surface of the palms or the soles.

Pharmacotherapy may be used to treat pain, ischaemia, dystrophy or hyperhidrosis. Pain relieving drugs, such a dyphenylhidantoin, carbamazapine, baclofen, amitriptyline, and mild analgesics may help to control pain and to facilitate activity of an affected extremity. Nonsteroidal anti-inflammatory drugs can help by controlling the inflammatory component of dystrophy. They also have nonspecific pain relieving properties. Peripheral vasodilators can be useful for the vasospastic disorders. Calcium channel blocking agents may be useful both for circulatory improvement and in reducing peripheral pain production. Alpha-1 adrenergic blocking agents may be effective in relieving pain by blocking the peripheral generation of nociceptive impulses mediated through the sympathetic nervous system. Most of the sympatholytic drugs that reduce perspiration cause excessive dryness of the mouth and have other side-effects. This limits their usefulness, but oxybutinin chloride can at times be both effective and well tolerated.

Sympathetic anaesthetic blocks given as a series may produce lasting benefit, especially in cases of recent onset. Thus, anaesthetic blockade should be carried out not only to help to determine whether the pain is sympathetically mediated but also in the hope of avoiding a surgical sympathectomy. Anaesthetic injections given early in a patient's clinical course have a much greater chance of producing long lasting or even permanent pain relief. In some patients, lasting cure is achieved even in chronically persistent states of sympathetically-mediated pain. Thus, if an anaesthetic block produces short-term useful relief, it should be repeated routinely at least once and more often if the resulting pain relief is prolonged and/or of increasing duration. As the literature on surgical sympathectomy amply documents, adequate or permanent relief of sympathetic or causalgic pain is notoriously difficult to achieve with sympathectomy, even if diagnostic blocks have provided excellent short-term relief. Although sympathetic fibres can be blocked at the level of the lumbar or the brachial plexus, the resultant associated somatic sensory blockade does not permit a conclusion regarding any possible sympathetic mediation of the pain. The most common anaesthetic blocks used are stellate ganglion and lumbar paravertebral blocks but injecting excessive amounts of local anaesthetics during a stellate block, or allowing the anaesthetic agent to reach nearby cervical nerve roots, can result in cutaneous sensory loss in the limb and confuse the interpretation of the test. Precise placement of the anaesthetic agent in individual upper thoracic ganglia is especially important in those patients whose pain persists despite partial sympathectomy. This is usually achieved by radiographic control and the injection of very small amounts of anaesthetic mixed with contrast medium.

Percutaneous alcohol or phenol sympathectomy offers the advantage of technical simplicity but carries a significant risk. Thoracic sympathectomy using alcohol has rarely been performed since Leriche and Fontaine (1932) described the inadvertent tracking of alcohol through a nerve root sheath into the subarachnoid space, causing paraplegia. Because the sympathetic ganglia are connected to the segmental nerves by rather short rami communicantes, especially in the thoracic region, and because the genitofemoral nerve courses in the retroperitoneal space near the lumbar sympathetic ganglia, somatic nerve or root injury, with consequent severe neuralgia, is a potential complication. In the lumbar area, damage to adjacent arteries, the ureter or veins may occur and, in the thoracic region, damage to the pleura poses significant risks. Ogawa (1992), who still performs both thoracic and lumbar alcohol sympathectomies, advocates preceding the injection of the sclerosing solutions by the injection of radiographic contrast medium to check for adequacy of the needle placement and to ensure that the sclerosing agent is less likely to reach and damage adjacent structures. Lumbar injections are made through a paravertebral needle placed at the level of the second or third lumbar vertebral body. Appropriate placement is confirmed by radiographic control. The chemicals injected are usually 7% aqueous phenol, 50% alcohol, or absolute alcohol. The volumes injected have varied, but volumes between 3 ml and 8 ml have been used.

Surgical treatment

Surgical upper thoracic sympathectomy is usually performed by one of three techniques (Wilkinson, 1996b,c). The posterior approach is through a midline interscapular incision, with removal of rib heads unilaterally or bilaterally. The ganglion chain is divided or resected. Wound pain is usually significant and intercostal pain not uncommon. The supraclavicular approach requires two incisions for bilateral sympathectomy but does not involve entry through the pleural space. The major risks are injury to the great vessels and the brachial plexus. Horner's syndrome, pneumothorax or other complications have been reported in as many as 60% of patients. The axillary transthoracic approach is often done in two parts for bilateral surgery. It is associated with a significant incidence of intercostal neuralgia and of brachial plexus injury. A variation of this approach uses endoscopic coagulation instead of resection of the ganglion chain. This technique was first described more than four decades ago (Kux, 1954) and has subsequently been reported by four different groups (Kux, 1980; Malone *et al.*, 1982; Rosner and Goldberg, 1979; Weale, 1980). Although it is simpler than thoracotomy, it still requires intubation and a general anaesthesic. Difficulty in visualization of the sympathetic ganglia, especially the second thoracic ganglion, and a high rate of recurrent symptoms have limited its adoption. Despite these problems, endoscopic sympathectomy is currently being reintroduced using modern endoscopic instruments and including resection of the sympathetic chain. At least one series has reported excellent long-term results (Byrne *et al.*, 1990).

In 1979, a technique for stereotactic percutaneous radiofrequency upper thoracic sympathectomy was reported (Wilkinson, 1984a,b). In the ensuing 7 years, two major modifications to the technique have been made, with considerable improvement in both initial and long-term results (Wilkinson, 1996a; Yarzebski and Wilkinson, 1987). The procedure is done on a day-surgery basis using local anaesthesia and neuroleptanalgesia. Two 18-gauge radiofrequency needle electrodes are used simultaneously. This reduces fluoroscopy time and minimizes the period of deep anaesthesia. To denervate the upper limb, the electrodes are most commonly placed at the T2 and T3 paravertebral ganglia. Bilateral procedures are commonly performed at a single session. At each site, a series of lesions are made in a rostrocaudal direction to destroy the entire ganglia in an attempt to reduce the frequency of late recurrences, although it is recognized that even following open surgical resection, some late recurrences will occur.

Surgically, the lumbar sympathetic chain is approached through a flank incision on each side to be treated. A muscle-splitting approach through the abdominal wall is used to reach the retroperitoneal space. The sympathetic chain is identified alongside the lumbar vertebrae and the sympathetic chain, ganglia and rami communicantes are segmentally resected. Access from the L2 to the L4 ganglia can readily be achieved. There has been considerable debate about which sympathetic ganglia should be included in the resection. The sympathetic preganglionic fibres arise from the lower thoracic cord and run downward to the lumbar ganglia. Many of the sympathetic efferents seem to originate in the second or third lumbar ganglia and then pass further caudally through the chain to exit with the postganglionic rami of L4 or even L5. Although the short-term results are good if ablation is directed to the L2 and L3 ganglia only, the long-term results appear to be improved by including L4 or even L5. Occasional patients have been reported in whom recurrent symptoms following L2 and L3 ganglion resection have then been abolished by resecting L4 or even L5.

Pernak and Berg (1985) have described an application of the radiofrequency stereotactic technique for lumbar sympathectomy. Although other authors have advocated multiple lesions and an extensive radiofrequency lumbar sympathectomy, they have achieved considerable success with a technique in which only single lesions are made, usually at the L3 level. A favourable early outcome is indicated by improved limb perfusion and increased skin temperature. Although a single lesion in the sympathetic chain is unlikely to result in a permanent sympathectomy, Pernak and Berg (1985) achieve excellent overall results by integrating the sympathectomy with an aggressive rehabilitation programme.

Evaluating the outcome of sympathectomy

The evaluation of the outcome of sympathectomy is complicated by two factors: the progress of the underlying disease, despite adequate sympathectomy, and the well-known capacity of the sympathetic nervous system to reorganize or regenerate.

Every large surgical series that include careful long-term follow-up (this information is not available in many of the series) includes an incidence of the delayed return of sympathetic function even following surgical resection of the ganglia. Haxton (1970) has reported that 22 of 35 patients (63%) had relapsed by 36 months after resection of the upper thoracic ganglia for Raynaud's disease, but severe relapse was 'rarely seen in the absence of demonstrable sympathetic activity'. Howng and Loh (1987) reported a 9.7% relapse rate after three to eight years in 41 patients who underwent open resection for hyperhidrosis. There are two documented cases in which actual regeneration has been identified at the time of surgical re-exploration. In those patients the recurrent symptoms resolved following resection of the regenerated material (Haxton, 1970; Mattassi *et al.*, 1981). In the thoracoscopic series published by Byrne *et al.* (1982), 15% of their patients had experienced 'complete' or 'partial' relapse by three years after surgery. Kao *et al.* (1994) performed a series of thoracoscopic laser sympathectomies for hyperhidrosis, generally limited to the T2 ganglia, but they included the T3 ganglia if there was also severe axillary hyperhidrosis. They did not report long-term results, but stated,

> It has been generally agreed that a recurrence of [hyperhidrosis] of clinical importance, after either open or endoscopic sympathectomy, would mostly develop within 1 year and almost always results from incomplete sympathectomy. ... It is believed if a recurrence has not developed by 1 year after an adequate sympathectomy, there is almost no tendency for a relapse of sweating to the point of clinical embarrassment or disability.

This impression is unsubstantiated and at variance with results reported following open sympathectomy. Late relapses were encountered in the author's series of radiofrequency sympathectomies. In fact, the risk of recurrence in this series was 5.3% in the fourth year and 2.2% in the fifth year after treatment. One recurrence developed at 6.5 years after treatment. As long ago as 1935, Telford, pioneer of sympathactomy, stated, 'I do not think that any operator who has had sufficient experience of sympathectomy and has followed up his cases for some years can regard the outcome of his work as entirely satisfactory.' The adequacy of sympathectomy can be determined either by the control of symptoms (elimination of excessive sweating, maintenance of adequate limb perfusion or control of causalgic pain), or by special tests of sympatholysis in patients in whom symptoms persist despite what may or may not be adequate sympathetic interruption.

Because pain and disability not uncommonly persist despite sympathectomy and because the sympathetic system has a propensity to regenerate, it is important in evaluating patients with persistent symptoms to determine whether or not they remain completely sympathectomized. A simple and fairly accurate bedside test is the starch iodine test. In this, the part of the patient's body to be tested is painted with an iodine solution, which is allowed to dry thoroughly. Powdered cornstarch is then dusted lightly over the entire area, and the patient is placed in a hot room or beneath hot lights and is given hot liquids to drink in order to induce perspiration. Light exercising can also help. The moisture produced allows the iodine and starch to interact, turning the white powder to black and thus delineating the areas where sweating has occurred. Bilateral measurement of skin temperature by thermography or thermistors and measurement of limb perfusion by plethysmography can also be used to quantitate differences in function btween the limbs. However, these techniques are subject to considerable variability and cannot confirm whether a sympathectomy is complete, especially if bilateral sympathectomy has been carried out. These variables include the extent of dystrophic and vascular changes in the limb, the ambient and body temperatures, and whether or not the patient has taken vasodilating medications. Diagnostic sympathetic blocks are the most reliable way of testing for the completeness of sympathectomy. These should be carried out with solutions containing radiographic contrast media that can be visualized under a fluoroscope or on permanent radiographs. Testing the completeness of sympathectomy usually begins with injections into the area of presumed sympathectomy and then proceeds to a blockade of the adjacent sympathetic ganglia. The outcome of these tests should be measured in terms not only of improvements in circulation and limb temperature but also in pain. Patients who continue to experience severe pain despite an already extensive sympathectomy will rarely obtain useful or lasting pain relief from its further enlargement or extension.

Outcome

The results of sympathectomy vary greatly according to the condition being treated. Sympathectomy for vascular spasm secondary to acute arterial occlusion will give nearly 100% long-term relief of the vasospastic component of the disorder. Sympathectomy for Raynaud's syndrome will initially give almost 100% relief of the painful ischaemic syndrome, but nearly 15% of those patients later develop a collagen vasculopathy. Symptoms recur in nearly 25% of patients despite sustained sympathectomy. Patients with ischaemic obliterative vascular disorders usually obtain transient relief of pain and improved healing of necrotic and ulcerated extremities, but the underlying disorder usually progresses, and further ischaemic symptoms eventually develop. Sympathectomy for Prinzmetal's angina has only been carried out in a relatively limited number of patients, although results have generally been quite good.

Sympathectomies carried out for disorders characterized principally by pain with or without dystrophic features have yielded only limited success. Most authors report sustained pain relief in only two-thirds to three-quarters of patients, regardless of the surgical technique. Dystrophic features may improve steadily but will usually require extensive secondary therapy. Because most of these disorders are initiated by some form of painful process, such as peripheral nerve injury, further therapy is usually necessary to restore these patients to their full functional status, to obtain relief from persistent somatic pain, and to rehabilitate these often chronically disabled patients.

The timing and extent of sympathectomy are also important in determining outcome. As has already been mentioned, anaesthetic sympathetic interruptions made shortly after the onset of pain not uncommonly provide long-term relief. Similarly, sympathectomy seems to provide a better chance of success in the patient with a syndrome characterized principally by pain when that surgery is performed earlier in its course rather than later. The extent of the sympathectomy necessary to control the pain is likewise not clear. In the lumbar area, sympathectomy has ranged from a single-level resection at L2 or L3 to a resection carried out from L2 to L5. In the thoracic region, the resection has most commonly been at T2 and T3, but recommendations have ranged from T1 to T5 to resection of T2 only.

References

Byrne J, Walsh TN, Hederman WP. (1982) Endoscopic transthoracic electrocautery of the sympathetic chain for palmar and axillary hyperhidrosis. *Br J Surg* 77: 1046–49.

Fine PG, Roberts WJ, Gillette RG, *et al.* (1994) Slowly developing placebo responses confound tests of intravenous phentolamine to determine mechanisms underlying idiopathic chronic low back pain. *Pain* 56: 235–42.

Haxton HA. (1970) Upper limb resympathectomy. *Br J Surg* 57: 106–108.

Howng S-L, Loh J-K. (1987) Long term follow-up of upper dorsal sympathetic ganglionectomy for palmar hyperhidrosis – a scale of evaluation. *Kaohsiung J Med Sci* 3: 704–707.

Kao M-C, Tasi J-C, Lai D-M, *et al.* (1994) Autonomic activities in hyperhidrosis patients before, during, and after endoscopic laser sympathectomy. *Neurosurgery* 34: 262–68.

Kux E. (1954) *Thorakoskopische Eingriffe am Nervensystem.* Stuttgart: Georg Thieme.

Kux M. (1980) Thoracic endoscopic sympathectomy by transthoracic electrocoagulation. *Br J Surg* 67: 71.

Leriche R, Fontaine R. (1932) Chirurgie des nerfs du coeur. *J Chir (Paris)* 40: 508–25.

Malone PS, Dingnan JP, Hederman WP. (1982) Transthoracic electrocoagulation (T.T.E.C.) – a new and simple approach to upper limb sympathectomy. *Jr Med J* 75: 20–21.

Mattassi R, Miele F, D'Angelo F. (1981) Thoracic sympathectomy: review of indications, results and surgical techniques. *J Cardiovasc Surg* 22: 336–39.

McGlone F, Dhar S, Dean J. (1992) Placebo controlled study of the effects of chemical sympathectomy on peripheral nerve function and pain. *Proceedings of 5th International Congress: The Pain Clinic.* Jerusalem: Israel Pain Association, 51.

Ogawa S. (1992) Sympathectomy with neurolytics. In Hyodo M, Oyama T, Swerdlow M, editors. *The pain clinic IV.* Utrecht: VSP, 138–46.

Pernak JM Berg HVD. (1985) Treatment of chronic low back pain following lumbar disc operations by using thermolesion of sympathetic ganglion. In: Erdmann W, editor. *The pain clinic I.* Rotterdam: VNU Science Press, 177–86.

Rosner K, Goldberg S. (1979) Der Stellewert der thorakoskopischen Sympathectomie bei der Behandlung des Raynaud-Syndrome. *Zi Gesamte Inn Med* 34: 127–28.

Schott GD. (1986) Mechanisms of causalgia and related clinical conditions: the role of the central and of the sympathetic nervous systems. *Brain* 109: 717–38.

Telford ED. (1935) The technique of sympathectomy. *Br J Surg* 23: 440–80.

Weale FE. (1980) Upper thoracic sympathectomy for transthoracic electrocoagulation. *Br J Surg* 67: 71–72.

Wilkinson HA. (1984a) Percutaneous radiofrequency upper thoracic sympathectomy: a new technique. *Neurosurgery* 15: 811–14.

Wilkinson HA. (1984b) Radiofrequency percutaneous upper thoracic sympathectomy: technique and review of indications. *N Engl J Med* 311: 34–36.

Wilkinson HA. (1996a) Percutaneous radiofrequency upper thoracic sympathectomy. *Neurosurgery* 38: 715–25.

Wilkinson HA. (1996b) Sympathectomy for pain. In: Youmans JR, editor. *Neurological surgery.* Philadelphia: Saunders.

Wilkinson HA. (1996c) Surgery of the sympathectic nervous system. In: Schmidek H, Sweet WH, editors. *Operative neurosurgical techniques.* Philadelphia: Saunders, 1573–83.

Yarzebski JL, Wilkinson HA. (1987) T2 and T3 sympathectic ganglia in the adult human: a cadaver and clinical-radiographic study and its clinical application. *Neurosurgery* 21: 339–42.

Index